# Current Management of Cerebral Aneurysms

AANS Publications Committee
Issam A. Awad, MD, Editor

## Neurosurgical Topics

American Association of
Neurological Surgeons

**ISBN: 1-879284-13-8**

**Neurosurgical Topics ISBN: 0-9624246-6-8**



Printed in U. S. A.



This publication is published under the auspices of the Publications Committee of the Amercian Association of Neurological Surgeons (AANS). However, this should not be construed as indicating endorsement or approval of the views presented, by the AANS, or by its committees, commissions, affiliates, or staff.

**Daniel L. Barrow, MD, Chairman**
AANS Publications Committee

Linda S. Miller, AANS Staff Editor

AANS2M1293

# Forthcoming Books in the *Neurosurgical Topics* Series

1993

*Interactive Image-Guided Neurosurgery*
Edited by Robert J. Maciunas, MD

1994

*Spinal Instrumentation*
Edited by Edward C. Benzel, MD

*Neurosurgical Emergencies, Volume I*
Edited by Christopher M. Loftus, MD

*Neurosurgical Emergencies, Volume II*
Edited by Christopher M. Loftus, MD

*Spinal Cord Injuries*
Edited by Edward C. Benzel and Charles H. Tator, MD

*Benign Cerebral Glioma*
Edited by Michael L.J. Apuzzo, MD

*Philosophy of Neurosurgery*
Edited by Issam A. Awad, MD

# Contents

# List of Contributors

**Arvind Ahuja, MD**
Clinical Instructor of Neurosurgery
State University of New York at Buffalo
Department of Neurosurgery
School of Medicine and Biomedical Sciences
Buffalo, New York

**Issam A. Awad, MD, MS, FACS**
Associate Professor of Surgery
Director, Neurovascular Surgery Program
Yale University School of Medicine
New Haven, Connecticut

**Gene H. Barnett, MD**
Vice Chairman of Neurological Surgery
(Formerly Director, Neurosurgical Intensive Care Unit)
Cleveland Clinic Foundation
Cleveland, Ohio

**Daniel L. Barrow, MD**
Associate Professor and Deputy Chief
Department of Neurosurgery
Emory University School of Medicine
Atlanta, Georgia

**H. Hunt Batjer, MD**
Professor, Department of Neurological Surgery
University of Texas, Southwest Medical Center
Dallas, Texas

**Douglas Chyatte, MD**
Associate Professor of Neurosurgery
Northwestern University School of Medicine
Chicago, Ilinois

**Fernando G. Diaz, MD, PhD**
Professor and Chairman
Neurological Surgery Department
Wayne State University School of Medicine
Detroit, Michigan

**J. Max Findlay, MD**
Associate Clinical Professor
Department of Surgery
University of Alberta
Edmonton, Canada

**Kevin J. Gibbons, MD**
Clinical Instructor of Neurosurgery
State University of New York at Buffalo
Department of Neurosurgery
School of Medicine and Biomedical Sciences
Buffalo, New York

**Lee R. Guterman, PhD, MD**
Clinical Instructor of Neurosurgery
State University of new York at Buffalo
Department of Neurosurgery
School of Medicine and Biomedical Sciences
Buffalo, New York

**Gregory Hariton, MD**
Department of Surgery
University of Alberta
Edmonton, Canada

**Roberto C. Heros, MD**
Lyle A. French Professor and Chairman
Department of Neurosurgery
University of Minnesota
Minneapolis, Minnesota

**Jonathan Hodes, MD**
Division of Neurological Surgery
University of Kentucky
College of Medicine
Lexington, Kentucky

**Leo N. Hopkins, MD**
Professor of Neurosurgery and Radiology
State University of New York at Buffalo
Department of Neurosurgery
School of Medicine and Biomedical Sciences
Buffalo, New York

**Neal F. Kassell, MD**
Professor and Vice Chairman
Department of Neurological Surgery
University of Virginia Health Sciences Center
Charlottesville, Virginia

**Thomas A. Kopitnik, MD**
Assistant Professor
Department of Neurological Surgery
University of Texas, Southwest Medical Center
Dallas, Texas

**Richard Leblanc, MSc, MD, FRCSC**
Associate Professor
Department of Neurology and Neurosurgery
McGill University and Montreal Neurological Institute
Head, Cerebrovascular Surgery Section
Montreal Neurological Hospital
Montreal, Quebec, Canada

**Kimberly Livingston, MD**
Clinical Instructor of Neurosurgery
State University of New York at Buffalo
Department of Neurosurgery
School of Medicine and Biomedical Sciences
Buffalo, New York

**Thomas J. Masaryk, MD**
The Cleveland Clinic Foundation
Department of Radiology
Section of Neuroradiology
Cleveland, Ohio

**Dan M. Meyer, MD, PhD**
Assistant Professor
Division of Cardiothoracic Surgery
Department of Surgery
University of Texas, Southwest Medical Center
Dallas, Texas

**Jacques J. Morcos, MD**
Resident in Neurosurgery
Department of Neursosurgery
University of Minnesota
Minneapolis, Minnesota

**Nelson Oyesiku, MD**
Department of Neurosurgery and Program in Neuroscience
Division of Biological and Biomedical Sciences
Emory University School of Medicine
Atlanta, Georgia

**John Perl II, MD**
The Cleveland Clinic Foundation
Department of Radiology
Section of Neuroradiology
Cleveland, Ohio

**Phillip D. Purdy, MD**
Associate Professor
Department of Radiology
University of Texas, Southwest Medical Center
Dallas, Texas

**Karen D. Rodman, MD**
Fellow, Cerebrovascular Diseases
Cleveland Clinic Foundation
Department of Neurology
Cleveland, Ohio

**Duke S. Samson, MD**
Clark Professor and Chairman
Department of Neurological Surgery
University of Texas, Southwest Medical Center
Dallas, Texas

**Armin Schubert, MD**
Chairman, Department of Anesthesiology
Cleveland Clinic Foundation
Cleveland, Ohio

**Christopher I. Shaffrey, MD**
Chief Resident
Department of Neurological Surgery
University of Virginia Health Sciences Center
Charlottesville, Virginia

**Mark E. Shaffrey, MD**
Chief Resident
Department of Neurological Surgery
University of Virginia Health Sciences Center
Charlottesville, Virginia

**Robert A. Solomon, MD**
Associate Professor of Clinical Neurosurgery
Columbia University College of Physicians and Surgeons
New York, New York

**Bernard Vellardo, MD**
Anesthesia Department
Wayne State University
School of Medicine
Detroit, Michigan

**Bryce Weir, MD**
Maurice Goldblatt Professor of Surgery and Neurology
Chief, Section of Neurosurgery,
Director of Brain Research Institute
University of Chicago
Chicago, Illinois

**Donald M. Whiting, MD**
Neurosurgery Resident
Cleveland Clinic Foundation
Cleveland, Ohio

# AANS Publications Committee

# Preface

Cerebral aneurysms remain a significant challenge to the neurological surgeon and continue to exact needless morbidity and mortality from patients. More than one million people, and possibly as many as five million harbor cerebral aneurysms in the United States alone, and more than 20,000 of these aneurysms bleed each year. Many patients do not survive long enough to reach a hospital, and half of the cases die or become severely disabled from sequelae of hemorrhage. In recent years, it has become clear that subarachnoid hemorrhage (SAH) may be a preventable disease; neurosurgeons are now faced with the novel challenge of screening for and managing unruptured aneurysms. This has occurred during a time of evolving diagnostic technology and ever-improving surgical outcome, as well as careful analysis of cost-effectiveness and resource utilization.

It has also become obvious that a prompt and accurate diagnosis is essential following SAH. Recent cooperative studies have revised old myths about the risk of rebleeding and have emphasized that such risk is greatest in the first hours following hemorrhage. Neurosurgeons have been entrusted with the important task of educating family and community health care providers, emergency room physicians, and patients themselves about the early symptoms and signs of SAH and the importance of prompt diagnosis. Epidemiologic information has repeatedly emphasized the terrible consequences, in morbidity and cost, of missed or delayed diagnosis of cerebral aneurysms and SAH.

Management strategies have also evolved in recent years. A consensus about the emergency management of aneurysm patients in the first hours following SAH has developed. Intensive care measures have been relatively standardized, and most centers have adopted a stance of emergency diagnosis and treatment. The decision to operate and the timing of surgery are now less dependent on arbitrary "clinical grades," but more on rational considerations of pathophysiology, lesion accessibility, and available facilities. Early surgical intervention has now become as safe as delayed surgery in experienced hands and in adequate facilities. This has dramatically minimized the dreadful risk of rebleeding and has allowed more aggressive and successful management of delayed sequelae of SAH. Microsurgical techniques have also evolved, with an increasing number of neurosurgeons mastering the skills which one decade ago belonged to the pioneers. Improved neuroanesthetic management, critical care, skull base exposure, and more recently, intraoperative angiography have all contributed to ever-improving surgical outcomes.

Management of the delayed sequelae of SAH has also changed dramatically in recent years. Calcium channel blockers have been shown to significantly decrease ischemic complications of vasospasm and have become a routine part of standard management of SAH. Serial monitoring of vasospasm is now possible at the bedside using transcranial Doppler (TCD). These advances, early surgical intervention, and judicious hemodynamic critical care management have all contributed to a continued decline in the devastating complications of vasospasm. Other cases, with intractable deterioration from vasospasm, are now benefiting at a few centers from novel treatment strategies, including intra-arterial papaverine and endovascular angioplasty. Intracisternal fibrinolysis and other pharmacologic manipulations are being intensely studied and may further dramatically affect management and outcome of cerebral vasospasm. Intense laboratory basic research was responsible for each of these advances and is likely to uncover more effective treatment strategies in the near future.

Endovascular techniques have evolved rapidly in the last decade. These currently represent an important option in the armamentarium of management of cerebral aneurysms. They have greatly enhanced the safety of parent vessel and temporary test occlusions and have contributed to more effective diagnosis and treatment through selective and intraoperative angiography. For inoperable cases, primary aneurysm treatment with balloons and coils is now routinely attempted and is frequently successful. Other endovascular techniques are on the horizon, including stents, glues, and safer and more effective coils. While there is no agreement about the specific indication of each of these emergent technologies in the management of individual aneurysms, a consensus is emerging about their general advantages and shortcomings.

Much of the above information is being presented and published by subspecialists from a handful of major neurovascular centers in specialized journals. General neurosurgeons, residents-in-training, and other physicians have frequently been denied practical and useful synthesis of this information. This book attempts to compile current knowledge on the pathology, clinical presentation, latest diagnostic techniques, and treatment strategies for cerebral aneurysms. Leading experts in the field have been invited to contribute their respective perspectives on various facets of this disease. All have presented clear, concise, and up-to-date surveys of the state-of-the-art treatment for cerebral aneurysms. They have outlined areas of remaining controversy, technical challenges, and unsettled problems. They have also highlighted useful and practical advances and technical recommendations that have worked for them or that have been shown to be effective in the literature.

This book attempts to go beyond the coverage of cerebral aneurysms in traditional neurosurgical texts while avoiding the burden of voluminous and often contradictory information in the more specialized journals and textbooks. The book is aimed primarily at providing the practicing neurosurgeon and the resident-in-training with a useful and practical body of knowledge about cerebral aneurysms, including the latest advances and remaining challenges. It is hoped that physicians of all specialties might use it as a source of practical, readable, and accessible information about this complex topic.

*Issam A. Awad, MD, MS, FACS*
*New Haven, Connecticut*
*1993*

# Dedication and Acknowledgments

*This book is dedicated to our patients with cerebral aneurysms.*

*The Editor is grateful for the trust that our patients and their families have placed in our neurosurgical team, and for the august privilege of seeing them through the many facets and hurdles of their illness. Those who prevailed through their ordeal inspired us to further advance the horizons of management of these lesions. The memory of those others who were devastated by cerebral aneurysms gives us further motivation to resolve numerous remaining clinical problems.*

*All members of neurovascular surgical teams are owed an integral share in the credit for any clinical success with cerebral aneurysms. Neuroradiologists, neurologists, neuroanesthesiologists, critical care specialists, and primary care physicians all play indispensable roles in the management of each case. The credibility and performance of the neurovascular surgical team is also greatly enhanced by the dedication of neurosurgical residents and the compassion and competence of nursing colleagues. No clinical success could have been accomplished without them, and no failure or complication could have been avoided without their help. These numerous members of the "team" also share in deserving the intellectual credit for identification of problems, discussion of alternative techniques, and multidisciplinary advancement of state-of-the-art intervention and management techniques for cerebral aneurysms.*

*Our own work would not have been possible without the solid foundation of scientific information, rational thinking, and technical advances introduced by countless neurosurgical pioneers. Other neurosurgeons have carried the torch, and have made further contributions to the advancement of knowledge and technique relevant to cerebral aneurysms. Many of these leaders have graciously contributed chapters to this book, and have each enhanced, through their respective contributions, the overall quality and comprehensiveness of this work.*

*This project would not have been completed without the understanding and encouragement from my wife Catherine, and the continued inspiration and support from the rest of my family. I wish to acknowledge the patient and expert secretarial assistance of Ms. Shirley McDaniel, who followed through the various stages of manuscript preparation with thoroughness and care. I am grateful to Ms. Linda Miller, Mr. Jeremy Longhurst, and Mr. Steven Serfling, of the American Association of Neurological Surgeons, for their expert and professional guidance through various phases of planning, budgeting, marketing, manuscript preparation, and editing. Lastly, I wish to thank Drs. Robert Wilkins and Daniel Barrow, and also all the members of the Publications Committee of the American Association of Neurological Surgeons for their inspiration, assistance, and support in the conceptualization and preparation of this work.*

*Numerous advances have occurred in the understanding of cerebral aneurysms and subarachnoid hemorrhage in recent years. There have also been major strides in management strategies and techniques, with many myths revisited, many approaches reconsidered, and many "forbidden frontiers" successfully conquered. In this book, the contributors have attempted to compile some of this information in a practical way to aid practicing neurosurgeons, residents-in-training, and other physicians who are not primary specialists in neurovascular surgery. This book does not shy away from areas of controversy, but attempts to reach a consensus whenever possible. I am indebted to each of the contributors—true experts in their field—for simplifying, clarifying, and synthesizing a vast body of complex, controversial, and evolving information. It has been a pleasure to work with each one of them, and I am particularly thankful for the concise, clear, and articulate synthesis of their respective topics.*

*The Editor*

# CHAPTER 1

# The Epidemiology, Genetics, and Clinical Behavior of Intracranial Aneurysms

Douglas Chyatte, MD

The conditions that lead to intracranial aneurysm formation occur commonly. Those that lead to rupture are considerably less frequent. Available evidence is consistent with the hypothesis that intracranial saccular aneurysms form when the mechanisms for arterial repair cannot compensate for pre-existing arterial weakness or ongoing arterial injury. Considerably less is known about the conditions associated with aneurysm rupture; however, it may be that rupture is associated with enzymatic injury to the aneurysm dome. An understanding of aneurysm formation and rupture may eventually allow us to identify individuals at risk for aneurysmal subarachnoid hemorrhage (SAH) and to prescribe preventive treatment before a devastating hemorrhage occurs.

## Historic Perspective

The word aneurysm comes from the Greek *aneurysma—ana* meaning "across" and *eurys* meaning "broad."[51] Aneurysms are not a disease unique to modern society. Both ancient literature and bony artifacts dating back to ancient Egypt indicate that aneurysms existed and at least some extracranial aneurysms were treated.[51,217]

Despite occasional reports, cerebral aneurysms were not well recognized as a cause of human illness until the end of the 19th century.* Initially, the diagnosis was made only after death. In 1872 Quincke[193] described the technique for lumbar puncture, and by 1891[194] the diagnosis of SAH could be made before death. Wichern[256] in 1911 correctly diagnosed SAH in 15 out of 22 living patients.

Although the clinical syndrome of SAH could be recognized, localization of the source of hemorrhage was not possible until Egaz Moniz developed cerebral angiography in 1928.[147-149] Although risky at first, angiography was performed at relatively low risk by the 1940s. As transfemoral techniques developed in the 1950s along with refinements in contrast agents, the use of diagnostic angiography for aneurysmal SAH increased.[127]

In 1937 Walter Dandy performed the first surgical repair of an intracranial aneurysm using a metallic clip.[49] The frequency and safety of direct surgical repair increased and improved as experience grew. The introduction of the operating microscope and microsurgical techniques in the late 1960s and 1970s served to further improve management results.

Despite these advances, aneurysmal SAH remains a devastating disease. It is estimated that about one third of all SAH patients die

*References 11,17–19,21,24,25,28,60,74,77,80,102,151 211,257,258

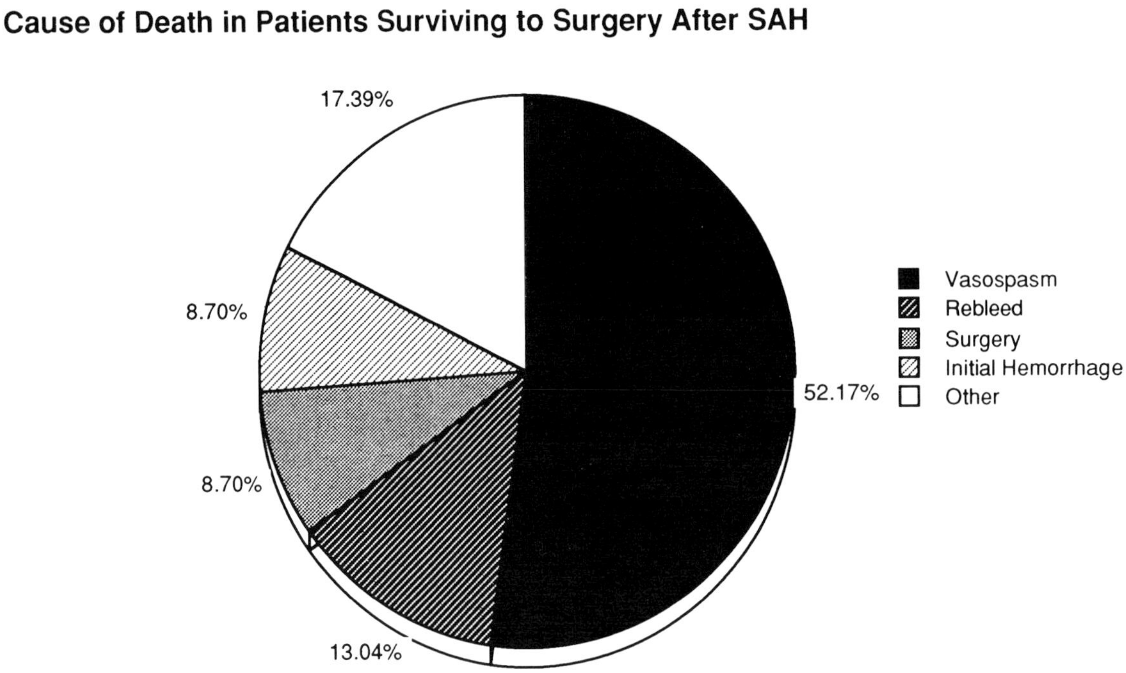


*Figure 1. Causes of mortality in patients with aneurysmal SAH.*[38]

before reaching medical attention. Of those reaching hospitals, only 30% to 40% recover sufficiently enough to be discharged.* Although delayed cerebral ischemia from vasospasm, rebleeding, and surgical misadventures take their toll, most morbidity and mortality occur as a direct result of a severe initial hemorrhage (Figure 1).[38] Consequently, further refinements in surgical or endovascular techniques, aggressive early surgery, or new treatments for vasospasm will have only a modest impact on overall management results. The greatest challenge for the present generation of aneurysm surgeons is the ability to identify asymptomatic individuals at high risk for aneurysmal SAH and provide treatment prior to the occurrence of hemorrhage. At first, this task seems overwhelming; however, existing epidemiologic and laboratory studies suggest directions for future research.

# Incidence

The incidence of cerebral aneurysms is unknown, as most aneurysms remain asymptomatic until rupture occurs, and because no prospective, large-scale screenings for aneurysms have been done. Most autopsy studies estimate that about 5% of the adult population have cerebral aneurysms.[34,50,53,101,226] More than half of the aneurysms identified were unruptured and unrecognized prior to death. In Western countries, the average annual incidence of aneurysmal SAH is approximately 10 in 100,000 per year.** Aneurysm rupture appears to be substantially rarer than aneurysm formation. Since the conditions that favor aneurysm formation only rarely lead to rupture, there appear to be some factors that are associated specifically with aneurysm formation, while others predispose to aneurysm rupture. Identifying the conditions that lead to aneurysm formation has been difficult. Identifying the factors that lead to aneurysm rupture has been even more challenging. Because most aneurysm patients come to medical attention only after an SAH has occurred, it is difficult if not impossible

*References 23,37,63,103,129,156,186,196,197,200

**References 37,129,169,178,186,199,222,224,252

in many situations to distinguish factors related to aneurysm formation from those that lead to rupture.

Many risk factors have been implicated in the pathogenesis of aneurysmal SAH. These include arterial hypertension,* atherosclerosis,[18,44,47,163,164,251] female gender,** age,*** cigarette smoking,[22,199] use of oral contraceptives,[126,185] analgesic use,[50] alcohol intoxication,[50,99] arterial deficiencies of reticular fibers and type III collagen,† asymmetry of the circle of Willis,[50,119] extracranial carotid artery kinks, coils, and fibromuscular dysplasia,[125,142,177,218] cerebral arteriovenous malformations,[9,52,87,157,247,249] and genetics.†† Potential factors related to aneurysm formation and rupture can be grouped into: (1) vascular factors, (2) genetic factors, (3) arterial hypertension, (4) hemodynamic factors, (5) age, and (6) gender (Table 1).[46,47,50,169,209,224,228] Arterial weakness sufficient to favor aneurysm formation may result when pre-existing arterial weakness (i.e. collagen deficiency) or ongoing vascular injury (i.e. mechanical damage due to hypertension or hemodynamic stress) cannot be balanced by arterial repair mechanisms.[50,191,192]

**TABLE 1**
**Factors Related to Aneurysm Formation and Rupture**

| |
|---|
| Vessel wall weakness |
|   Injury |
|     Chemical |
|     Mechanical |
|     Metabolic derangement |
|   Congonital |
|     Morphologic |
|     Genetic |
|     Metabolic derangement |
| Hemodynamic |
| Hypertensive |
| Other Genetic |
| Other |

*References 6,22,23,47,50,122,172,199,224,225,228
**References 23,172,199,251
***References 22,23,188,202,236,237,254
†References 40,90–91,92–95,97,124,155,169,173,175,174,188,190,192,228
††References 50,65,67,72,111,132,135,140,159,160,167,169–171,177,192,200,206,237

## Arterial Hypertension

Epidemiologic studies associate arterial hypertension with aneurysmal SAH.††† Increased hemodynamic stresses caused by arterial hypertension may aggravate existing or acquired structural weakness in cerebral arteries. Hypertension may induce mechanical injury of the vessel wall as the relatively unsupported cerebral arteries traverse the subarachnoid space. Animal experiments confirm epidemiologic observations by causally relating arterial hypertension to, at the very least, aneurysm formation.* In animals, hypertension coupled with the added hemodynamic stress of carotid ligation appear to be the minimal requirements for aneurysm formation.[88,120,191] Spontaneous production of cerebral aneurysms becomes more efficient if animals are also made lathyritic by $\beta$-aminopropionitrile feeds. Repair of mechanical arterial injury induced by hypertension and carotid ligation may be less efficient in lathyritic animals.

The actual incidence of premorbid arterial hypertension in patients with aneurysmal SAH is difficult to determine because hypertension often remains undiagnosed.** The Framingham study, one of the few sources of prospective information,[199] followed 5,184 patients for 26 years. All patients had biennial examinations which included blood pressure measurement. Patients who had two blood pressure recordings greater than 160 mm Hg systolic or 95 mm Hg diastolic during one visit were considered to be hypertensive. Patients were considered normotensive if blood pressure remained below 140/90 mm Hg, while intermediate patients were classified as having borderline hypertension. An-

†††References 6,22,23,47,50,122,172,199,224,225,228
*References 82,84,85,88,120,191,262
**References 22,23,50,86,139,207,215,220

eurysmal SAH occurred in 28 patients in100,000 per year (36 patients). When each aneurysm patient was compared to four controls matched for age and sex, arterial hypertension appeared to be significantly more common in the aneurysm cases than in the controls. This relationship held regardless of when patients were first noted to be hypertensive during the study. These results imply that more effective control of arterial hypertension may decrease the risk of future aneurysmal SAH.[22] From this type of study, however, it is impossible to determine whether arterial hypertension represents a risk factor for aneurysm formation, aneurysm rupture, or both.

The relationship between arterial hypertension and cerebral aneurysms also can be investigated by correlating the number of aneurysms found in a particular patient with the presence or absence of high blood pressure. Ostergaard[172] correlated arterial hypertension with the number of aneurysms in each of 737 aneurysm patients. Hypertension was found in 21.1% of patients with a single aneurysm, but in 41.3% of patients with multiple aneurysms. These results support the hypothesis that hypertension is important for aneurysm formation.

No studies have focused on the relationship of arterial hypertension to initial aneurysm rupture. Although hypertension is believed to play a role in aneurysmal rebleeding,[248] its role in primary rupture remains uncertain. The critical diameter for aneurysm rupture is not significantly related to arterial blood pressure, being directly proportional to only the cubed root of the inverse of blood pressure.[169] Epidemiologic studies of unruptured intracranial aneurysms[252,253] provide further evidence that arterial hypertension may not cause primary aneurysm rupture. In these studies, multivariate discriminant analysis failed to associate arterial hypertension with an increased risk of rupture. Arterial hypertension does appear to be related to aneurysmal SAH, perhaps as a risk factor for aneurysm formation. The importance of arterial hypertension in initial aneurysm rupture is less clear.

## Hemodynamic Stress

Like hypertension, hemodynamic imbalance resulting in increased flow in cerebral arteries has been associated with cerebral aneurysms.[50,61,119,223,224,247] Aneurysms of the anterior communicating artery are associated with inequalities in the size of the proximal segments of the anterior cerebral arteries (A1 segments).[106,119,216,223,259] Hemodynamic stresses associated with flow imbalances may cause mechanical damage to the vessel wall. Hemodynamic stresses produced by carotid artery ligation are a required condition for aneurysm formation in animal models.[82,84,85,88,120,191]

Intracranial arteriovenous malformations (AVMs) increase cerebral blood flows and provide another circumstance to explore in the relationship between hemodynamic stress and cerebral aneurysms. Intracranial aneurysms occur in 10% to 15% of patients with intracranial AVMs.* Enhanced flow in the afferent arteries has been blamed for many of these aneurysms. Aneurysms associated with AVMs fall into three broad groups: (1) those found on enlarged arteries that ultimately feed the AVM in common locations for berry aneurysms; (2) those occurring on feeding vessels near an AVM in unusual locations for berry aneurysms; and (3) those arising at locations seemingly unrelated to the AVM. Perret et al[184] found 37% of aneurysms to be located on major feeding vessels to the AVM, 21% proximal on feeding vessels, and 42% seemingly unrelated to the AVM. These data suggest that hemodynamic factors alone may not be responsible for the association of AVMs and aneurysms.

To explore the relationship between AVMs and aneurysms further, Yasargil[261] studied the correlation of the estimated degree of AVM blood flow with the incidence of cerebral aneurysms. No correlation was found. None of the very high-flow fistulas studied were associated with intracranial arterial aneurysms.

---

*References 9,52,87,145,157,181,184,235,247,249,261

If increased flow alone is important in the etiology of concurrent aneurysms, more aneurysms should have been found associated with high-flow fistulas or large AVMs than low-flow lesions. Yasargil[264] concluded that hemodynamic factors played only a small role in aneurysm development as related to AVMs, perhaps by acting upon some pre-existing vascular disorder.

Extracranial arterial abnormalities provide another means to study the relationship between hemodynamic stress and intracranial saccular aneurysm formation because they increase hemodynamic stresses on cerebral arteries by inducing flow imbalances. Spallone and Cantore[218] retrospectively reviewed angiograms from 76 consecutive aneurysm patients for the presence of extracranial carotid kinks, coils, and stenoses, and compared these findings to a group of 120 patients undergoing angiography for reasons other than aneurysm or occlusive disease. Extracranial carotid abnormalities occurred significantly more frequently in aneurysm patients than in the control group. Although the incidence of arterial kinks and coils was increased in the aneurysm group, no difference was found in the incidence of atherosclerotic carotid stenosis. Intracranial aneurysms occurred twice as often on the carotid contralateral to the extracranial abnormality as ipsilateral. Again hemodynamic factors alone do not appear to be sufficient to trigger the formation of intracranial aneurysms. Extracranial coils and kinks may merely be markers of a more generalized vascular disorder that also can lead to the formation of cerebral aneurysms.

Fibromuscular dysplasia (FMD) is an example of a generalized vascular disorder that is known to affect the extracranial arteries. FMD is a genetic disease that affects women more than men and may be inherited in a dominant fashion with variable penetrance. The incidence of cerebral aneurysms appears to be associated with FMD.[113,142,177] Mettinger and Ericson[142] retrospectively reviewed 4,000 cerebral angiograms in which FMD was commonly overlooked in the majority of patients when the arteriograms were read initially. More than half of the FMD patients had associated intracranial aneurysms, usually located on the same side as the more severely affected carotid artery. About half of the patients with aneurysms and FMD also had hypertension, which indicates that aneurysms in many patients developed in the absence of arterial hypertension. Cerebral aneurysms and FMD appear to be pathogenetically related.

Hemodynamic stresses are linked to the incidence of cerebral aneurysms. Hemodynamic factors alone, however, do not appear to be sufficient to induce aneurysm formation. The coexistence of other factors, such as an underlying vascular disorder, may be necessary for aneurysm formation.

## Age

The incidence of aneurysmal SAH increases with age, reaching a peak in the sixth decade.* Incidental aneurysms found on routine angiography or on postmortem examination in children are rare.[26,50,100,243] Symptomatic aneurysms in children, although more common, are also rare, constituting only a small part of clinical and epidemiologic aneurysm series.** The vast majority of saccular aneurysms appear to form after the first and second decade of life.

Because the majority of cerebral aneurysms appear to be acquired lesions, the time interval between aneurysm formation and rupture is an important concern. Little is known about this temporal relationship. Because age is a risk factor for aneurysm formation, one approach used has been to study the relationship between age and aneurysm size. Although growth of known aneurysms and development of new aneurysms is a well-documented phenomenon,*** patient age does not appear to be associated with aneurysm size.[34,138,252] Based on these data,

*References 5,20,23,38,79,117,169,178,186,196,199, 204,209,233,234,254,255

**References 12,62,63,73,98,130,143,176,180,186,196 197,233,234,243,261

***References 2,8,9,32,46,61,69,78,89,105,118,144, 154,163,168,208,229,247,260,263

Weibers et al[252] hypothesized that most intracranial aneurysms develop over a relatively short time. When the limits of aneurysm wall elasticity are reached, the aneurysm either ruptures or undergoes compensatory hardening. These authors concluded that increasing age itself was not a risk factor for aneurysm rupture.

The mechanisms that link both unruptured and ruptured aneurysms to age have not as yet been identified. Years of hypertension, hemodynamic stresses, or other means of vascular-injury may be required to induce enough weakness in the arterial wall to favor aneurysm formation.[114] Both epidemiologic and postmortem studies point to such an association between atherosclerosis and cerebral aneurysms.[44,50,100,114,205,248] These studies, however, represent a select group of patients dying from ruptured intracranial aneurysms, and are biased by the high case fatality rate in aneurysm patients with concomitant coronary artery disease[231] or hypertension.[7,79,128,248] Because of this, the significance of atherosclerosis in the formation or rupture of cerebral aneurysms remains unclear.

Intracranial aneurysms in children or adolescents differ from those in adults, indicating that they may represent a distinct pathogenetic subgroup.[3,12,62,73,98,137,143,176,243] In pediatric series, males outnumber females 3 to 1 while nearly the reverse is true in adults.[3,62,137,143,176,180] Aneurysms in children, unlike those in adults, are rarely incidental in postmortem or angiographic findings; the risk of rupture is higher as well.[26,100,243] Also, they have a propensity to reach giant size, expand rapidly, and involve the posterior circulation or peripheral arterial branches.*

The incidence of both ruptured and unruptured saccular aneurysms increases with age, although age itself may not be a risk factor for rupture alone. Pediatric and adult aneurysms may be governed by different pathogenic mechanisms.

*References 3,12,62,73,98,137,143,176,243

## Gender

Adult women are affected by aneurysmal SAH more than men by a ratio of 60 to 40.** In children and adolescents this gender ratio is reversed, with males predominating nearly 3 to 1.[3,62,137,143,176,180] The reversal in ratio cannot be explained by numeric differences in gender at various ages or by the presence of gender-related hypertension or other known gender-related risk factors.[23,130,199]

Efforts to determine whether gender is related to aneurysm formation, rupture, or both have produced conflicting results. In a large, planned postmortem series of 2,786 consecutive autopsies, 137 patients (4.9%) were identified with at least one intracranial aneurysm.[34] Aneurysms were found in 7.2% of all females and 3.5% of males. There was no difference between the sexes in the proportion of ruptured and unruptured aneurysms. In a retrospective autopsy series of similar size, ruptured aneurysms occurred more commonly in females than males (1.7 to 1) but unruptured aneurysms occurred equally in both sexes.[50] Multiple aneurysms are more common in women than men, suggesting that gender is at least a risk factor for aneurysm formation.[6,172]

Little is known about the links between gender and aneurysmal SAH. Because gender ratio reversal occurs after the first two decades, hormonal factors have been considered.[227] Both former and current users of oral contraceptives are at increased risk for aneurysmal SAH.[185,195] Similarly, unmarried women have a lower incidence of SAH than either married or divorced women.[127] In pregnant women, the incidence of aneurysmal SAH increases with increasing gestational age.[67] Studies of aneurysm formation in animals, however, have not confirmed the significance of estrogen.[48,236]

In adults, aneurysmal SAH is more common in women than men. Gender is probably

**References 23,37,38,50,63,79,129,130,169,184,186, 199,204,233,234,252,253,255

related at least to aneurysm formation; however, its importance as a risk factor for rupture is not clear.

## Genetics

Genetic factors play a role in aneurysmal SAH. One large autopsy series reported that 11% of patients with either a ruptured or unruptured aneurysm had a family history of cerebrovascular disease as compared with 4% of matched controls.[50] A Swedish study of nearly 500 consecutively treated aneurysm patients revealed a higher incidence of blood relatives with aneurysmal SAHs than expected in the general population.[159]

In rare cases, aneurysmal SAH occurs in patients with clearly defined genetic disorders.* In most situations these genetic conditions are associated with existing weakness, ongoing injury, or degeneration of the arterial wall. Most aneurysms, however, are not associated with clearly defined genetic abnormalities, and other approaches have been used to study the importance of genetic factors.

The HLA region of chromosome 6 is a highly polymorphic gene region that specifies the various HLA factors: (1) HLA-ABC antigens, (2) HLA-DR and related antigens, and (3) some complement factors. Because the HLA region is so highly polymorphic (i.e. several different genes or alleles are available to occupy each gene locus), it has been used as a genetic marker for a variety of diseases.[247] HLA factors and certain complement genes are linked to aneurysmal SAH.** Norrgard et al[161] found a higher incidence of the HLA antigen A28, and a significantly decreased frequency of the HLA antigen B40 and the complement factor C4B2 among aneurysm patients when compared to controls from the same geographic region. Ostergaard et al[175] found an increased B7 homozygosity and BfS phenotype in aneurysm patients. No association has been found between blood group or serum proteins and cerebral aneurysm disease.[161] Familial studies tracing the link between inheritance of HLA factors and intracranial aneurysms have not been performed. It is not known whether HLA and complement factors are related to aneurysm formation, or rupture, or both. The mechanisms that link HLA to aneurysm disease are not known. It is generally believed that the HLA system participates in the regulation not only of the immune system[175,247] but also of some nonimmunologic areas such as the endocrine system.[173,175,247]

Although the majority of cerebral aneurysms appear to be "sporadic," many families have been reported that appear to have an autosomal dominant pattern of disease transmission.* Familial patients differ from "sporadic" aneurysm patients in several ways. In the former, aneurysm rupture tends to occur from smaller aneurysms at younger ages, and the distribution of aneurysms around the circle of Willis is different. In some families, multiple, broad-based, or fusiform aneurysms are common. These clinical differences suggest that familial aneurysms, like pediatric aneurysms, may represent a distinct pathogenetic subset.

The author[35] has studied the secretion of proteolytic enzymes by skin fibroblasts from one patient with multiple broad-based intracranial aneurysms and a family history of both intracranial and aortic aneurysm diseases. Although the secretion of collagenase by "sporadic" intracranial aneurysm patients was the same as for controls, the familial patient's fibroblasts secreted significantly more collagenase activity. Secretion of endoproteinase activity was also increased in the familial patient when compared to normal controls or "sporadic" cerebral aneurysm patients. Aneurysm formation may have occurred in this

*References 65,67,72,111,135,146,169,192,200,228, 229,237,238

**References 132,133,140,160,170,171,206

*References 1,4,6,10,15,16,29,30,33,41,42,45,56–58, 66,68,71,77,81,83,104,107–109,112,121,124,131,136, 140,152,153,158,161,162,167,179,182,187,189,201–203,212–214,219,221,238–240,242,245,246,250

patient because enzymatic injury induced weakness of the arterial wall.

Genetic factors appear to influence the occurrence of aneurysmal SAH. Although most aneurysms appear to arise "sporadically," familial intracranial saccular aneurysms, as with pediatric aneurysms, may be a distinct pathogenetic group.

## Vascular Factors

Saccular aneurysms are unique to the intracranial cerebral vessels, as aneurysms affecting the aorta or other extracranial arteries are usually fusiform.[191,192,227] Unlike somatic arteries, cerebral vessels are thin-walled and remain relatively unsupported as they tra-verse the subarachnoid space. This may place increased mechanical demands on the tissues of cerebral arteries when compared with extracranial arteries. Cerebral arteries are composed of four distinct microscopic layers: (1) the adventitia, (2) the media, (3) an internal elastic lamina (cerebral arteries have no external elastic lamina), and (4) an intima lined by endothelial cells. Disorders, whether congenital or acquired, of nearly every layer alone or in combination have been hypothesized to be important to the formation of cerebral aneurysms. Forbus[64] proposed that focal areas of weakness due to gap defects of the media ("loci minoris resistentiae") eventually developed into cerebral aneurysms. These gaps, however, occur commonly in normal individuals and may increase in size and frequency with age.* No evidence exists indicating that these gaps enlarge to become aneurysms. Glynn[75] proposed that focal degeneration of the internal elastic lamina was related to aneurysm formation, while Carmichael[31] believed that focal defects of both the internal elastic lamina and media must be present before aneurysms could form.

More recently, interest has focused on relating aneurysmal SAH to more generalized disorders of the cerebral blood vessels. Microscopically, even nonaneurysmal portions of cerebral arteries taken from aneurysm patients show clear structural derangements. Examination of cerebral arteries from normal individuals reveals a dense, uniformly distributed network of fine reticular fibers in the arterial media (Figure 2A). This pattern does not appear to be influenced by aging or intimal proliferation.[93] Several studies show that the total amount of reticular fibers are reduced in the media of cerebral arteries of aneurysm patients.[36,40,94–97,174,175] Reticular fibers in these patients are irregularly distributed and shorter than normal (Figure 2B). Somatic arteries of patients with cerebral aneurysms also appear to be deficient in reticular fibers.[171] In both aneurysm and control patients, no differences are observed in the-appearance or content of elastin fibers which are limited almost exclusively to the internal elastic lamina.[36,40]

Reticular fibers are, at least in part, composed of type III collagen,[115,116,150] a major collagen of arterial tissue. Immunohistochemical staining of cerebral arteries for type III collagen shows reduced amounts in aneurysm patients.[36] It is possible that deficient structural elements undermine the mechanical integrity of the cerebral arterial wall and thus promote aneurysm formation and rupture.

Pope et al[190] were the first to link abnormalities in type III collagen metabolism with the occurrence of cerebral aneurysms. Using polyacrylamide gel electrophoresis of pepsin-digested skin biopsy specimens, and carboxymethyl cellulose chromatography of radioactively labeled collagens produced by cultured fibroblasts, they observed a relative deficiency of type III collagen with respect to type I collagen in 7 of 12 aneurysm patients. Although not definitive, Pope's data suggested that these differences were due to decreased amounts of type III collagen rather than increased amounts of type I collagen. Based on these results, they speculated that: (1) some cerebral aneurysms resemble various inherited defects of connective tissue (i.e. Ehlers-Danlos syndrome type IV); (2) type III

*References 75,88,134,141,192,209,229,262

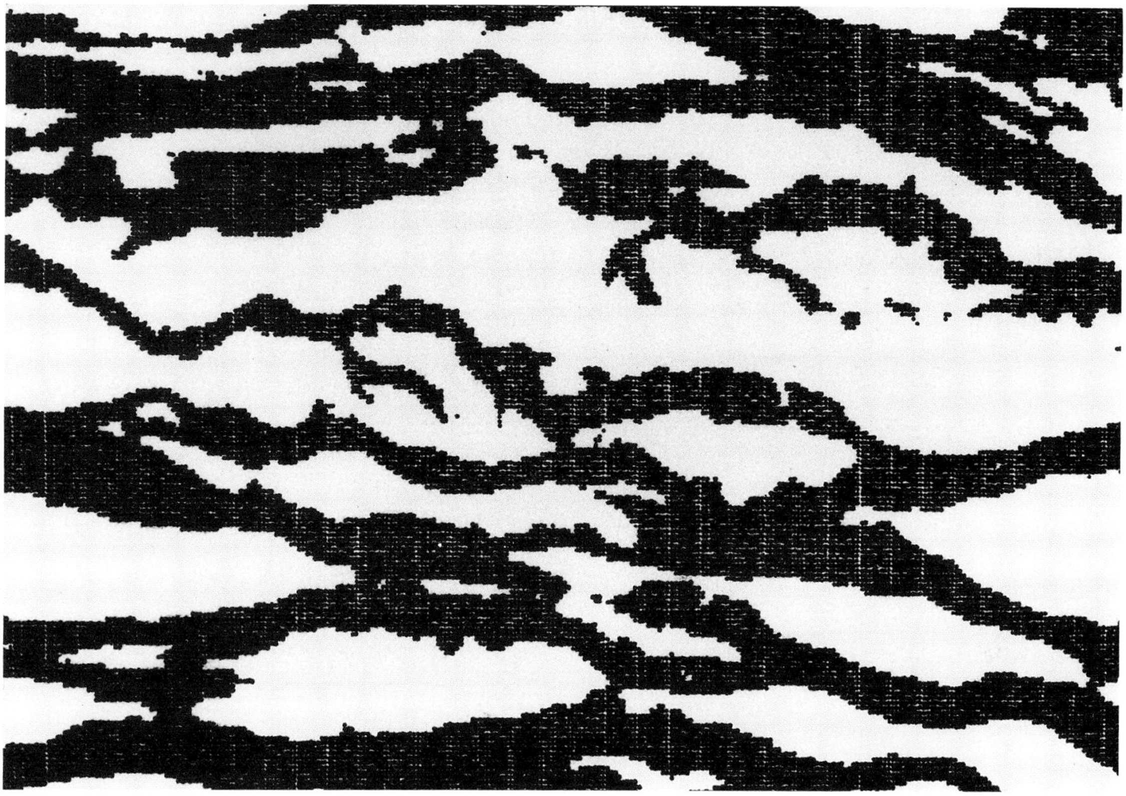

*Figure 2A. Computerized digital image of a photomicrograph of the media of a cerebral artery taken from a control patient (stained by Laidlaw's Silver Impregnation method for reticular fibers) generated for the purpose of morphometric analysis. Reticular fibers are displayed as the black areas. The reticular fibers are uniformly distributed and form a dense network.*[40]

collagen deficiencies directly interfere with the mechanical properties of biologic tissues; and (3) the collagen deficiencies observed in some aneurysm patients influence the properties of the arterial wall in such a way as to promote aneurysm formation (the "collagen hypothesis"). Several years later, the same group[155] reported a similar set of experiments performed on skin and temporal artery specimens collected at the time of surgery from 17 aneurysm patients. Eleven of these 17 patients studied appeared to be type III collagen-deficient. In this report, measurement of pepsin-released tissue collagen did not appear as easy to interpret as in the earlier report, and most conclusions were based on ratios of radioactive labeled collagens estimated by slab gel autoradiography and scanning densitometry, or chromatographic separation of radioactive collagens produced by cultured fibroblasts. It also appeared that there were variations in the severity of type III collagen deficiency. No obvious clinical differences distinguished type III collagen-deficient aneurysm patients from those who were not; however, there were more women than men in the former group. In neither study did these researchers comment on the family histories of the patients studied.

Recently Ostergaard and Oxlund[170] used gel electrophoresis to study the ratio of type I to type III collagen in cyanogen-bromide digests prepared from middle cerebral and brachial arteries collected at autopsy from patients who died from aneurysmal SAH, and control patients who were not believed to have had cerebral aneurysms. A decrease in the amount of type III collagen relative to type I

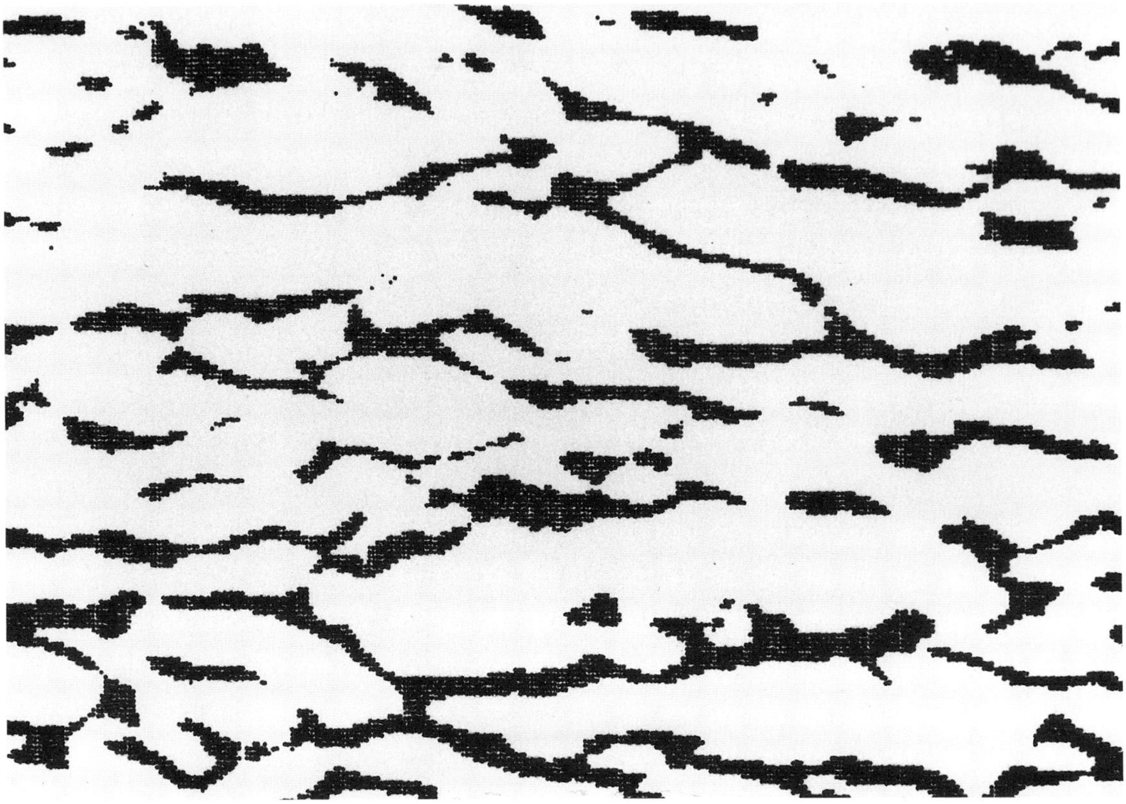

*Figure 2B. Computerized digital image of a photomicrograph of the media of a cerebral artery taken from an aneurysm patient (stained by Laidlaw's Silver Impregnation method for reticular fibers) generated for the purpose of morphometric analysis. Reticular fibers are displayed as the black areas. Reticular fibers are sparse, irregularly distributed, and shortened.*[40]

collagen was noted in both the middle cerebral and brachial arteries in 6 of the 14 aneurysm patients studied. As in the previous studies, it was not clear whether this represented a relative deficiency of type III collagen (i.e. type I collagen was increased) or an absolute deficiency of type III collagen. Again, deficient patients were predominantly female. In addition to this biochemical analysis, the biomechanical properties of these arteries were also studied. Type III collagen-deficient middle cerebral arteries showed normal mechanical strength. However, a significant increase in arterial extensibility was noted at physiologically relevant stresses (corresponding to blood pressures between 100–200 mm Hg). No differences were observed in the biomechanical properties of collagen-deficient brachial arteries.

The "collagen hypothesis," however, has remained controversial.[123,124,188,189] Deficiencies in type III collagen have been observed in some but not all aneurysm patients, with the degree of deficiency being small in most instances. One recent report failed to identify abnormalities of type III collagen synthesis by skin fibroblasts taken from a patient with multiple cerebral aneurysms and a strong family history for aneurysm disease.[124]

A deficiency of type III collagen can be the result of depressed synthesis or accelerated degradation. The author[39] used Southern blots to explore the possibility that differences associated with the type III collagen gene are related to type III collagen deficiency and the occurrence of cerebral aneurysms. Normal control subjects showed a simple two-allele polymorphism associated with the type III col-

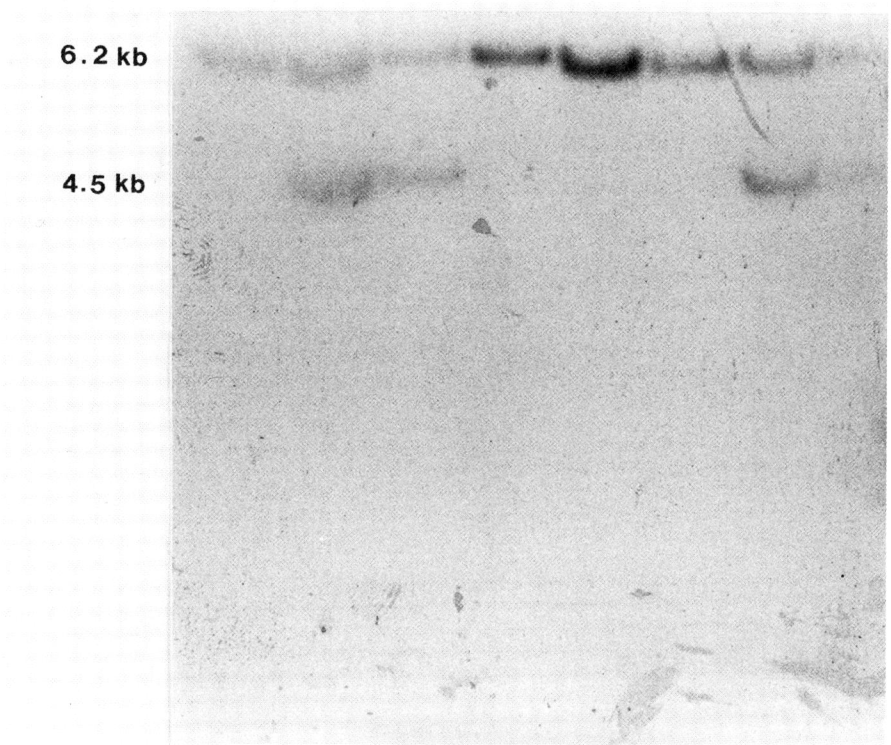


*Figure 3A. Southern blot of an Ava II digest of genomic DNA extracted from eight normal control subjects probed with pPB-1, a genomic DNA probe to the 3'-flanking region of the type III collagen gene. A simple two-allele polymorphism associated with the type III collagen gene was identified in all normal control subjects with a band at either 6.2 kb ($A_1$) or 4.5 kb ($A_2$) or both.*[39]

lagen gene ($A_1$ = 6.2 kb and $A_2$ = 4.5 kb after Ava II digestion) (Figure 3A). In five of the ten aneurysm patients studied, however, novel restriction fragment length polymorphisms associated with the type III collagen gene were found that were not present in any of the control subjects examined (Figure 3B). Based on the pattern of banding, a "recessive" model was proposed in which abnormal genes associated with the type III collagen gene inherited from both parents were required for aneurysm formation. The five remaining aneurysm patients had Southern blots similar to normal control subjects. Cerebral aneurysms may have developed in these patients by mechanisms other than those associated with the type III collagen gene. Alternatively, these patients may harbor small changes associated with this gene that remain below the resolution of Southern blot analysis.

These observations provide evidence that cerebral aneurysms, at least in some patients, are related to genetic differences associated with the type III collagen gene. It is conceivable that in these patients a defective type III collagen gene results in impaired production of this protein, undermining the mechanical integrity of the cerebral vessel wall and producing conditions that promote the formation and rupture of cerebral aneurysms.

## Factors Related to Aneurysm Rupture

Little is known about the factors immediately related to aneurysm rupture. Rupture usually occurs at the aneurysm's apex,[46] though less commonly, bleeding will occur from the body. Only rarely will bleeding come

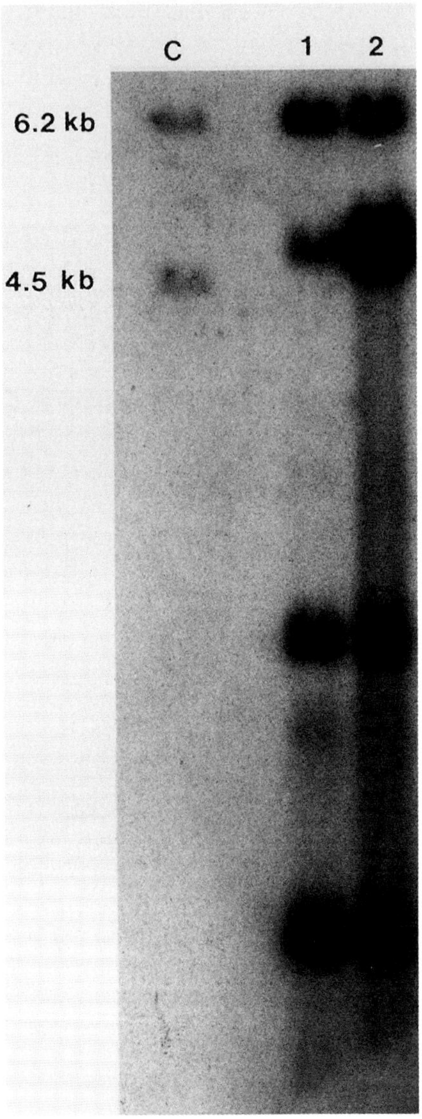


*Figure 3B. Southern blot similar to Figure 3A showing a normal control (C) for reference and novel restriction fragment length polymorphisms associated with the type III collagen gene in aneurysm patients 1 and 2. The control patient shows a band at 6.2 kb ($A_1$) and 4.5 kb ($A_2$). Both aneurysm patients show fragments at 6.2 kb, similar to $A_1$ found in normal controls, and fragments at 4.8 kb, 3.4 kb, and 2.6 kb. These latter three fragments are novel restriction fragment polymorphisms associated with cerebral aneurysm disease not observed in any normal control subjects.*[39]

from the aneurysm neck. Multiple loculations are more common in ruptured than unruptured aneurysms, and in many cases may be the source of hemorrhage.[46] Multiple aneurysms are more common in patients with SAH than those with unruptured lesions.[50] In most multiple aneurysms, the aneurysm with the largest external diameter will be the source of hemorrhage.[46]

Crompton[46] was the first to hypothesize that enzymatic injury to the aneurysm wall may immediately precede aneurysm rupture. Mural deposition of fibrin was found within many aneurysms after rupture. Numerous polymorphonuclear leukocytes, plasma cells, and small round cells also were seen throughout the aneurysm wall. Initially, Crompton suggested that these changes were the result of the aneurysm rupture. However, the finding of these prominent changes along with necrosis of the aneurysm wall immediately after aneurysm rupture suggested that they may have occurred before aneurysm rupture. A study of cases of unruptured aneurysms revealed similar changes in 23 of 79 unruptured aneurysms. Crompton concluded that cellular and fibrinoid infiltration of the unruptured aneurysm wall resulted in weakening of the wall, creating conditions that may lead to rupture.

Hashimoto et al[85] reported similar changes in experimental aneurysms occurring with carotid ligation in hypertensive, lathyritic rats. Initially, endothelial cells show regressive changes such as balloon-like protrusions and crater-like depressions. Gaps formed at the junctions between endothelial cells suggest that it may be beyond the ability of the endothelial cells to transform and cover the whole surface of the aneurysm. Many leukocytes were found adhering to the interendothelial gaps, providing the opportunity for enzymatic damage of the aneurysm wall. Supporting this hypothesis, increased acid phosphatase activity was found to be associated with the aneurysm wall.

Cigarette smoking may further increase enzymatic injury. Cigarette smoking is associated with aneurysmal SAH and is also known to increase circulating protease activity and decrease protease inhibitors.*

---

*References 13,14,22,27,43,55,110,166,185,241

Because of the complex composition of blood, its pulsatile flow, and the architectural and biomechanical properties of the cerebral arteries, rheologic factors other than simple blood pressure and hemodynamic flow may be related to aneurysmal SAH. Distinct fluctuations of flow superimposed on the pulse wave have been identified within spontaneous human and experimental aneurysms.* In some patients, these fluctuations appear to be periodic, with measured period lengths of 60–150 msec.[230] These flow fluctuations may induce vibrations of the aneurysm wall that contribute to aneurysm progression and eventual rupture.

## Natural History of Unruptured Aneurysms

Although Weibers et al[252] postulated thataneurysms develop over a relatively short time, followed by either rupture or stabilization, hemorrhage from existing unruptured lesions is common.[59,198,252,253] Rosenorn et al[198] estimated that the minimum annual risk of hemorrhage from previously identified unruptured lesions was at least 2%. Weibers et al[253] found that aneurysm size was the single most important variable related to subsequent rupture. When multiple variables were considered, aneurysm size coupled with patient's age was more significant than size alone. Among patients with aneurysms 10 mm or larger in diameter, actuarial analyses using aneurysm rupture as an endpoint showed a rupture rate of 24% at 7 years after diagnosis for patients younger than the median age (59 years), and a rupture rate of 48% at 7 years after the diagnosis for patients of the median age or older.

Unruptured giant aneurysms present a special problem, largely because the risk of surgical repair is greater than with smaller lesions.[54,183,233,234] Little is known about the natural history of unruptured giant aneurysms; however, the available evidence suggests that the natural history is quite poor, making consideration of repair reasonable.[70]

*References 101,210,230,232

## Conclusion

Aneurysmal SAH remains a devastating disease. One-third of all patients who suffer an aneurysmal SAH will not survive long enough to reach medical attention. Of those who do survive to hospital admission, nearly one half will die or be left neurologically devastated. This unacceptable morbidity and mortality occur primarily as a direct result of the initial hemorrhage, and in many situations cannot be altered by modern therapy. An understanding of aneurysm formation and rupture may allow us to identify individuals at risk for aneurysmal SAH and to prescribe preventive treatment before the devastating effects of hemorrhage.

## References


1. Acosta-Rua GJ. Familial incidence of ruptured intracranial aneurysms. report of 12 cases. *Arch Neurol.* 1978;35:675–677.
2. Allcock JM, Canham PB. Angiographic study of the growth of intracranial aneurysms. *J Neurosurg.* 1976;45:617–621.
3. Amacher AL, Drake CG. The results of operating upon cerebral aneurysms and angiomas in children and adolescents. I: Cerebral aneurysms. *Childs Brain.* 1979;5:151 165.
4. Ambrosetto P, Galassi E. Familial occurrence of multiple intracranial aneurysms. case reports and review of the literature. *Acta Neurochir (Wein).* 1981;56:233–238.
5. Andrews RJ. Familial intracranial aneurysms. *Arch Neurol.* 1979;36:524. Letter.
6. Andrews RJ, Spiegel P. Intracranial aneurysms: Age, sex, blood pressure, and multiplicity in an unselected series of patients. *J Neurosurg.* 1979; 51:27–32.
7. Artiola i Fortuny L, Prieto-Valiente L. Long-term prognosis in surgically treated intracranial aneurysms, I: mortality. *J Neurosurg.* 1981;54:26–34.
8. Asari S, Kunishio K, Sunami N, et al. Rapid growth and rupture of a newly originated aneurysm near the clipped middle cerebral artery aneurysm [In Japanese]. *No Shinkei Geka.* 1986;14:587–591. English abstract.
9. Azzam CJ. Growth of multiple peripheral high flow aneurysms of the posterior inferior cerebellar artery associated with a cerebellar arteriovenous malformation. *Neurosurgery.* 1987;21:934–939.

10. Bannerman RM, Ingall GB, Graf CJ. The familial occurrence of intracranial aneurysms. *Neurology.* 1970;20:283–292.
11. Beadles CF. Aneurisms of the larger cerebral arteries. *Brain.* 1907;30:285–336.
12. Becker DH, Silverberg GD, Nelson DH, et al. Saccular aneurysm of infancy and early childhood. *Neurosurgery.* 1978;2:1–7.
13. Bell BA, Ambrose J. Smoking and the risk of stroke. *Acta Neurochir (Wein).* 1982;64:1–7.
14. Bell BA, Symon L. Smoking and subarachnoid hemorrhage. *Br Med J.* 1979;1:577–578.
15. Bentzen N. Family incidence of intracranial aneurysms: case reports. *N Z Med J.* 1972;75:153–155.
16. Beumont PJ. The familial occurrence of berry aneurysm. *J Neurol Neurosurg Psychiatry.* 1968; 31: 399–402.
17. Biumi F. Observations anatomicae, scholiis illustratae. Observatio V. In: Sandifort E, *Thesaurus Dissertationum.* Milan: S and J Luchtmans; 1765:373–379.
18. Blackhall L. In: *Observations on the Nature and Cure of Dropsies.* 2nd ed. London: Longman, Hurst, Rees, Orme and Brown; 1814:126–135.
19. Blane G. History of some cases of disease in the brain, with an account of the appearances upon examination after death, and some general observations on complaints of the head. *Trans Soc Improve Med Chir Knowledge.* 1800;2:192–198.
20. Bolander HG, Kourtopoulos H, West KA. Retrospective analysis of 162 consecutive cases of ruptured intracranial aneurysms. *Acta Neurochir.* 1984; 70:31–41.
21. Bonet T. *Sepulcretum Anatomicum.* Geneva:1679.
22. Bonita R. Cigarette smoking, hypertension and the risk of subarachnoid hemorrhage: a population based case-control study. *Stroke.* 1986; 17:831–835.
23. Bonita R, Thomson S. Subarachnoid hemorrhage: epidemiology, diagnosis, management and outcome. *Stroke.* 1985;16:591–594.
24. Bramwell B. Clinical and pathological memoranda, IV: case of aneurism of the right internal carotid artery. *Edinburgh Med J.* 1886;32:97–108.
25. Bramwell B. Two enormous intracranial aneurisms. *Edinburgh Med J.* 1887;32:911–922.
26. Bremer JL. Congenital aneurysms of the cerebral arteries. *Arch Pathol.* 1943;35:819–831.
27. Bridges RB, Wyatt RJ, Rehm SR. Effect of smoking on peripheral blood leukocytes and serum antiproteases. *Eur J Respir Dis Suppl.* 1985;139: 24–33.
28. Brinton W. Report on cases of cerebral aneurisms. *Trans Pathol Soc Lond.* 1850–52;3:47–49.
29. Brisman R, Abbassioun K. Familial intracranial aneurysms. *J Neurosurg.* 1971;34:678–682.
30. Brodsky MC, Frenkel REP, Spoor TC. Familial intracranial aneurysm presenting as a subtle stable third nerve palsy. Letter. *Arch Ophthalmol.* 1988; 106:173.
31. Carmichael R. The pathogenesis of non-inflammatory cerebral aneurysms. *J Pathol Bact.* 1950;62: 1–19.
32. Cecotto C, Janes PP, De Nardi F. Origin and growth of cerebral aneurysms: report of two cases. *Acta Neurochir Suppl (Wien).* 1979; 28:627.
33. Chakravorty BG, Gleadhill CA. Familial incidence of cerebral aneurysms. *Br Med J.* 1966;1:147–148.
34. Chason JL, Hindman WM. Berry aneurysms of the circle of Willis. *Neurology.* 1958;8:41–44.
35. Chyatte D, Brophy C, Reilly J, et al. Metabolism of the extracellular matrix in cerebral aneurysm disease. *American Association of Neurological Surgeons,* Nashville, Tenn: American Association of Neurological Surgeons 58th Annual Meeting; 1990: 321.
36. Chyatte D, Brophy C, Reilly J, et al. Morphometric analysis of reticular, elastin and type III collagen fibers in the cerebral arteries of patients with intracranial aneurysms. *Stroke.* 1990;21:161. Abstract
37. Chyatte D, Chen TL, Brass L. Seasonal variation in the incidence of aneurysmal subarachnoid hemorrhage in Connecticut during the last decade. *American Association of Neurological Surgeons.* New Orleans: American Association of Neurological Surgeons; 1991:306.
38. Chyatte D, Fode NC, Sundt TM Jr. Early versus late intracranial aneurysm surgery in subarachnoid hemorrhage. *J Neurosurg.* 1988;69:326–331.
39. Chyatte D, Mierzejewski C. Novel restriction fragment length polymorphism associated with the gene for type III collagen (COL3A1) in patients with cerebral aneurysms. *Congress of Neurological Surgeons.* Orlando, Fla: Congress of Neurological Surgeons; 1991:163.
40. Chyatte D, Reilly J, Tilson MD. Morphometric analysis of reticular and elastin fibers in the cerebral arteries of patients with intracranial aneurysms. *Neurosurgery.* 1990;26:939–943.
41. Colafranceshi M, Mennonna P. Unusual observation of a familial aneurysm of the anterior communicating artery [In Italian]. *Arch De Vecchi Anat Patol.* 1967; 50:789–807. English abstract.
42. Coppola AR. Familial intracranial aneurysm. *Int Surg.* 1973;58:508.
43. Cox DW, Billingsley GD. Oxidation of plasma alpha 1-antitrypsin in smokers and nonsmokers and by an oxidizing agent. *Am Rev Respir Dis.* 1984; 130:594–599.
44. Crawford T. Some observations on the pathogenesis and natural history of intracranial aneurysms. *J Neurol Neurosurg Psychiatry.* 1959;22:259-266.
45. Crompton M. Familial incidence of cerebral aneurysms. *Br Med J.* 1979;1:292.
46. Crompton MR. Mechanism of growth and rupture in cerebral berry aneurysms. *Br Med J.* 1966; 1: 1138–1142.
47. Crompton MR. The pathogenesis of cerebral aneurysms. *Brain.* 1966;89:797–814.
48. Dai Z, Yao-dong B, Zi-Wei D, et al. Experimental cerebral aneurysms in rats: experimental method and effect of estradiol. *Chinese Med J Engl.* 1985;98: 421–426.
49. Dandy WE. Intracranial aneurysm of the internal carotid artery cured by operation. *Ann Surg.* 1938; 107:654–659.
50. de la Monte SM, Moore GW, Mong MA, et al. Risk factors for the development and rupture of intracranial berry aneurysms. *Am J Med.* 1985;78:957–964.
51. de Moulin D. Aneurysms in antiquity. *Arch Chir Neerl.* 1961;13:49–63.
52. Deruty R, Mottolese C, Soustiel JF, et al. Association of cerebral arteriovenous malformation and cerebral aneurysm: Diagnosis and management. *Acta Neurochir (Wien).* 1990;107:133–139.
53. Di Bonito L, Giarelli L. Pathogenesis of cerebral

hemorrhage in the light of objective lesions in the encephalic arteries observed in 226 necropsies. [In Italian.] *Minerva Med.* 1975;66:4391–4398. English abstract.
54. Drake CG. Giant intracranial aneurysms: experience with surgical treatment in 174 patients. *Clin Neurosurg.* 1979;26:12–95.
55. Dubick MA, Conteas CN, Billy HT, et al. Raised serum concentrations of pancreatic enzymes in cigarette smokers. *Gut.* 1987;28:330–335.
56. Edelsohn L, Caplan L, Rosenbaum AE. Familial aneurysms and infundibular widening. *Neurology.* 1972;22:1056–1060.
57. Eishunnar KS, Whittle IR. Familial intracranial aneurysms: report of five families. *Br J Neurosurg.* 1990;4:181–186.
58. Endtz LJ. Familial incidence of intracranial aneurysms. *Acta Neurochir (Wien).* 1968;19:297–305.
59. Eskesen V, Rosenorn J, Schmidt K, et al. Clinical features and outcome in 48 patients with unruptured intracranial saccular aneurysms: a prospective consecutive study. *Br J Neurosurg.* 1987;1: 47–52.
60. Fearnsides EG. Intracranial aneurysms. *Brain.* 1916;39:224–296.
61. Ferguson GG. Physical factors in the initiation, growth and rupture of human intracranial saccular aneurysms. *J Neurosurg.* 1972;37:666–677.
62. Ferrante L, Fortuna A, Celli P, et al. Intracranial arterial aneurysms in early childhood. *Surg Neurol.* 1988;29:39–56.
63. Fogelholm R. Subarachnoid hemorrhage in Middle-Finland: incidence, early prognosis and indications for neurosurgical treatment. *Stroke.* 1981;12:296–301.
64. Forbus WD. On the origin of miliary aneurysms of the superficial cerebral arteries. *Bull Johns Hopkins Hosp.* 1930;47:239–284.
65. Forrai G, Tauszik T, Tauszik N, et al. A high incidence of PKD in a large geographic area of southwestern Hungary: a medical genetic study. *Prog Clin Biol Res.* 1989;305:89–94.
66. Fox JL. Familial intracranial aneurysms: case report. *J Neurosurg.* 1982;57:416–417.
67. Fox JL. *Intracranial Aneurysms.* New York: SpringerVerlag; 1983.
68. Fox JL, Ko JP. Familial intracranial aneurysms: six cases among 13 siblings. *J Neurosurg.* 1980;52: 501–503.
69. Fujii H, Nozaki J, Ito H, et al. New growth aneurysm in an adult whose multiple aneurysms were operated on two years ago: a case report. [In Japanese.] *Rinsho Hoshasen.* 1981;26:295–298. English abstract.
70. Fujita K, Yamashita H, Masumura M, et al. Natural history of giant intracranial aneurysms. *No Shinkei Geka.* 1988;16:225–231.
71. Fukawa O, Aihara H. [Familial intracranial aneurysms—report of 20 cases in eight families and review of the literature]. [In Japanese.] *No Shinkei Geka.* 1987;15: 911–919. English abstract.
72. Gabow PA. Autosomal dominant polycystic kidney disease—more than a renal disease. *Am J Kidney Dis.* 1990;16:403–413.
73. Gerosa M, Licata C, Fiore DL, et al. Intracranial aneurysms of childhood. *Childs Brain.* 1980;6: 295–302.
74. Gillingham FJ. The management of ruptured intracranial aneurysm: Hunterian lecture delivered at the Royal College of Surgeons of England on 24th January, 1957. *Ann R Coll Surg Engl.* 1958;23:89–117.
75. Glynn LE. Medial defects in the circle of Willis and their relation to aneurysm formation. *J Pathol Bact.* 1940;51:213–222.
76. Gowers WR. *A Manual of Diseases of the Nervous System.* 2nd ed. London: Churchhill; 1893.
77. Graf CJ. Familial intracranial aneurysms. *J Neurosurg.* 1966;25:304–308.
78. Graf CJ, Hamby WB. Report of a case of cerebral aneurysm in an adult developing apparently de novo. *J Neurol Neurosurg Psychiatry.* 1964; 27:153–156.
79. Graf CJ, Nibbelink DW. Cooperative study of intracranial aneurysms and subarachnoid hemorrhage: report on a randomized treatment study, III: intracranial surgery. *Stroke.* 1974;5:559–601.
80. Gull W. Cases of aneurism of cerebral vessels. *Guy's Hosp Rep.* 1859;5:281–304.
81. Halal F, Mohr G, Toussi T, et al. Intracranial aneurysms: a report of a large pedigree. *Am J Med Genet.* 1983;15:89–95.
82. Handa H, Hashimoto N, Nagata I, et al. Saccular aneurysms in rats: A newly developed animal model of the disease. *Stroke.* 1983;14:857–866.
83. Hashimoto I. Familial intracranial aneurysms and cerebral vascular anomalies. *J Neurosurg.* 1977;46: 419–427.
84. Hashimoto N, Handa H, Nagata I, et al. Experimentally induced cerebral aneurysms in rats, Part V: relation of hemodynamics in the circle of Willis to formation of aneurysms. *Surg Neurol.* 1980;13: 41–45.
85. Hashimoto N, Handa H, Nagata I, et al. Animal model of cerebral aneurysms: pathology and pathogenesis of induced cerebral aneurysms in rats. *Neurol Res.* 1984;6:33–40.
86. Hawthorne VM, Greaves DA, Beevers DG. Blood pressure in a Scottish town. *Br Med J.* 1974;3:600–603.
87. Hayashi S, Arimoto T, Itakura T, et al. The association of intracranial aneurysms and arteriovenous malformation of the brain: case report. *J Neurosurg.* 1981;55:971–975.
88. Hazama F, Hashimoto N. An animal model of cerebral aneurysms. *Neuropathol Appl Neurobiol.* 1987;13:77–90.
89. Hecht ST, Horton JA, Yonas H. Growth of a thrombosed giant vertebral artery aneurysm after parent artery occlusion. *AJNR.* 1991;12:449–451.
90. Hegedüs K. Dissecting intracranial aneurysm. *Arch Psychiatr Nervenkr.* 1982;232:25–32.
91. Hegedüs K. Ectasia of the basilar artery with special reference to possible pathogenesis. *Surg Neurol.* 1985;24:463–469.
92. Hegedüs K. Reticular fiber deficiency in the intracranial arteries of patients with dissecting aneurysm and review of the possible pathogenesis of previously reported cases. *Eur Arch Psychiatry Neurol Sci.* 1985;235:102–106.
93. Hegedüs K. Pattern of reticular fibers of the major cerebral arteries in cases of unexplained subarachnoid hemorrhage. *J Neurol.* 1986;233:44–47.
94. Hegedüs K. Some observations on reticular fibers in the media of the major cerebral arteries: a comparative study of patients without vascular diseases and those with ruptured berry aneurysms. *Surg Neurol.* 1984;22:301–307.

95. Hegedüs K, Molnár L. Anatomical patterns of hypoplastic posterior communicating arteries and their implications for cerebrovascular diseases. *Eur Arch Psychiatry Neurol Sci.* 1987;236:241–246.
96. Hegedüs K, Molnár P. Histopathological study of major intracranial arteries in premature infants related to intracranial hemorrhage. *J Neurosurg.* 1985;62:419–424.
97. Hegedüs K, Molnár P. On the pattern of reticular fibers in the intracranial arteries of mature newborns with and without intracranial hemorrhage. *Childs Nerv Syst.* 1986;2:2–4.
98. Heiskanen O, Vilkki J. Intracranial arterial aneurysms in children and adolescents. *Acta Neurochir* (Wien). 1981;59: 55–63.
99. Hillbom M, Kaste M. Alcohol intoxication: A risk factor for primary subarachnoid hemorrhage. *Neurology.* 1982;32:706–711.
100. Housepian EM, Pool JL. A systematic analysis of intracranial aneurysms from the autopsy file of the Presbyterian Hospital, 1914 to 1956. *J Neuropathol Exp Neurol.* 1958;17:409–423.
101. Hung EJN, Botwin MR. Mechanics of rupture of cerebral saccular aneurysms. *J Biomech.* 1975;8: 385–392.
102. Hutchinson J. Aneurysms of the internal carotid within the skull diagnosed 11 years before patient's death. Spontaneous cure. *Trans Clin Soc (Lond).* 1875;8:127–131.
103. Iganava T, Takahashi M, Aoki H, et al. Aneurysmal subarachnoid hemorrhage in Izumo City and Shimane Prefecture of Japan: outcome. *Stroke.* 1988;19:176–180.
104. Ikeda H, Sakugawa H, Ueda S, et al. Familial cases of cerebral aneurysm. [In Japanese.] *No To Shinkei.* 1971;23: 201–205. English abstract.
105. Ikeda K, Hayase H, Hayashi M, et al. Aneurysm growth and enlargement of pre-aneurysmal lesions. [In Japanese.] *No Shinkei Geka.* 1984;12: 1151–1158. English abstract.
106. Jacques L. Aneurysm and anomaly of the circle of Willis. *Arch Pathol.* 1926;1:213–220.
107. Jain KK. Familial intracranial aneurysms: review of literature and presentation of six new cases. *Acta Neurochir (Wien).* 1974;30:129–137.
108. Jaksche H. Familial aneurysms. 4 carotid artery aneurysms in a family with 10 members. [In German.] *Zentralbl Neurochir.* 1986;47:351–353. English abstract.
109. Jankowicz E, Banach S, Pikiel L. [Familial occurrence of congenital intracranial aneurysm associated with cystic degeneration of the kidneys]. [In Polish.] *Neurol Neurochir Pol.* 1971;5:263–265.
110. Janoff A, Carp H. Possible mechanisms of emphysema in smokers: cigarette smoke condensate suppresses protease inhibition in vitro. *Am Rev Respir Dis.* 1977;116:65–72.
111. Kahn E, Markowitz J, Duffy L, et al. Berry aneurysms, cirrhosis, pulmonary emphysema, and bilateral symmetrical cerebral calcifications: a new syndrome. *Am J Med Genet Suppl.* 1987; 3:343–356.
112. Kak VK, Gleadhill CA, Bailey IC. The familial incidence of intracranial aneurysms. *J Neurol Neurosurg Psychiatry.* 1970;33:29–33.
113. Kalyanaraman UP, Elwood PW. Fibromuscular dysplasia of intracranial arteries causing multiple intracranial aneurysms. *Hum Pathol.* 1980;11: 481–484.
114. Kannel WB, Wolf PA, McGee DL, et al. Systolic blood pressure, arterial rigidity, and risk of stroke: the Framingham study. *JAMA.* 1981;245: 1225–1229.
115. Karttunen T, Alavaikko M, Apaja-Sarkkinen M, et al. An immunohistochemical study of laminin, type-IV collagen and type-III pN-collagen with relation to reticular fibres in Hodgkin's disease. *Int J Cancer.* 1988;41:52–58.
116. Karttunen T, Sormunen R, Risteli L, et al. Immunoelectron microscopic localization of laminin, type IV collagen and type III pN-collagen in reticular fibers of human lymph nodes. *J Histochem Cytochem.* 1989;37:279–286.
117. Kasseli NF, Adams HP Jr, Torner JC, et al. Influence of timing of admission after aneurysmal subarachnoid hemorrhage on overall outcome: report of the Cooperative Aneurysm Study. *Stroke.* 1981; 12:620–623.
118. Katayama Y, Tsubokawa T, Miyazaki S, et al. Growth of totally thrombosed giant aneurysm within the posterior cranial fossa: diagnostic and therapeutic considerations. *Neuroradiology.* 1991; 33:168–170.
119. Kayembe KNT, Sasahara M, Hazama F. Cerebral aneurysms and variations in the circle of Willis. *Stroke.* 1984;15:846–850.
120. Kim C, Kikuchi H, Hashimoto N, et al. Establishment of the experimental conditions for inducing saccular cerebral aneurysms in primates with special reference to hypertension. *Acta Neurochir (Wien).* 1989;96:132–136.
121. Kunishio K, Kuyama H, Asari S, et al. Unruptured cerebral aneurysms in two siblings screened by cerebral computed angiotomography. [In Japanese.] *No Shinkei Geka.* 1988;16:1267–1271.
122. Kwak R, Mizoi K, Katakura R, et al. The correlation between hypertension in past history and the incidence of cerebral aneurysms. *Tohoku J Exp Med.* 1979;128:267–271.
123. Leblanc R, Lozano A, van Der Rest M. Collagen deficiency in cerebral aneurysms Letter. *Stroke.* 1989;20:561.
124. Leblanc R, Lozano A, van Der Rest M, et al. Absence of collagen deficiency in familial cerebral aneurysms. *J Neurosurg.* 1989;70:837–840.
125. Lie JT, Kim HSS. Fibromuscular dysplasia of the superior mesenteric artery and coexisting cerebral berry aneurysms. *Angiology.* 1977;28:256–260.
126. Lindegård B, Hillbom M, Brody S. High-dose estrogen-progestogen oral contraceptives: a risk factor for aneurysmal subarachnoid hemorrhage? *Acta Neurol Scand.* 1987;76:37–45.
127. Lindgren E. A history of neuroradiology. In: Newton TH, Potts DG, eds. *Radiology of the Skull and Brain.* St. Louis, Mo: C.V. Mosby; 1971,1:25.
128. Ljunggren B, Säveland H, Brandt L. Causes of unfavorable outcome after early aneurysm operation. *Neurosurgery.* 1983;13:629–633.
129. Ljunggren B, Säveland H, Brandt L, et al. Early operation and overall outcome in aneurysmal subarachnoid hemorrhage. *J Neurosurg.* 1985;62: 547–551.
130. Locksley HB. Report on the cooperative study of intracranial aneurysms and subarachnoid hemorrhage, section V, part 1: natural history of subarachnoid hemorrhage, intracranial aneurysms and arteriovenous malformations. *J Neurosurg.* 1966; 25:219–239.

131. Lozano AM, Leblanc R. Familial intracranial aneurysms. *J Neurosurg.* 1987;66:522–528.
132. Lye RH, Dyer PA. Intracranial aneurysm and HLA-DR2. *J Neurol Neurosurg Psychiatry.* 1989; 52;291. Letter.
133. Lye RH, Dyer PA, Sheldon S, et al. Are HLA antigens implicated in the pathogenesis of non-haemorrhagic deterioration following aneurysmal subarachnoid haemorrhage. *J Neurol Neurosurg Psychiatry.* 1989;52:1197–1199.
134. Macfarlane TW, Canham PB, Roach MR. Shape changes at the apex of isolated human cerebral bifurcations with changes in transmural pressure. *Stroke.* 1983;14:70–76.
135. Makos MM, McComb RD, Hart MN, et al. Alpha-glucosidase deficiency and basilar artery aneurysm: report of a sibship. *Ann Neurol.* 1987;22:629–633.
136. Maroun FB, Murray GP, Jacob JC, et al. Familial intracranial aneurysms: report of three families. *Surg Neurol.* 1986;25:85–88.
137. Matson DD. Intracranial arterial aneurysms in childhood. *J Neurosurg.* 1965;23:578–583.
138. McCormick WF, Acosta-Rue GJ. The size of intracranial saccular aneurysms: an autopsy study. *J Neurosurg.* 1970;33:422–427.
139. McCormick WF, Schmalstieg E. The relationship of arterial hypertension to intracranial aneurysms. *Arch Neurol.* 1977;34:285–287.
140. Mellergard P, Ljunggren B, Brandt L, et al. HLA-typing in a family with six intracranial aneurysms. *Br J Neurosurg.* 1989;3:479–485.
141. Merei FT, Gallyas F. Role of the structural elements of the arterial wall in the formation and growth of intracranial saccular aneurysms. *Neurol Res.* 1980; 2:283–303.
142. Mettinger KL, Ericson K. Fibromuscular dysplasia and the brain: observations on angiographic, clinical and genetic characteristics. *Stroke.* 1982; 13: 46–52.
143. Meyer FB, Sundt TM Jr, Fode NC, et al. Cerebral aneurysms in childhood and adolescence. *J Neurosurg.* 1989;70:420–425.
144. Miller CA, Hill SA, Hunt WE. "De novo" aneurysms: a clinical review. *Surg Neurol.* 1985;24: 173–180.
145. Miyasaka K, Wolpert SM, Prager RJ. The association of cerebral aneurysms, infundibula, and intracranial arteriovenous malformations. *Stroke.* 1982; 13:196–203.
146. Mohr T, Tunyogi CM, Mehes K. Family studies in cases of polycystic kidney and cerebral aneurysm. [In Hungarian.] *Orv Hetil.* 1986;127:1513–1516. English abstract.
147. Moniz E. Aneurysme intra-cranien de las carotide inferne droite rendu visible par l'arteriographie cerebrale. *Rev Oto Neuro Ophtal.* 1933;11:746–748.
148. Moniz E. *L'Angiographie Cerebrale.* Paris: Masson et Cie; 1934.
149. Moniz E, Dias A, Lima A. La radio-artériographie et la topagraphie cranio-encéphalique. *J Radiologie.* 1928; 12:72–82.
150. Montes GS, Krisztan RM, Shigihara KM, et al. Histochemical and morphological characterization of reticular fibers. *Histochemistry.* 1980;65:131–141.
151. Morgagni JB. *De Sedibus et Causis Morborum per Anatonem Indagatis, Book 1, letters 3 and 4. Venetis, ex typog. Remodiniana, 1769.* New York: Hafner; 1960.
152. Morooka Y, Waga S. Familial intracranial aneurysms: report of four families. *Surg Neurol.* 1983; 19:260–262.
153. Nagae K, Goto I, Ueda K, et al. Familial occurrence of multiple intracranial aneurysms: case report. *J Neurosurg.* 1972;37:364–367.
154. Nagata I, Kikuchi H, Yamagata S, et al. Intraluminal thrombosis and growth-mechanism of giant intracranial aneurysms. [In Japanese.] *No Shinkei Geka.* 1990; 18:1115–1120. English abstract.
155. Neil-Dwyer G, Bartlett J, Nicholls A, et al. Collagen deficiency and ruptured cerebral aneurysms: a clinical and biochemical study. *J Neurosurg.* 1983; 59: 16–20.
156. Nibbelink DW, Torner JC, Henderson WG. Intracranial aneurysms and subarachnoid hemorrhage: report on a randomized treatment study, IV-A: regulated bed rest. *Stroke.* 1977;8:202–218.
157. Niiro M, Awa H, Kobayashi E, et al. Cerebral arteriovenous malformation co-existed with a cerebral aneurysm at the territory of the posterior choroidal artery: a case report with a special reference to considerations of the occurrence. [In Japanese.] *No Shinkei Geka.* 1980;8:659–665. English abstract.
158. Norrgård Ö, Ångquist KA, Fodstad H, et al. Coexistence of abdominal aortic aneurysms and intracranial aneurysms. *Acta Neurochir (Wien).* 1987; 87:34–39.
159. Norrgård Ö, Ångquist KA, Fodstad H, et al. Intracranial aneurysms and heredity. *Neurosurgery.* 1987;20:236–239.
160. Norrgård Ö, Beckman G, Beckman L, et al. Genetic markers in patients with intracranial aneurysms. *Hum Hered.* 1987;37:255–259.
161. Norrgård Ö, Rais O, Ångquist KA. Familial occurrence of abdominal aortic aneurysms. *Surgery.* 1984;95:650–656.
162. Novaes V, Campos JS, Pereira GA. Familial incidence of intracranial aneurysms. [In Spanish.] *Arq Neuropsiquiatr.* 1973;31:171–179. English abstract.
163. Nyström SHM. On factors related to growth and rupture of intracranial aneurysms. *Acta Neuropathol (Berl).* 1970;16:64–72.
164. Nyström SH. On factors related to spontaneous healing of ruptured intracranial aneurysms. *Acta Pathol Microbiol Scand [a].* 1972;80:566–572.
165. Ohara H, Suzuki J. Clinico-pathological study of cerebral aneurysms—origin, rupture, repair and growth. [In Japanese.] *No To Shinkei.* 1977; 29: 1103–1114. English abstract.
166. Ohlsson K, Fryksmark U, Tegner H. The effect of cigarette smoke condensate on alpha 1-antitrypsin, antileukoprotease and granulocyte elastase. *Eur J Clin Invest.* 1980;10:373–379.
167. Oorthuys JW. [Clinico-genetic aspects, early diagnosis and neurosurgical treatment of familial intracranial aneurysms]. [In Polish.] *Ned Tijdschr Geneeskd.* 1987;131:1016. Letter.
168. Østergaard JR. A long-term follow-up study of juvenile aneurysm patients. *Acta Neurochir.* 1985;77: 103–109.
169. Østergaard JR. Risk factors in intracranial saccular aneurysms: aspects on the formation and rupture of aneurysms, and development of cerebral vasospasm. *Acta Neurol Scand.* 1989;80:81–98.
170. Østergaard JR, Brunn-Petersen G, Kristensen BØ. The C3-F gene in patients with intracranial saccular aneurysms. *Acta Neurol Scand.* 1986;74:356–359.

171. Østergaard JR, Bruun-Petersen G, Lamm LU. HLA antigens and complement types in patients with intracranial saccular aneurysms. *Tissue Antigens.* 1986; 28:176–181.
172. Østergaard JR, Høg E. Incidence of multiple intracranial aneurysms. Influence of arterial hypertension. *J Neurosurg.* 1985;63:49–55.
173. Østergaard JR, Oxlund H. Collagen type III deficiency in patients with rupture of intracranial saccular aneurysms. *J Neurosurg.* 1987;67:690–696.
174. Østergaard JR, Reske-Nielsen E, Buhl J. Deficiency of reticular fibers in cerebral arteries. On the etiology of saccular aneurysms in childhood. *Br J Neurosurg.* 1989;3:113–115.
175. Østergaard J, Reske-Nielsen E, Oxlund H. Histological and morphometric observations on the reticular fibers in the arterial beds of patients with ruptured intracranial saccular aneurysms. *Neurosurgery.* 1987;20:554–558.
176. Østergaard JR, Boldby B. Intracranial aneurysms in children and adolescents. *J Neurosurg.* 1983;58: 832–837.
177. Ouchi Y, Tagawa H, Yamakado M, et al. Clinical significance of cerebral aneurysm in renovascular hypertension due to fibromuscular dysplasia: two cases in siblings. *Angiology.* 1989;40:581–588.
178. Pakarinen S. Incidence, aetiology and prognosis of primary subarachnoid hemorrhage. *Acta Neurol Scand.* 1967;43:234–254.
179. Pascu I, Sipos C, Piros F, et al. [Multiple and familial cerebral aneurysms]. *Rev Med Interna Neurol Psihiatr.* [In Rumanian.] 1974;19:411–416. English abstract.
180. Patel AN, Richardson AE, Ruptured intracranial aneurysms in the first two decades of life: a study of 58 patients. *J Neurosurg.* 1971;35:571–576.
181. Paterson JH, McKissock W. A clinical survey of intracranial angiomas with special reference to their mode of progression and surgical treatment: a report of 110 cases. *Brain.* 1956;79:233–266.
182. Patrick D, Appleby A. Familial intracranial aneurysm and infundibular widening. *Neuroradiology.* 1983;25:329–334.
183. Peerless SJ, Drake CG. Treatment of giant cerebral aneurysms of the anterior circulation. *Neurosurg Rev.* 1982;5:149–154.
184. Perret G, Nishioka H. Report on the cooperative study of intracranial aneurysms and subarachnoid hemorrhage, section VI: arteriovenous malformations: an analysis of 545 cases of cranio-cerebral arteriovenous malformations and fistulae reported to the cooperative study. *J Neurosurg.* 1966;25: 467–490.
185. Petitti DB, Wingerd J. Use of oral contraceptives, cigarette smoking, and the risk of subarachnoid hemorrhage. *Lancet.* 1978;2:234–236.
186. Phillips LH II, Whisnant JP, O'Fallon WM, et al. The unchanging pattern of subarachnoid hemorrhage in a community. *Neurology.* 1980;30:1034–1040.
187. Pizzedaz C, Ferrari G. Familial intracranial aneurysms. [In Italian.] *Riv Neurobiol.* 1980;26:193–198. English abstract.
188. Pope FM, Type III collagen mutations and cerebral aneurysms. *Stroke.* 1989;20: 1432–1433. Letter.
189. Pope FM, Limburg M, Schievink WI. Familial cerebral aneurysms and type III collagen deficiency. *J Neurosurg.* 1990;72:156–158. Letter.
190. Pope FM, Nicholls AC, Narcisi P, et al. Some patients with cerebral aneurysms are deficient in type III collagen. *Lancet.* 1981;1:973–975.
191. Powell J. Models of arterial aneurysm: for the investigation of pathogenesis and pharmacotherapy: a review. *Atherosclerosis.* 1991;87:93–102.
192. Powell J, Greenhalgh RM. Cellular, enzymatic, and genetic factors in the pathogenesis of abdominal aortic aneurysms. *J Vasc Surg.* 1989;9:297–304.
193. Quincke H. Zur Physiologie der Cerebrospinalflussigheit. *Arch Anat Physiol.* 1872;153–177.
194. Quincke H. Die lumbalpunction des hydrocephalus. *Berl Klin Wochenschr.* 1891;28:929–933.
195. Royal College of General Practitioners' Oral Contraception. Further analyses of mortality in oral contraceptive users. *Lancet.* 1981;1:541–546.
196. Rasmussen P, Busch H, Haase J, et al. Intracranial saccular aneurysms: results of treatment in 851 patients. *Acta Neurochir (Wien).* 1980;53:1–17.
197. Rosenorn J, Eskesen V, Schmidt K, et al. Clinical features and outcome in 1076 patients with ruptured intracranial saccular aneurysms: a prospective consecutive study. *Br J. Neuro Surg.* 1987;1: 33–46.
198. Rosenorn J, Eskesen V, Schmidt K. Unruptured intracranial aneurysms: an assessment of the annual risk of rupture based on epidemiological and clinical data. *Br J Neurosurg.* 1988;2:369–377.
199. Sacco RL, Wolf PA, Bharucha NE, et al. Subarachnoid and intracerebral hemorrhage: natural history, prognosis, and precursive factors in the Framingham study. *Neurology.* 1984;34:847–854.
200. Saifuddin A, Dathan JR. Adult polycystic kidney disease and intracranial aneurysms. *Br Med J Clin Res.* 1987;295:526.
201. Sakai N, Miwa M, Takada M, et al. Familial occurrence of intracranial aneurysm. Report of 3 sibling cases and review of literature. [In Japanese.] *No Shinkei Geka.* 1974;2:161–167. English abstract.
202. Sakai N, Sakata K, Yamada H, et al. Familial occurrence of intracranial aneurysms. *Surg Neurol.* 1974;2:25–29.
203. Salvati M, Cosentino F, Ferrari M, et al. Familial cerebral aneurysms: case report and review of the literature. [In Italian.] *Riv Neurol.* 1989;59:66–70. English abstract.
204. Sano K, Saito I. Timing and indication of surgery for ruptured intracranial aneurysm with regard to cerebral vasospasm. *Acta Neurochir (Wien).* 1978; 41:49–60.
205. Sarner M, Crawford MD. Ruptured intracranial aneurysm: clinical series. *Lancet.* 1965;2: 1251–1254.
206. Schievink WI, De Waal LP, Hageman LM, et al. Intracranial aneurysm and HLA-DR2. *J Neurol Neurosurg Psychiatry.* 1988;51:883. Letter.
207. Schroll M. Blood pressure as a cardiovascular risk factor in a 10-year prospective study of men and women born in 1914 and examined in 1964 and 1974 in Glostrup. *Dan Med Bull.* 1981;28:154–164.
208. Schubiger O, Valavanis A, Wichmann W. Growth mechanism of giant intracranial aneurysms; demonstration by CT and MR imaging. *Neuroradiology.* 1987;29:266–271.
209. Sekhar LN, Heros RC. Origin, growth, and rupture of saccular aneurysms: a review. *Neurosurgery.* 1981;8:248–260.
210. Sekhar LN, Sun M, Bonaddio D, et al. Acoustic

recordings from experimental saccular aneurysms in dogs. *Stroke.* 1990;21:1215–1221.
211. Serres ERA. *L'Annuare des hopitaux (Paris).* Paris: 1819.
212. Shigemori M, Nakayama K, Ohshima Y, et al. Familial intracranial aneurysms. *Kurume Med J.* 1985; 32:209–213.
213. Shigemori M, Nakayama K, Oshima Y, et al. Familial cerebral aneurysms in three families, with two sibling pairs. [In Japanese.] *No Shinkei Geka.* 1986;14:189–194. English abstract.
214. Shigemori M, Shirahama M, Tokutomi T, et al. Familial intracranial aneurysms associated with rare cerebrovascular anomalies: case reports. *Neurol Med Chir (Tokyo).* 1982;22:77–80.
215. Sigurdsson JA, Bengtsson C. Prevalence and management of arterial hypertension in a population sample of Swedish women. *Scand J Soc Med.* 1981; 9:41–47.
216. Slany A. Anomalien des circulus arteriosus Willisi in iher beziehung zur aneurysmenbildung an der hirnbasis. *Virchows Arch.* 1938;301:62–71.
217. Smith EG, Jones WF. Report on the human remains. In: *The Archaeological Survey of Nubia. Report for 1907-1908.* Cairo: National Printing Department; 1910:270.
218. Spallone A, Cantore G. The role of extracranial carotid abnormalities in the genesis of cerebral aneurysms. *J Neurosurg.* 1981;55:693–700.
219. Spissu A, Giagheddu M. Familial intracranial-aneurysms and otosclerosis. [In Italian.] *Riv Neurol.* 1973; 43: 229–235.
220. Stamler J, Stamler R, Riedlinger WF, et al. Hypertension screening of 1 million Americans: community Hypertension Evaluation clinic (CHEC) program, 1973-1975. *JAMA.* 1976;235:2299-2306.
221. Stavenow L. Familial occurrence of intracranial aneurysms. *Acta Med Scand.* 1979;206:197–200.
222. Stehbens WE. Aetiology of cerebral aneurysms *Lancet.* 1981;2:524–525. Letter.
223. Stehbens W. Aneurysms and anatomical variation of cerebral arteries. *Arch Path.* 1963;75:45–64.
224. Stehbens WE. Etiology of intracranial berry aneurysms. *J Neurosurg.* 1989;70:823–831.
225. Stehbens WE. Hypertension and cerebral aneurysms. *Med J Aust.* 1962;2:8–10.
226. Stehbens WE. Medial defects of the cerebral arteries of man. *J Pathol Bacteriol.* 1959;78:179–185.
227. Stehbens WE. *Pathology of the Cerebral Blood Vessels.* St. Louis, Mo: C.V. Mosby; 1972.
228. Stehbens WE. Pathology and pathogenesis of intracranial berry aneurysms. *Neurol Res.* 1990;12:29–34.
229. Steiger HJ, Aaslid R, Keller S, et al. Growth of aneurysms can be understood as passive yield to blood pressure: an experimental study. *Acta Neurochir (Wien).* 1989;100:74–78.
230. Steiger H-J, Reulen HJ. Low frequency flow fluctuations in saccular aneurysms. *Acta Neurochir (Wien).* 1986;83:131–137.
231. Stemmermann GN, Hayashi T, Resch JA, et al. Risk factors related to ischemic and hemorrhagic cerebrovascular disease at autopsy: the Honolulu heart study. *Stroke.* 1984;15:23–28.
232. Sun M, Sekhar LN, Sclabassi RJ, et al. Recording and processing aneurysmal vibration signals in dogs. *J Biomed Eng.* 1988;10:336–342.
233. Sundt TM Jr, Whisnant J. Subarachnoid hemorrhage from intracranial aneurysms: surgical management and natural history of disease. *N Engl J Med.* 1978; 299:116–122.
234. Sundt TM Jr, Kobayashi S, Fode NC, et al. Results and complications of surgical management of 809 intracranial aneurysms in 722 cases: related and unrelated to grade of patient, type of aneurysm, and timing of surgery. *J Neurosurg.* 1982;56:753–765.
235. Suzuki J, Ohara H. Clinicopathological study of cerebral aneurysms: origin, rupture, repair, and growth. *J Neurosurg.* 1978;48:505–514.
236. Suzuki S, Robertson JT, White RP, et al. Experimental intracranial aneurysms in rats: a gross and microscopic study. *J Neurosurg.* 1980;52: 494–500.
237. Takahashi H, Calvert JP, Dittemore-Hoover D, et al. A hereditary model of slowly progressive polycystic kidney disease in the mouse. *J Am Soc Nephrol.* 1991;1:980–989.
238. ter Berg HM, Bijlsma JB, Veiga-Pires JA, et al. Familial association of intracranial aneurysms and multiple congenital anomalies. *Arch Neurol.* 1986; 43:30–33.
239. ter Berg HWM, Dippel DWJ, Habbema JDF, et al. Treatment of intact familial intracranial aneurysms: a decision-analytical approach. *Neurosurgery.* 198;23:329–334.
240. ter Berg JWM, Overtoom TMD, Ludwig JW, et al. Detection of unruptured familial intracranial aneurysms by intravenous digital subtraction angiography. Screening of two affected families. *Neuroradiology.* 1987;29:272–276.
241. Tetley TD, Smith SF, Burton GH, et al. Effects of cigarette smoking and drugs on respiratory tract proteases and antiproteases. *Eur J Respir Dis Suppl.* 1987;153:93–102.
242. Thierry A, Ballivet J, Dumas R, et al. Familial cases of intracranial aneurysms: review of the medical literature and report on one case. [In French.] *Neurochir.* 1972;18:267–276. English abstract.
243. Thompson JR, Harwood-Nash DC, Fitz CR. Cerebral aneurysms in children. *AJR.* 1973;118:163–175.
244. Tiwari JL, Terasaki PI. *HLA and Disease Association.* New York, NY: Springer-Verlag; 1985.
245. Toglia JU, Samil AR. Familial intracranial aneurysms. *Dis Nerv Syst.* 1972;33:611–613.
246. Tognetti F, Andreoli A, Testa C. 'Twin' familial aneurysms of the anterior communicating artery. *Neurol Res.* 1985;7:166–167.
247. Tognetti F, Limoni P, Testa C. Aneurysm growth and hemodynamic stress. *Surg Neurol.* 1983;20: 74–78.
248. Torner JC, Kassel NF, Wallace RB, et al. Preoperative prognostic factors for rebleeding and survival in aneurysm patients receiving antifibrinolytic therapy: report on the cooperative aneurysm study. *Neurosurgery.* 1981;9:506–513.
249. Tran-Dinh, Williams LM, Jayasinghe LS. Association of intracranial aneurysm and arteriovenous malformation. *Med J Aust.* 1983;1:521–523.
250. Verdura J, Resnikoff S, Rosenthal J, et al. Familial intracranial aneurysms, with two occurring at the distal anterior cerebral artery. *Neurosurgery.* 1983; 12:214–216.
251. Walker AE, Allegre GE. The pathology and pathogenesis of cerebral aneurysms. *J Neuropathol Exp Neurol.* 1954;13:248–259.
252. Weibers DO, Whisnant JD, O'Fallon WM. The

natural history of unruptured intracranial aneurysms. *N Eng J Med.* 1981;304:696–698.
253. Weibers DO, Whisnant JP, Sundt TM Jr, et al. The significance of unruptured intracranial saccular aneurysms. *J Neurosurg.* 1987;66:23–29.
254. Weir B, Aronyk K. Management mortality and the timing of surgery for supratentorial aneurysms. *J Neurosurg.* 1981;54:146–150.
255. Whisnant JP, Phillips LH II, Sundt TM Jr. Aneurysmal subarachnoid hemorrhage: timing of surgery and mortality. *Mayo Clin Proc.* 1982;57:471–475.
256. Wichern H. Zur diagnose perforierender aneurysmen der hirnarterien. *Munchen Med Wochenschr.* 1911;58:2724–2729.
257. Wilkins RH. Neurosurgery classics: XXIV. *J Neurosurg.* 1964;21:892–905.
258. Wilks S. Sanguineous meningeal effusion (apoplexy); spontaneous and from injury. *Guy's Hosp Rep.* 1859;5:119–127.
259. Wilson G, Riggs HE, Rupp C. The pathologic anatomy of ruptured cerebral aneurysms. *J Neurosurg.* 1954;11:128–134.
260. Yamaki T, Yoshino E, Higuchi T. Rapidly growing aneurysm. *Surg Neurol.* 1986;26:301–305.
261. Yasargil MG. *Microneurosurgery.* New York, Ny: Thieme-Stration; 1987.
262. Yong-Zhong G, van Alpher HAM. Pathogenesis and histopathology of saccular aneurysms: review of the literature. *Neurol Res.* 1990;12:249–255.
263. Yoshimoto T, Suzuki J. Eight year documented study of an aneurysm growth at the origin of the posterior communicating artery. [In Japanese.] *No Shinkei Geka.* 1974;2:571–573. English abstract.

# CHAPTER 2

# Clinical Presentation

Karen D. Rodman, MD, and Issam A. Awad, MD, MS, FACS

## Subarachnoid Hemorrhage

The rupture of saccular intracranial aneurysms represents the most common cause of subarachnoid hemorrhage (SAH) and results in significant neurologic disability or death. Saccular aneurysms occur at the bifurcations of large arteries at the base of the brain, and about 80% to 85% involve the anterior circulation.[16,144] Sahs et al,[161] and Popovic et al[156] found that peak age for aneurysm rupture was 55–60 years of age.

The classic clinical presentation for SAH is the sudden onset of an explosive "worst headache of one's life" associated with meningismus, and impaired level of consciousness. In 4 prospective studies involving 949 patients,[1,12,65,215] 50% to 80% reported an explosive, unremitting, acute, frequently nonlateralizing headache radiating to either the neck or the eyes. The headache is typically localized to the frontal and occipital areas.[1,63] Nausea with or without vomiting, meningismus, and transient loss of consciousness are the next most common clinical presentations.[1,77,215] The transient loss of consciousness occurring in 20% to 80% of subjects,[215] and lasting between 10–30 minutes,[63] can be preceded by a severe headache; or the headache can occur upon regaining consciousness in up to 45% of cases.[63] When an aneurysm ruptures, increased intracranial pressure (ICP) with a secondary decrease in cerebral perfusion pressure might explain transient loss of consciousness.[16] During lapsed consciousness the "aneurysmal blackout phenomenon" can occur,[63,65,134] involving generalized extension and stiffening of all extremities, and accompanied by dilated pupils and temporary respiratory arrest. This transient decerebrate state is believed to reflect the flooding of the subarachnoid space with blood at high ICPs.

Meningismus, or neck pain, occurs in up to 40% of patients, and can be associated with a positive Brudzinski's manifesting as flexion of the neck with involuntary hip flexion.[77]

Subhyaloid, preretinal hemorrhages, or extension of blood into the vitreous humor (5% to 30%) are additional manifestations of SAH.[1,65,77] Subhyaloid hemorrhages should be looked for with the patient in the sitting position; they will have a cup-shaped appearance with a meniscus. Other early ocular signs include an oculomotor (III) nerve palsy with adduction palsy and a dilated, fixed pupil with posterior communicating artery aneurysms. An abducens (VI) nerve palsy may reflect increased ICP or, less often, direct aneurysm compression anywhere along its course.

Less common (≤ 15%) presentations of SAH include hypercusis, photophobia, coma, fever, chest and back pain, and focal neurologic deficit.[1,2,19,65,210] Focal deficits such as contralateral paresis (e.g. middle cerebral artery [MCA] aneurysm), or paraparesis (e.g. anterior communicating artery aneurysm) can reflect the locale of the ruptured aneurysm. Chest pain can be a misleading sign: several case reports have described chest pain associated with abnormal electrocardiogram (EKG) rhythms (e.g. premature ventricular contractions) as the initial presentation of a SAH.[19,190] Subarachnoid blood can produce a sudden "adrenergic storm," which causes arrhythmias and accelerated cardiac pacing.

Among the abnormal EKG patterns recorded in patients following SAH are the following: inverted T waves, prolonged Q-T interval, ST depression, and occasional Q waves.[5,128,146] The prolongation of the Q-T interval enhances the possibility of ventricular fibrillation by delaying ventricular repolarization. Sudden death from a malignant arrhythmia can be the result.[59,190]

Reichenbach[158] coined the term "myofibrillar degeneration" to describe scattered areas of microscopic necrosis in the myocardium post-SAH. A subarachnoid-induced increased ICP,[139] and massive central nervous system (CNS) release of catecholamines, or "adrenergic storm," are believed to be the reasons for the pathology.[190,192] This release of catecholamines could cause direct myocardial damage,[158,188] and potentially trigger malignant arrhythmias, which may lead to cardiac arrest.[59,146,190]

In the setting of suspected myocardial dysfunction, a clinician should consider the possibility of SAH if the following parameters are present: (1) a persistent severe headache post–cardiac arrest, and (2) retinal hemorrhages with or without papilledema associated with a new focal neurologic deficit.

SAH can occur during both exertional and nonexertional activities. Aneurysmal rupture occurs in 21% to 57% of people during activities such as lifting, bending, defecating, and sexual intercourse. The remainder of ruptured aneurysms occur during quiescent periods such as sleep and sitting.[1,16,63,65,77]

Despite advances in medical treatment, the mortality rate in SAH remains high (50%).[16,34] The time from onset of SAH to definitive treatment and the initial clinical grade of the patient are the two main early factors related to prognosis. The Hunt–Hess and World Federation of Neurologic Surgeons classifications (in Tables 1 and 2) are used prognostically in patients initially presenting with SAH. As illustrated in the tables, an increased grade indicates more severe neurologic deficits and correlates with a poorer prognosis.[16,34,77,156,161]

Delayed manifestations of SAH such as rebleeding, vasospasm, and hydrocephalus are common. Rebleeding is highest within the first 3 weeks after a subarachnoid bleed. Within the first 14 days, 15% to 20% will have rebled, and up to 50% will have rebleeding within 6 months.[16,77,156] Clinically, rebleeding is heralded by a sudden severe headache accompanied by nausea, vomiting, and possibly focal neurologic deficits. Vasospasm, either local or diffuse, is a major cause of mortality and morbidity following SAH, and occurs in 30% to 40% of patients, usually presenting during the first 4–14 days.[81,101] The occurrence of new, uni- and/or multifocal neurologic deficits (e.g. hemiparesis, aphasia, or cranial nerve palsies) are hallmark signs of the presentation of vasospasm. Hydrocephalus occurs 5–20 days following aneurysmal rupture in up to 32% of patients. It can present clinically as lethargy, incontinence, ataxic gait, and vertical gaze palsy.[16,63,156]

The presentation and medical management of vasospasm, rebleeding, and hydrocephalus will be more extensively covered in other chapters.

## *Warning Headaches and Warning Leaks*

Neurosurgeons and neurologists now recognize that a major SAH is frequently preceded by a warning headache of variable localizing value, with or without other neurologic deficits.[49,112] If warning signs are missed, patients suffer a higher mortality rate (40% to 50%).[34,161,197] The initial symptoms of warning headache are often erroneously attributed to migraine: sinusitis, meningitis, seizure, or hypertension.[34,46,49,147] Gillingham[75] coined the term "warning leak" to describe this situation. Hauerberg et al[82] studied 1,076 patients with aneurysmal SAH over a 5-year

TABLE 1
**Hunt–Hess Clinical Grading Post–Subarachnoid Hemorrhage***

| Grade | Description of Patient's Condition |
|---|---|
| 1 | Asymptomatic, or mild H/A and mild nuchal rigidity |
| 2 | Cranial nerve palsy, nuchal rigidity, and moderate to severe H/A |
| 3 | Drowsy, confused, or mild focal deficit (e.g., hemiparesis, hemianesthesia) |
| 4 | Stupor, moderate to severe hemiparesis, early decerebrate rigidity |
| 5 | Comatose and decerebrate rigidity |

Abbreviation: H/A = Headache
*Revised from Reference 16

period for warning leak symptomatology and found that severe, acute headache was the most common (83%) warning leak symptom. Other SAH series report an incidence of warning headache in 25% to 75% of patients.[65,113,145] However, it is not known how often such a headache may have represented a true "leak" (minor SAH) or whether it represented nonhemorrhagic pain preceding aneurysm rupture. The term "warning headache" or "sentinel headache" may be more accurate than "warning leak," since such headache may not always represent a true "leak."

The warning headache is often unremitting and lasts 1–2 days, and sometimes as long as 2 weeks.[49,148] This "sentinel headache" can have some localizing value. A periorbital, hemifacial headache ipsilateral to the aneurysm occurs in up to 53% of posterior communicating artery aneurysms.[112,145,148] Anterior communicating artery aneurysms can be associated with a severe bifrontal headache which radiates bicipitally in 5% to 40% of patients.[112,208] MCA aneurysms can be associated with a hemicranial headache ipsilateral to the aneurysms in 30% of cases. Posterior circulation aneurysms can present with a sudden, severe occipital headache in up to 60% of cases.[29,43,51,208]

Other symptomatology can accompany the "sentinel headache." Nausea with or without vomiting (18% to 50%), neck pain (6% to 30%), and lethargy with or without loss of consciousness (8% to 40%) are the next most frequently reported early warning

TABLE 2
**World Federation of Neurologic Surgeons (WFNS) Clinical Grading Post–Subarachnoid Hemorrhage (SAH)***

| WFNS Grade | Glasgow Coma Score (GCS) | Motor Deficit (e.g. Aphasia and/or Hemiparesis or Hemiplegia) | Comment |
|---|---|---|---|
| 0 | 15 | Absent | Unruptured |
| 1 | 15 | Absent | |
| 2 | 13–14 | Absent | |
| 3 | 13–14 | Present | |
| 4 | 7–12 | Present or Absent | |
| 5 | 3–6 | Present or Absent | |

*Revised from Reference 77

signs.[11,34,65,113,148,208] Less commonly reported (< 11%) are transient neurologic signs including visual loss, ptosis, amaurosis fugax, photophobia, diarrhea, and hemiparesis.[49,65,113,162,208] These uncommon clinical presentations can have some localizing value. Warning headaches of an MCA aneurysm can present with transient contralateral hemiparesis. In such cases embolism, rather than bleeding, may be the mechanism producing the transient focal deficit. Transient diarrhea and paraparesis can accompany warning headaches of an anterior communicating artery aneurysm.[145,208]

The true incidence of sentinel headache or of true leaks preceding SAH is difficult to determine. Certain factors (e.g. locale of the aneurysm) seem to predispose to their occurrence. Young adults in the third and fourth decades have the highest incidence of warning symptoms. Okawara[145] found that in 112 cases of aneurysms presenting with warning signs, young males in their thirties had the highest percentage (99%) of warning headaches. Young females of similar age had the next highest percentage (66%). Once patients reached the seventh decade, the percentage of warning symptoms declined to 33% in males and 47% in females. Other reports refute Okawara's conclusions, finding that women in all age groups had the highest percentage of warning headaches.[55,208]

Location of aneurysms can be correlated with the development of warning headaches. Aneurysms of the internal carotid artery (ICA) were the most common, while anterior communicating artery and MCA aneurysms had the second most frequent correlation. Posterior circulation aneurysms had the least association with warning headaches.[82,145,208]

In reviewing five large series comprising over 600 patients, warning signs appear in 28% to 60% of those studied.[55,112,145,208] One small study[27] reports a 60% to 70% occurrence of premonitory symptoms prior to a major SAH. The average interval between the presentation of the warning headache and the onset of major SAH is 2–20 days.[112,145,208] The interval, however, can be as short as several hours,[49] or as long as 3–6 months.[11]

Pathologic examination of the aneurysms of patients with warning headache may reveal minor bleeds in the aneurysmal walls.[11,148] Expansion of the aneurysm with adjacent neural or dural compression, or ischemia due to localized cerebral vasospasm, are alternate theories possibly explaining the pathogenesis of warning headache.[145,148]

The diagnostic evaluation of a suspected warning headache includes computed tomography (CT) of the brain and cerebrospinal fluid (CSF) examination. If the warning headache is misdiagnosed and a major SAH occurs, mortality and morbidity are high. Although CT sensitivity approaches 90% for detecting a major SAH,[14,83,142] CT is unreliable for detecting minor bleeds associated with warning headaches. The CT detects subarachnoid blood in 12% to 75% of patients with warning headache.[55,82,112] Xanthochromic spinal fluid is more sensitive (80% to 96%) in detecting subarachnoid blood 10 hours post-warning headache.[210] Therefore, normal CT coupled with a normal spinal fluid within the first 12 hours after symptom-onset effectively rules out a minor subarachnoid bleed. If the index of suspicion is sufficiently high, a CT with contrast, magnetic resonance angiogram (MRA) or formal angiography should be considered.

## *Cerebrospinal Fluid Findings*

The examination of the CSF is an important adjunct in the diagnosis of SAH. Barrows[17] first documented changes in red blood cells, protein, and pigment in the CSF over an 18-day period following SAH. There was an early rise in red blood cells (RBCs) in excess of 1.1 million cells per cubic ml in the first 24 hours postictus. The RBC then declined over a 2-week period. Protein concentrations up to 224 mg/dl were seen in the first three days following SAH. The protein concentration then declined to normal ranges over a 2-week period.

Recent literature[77,212,215] has more clearly delineated the CSF changes in SAH. The opening pressure is normal, or frequently elevated up to 300 mm $H_2O$ in 38% to 60% of patients.[3,63,64,206] It then falls over 2–3 days but remains elevated for up to 3 weeks in 80% of patients.[63,64] The increase in opening pressure is secondary to obstruction of the subarachnoid cerebral fluid pathway by blood.[58,206]

The CSF is bloody to the naked eye in the first 2 hours postictus if at least 6,000 RBCs per cubic ml are present. If between 500 and 6,000 RBCs per cubic ml are present, the spinal fluid will appear cloudy and pinkish-tinged.[3,115] The CSF becomes clear by 3 weeks after the SAH.

There is a rapid rise in RBCs (up to 1 million/mL[3]) occurring several hours postictus, reaching its peak in 2 days, and followed by a rapid decline of the RBCs over the next 7–14 days.[64,212,215] Both leukocyte and protein concentrations increase proportionally to the RBCs in the first several hours after the bleed.[15,77,212,215] Within the next 24–48 hours, there is a secondary increase in white blood cells (WBCs) (50 to 3,600/mm) and protein (100 to 2,200 mg/dl).[3,15,64,77,215] The WBC and protein concentrations then decline toward normal ranges over the next 7–14 days. (See Table 3.)

The differential of WBCs in the spinal fluid postictus shows a distinct pattern. At day 4 to day 6, there is an initial increase in neutrophils. By day 21, these have declined, and lymphocytes and mononuclear cells predominate.[93] The WBC elevation possibly reflects a meningeal reaction to the subarachnoid blood, while increase in protein concentration indicates an influx of serum proteins across a damaged blood-brain barrier (BBB).[13]

CSF glucose is often normal[77] post-SAH. Older studies, however, have documented hypoglycorrachia (20–40 mg/dl) in the absence of CNS infection in 6% to 14% of adult subjects 6 days postictus.[125,199] Later studies have verified hypoglycorrachia following SAH.[64,151,203] Troost[199] and Sambrook[164] detailed CSF glucose in the range of 13–30 mg/dl at 5–10 days following an SAH. Both authors postulated that excessive RBC glycolysis, coupled with impaired glucose transport into the spinal fluid, were possible mechanisms for this phenomenon.

Barrows[17] was one of the first investigators to measure and document pigments such as oxyhemoglobin and bilirubin in the spinal fluid following SAH. The pigment of oxyhemoglobin appears at the onset of the bleed, reaches peak concentration in 3–4 days, and then declines to normal concentration over the next 7 days. Oxyhemoglobin imparts a

TABLE 3
**CSF Findings in SAH and in Traumatic Tap (Adult Values)***

| Condition | OP (cm $H_20$) | Appearance | Cells | Protein (mg/dl) | Glucose (mg/dl) | Miscellaneous |
|---|---|---|---|---|---|---|
| Normal | 7–18 | Clear | No RBC or WBC | 15–45 | 50 | |
| Traumatic (Bloody) | Nl | Bloody, supernatant clear | RBC:WBC ratio as in peripheral blood count | Slight ↑ | Nl | Blood ↓ in successive tubes; xanthochromia takes hours |
| SAH | ↑ | Bloody, supernatant xanthochromic | Early ↑ RBCs<br>Late ↑ WBCs | 50–400<br>100–800 | Nl or ↓ | RBCs disappear in 2 weeks; xanthochromia may persist for weeks |

Abbreviations in Table:
OP = Opening Pressure
Nl = Normal
↑ = Increased
↓ = Decreased
SAH = Subarachnoid Hemorrhage
RBC = Red Blood Cell
WBC = White Blood Cell
*Revised from Reference 77

reddish-pink coloring to the spinal fluid. Bilirubin appears 1–2 days following SAH and confers a yellow coloring to the spinal fluid, referred to as xanthochromia, and then declines over the next 3 weeks.

Later investigators confirmed and expanded Barrows' findings on the production of oxyhemoglobin post-SAH. Hemoglobin is enzymatically degraded by heme-oxygenase to produce bilirubin. In contrast to Barrows' findings, bilirubin is detected earlier in the CSF (6–15 hours), reaching its peak concentration 2–3 days postictus. It then declines over the next 2–3 weeks.[15,64]

Pigments such as oxyhemoglobin and bilirubin are present following an SAH but not in the case of traumatic lumbar puncture, thus helping to distinguish the one from the other. CSF that doesn't clear and has similar RBC counts in all tubes collected during a lumbar puncture points to an SAH rather than a traumatic lumbar puncture.[93,201,215] (See Table 4.)

A recent test called the D-dimer assay shows promise in its ability to distinguish between SAH and a traumatic tap. By using a monoclonal fibrin derivative, the D-dimer assay detects subarachnoid blood in the spinal fluid. This assay is negative in a specimen from a traumatic tap.[110]

CSF can be used to assess the clinical course and possibly predict the prognosis in patients following an SAH. The chemical composition of the spinal fluid may have prognostic importance following SAH. The potassium ($K^+$) concentration is low (2.8 mEq/l) in normal spinal fluid.[64] Sambrook[164] illustrated a decline in spinal fluid $K^+$ over a 2-week period following an SAH. There was a mild decrease in CSF $K^+$ (2.5–2.6 mEq/l) over day 1, followed by a precipitous decrease in the ion (1.8–2.2 mEq/l) from day 5 to day 10 postictus. The CSF $K^+$ then returned to normal values over 2–3 weeks. When this ion was at its lowest concentration, there was a decline in mental status (e.g. comatose), which rapidly improved upon normalization of the CSF $K^+$ levels. The lowered CSF $K^+$ concentrations are believed to reflect pial and ependymal ventricular transport system damage, which were incurred during an SAH.

Correlations between CSF lactic acidosis and clinical outcome have been postulated. Sambrook[163] found that patients with the greatest CSF lactic acidosis (e.g. pH $\leq$ 7.25 at days 3–5 postictus) had the poorest clinical outcome. More current literature supports this observation.[97,172]

Cerebral vasospasm is a frequent cause of delayed morbidity and mortality 5–10 days following an SAH. Within the past 5 years, levels of vasoactive proteins in the spinal fluid have been used to predict vasospasm. Elevated levels of CSF prostaglandins, serotonin, thromboxane $A_2$, endothelin, and complement components have been correlated with the development of delayed cerebral vaso-

TABLE 4
**Differential Features of Subarachnoid Hemorrhage and Traumatic Tap: The Three Tube Test***

| CSF Finding | Subarachnoid Hemorrhage | Traumatic Tap |
|---|---|---|
| Pressure | Increased or normal | Normal |
| Appearance | Equal blood in all tubes | First or last tube is bloodier, others are clearer |
| Supernatant fluid color | Pigment in excess of protein level | Clear |
| RBC count and hematrocrit | Similar in all tubes | Variable in different tubes |
| WBC count | Proportional to RBC in earliest stages, relatively increased later | proportional to RBC count RBC count |
| Clot formation | Absent | Occurs rarely |
| Repeat puncture | Findings similar to those at initial tap | Usually clear |

Revised from Reference 64

spasm by day 6 following an SAH.[37,99,189] These variables might have a role in following the clinical course of vasospasm.

## Specific Aneurysm Syndromes

Ruptured and unruptured aneurysms have such varied clinical presentations including acute focal deficits (e.g. hemiparesis and/or hemiplegia, cranial nerve palsies, and/or aphasia); subacute and even chronic focal deficits secondary to aneurysmal mass effect or thromboembolic phenomena. In the following sections, we shall describe the clinical presentations of both ruptured and unruptured aneurysms in common locations in the anterior and posterior circulations.

### *Intracavernous-Carotid Artery Aneurysms*

Intracavernous-carotid artery aneurysms represent 3% to 5% of all intracranial aneurysms,[23,66,141,166] showing a marked female preponderance (53% to 80%).[23,106,120,153] The mean age range is 51–58 years in several studies.[28,50,74] Six percent to 51% of cavernous-carotid artery aneurysms can be associated with hypertension.[153]

Ruptured intracavernous-carotid artery aneurysms less commonly (≤ 10%) present as an SAH.[120,135,159] The acute onset of retro-orbital eye pain ipsilateral to the aneurysm, associated with ophthalmoplegia is the hallmark of a ruptured intracavernous aneurysm. The common extraocular palsies include the oculomotor (III), trochlear (IV), and abducens (VI) cranial nerves.[141,209] Rupture of a cavernous aneurysm can produce a carotid-cavernous fistula. On exam, the eye ipsilateral to the ruptured cavernous artery aneurysm reveals injection of the sclera, chemosis, pulsating exophthalmos with or without a periorbital bruit, and blindness.[16,28,117] Rarely, ruptured cavernous aneurysms can be associated with acute epistaxis due to erosion into the sphenoid sinus.[118,159]

Unruptured large (10–24 mm) or giant (≥ 25 mm) intracavernous aneurysms compress adjacent neurologic structures over a chronic period of months to years.[118,135,159] Unruptured cavernous aneurysms are often associated with ipsilateral ocular and upper facial pain secondary to aneurysmal compression of the ophthalmic division of the trigeminal (V) nerve in over 60% of the cases. A partial oculomotor nerve palsy with ptosis, vertical diplopia, and a dilated pupil occurs in 20% to 40% of patients.[74,118,141,159] Intracavernous aneurysm can also be associated with trochlear nerve palsy (inability to look down and in) and abducens nerve palsy (horizontal gaze palsy).[74,118,141] If the sympathetic fibers are involved in the cavernous sinus, a Horner's syndrome can occur with an associated ptosis and miosis in a small number of patients.

As an untreated intracavernous artery aneurysm expands laterally, it can involve the superior orbital fissure and cause exophthalmos.[159] If the aneurysm expands upward and medially to the level of the anterior clinoid process, it may compress the optic nerve and/or chiasm.[74,118] Involvement of the optic nerves and chiasm is rarely associated with ipsilateral field defects, blindness, and bitemporal hemianopias—symptoms which are more prevalent among the more distal carotid-ophthalmic aneurysms. Traction on the facial nerve at the petrous ridge, and compression of the greater petrosal nerve with loss of taste occur infrequently.[159]

Aneurysms of the intracavernous ICA can be associated with thrombosis of the parent vessel. This can produce, in rare instances, aphasia and/or contralateral hemiparesis.[28,118,200]

### *Carotid-Ophthalmic Aneurysms*

Carotid-ophthalmic artery aneurysms were first reported as a separate entity in a series of 14 patients by Drake et al in 1968.[54] These aneurysms arise from the ICA at or near the origin of the ophthalmic artery, representing from 2% to 8% of all intracranial aneurysms.[120,141,213,219] In several series, which together comprise a total of over 500 patients, carotid-ophthalmic aneurysms had a 50% to 85% female preponderance[45,169,194,205] with a mean age at presentation of 36 to 55 years.[62,96,169,205] Ophthalmic aneurysms have a high association with multiple aneurysms (30% to 60%),[4,45,62,169,213] which often occur in the contralateral carotid-ophthalmic and internal carotid arteries.[45,62,169,213,219]

Carotid-ophthalmic artery aneurysms can present as either an acute SAH (22% to 47%),[4,45,77,96,169,213,219] or as an unruptured compressive mass (53% to 78%) involving the optic nerve or chiasm.[40,62,121,213] Ruptured carotid-ophthalmic aneurysms present with an acute, retro-orbital pain, ipsilateral to the aneurysm associated with varying degrees of blindness.[4,108,141,219] Ipsilateral central scotomatas, altitudinal and nasal hemianopsias, and distortions of color vision are other common presentations of ruptured carotid-ophthalmic aneurysms.[40,77,108,135,141,209] The remainder of the clinical exam reflects symptoms of SAH.

Unruptured large (10–24 mm) or giant (≥ 25 mm) carotid-ophthalmic aneurysms present with slowly progressive visual symptoms reflecting varying degrees of involvement of the optic nerves and/or chiasm. The duration of visual symptomatology can vary from 1 month to 6 years.[62,141,169] Initially, the unruptured aneurysm compresses the ipsilateral optic nerve from behind, causing an ipsilateral central scotomata. This defect then progresses to an ipsilateral-inferior nasal hemianopia,[50,104] which is then followed by a complete nasal hemianopia.[40,45] If the aneurysm continues to expand, it often extends medially to compress both the optic nerves and chiasm. When this occurs, a superior temporal defect of the contralateral eye, followed by end-stage blindness of the ipsilateral eye, becomes apparent.[45,50,104] If the optic chiasm is primarily involved, visual field defects such as bitemporal and contralateral hemianopias predominate.[45,62,74]

On physical exam, the eye ipsilateral to the unruptured aneurysm will show some or all of the following: (1) optic atrophy, (2) papilledema, (3) afferent pupil defect (e.g. Marcus-Gunn pupil), and (4) varying degrees of decreased visual acuity. These findings on exam reflect optic nerve injury.[4,40,62,74,160] (See Table 5 for clinical data, and signs and symptoms of carotid-ophthalmic aneurysms.)

In a very small number of cases, a thrombosed carotid-ophthalmic artery aneurysm is associated with embolism or even carotid occlusion. This can lead to ischemic symptoms in the ICA distribution including aphasia and contralateral hemiparesis.[62,74]

## *Posterior Communicating Artery Aneurysms*

Posterior communicating-ICA aneurysms represent 4% to 11% of all intracranial aneurysms.[105,222] These commonly present as an acute oculomotor palsy with ptosis, dilated and unreactive pupil, and ophthalmoplegia at the onset of SAH. The subarachnoid blood is postulated to dissect into the oculomotor nerve fascicles causing subsequent dysfunction.[63,91,213] Other signs of SAH such as headache, meningismus, and, rarely, hypothalamic dysfunction can accompany the oculomotor palsy.

Hypothalamic micro- and macrohemorrhages due to posterior communicating aneurysms have been described.[41] Ruptured posterior communicating aneurysms may cause secondary hypothalamic lesions leading to variable neurologic dysfunction. Hypothalamic damage can lead to a massive outpouring of catecholamines, subsequently resulting in cardiac dysfunction.[188] Priapism has been reported after rupture of a posterior communicating aneurysm,[191] possibly due to autonomic dysfunction caused by a lesion in the hypothalamus.

Unruptured posterior communicating aneurysms may exert mass effect on the adjacent oculomotor nerve and other neural structures. The occurrence of oculomotor palsy with unruptured posterior communicating aneurysms occurs in 14% to 56% in several smaller studies.[145,152] Some larger series report a 50% to 80% incidence of complete oculo-

TABLE 5
**Comparison of Published Series of Carotid-Ophthalmic Aneurysms***

| | No. of Cases | Sex | | SAH | Multiple Aneurysms | Visual Changes |
|---|---|---|---|---|---|---|
| | | Male | Female | | | |
| Cooperative Study (121) | 143 | 36 | 107 | 101 | | |
| Drake et al, 1968(54) | 14 | 3 | 11 | 13 | 9 | 1 |
| Kothandaram et al, 1971(104) | 19 | 4 | 15 | 15 | 4 | 4 |
| Thurel et al, 1974(194) | 17 | 6 | 11 | 14 | 4 | 3 |
| Almeida et al, 1976(4) | 8 | 3 | 5 | 7 | 3 | 1 |
| Day, 1990 (45) | 80 | 11 | 69 | 23 | 36 | 24 |
| TOTAL | 281 | 63 (22%) | 218 (78%) | 173 (62%) | 56 (20%) | 33 (12%) |

*Revised from Reference 219 and updated

motor palsy with posterior communicating artery aneurysms.[100,162] Compression of the oculomotor nerve often causes a complete ipsilateral ptosis with a dilated, unreactive pupil,[76,78,196,209] followed by paralysis of extraocular muscles controlled by the oculomotor nerve. With oculomotor paresis, only lateral abduction of the affected eye remains intact.[63,80,98,100,162] Although a dilated, unreactive pupil remains the hallmark of these aneurysms, there are case reports of pupillary-sparing posterior communicating aneurysms.[98,100]

Prognosis for full recovery of oculomotor nerve function depends on such factors as the timing of surgery. If surgery is performed within 10 days of onset of oculomotor nerve palsy, prognosis for recovery of oculomotor nerve function is excellent. This fact has been illustrated in 4 major series comprising over 500 patients.[61,68,80,152] The levator palpebrae and parasympathetic fibers tend to recover the earliest. The extraocular muscles such as the inferior oblique and recti muscles often recover last.[80,152]

Ipsilateral orbital pain radiating to the forehead is reported in several large series in 31% to 59% of patients with posterior communicating artery aneurysms.[121,145,162] However, ipsilateral orbital and forehead pain can have variable localizing value, and have also been described with carotid-ophthalmic and cavernous artery aneurysms.[45,118,131,169]

Seizures and trigeminal neuralgia are less frequent manifestations of unruptured posterior communicating aneurysms. A major cooperative study by Sahs et al[162] reported only 7 cases (≤ 1%) of unruptured posterior communicating aneurysms associated with seizures. Other isolated case studies[29,131] report complex partial seizures in unruptured posterior communicating aneurysms. Pathogenesis is felt to be secondary to aneurysmal compression of, or minor "leak" into, the adjacent temporal lobe.

Trigeminal neuralgia over a chronic (18-month) period has been reported from a giant, unruptured posterior communicating aneurysm impinging on the pontine cistern.[116]

## *Other Internal Carotid Artery Aneurysms*

Aneurysms arising from the ICA proper at or before its intracranial bifurcation represent 2.6% to 8% of all aneurysms (excluding the categories of intracavernous, carotid-ophthalmic, and posterior communicating artery aneurysms).[111,120,170] They commonly present with SAH or as an unruptured suprasellar mass causing neurologic symptoms as the aneurysm slowly enlarges.[205]

A ruptured intracranial aneurysm of the ICA can present as a typical SAH.[92,150,205] Acute amaurosis fugax ipsilateral to the aneurysm, associated with contralateral hemiparesis, may be a useful lateralizing sign in any ICA aneurysm.[29,89,135]

Similar to other anterior circulation aneurysms, ICA aneurysms may result in subdural, intracerebral, and intraventricular bleeds.[111,154] Pasqualin et al[150] found a high incidence of such bleeds associated with ICA aneurysms among 899 patients with various intracranial aneurysms. Temporal lobe (50%) and frontal lobe (27%) hematomas were the most commonly reported sites of intracerebral bleeds with ICA aneurysms. There was an unusually high percentage (35%) of subdural hematomas associated with the aneurysms in this series. Barnett et al[13] found a smaller incidence of subdural hematomas (9%) with ICA aneurysms. Inagawa's autopsy series of 133 patients was also consistent with a smaller percentage (4%) of subdural hematomas.[92]

Aphasia with or without contralateral hemiparesis and contralateral hemisensory loss are common presentations of unruptured, slowly expanding ICA aneurysms.[6,29,44,89,135,154] These symptoms develop gradually over months or years.[6,29,44,184]

Unruptured ICA aneurysms can radiographically appear as suprasellar masses simulating tumors. Lodge[122] was among the early investigators to report a large internal carotid aneurysm simulating a pituitary tumor with secondary hypopituitarism. Later studies[13,73] have verified pituitary and hypothalamic derangements associated with these aneurysms. Prolactinemia, galactorrhea, and diabetes insipidus are symptoms of pituitary-hypothalamic axis dysfunction.

The optic nerve–chiasm syndrome is well recognized with internal carotid unruptured aneurysms. Older, smaller studies[29,63,94] and a large prospective study[74] verified optic nerve–chiasm derangements with secondary visual changes. The visual abnormalities included ipsilateral arcuate defects, central scotomatas, optic atrophy, and blindness due to optic nerve compression by the aneurysm. Bitemporal hemianopias and contralateral visual field defects reflect involvement of the optic nerve chiasm. Visual symptoms are often chronic in nature, ranging from months to years.[29] If the ICA aneurysm is more posteriorly situated, both the optic (II) and oculomotor cranial nerves can be compressed,[154] producing an oculomotor palsy (ptosis, dilated pupil, extraocular palsy) with large ICA aneurysms.

Giant ($\geq$ 25 mm) ICA aneurysms can obstruct the foramen of Monro and cause secondary hydrocephalus.[29,137] The hydrocephalus may present as an insidious dementia with associated gait ataxia/apraxia and urinary incontinence.

## *Middle Cerebral Artery Aneurysms*

Saccular and fusiform MCA aneurysms comprise 20% of all intracranial aneurysms,[77,213,222] greater than 50% arising at the bifurcation of the first main division (M1 trunk).[144,213] There is a tendency toward a female preponderance for these aneurysms,[120,213,222] the majority presenting as SAH. Unruptured MCA aneurysms, however, give rise to neurologic symptoms through mass effect, infarction, or distant emboli.[7,168]

The clinical presentation of middle cerebral aneurysms is often that of an acute subarachnoid bleed clinically indistinguishable from ruptured aneurysms in other territories. The rupture of MCA aneurysms, however, can have distinct clinical features. A contralateral hemiparesis coupled with an aphasia (if the dominant lobe is involved), contralateral visual field defect, seizures, and contralateral facial paresis have been described with middle cerebral aneurysmal rupture in 50% to 80% of cases.[3,63,135,208,213]

Several prospective case studies and autopsy series illustrate that ruptured MCA aneurysms are associated with intracerebral bleeds in 39% to 55% of their study population.[13,92,144,150,213] These hematomas are invariably located in the temporal, frontal, and parietal areas, with some secondary extension into the basal ganglia.[33,63,92,150] Temporal lobe hematomas represent 83% of the intracerebral bleeds in several studies.[150,213] Hematomas induced by middle cerebral aneurysms can cause seizure activity in 5% to 25% of patients.[135,144,208,213]

Unruptured MCA aneurysms can present with unique clinical syndromes and can give rise to neurologic symptomatology due to mass effect, emboli, or infarction. Large (10–24 mm), or giant (≥ 25mm) unruptured middle cerebral aneurysms in the sylvian fissure can exert compressive effects on the fronto-parietal-temporal lobes and the underlying basal ganglia. This in turn can cause seizures, contralateral hemiparesis, and sensory loss over a subacute (1-month) to chronic (5-year) period.[29,144,184] As the aneurysm expands over variable time periods, it compresses the above neural structures, causing increasing, progressive symptoms.[29]

Unruptured aneurysms with intraluminal thrombosis can give rise to distal thromboemboli from the aneurysm sac, and these in turn may cause cerebral infarction and/or transient ischemic attacks (TIAs).[7,9,56,144,184,213] Distal embolic events are more commonly seen in middle cerebral aneurysms. Aphasia,[25,38,184] contralateral hemiparesis, and contralateral cortical hemisensory loss[38,71,87,209] are common TIA-like syndromes associated with aneurysmal emboli from the MCA. The TIAs cease once the aneurysm is successfully resected.

A small subset of giant MCA aneurysms called "serpentine aneurysms" are described in the literature. These are giant, partially thrombosed MCA aneurysms with tortuous (e.g. serpentine), vascular channels running through them.[123,182] They can exert symptoms over a chronic period (2 months to 5 years) due to compressive effects on adjacent neural structures. Aphasia, hemiplegia, depression, and dementia were the commonly described frontoparietal lobe dysfunctions linked with serpentine, MCA aneurysms.[123,193]

The blood supply through the tortuous "serpentine" vascular channel of the aneurysm is important for circulation to territories distal to the aneurysm. Surgical resection of the aneurysm disrupts circulation through these abnormal channels and sometimes causes cerebral infarction. The incidence of immediate postoperative stroke increases if the main trunk of the MCA was the major vessel feeding the "serpentine" channels.*

## *Anterior Communicating Artery Aneurysms*

Anterior communicating artery aneurysms comprise about 30% of all intracranial aneurysms, and are the most common site of aneurysmal SAH.[77,120,141] Rupture of this type of aneurysm often has nonlocalizing features. However, a localizing transient paraparesis lasting several minutes to several hours can occur with rupture of these aneurysms.[3,63,126,144,208]

An older autopsy series comprising 106 patients showed anterior hypothalamic damage due to rupture of anterior communicating artery aneurysms. Microhemorrhages, infarcts, and massive bleeds into the hypothalamus were the cause of pathology.[41] Later studies have verified hypothalamic-pituitary adrenal dysfunction occurring when ruptured anterior communicating aneurysms bleed into the diencephalon, causing autonomic instability such as fluctuating hypo-hypertension and hypo-hyperthermia.[144] Diabetes insipidus[77,120,130] is a common manifestation of hypothalamic-pituitary dysfunction. Manifestations of adrenal malfunction, including abnormal diurnal cortisol levels, and abnormal responses to dexamethasone tests, have been documented.[120,130]

Norlen[140] was an early investigator who reported amnesia in association with anterior communicating artery aneurysms. Recent case series have demonstrated Korsakoff-like amnestic syndromes after rupture of these aneurysms into the medial frontal lobes, anterior commissure, and septal and basal ganglia areas.[42,60,70,109,174]

The surgery involved in clipping anterior communicating aneurysms can lead to some peculiar neurologic syndromes, including subacute to chronic amnesia.[72,88,206] Yasargil et al[221] postulated that perforating arteries off the anterior communicating artery were damaged during the surgical resection of such aneurysms. Damage to these vessels could

*References 123,168,193,195

produce infarction in areas of the brain (e.g. fornix, anterior commissure), which are important to memory function.

Wrapping ruptured[32,127] and unruptured[129] anterior communicating aneurysms can cause an "optico-chiasmal arachnoiditis." Patients typically present with a sudden decrease in visual acuity, and/or visual field cuts several months postaneurysm clipping. Surgical reintervention has demonstrated adhesions and mononuclear infiltrates in the visual centers. Visual acuity improves with lysis of adhesions and removal of the wrapping. Fortunately, with techniques of microsurgical dissection and temporary vessel occlusion, clipping of most aneurysms is technically possible, thereby avoiding these sequelae of wrapping.

Ruptured anterior communicating artery aneurysms have a high percentage (20% to 65%) of frontal lobe hematomas.[77,144,150,223] Less commonly, rupture of these aneurysms can spread laterally to form subcortical internal capsular hematomas.[144] Anterior communicating artery aneurysms rupture into the intraventricular areas in a high percentage of cases (53% to 79%).[92,150,213] Aneurysmal blood often dissects through the medial frontal lobe[119,133,175] or through the corpus callosum[92] into the frontal horns of the lateral ventricles. Anterior communicating aneurysms may also bleed through the lamina terminalis into the third ventricle.[84,181] Intraventricular hemorrhage associated with these aneurysms can cause acute or subacute hydrocephalus in 25% of cases.[13,63,77,135]

Unruptured anterior communicating artery aneurysms present less frequently as space-occupying lesions with slowly progressive neurologic symptoms. Large (10–24 mm in diameter) anterior communicating artery aneurysms can expand medially to compress the optic nerves and/or chiasm. A subacute-to-chronic visual loss (2 weeks to 2 months) heralded by blindness ipsilateral to the aneurysm with or without field cuts[8,31,67,165,185] is common. Anterior communicating artery aneurysms can compress the frontal lobes on a chronic basis (e.g. 7 years) and cause a dementia with a schizophrenic, abulic state.[26,135,144]

## *Distal Anterior Cerebral Artery Aneurysms*

The ACA divides into the frontopolar artery and orbital branches as it ascends over the genu of the corpus callosum. The distal ACA then divides into the callosomarginal and pericallosal arteries. The callosomarginal artery gives off various internal frontal arteries before terminating as the paracentral artery. The pericallosal artery gives off the precuneal artery before terminating as the posterior pericallosal artery.

Distal ACA aneurysms can occur at various bifurcation points (e.g. origin of callosomarginal artery, origin of the frontopolar artery) along the course of the aneurysms.[176] Saccular aneurysms of the distal ACA represent 2% to 4.5% of all intracranial aneurysms.[186,213,214,220] They have a high percentage (30% to 70%) of associated anomalies such as arteriovenous malformation (AVM), azygous ACA, and coarctation of the aorta.[21,143,214]

The clinical presentation of a ruptured ACA aneurysm includes a sudden severe headache with meningismus, and possible contralateral lower extremity monoparesis.[21,176,213] Transient diarrhea or incontinence due to superior frontal lobe or paracentral lobule dysfunction can appear after aneurysmal rupture of this artery.[145,213] Ruptured distal anterior cerebral aneurysms can be associated with frontal lobe and/or corpus callosal hematomas in 30% to 48% of various studies.[176,214,224] A hematoma in the rostral frontal lobe can lead to contralateral and/or bilateral frontal release signs of grasping and groping, abulia, and akinetic mutism.[213] Blood in the corpus callosum can dissect into the frontal horns of the lateral ventricle in 2% to 13% of case series.[92,119,133,150] By this mechanism, these particular aneurysms can cause intraventricular hemorrhage.

Unruptured distal ACA aneurysms can present with embolic TIAs, or exert mass effect upon the adjacent frontal lobes or optic nerves and chiasm. Emboli to other distal branches of the ACA aneurysms can cause contralateral leg weakness.[202,214,220] A progressive frontal-lobe dysfunction with abulia, short-term memory loss, dementia, and spastic gait can occur anywhere from several months up to 13 years as a result of these aneurysms.[21,136] ACA aneurysms can exert a mass effect upon the optic nerves and cause a visual loss ipsilateral to the aneurysm.[21,141,202,213]

## Basilar Artery Aneurysms

Posterior circulation aneurysms, which include the vertebral and basilar arteries and their branches, comprise 8% to 15% of intracranial aneurysms.[30,52,144,225] Saccular aneurysms of the basilar bifurcation commonly present with symptoms of SAH. Fusiform aneurysms of this vessel are associated with tortuous dilatation and elongation of the artery. These types of aneurysms often are seen in advanced atherosclerosis in the vertebrobasilar system.[39,209,217] Insidious, chronic, progressive neurologic symptoms due to slowly expanding fusiform aneurysms are a common clinical presentation.

Rupture of basilar bifurcation aneurysms presents with clinical signs such as sudden occipital headache, impaired consciousness, hemiparesis, coma, and isolated cranial nerve palsies in over one third of cases.[20,43,63,89,206] Oculomotor and abducens nerve palsies, with or without ocular bobbing, represent involvement of the midbrain-pontine area during rupture of basilar bifurcation aneurysms.[43,63] Hemiparesis and/or quadriparesis reflect both unilateral and bilateral involvement of pyramidal tracts in the upper brain stem.[13,29,43] Rupture of basilar bifurcation aneurysms produces an intraventricular bleed into the third ventricle in 25% to 40% of cases.[63,92,103,150,213]

Unruptured basilar bifurcation aneurysms give rise to chronic (3 months to 2 years), progressive, neurologic symptoms synonymous with a slowly expanding space-occupying lesion.[24] Ocular palsies involving the oculomotor and abducens nerves are well documented in unruptured basilar bifurcation aneurysms. An oculomotor palsy causing ptosis, vertical diplopia, and a dilated, unreactive pupil have been cited in both small and large case series.[18,51,198,209] In some studies, pupillary-sparing oculomotor palsies occurred.[24,124,179] Supranuclear gaze palsies correlated with vertical and horizontal gaze impairments[63,103,180] and internuclear ophthalmoplegia[29,86] have been cited. Stark[180] postulated that large, unruptured basilar aneurysms exerted upward pressure on the pretectal midbrain region.

Unruptured basilar aneurysms may cause bulbar signs of dysphagia and hoarseness, frequently coupled with a hemi- and/or quadriparesis over a period of several months. Compression of the pontine corticobulbar and corticospinal tracts by the aneurysm is the presumed mechanism of pathology.[29,51,144] Radiologic and surgical studies have also documented obstruction of the third ventricle with secondary hydrocephalus by giant basilar artery (BA) aneurysms.[29,47,57,144]

Unruptured BA aneurysms can cause TIA-like syndromes months or years prior to fatal rupture of the aneurysm. Clinically, the patients presented with ipsilateral abducens and facial nerve palsies coupled with contralateral hemiparesis and/or hemiataxia.[86,213] Thromboembolism or compressive damage of brain stem perforating blood vessels are proposed mechanisms of pathogenesis.[86]

## Superior Cerebellar Artery Aneurysms

The superior cerebellar artery (SCA) is one of the terminal branches of the BA bifurcation. SCA aneurysms commonly arise at the junction of superior cerebellar and basilar arteries, project laterally and posteriorly, and are embedded in the cerebral peduncle. The fundus of the aneurysm has close contact with the oculomotor nerve.[213] These rare aneurysms can present equally as an SAH or an unruptured mass causing compressive neurologic symptoms.[85,171] Rupture of SCA aneurysms can be associated with an immediate comatose state with subsequent decorticate/decerebrate posturing and ocular bobbing.[171] These signs reflect damage at the midbrain-pontine junction.

With unruptured SCA aneurysms, deformity of the oculomotor nerve as well as compression of the cerebral peduncle produces a Weber's syndrome.[204,209,213] On exam, the patient has an oculomotor nerve palsy on the side of the aneurysm, coupled with a contralateral hemiparesis. Further compression of midbrain structures, such as the abducens nerve and the superior cerebellar peduncles, by this aneurysm causes a slowly progressive diplopia, superior oblique extraocular palsy, and hemiataxia.[85,149] Rarely, aneurysms may be encountered along the distal SCA, and may present with SAH or, less commonly, with trochlear nerve palsy.

## *Posterior Cerebral Artery Aneurysms*

The BA terminates at the pontomesencephalic junction as the paired posterior cerebral arteries (PCAs). In large cooperative studies by Locksley[120,121] involving over 6,000 cases, it was found that posterior cerebral aneurysms represented about .8% of all intracranial aneurysms. Several smaller, more recent series found that PCA aneurysms represented 1% to 1.3% of all intracranial aneurysms,[22,36,155] with saccular aneurysms of the PCA comprising about 60% to 70% of these. Giant aneurysms comprise 20%, and fusiform aneurysms represent 10% of the posterior cerebral aneurysms.[69,155]

PCA aneurysms can present as SAH in 50% to 80% of cases.[36,120,155] This can result in debilitating brain stem syndrome and deep coma, with very poor prognosis.[35,155,167] Other less dramatic presentations of ruptured PCA aneurysms include an ipsilateral oculomotor palsy coupled with a contralateral hemiparesis.[36,48,155] A ruptured PCA aneurysm can be clinically indistinguishable from other ruptured aneurysms.

Unruptured PCA aneurysms present as mass lesions which can radiographically appear as parieto-temporal-occipital lobe tumors.[36,70,155] Symptomatology with these aneurysms can occur anywhere from months to years.[22,36,48,69] As the posterior cerebral aneurysms enlarge and compress the aforementioned lobes, the result is memory loss, seizures, visual hallucinations, and contralateral hemiplegia and hemianopias.[36,63,69,155,209]

## *Anterior-Inferior Cerebellar Artery Aneurysms*

The anterior-inferior cerebellar artery (AICA) arises as the first main branch of the BA.[209] This artery then gives off various branches to supply the pons and pontomedullary junction. Basilar-AICA aneurysms represent a very small group of aneurysms. They present equally as either SAH or as an unruptured cerebellopontine angle (CPA) mass simulating an acoustic neuroma.[30,44,138,226]

An acute occipital headache coupled with vertigo, tinnitus, deafness, and facial paresis ipsilateral to the aneurysm are hallmarks of ruptured AICA aneurysms.[44,102,138,225]

Unruptured AICA aneurysms often occur at the CPA and may cause fluctuating neurologic symptoms over a period of weeks or months. The common scenarios are facial numbness, facial paralysis, pulsatile tinnitus, hypercusis, progressive deafness, and a horizontal nystagmus ipsilateral to the aneurysm. Ipsilateral hemiataxia, or a contralateral hemiparesis can also occur.[30,89,226]

## *Vertebral and Posterior Inferior Cerebellar Artery Aneurysms*

Vertebral artery aneurysms are quite uncommon and frequently are linked with anomalous development of the vertebral artery (e. g. congenital absence of the contralateral vertebral artery, vertebral artery ending in the posterior inferior cerebellar artery [PICA] and fenestration of the BA). [213] Aneurysms of the vertebral artery commonly arise at or beyond the origin of the PICA. Vertebral-PICA junction aneurysms represent 1% of all intracranial aneurysms.[53,95] Other vertebral artery aneurysms documented in the literature include those of the vertebral artery/basilar artery junction or arising from the vertebral artery immediately as it enters the subarachnoid space.

Rupture of vertebral aneurysms occurs in up to 80%[51,114,157,177,218] of reported cases. Patients commonly present with acute occipital headache, and transient loss of consciousness, sometimes followed by a comatose state. Transient brain stem signs such as dysarthria, hemiataxia, quadriparesis, and lower cranial nerve palsies can accompany the rupture of vertebral aneurysms.[51,90,95]

Unruptured intracranial vertebral aneurysms can present as compressive mass lesions giving rise to lower brain stem/upper cervical cord symptomatology or, rarely, with distal embolic phenomena to other vascular territories.[10,157,211,216] Unruptured vertebral artery, PICA, and vertebral/basilar artery junction aneurysms commonly impinge on the lower medulla oblongata and pontomedullary-cerebellar junction respectively. Unruptured vertebral/basilar artery aneurysms commonly present with abducens nerve (horizontal nystagmus), facial nerve (peripheral facial palsy), and vestibulocochlear nerve (vertigo, deafness) palsies ipsilateral to the aneurysm. An ipsilateral hemiataxia or a contralateral hemiparesis often accompanies these cranial nerve palsies.[107,157,178,209]

Unruptured vertebral aneurysms at the level of the foramen magnum rarely have been reported in the literature. They cause progressive spinal cord dysfunction at the upper cervical level, sometimes producing a Brown-Seguard syndrome. The syndrome begins with a hemiparesis and hemisensory loss involving the arm and leg, but sparing the face ipsilateral to the aneurysm. As the aneurysm grows, there is involvement of the spinothalamic tract which causes a decrease to pain or pinprick in the contralateral arm and leg.[29,132]

The more common vertebral-PICA aneurysms act as posterior fossa lesions compressing the medulla. Patients frequently complain of a chronic, occipital headache (months to years), which often worsens on recumbency.[79,90,177,211] Distortion of the medulla leads to facial numbness, dysphagia, decreased gag reflex, hoarseness, vertigo, tongue atrophy, and ataxia with progressive contralateral hemiparesis. These physical findings have been demonstrated in several smaller series of vertebral-PICA aneurysms, each comprising fewer than 20 patients.* Such symptoms were of a progressive nature and occurred over a 6-month to 2-year period.[29,79,187]

Emboli from unruptured thrombosed vertebral-PICA aneurysms can lodge in the upper BA and cause a fatal upper brain stem infarction.[51] The surgery involved in treating an unruptured vertebral artery aneurysm can cause embolic events.[216] The clipping of a parent vertebral artery proximal to the thrombosed vertebral aneurysm can cause immediate postoperative or delayed infarction in the distal PICA territory or upper brain stem. Infarction in the distal PICA territory may result in a Wallenberg syndrome with ipsilateral hemiataxia, hemisensory loss, and dysphagia, hoarseness, or vertigo. Upper brain stem infarction often presents with quadriparesis, upper cranial nerve signs, and ophthalmoparesis.** Other aneurysms rarely arise along the distal course of the PICA. These can present with SAH and fourth ventricular hemorrhage. Unruptured distal PICA aneurysms may present as mass lesions, and should be considered in the differential diagnosis of posterior fossa, cerebellar, and fourth ventricular tumors.

## Summary

The clinical presentation of intracranial cerebral aneurysms is most commonly as SAH. Features of this syndrome are highly characteristic, and the distribution of subarachnoid blood or any associated parenchymal hematoma may assist in localizing the ruptured aneurysm. A high index of clinical suspicion must accompany the evaluation of any severe headache, so as to consider and exclude aneurysmal bleeding.

Syndromes of unruptured cerebral aneurysms are highly diverse, and relate to location

*References 10,29,51,132,157,216
**References 51,173,183,207,216

of the aneurysm, adjacent neural structures, and the vascular territory of the parent vessel. These syndromes can be quite typical and characteristic in more common aneurysm locations.

## References


1. Adams HP Jr, Jergenson DD, Kassell NF, et al. Pitfalls in the recognition of subarachnoid hemorrhage. *JAMA.* 1980;244:794–796.
2. Adams HP Jr, Kassell NF, Kongable G, et al. Atypical features of subarachnoid hemorrhage. *Ann Neurol.* 1985;18:123. Abstract.
3. Adams RD, Victor M. *Principles of Neurology.* 4th ed. New York, NY: McGraw Hill Inc.; 1989:666–673.
4. Almeida GM, Shibata MK, Bianco E. Carotid-ophthalmic aneurysms. *Surg Neurol.* 1976;5:41–45.
5. Aminoff MJ. *Neurology and General Medicine.* New York, NY: Churchill Livingstone; 1989:161–165.
6. Anson JA, Stone JL, Crowell RM. Rupture of giant carotid aneurysm after extracranial-to-intracranial bypass surgery. *Neurosurgery.* 1991;28:142–147.
7. Antunes JL, Correll JW. Cerebral emboli from intracranial aneurysms. *Surg Neurol.* 1976;6: 7–10.
8. Aoki N. Partially thrombosed aneurysm presenting as the sudden onset of bitemporal hemianopsia. *Neurosurgery.* 1988;22:564–566.
9. Auld AW, Shafey S. Transient ischemic attacks not produced by extracranial vascular disease: a plea for complete and early angiographic investigation. *South Med J.* 1976;69:722–724.
10. Ausman JI, Diaz FG, Mullan S, et al Posterior inferior to posterior inferior verebellar artery anastomosis combined with trapping for vertebral artery aneurysm: case report. *J Neurosurg.* 1990; 73:462–465.
11. Ball MJ. Pathogenesis of the "sentinel headache" preceding berry aneurysm rupture. *Can Med Assoc J.* 1975;112:78–79.
12. Bamford J, Sandercock P, Dennis M, et al. A prospective study of acute cerebrovascular disease in the community: the Oxfordshire Community Stroke Project 1981-1986, II: incidence, case fatality rates and overall outcome at one year of cerebral infarction, primary intracerebral and subarachnoid hemorrhage. *J Neurol, Neurosurg Psychiatry.* 1990;53: 16–22.
13. Barnett HJM. Some clinical features of intracranial aneurysms. *Clin Neurosurg.* 1968;16:43–72.
14. Barnett HJM. Spontaneous intracranial hemorrhage. In: Wyngaard JB, Smith LH Jr, eds. *Cecil Textbook of Medicine.* 18th ed. Philadelphia, Pa: WB Saunders; 1988:2:2173–2180.
15. Barnett HJM, Mohr JP, Stein BM, et al *Stroke: Pathophysiology, Diagnosis and Management.* New York, NY: Churchill Livingstone; 1986;1: 109–113.
16. Barnett HJM, Mohr JP, Stein BM, et al *Stroke: Pathophysiology Diagnosis and Management.* Volume II. New York, NY: Churchill Livingstone; 1986:643–1658.
17. Barrows LJ, Hunter FT, Banker BQ. The nature and clinical significance of pigments in the cerebrospinal fluid. *Brain.* 1955;78:59–80.
18. Bartleson JD, Trautman JC, Sundt TMJ. Minimal oculomotor nerve paresis secondary to unruptured intracranial aneurysm. *Arch Neurol.* 1986;43: 1015–1020.
19. Barton CW. Subarachnoid hemorrhage presenting as acute chest pain: a variant of le coup depoignard. *Ann Emer Med.* 1988;17:977–978.
20. Batjer H, Mickey B, Samson D. Enlargement and rupture of distal basilar artery aneurysm after iatrogenic carotid occlusion. *Neurosurgery.* 1987;20: 624–628.
21. Becker DH, Newton TH. Distal anterior cerebral artery aneurysm. *Neurosurgery.* 1979;4:495–503.
22. Belec L, Cesaro P, Brugieres P, et al. Tumor-simulating giant serpentine aneurysm of the posterior cerebral artery. *Surg Neurol.* 1988;29:210–215.
23. Berenstein A, Ransohoff J, Kupersmith M, et al. Transvascular treatment of giant aneurysms of the cavernous carotid and vertebral arteries. *Surg Neurol.* 1984;21:3–12.
24. Boccardo M, Ruelle A, Banchero MA. Isolated oculomotor palsy caused by aneurysm of the basilar artery bifurcation. *J Neurol.* 1986; 233:61–62.
25. Bojanowski WM, Spetzler RF, Carter LP. Reconstruction of MCA bifurcation after excision of a giant aneurysm. *J Neurosurg.* 1988; 68:974–977.
26. Bokemeyer C, Frank B, Brandis A, et al. Giant aneurysm causing frontal lobe syndrome. *J Neurol.* 1990;237:47–50.
27. Bouzarth WF, Goldman HW. Subarachnoid hemorrhage. In: Callaham ML, ed. *Current Therapy in Emergency Medicine.* Philadelphia, Pa: Deckern; 1987:302–305.
28. Brihaye J. Intracavernous carotid aneurysms. In: Pia HW, Langmaid C, Zierski J, eds. *Cerebral Aneurysms: Advances in Diagnosis and Therapy.* New York, NY: Springer-Verlag; 1979:67–78.
29. Bull J. Massive aneurysms at the base of the brain. *Brain.* 1969;92:535–570.
30. Cantore GP, Ciapetta P, Vagnozzi R, et al Giant aneurysm of the anterior inferior cerebellar artery simulating a cerebellopontine angle tumor. *Surg Neurol.* 1982;18:76–78.
31. Caprioli J, Fagadau W, Lesser R. Acute monocular visual loss secondary to anterior communicating artery aneurysm in a patient with sickle cell disease. *Ann Opthalmol.* 1983;15:873–876.
32. Carney PG, Oatey PE. Muslin wrapping of aneurysms and delayed visual failure: a report of three cases. *J Clin Neuroophthalmol.* 1983;3:91–96.
33. Cedzich C, Schramm J, Röckelein G. Multiple cerebral artery aneurysms in an infant. *J Neurosurg.* 1990;72:806–809.
34. Chan BSH, Dorsch NWC. Delayed diagnosis in subarachnoid hemorrhage. *Med J Aust.* 1991;154: 509–511.
35. Chang HS, Fukushima T, Miyazaki S, et al. Fusiform posterior cerebral artery aneurysm treated with excision and end-to-end anastomosis: case report. *J Neurosurg.* 1986;6 4:501–504.
36. Chang HS, Fukushima T, Takakura K, et al. Aneurysms of the posterior cerebral artery: a report of 10 cases. *Neurosurgery.* 1986;19:1006–1011.
37. Chehrazi BB, Giri S, Joy RM. Prostaglandins and

vasoactive amines in cerebral vasospasm after aneurysmal subarachnoid hemorrhage. *Stroke.* 1989; 20:217–224.
38. Cohen MM, Hemalatha CP, D'Addario RT, et al. Embolization from a fusiform middle cerebral artery aneurysm. *Stroke.* 1980;11:158–161.
39. Constans JP, Viscot A, Fredy D, et al. Anéurysme géant du tronic basilaire révélé par une néuralgie faciale essentielle. *Neurochir.* 1976;22:493–502.
40. Cox TA, Corbett JJ, Thompson HS, et al. Unilateral nasal hemianopia as a sign of intracranial optic nerve compression. *Am J Ophthalmol.* 1981;92: 230–232.
41. Crompton MR. Hypothalamic lesions following the rupture of cerebral berry aneurysms. *Brain.* 1963; 86:301–314.
42. Crowell RM, Morawetz RB. Anterior communicating artery has significant branches. *Stroke.* 1977; 8:272–273.
43. Cruciger MP, Hoyt WF, Wilson CB. Peripheral and midbrain oculomotor palsies from operations for basilar bifurcation aneurysm in a series of 31 cases. *Surg Neurol.* 1981;15:215–216.
44. Dalley RW, Robertson WD, Nugent RA. Computerized tomography of anterior inferior cerebellar artery aneurysm mimicking an acoustic neuroma. *J Comput Assist Tomogr.* 1986;10:881–884.
45. Day AL. Aneurysms of the ophthalmic segment: a clinical and anatomical analysis. *J Neurosurg.* 1990; 72:677–691.
46. Day JW, Raskin NH. Thunderclap headache: symptom of unruptured cerebral aneurysm. *Lancet.* 1986; 2:1247–1248.
47. Depierreux M, Retif J, Flament-Durand J. Hydrocephalus due to a large aneurysm in the basilar artery [in French]. *Acta Neurol Belg.* 1980;80:80–85. English abstract.
48. Deruty R, Mottolese C, Bascoulergue Y, et al Spontaneous progressive thrombosis and surgical resection of a giant aneurysm of the posterior cerebral artery in an 18-year-old. *Neurol Res.* 1987;9:169–176.
49. Dorsch NW. Cerebral aneurysms and the "missed" hemorrhage. *Aust NZ J Med.* 1986;16: 486–490.
50. Drake CG. Giant intracranial aneurysms: experience with surgical treatment in 174 patients. *Clin Neurosurg.* 1979;26:12–95.
51. Drake CG. Ligation of the vertebral (unilateral or bilateral) or basilar artery in the treatment of large intracranial aneurysms. *J Neurosurg.* 1975;43: 255–274.
52. Drake CG. Management of aneurysms of the posterior circulation. Youmans JR, ed. *Neurological Surgery*. Philadelphia, Pa: WB Saunders Co; 1973: 2:787–806.
53. Drake CG. The treatment of aneurysms of the posterior circulation. *Clin Neurosurg.* 1979;26: 96–144.
54. Drake CG, Vanderlinden RG, Amacher AL. Carotid-ophthalmic aneurysms. *J Neurosurg.* 1968;29: 24–31.
55. Duffy GP. The "warning leak" in spontaneous subarachnoid hemorrhage. *Med J Aust.* 1983;1:514–516.
56. Duncan A, Caplan LR, Rumbaugh C. Aneurysms: a source of cerebral emboli. *Neurology.* 1979;29: 592. Abstract.
57. Ekbom K, Greitz T. Syndrome of hydrocephalus caused by saccular aneurysms of the basilar artery. *Acta Neurochir (Wien).* 1971;24:71–77.
58. Ellington E, Margolis G. Block of arachnoid villus by subarachnoid hemorrhage. *J Neurosurg.* 1969; 30:651–657.
59. Estanol BV, Marin OSM. Cardiac arrhythmias and sudden death in subarachnoid hemorrhage. *Stroke.* 1975;6:382–386.
60. Fasanaro AM, Valiani R, Russo G, et al Memory performances after anterior communicating artery aneurysm surgery. *Acta Neurol Napoli.* 1989;11: 272–278.
61. Feely M, Kapoor S. Third nerve palsy due to posterior communicating artery aneurysm: the importance of early surgery. *J Neurol Neurosurg Psychiatry.* 1987;50:1051–1052.
62. Ferguson GG, Drake CG. Carotid-ophthalmic aneurysms: visual abnormalities in 32 patients and the results of treatment. *Surg Neurol.* 1981;16:1–8.
63. Fisher CM. Clinical syndromes in cerebral thrombosis, hypertensive hemorrhage and ruptured saccular aneurysm. *Clin Neurosurg.* 1975;22: 117–147.
64. Fishman RA. *Cerebrospinal Fluid in Diseases of the Nervous System.* Philadelphia, Pa: WB Saunders; 1980:170–220.
65. Fontanarosa PB. Recognition of subarachnoid hemorrhage. *Ann Emerg Med.* 1989;18:1199–1205.
66. Fox AJ, Viñuela F, Pelz DM, et al. Use of detachable balloons for proximal artery occlusion in treatment of unclippable cerebral aneurysms. *J Neurosurg.* 1987;66:40–46.
67. Fox JL. *Intracranial Aneurysms.* New York, NY: Springer Verlag; 1983:133–162.
68. Fujiwara S, Fujii K, Nishio S, et al. Oculomotor nerve palsy in patients with cerebral aneurysms. *Neurosurg Rev.* 1989;12:123–132.
69. Fukamachi A, Hirato M, Wakao T, et al. Giant serpentine aneurysm of the posterior cerebral artery. *Neurosurgery.* 1982;11:271–276.
70. Fukamachi A, Horikoshi T, Nagaseki Y, et al. Symmetrical bilateral low-density lesions in the areas of supply by Heubner's arteries after aneurysm surgery. *Acta Neurochir (Wien).* 1987;84:89–92.
71. Fukuoka S, Suematsu K, Nakamura J, et al. Transient ischemic attack caused by unruptured intracranial aneurysms. *Surg Neurol.* 1982;17: 464–467.
72. Gade A. Amnesia after operations on aneurysms of the anterior communicating artery. *Surg Neurol.* 1982;18:46–49.
73. Garg SK, Dash RJ. Galactorrhea/amenorrhea syndrome due to an internal carotid artery aneurysm. *Postgrad Med J.* 1985;61:611–613.
74. Gelber BR, Sundt TM Jr. Treatment of intracavernous and giant carotid aneurysms by combined internal carotid ligation and extra- to intracranial bypass. *J Neurosurg.* 1980;52:1–10.
75. Gillingham FJ. The management of ruptured intracranial aneurysms. *Scott Med J.* 1967;12:377–383.
76. Good EF. Ptosis as the sole manifestation of compression of the oculomotor nerve by an aneurysm of the posterior communicating artery. *J Clin Neuroophthalmol.* 1990;10:59–61.
77. Greenberg MS. *Handbook of Neurosurgery.* Syracuse, NY: Greenberg Graphics Inc.; 1990:129–583.
78. Greenspan BN, Reeves AG. Transient partial oc-

ulomotor nerve paresis with posterior communicating artery aneurysms: a case report. *J Clin Neuroophthalmol.* 1990;10:56–58.
79. Hahn FJ, Ong E, McComb R, et al. Peripheral signal void ring in a giant vertebral aneurysm: MR and pathology findings. *J Comput Assist Tomog.* 1986;10:1036–1038.
80. Hamer J. Prognosis of oculomotor palsy in patients with aneurysms of the posterior communicating artery. *Acta Neurochir (Wien).* 1982;66:173–185.
81. Hamer J, Penzholz H, Gotte B. Time course and clinical significance of cerebral vasospasm after aneurysmal subarachnoid hemorrhage. *Acta Neurochir (Wien).* 1980;52:157–158. Abstract.
82. Hauerberg J, Andersen BB, Eskesen V, et al. Importance of the recognition of a warning leak as a sign of a ruptured intracranial aneurysm. *Acta Neurol Scand.* 1991;83:61–64.
83. Henry GL. Headache. In: Rosen P, Baker FJ III, Barkin RM, et al, eds. *Emergency Medicine: concepts and Clinical Practice.* 2nd ed. St. Louis, Mo: CV Mosby; 1988;1:279–293.
84. Hesselink JR. Aneurysm rupture and its complications. In: Fox JL, ed. *Intracranial Aneurysms.* New York, NY: Springer Verlag; 1983;1: 549–594.
85. Hirose Y, Nakamura T, Takamiya Y, et al. Fusiform superior cerebellar artery aneurysm presenting with contralateral abducens nerve paresis: case report. *Neurol Med-Chir (Tokyo).* 1990;30: 119–122.
86. Hirsch LF, Gonzalez CF. Fusiform basilar aneurysm simulating carotid transient ischemic attacks. *Stroke.* 1979;10:598–601.
87. Hoffman WF, Wilson CB, Townsend JJ. Recurrent transient ischemic attacks secondary to an embolizing saccular middle cerebral artery aneurysm. *J Neurosurg.* 1979;51:103–106.
88. Hori S, Suzuki J. Early and late results of intracranial direct surgery of anterior communicating artery aneurysms. *J Neurosurg.* 1979; 50:433–440.
89. Hosobuchi Y. Direct surgical treatment of giant intracranial aneurysms. *J Neurosurg.* 1979;51: 743–756.
90. Hudgins RJ, Day AL, Quisling RG, et al. Aneurysms of the posterior inferior cerebellar artery. *J Neurosurg.* 1983;58:381–387.
91. Huige WMM, van Vliet AGM, Bastiaensen LAK. Early symptoms of subarachnoid hemorrhage due to aneurysms of the posterior communicating artery. *Doc Ophthalmol.* 1988;70:251–256.
92. Inagawa T, Hirano A. Ruptured intracranial aneurysms: an autopsy study of 133 patients. *Surg Neurol.* 1990;33:117–123.
93. Ito U, Fukumoto T, Inaba Y. *Cerebrospinal Fluid Cytology After Subarachnoid Hemorrhage.* New York, NY: Plenum; 1980;2:541–557.
94. Jefferson G. Compression of chiasma, optic nerves and optic tracts by intracranial aneurysms. *Brain.* 1937;60:444–497.
95. Jewel KL. Bilateral extracranial vertebral artery aneurysms. *AJR.* 1977;128:324–325.
96. Jomin M, Lesoin F, Lozes G, et al. Surgical prognosis of unruptured intracranial arterial aneurysms: report of 50 cases. *Acta Neurochir (Wien).* 1987;84:85–88.
97. Jordan GW, Statland B, Halsted C. CSF lactate in diseases of the CNS. *Arch Int Med.* 1983;143:85–87.
98. Kasoff I, Kelly DL Jr. Pupillary sparing in oculomotor palsy from internal carotid aneurysm: case report. *J Neurosurg.* 1975;42:713–717.
99. Kasuya H, Shimizu T. Activated complement components C3a C4a in cerebrospinal fluid and plasma following subarachnoid hemorrhage. *J Neurosurg.* 1989;71:741–746.
100. Kissel JT, Burde RM, Klingele TG, et al. Pupil-sparing oculomotor palsies with internal carotid-posterior communicating artery aneurysms. *Ann Neurol.* 1983;13:149–154.
101. Kistler JP, Crowell RM, Davis KR, et al. The relation of cerebral vasospasm to the extent and location of subarachnoid blood visualized by CT scan. *Neurology.* 1983;33:424–436.
102. Kiya K, Uozumi T, Emoto K, et al. Anterior-inferior cerebellar artery aneurysm at the internal auditory meatus: case report. *Neurol Med Chir (Tokyo).* 1989;29:592–595.
103. Koga H, Mori K, Kawano T. Parinaud's syndrome and hydrocephalus due to a basilar artery aneurysm. *Surg Neurol.* 1983;19:548–553.
104. Kothandaram P, Dawson BH, Kruyt RC. Carotid-ophthalmic aneurysms: a study of 19 patients. *J Neurosurg.* 1971;34:544–548.
105. Kudo T. An operative complication in a patient with a true posterior communicating artery aneurysm. *Neurosurgery.* 1990;27:650–653.
106. Kupersmith MJ, Berenstein A, Choi I, et al. Percutaneous transvascular treatment of giant carotid aneurysms: neuro-ophthalmologic findings. *Neurology.* 1984;34:328–335.
107. Kurokawa Y, Okamura T, Watanabe K. Transcerebellar thrombectomy for the successful clipping of thrombosed giant vertebral artery-posterior inferior cerebellar artery aneurysm: case report. *Surg Neurol.* 1990;33:217–220.
108. Kuzniecky R, Melmed C, Schipper H. Carotid-ophthalmic aneurysm: an uncommon cause of acute monocular blindness. *Can Med Assoc J.* 1987;136: 727–728.
109. Laicona M, DeSantis A, Barbarotto R, et al. Neuropsychological follow-up of patients operated for aneurysms of anterior communicating artery. *Cortex.* 1989;25:261–273.
110. Lang DT, Berberian LB, Lee S, et al Rapid differentiation of subarachnoid hemorrhage from traumatic lumbar puncture using the D-dimer assay. *Am J Clin Pathol.* 1990; 93:403–405.
111. Laranjeira M, Sadasivan B, Ausman JI. Direct surgery for carotid bifurcation artery aneurysms. *Surgical Neurology.* 1990;34:250–254.
112. Leblanc R. The minor leak preceding subarachnoid hemorrhage. *J Neurosurg.* 1987;66:35–39.
113. Leblanc R, Winfield JA. The warning leak in subarachnoid hemorrhage and the importance of its early diagnosis. *Can Med Assoc J.* 1984;131:1235–1236.
114. Lee KS, Gower DJ, Branch CL Jr, et al. Surgical repair of aneurysms of the posterior inferior cerebellar artery: a clinical series. *Surg Neurol.* 1989; 31:85–91.
115. Lee MC, Heaney LM, Jacobson RL, et al. Cerebrospinal fluid in cerebral hemorrhage and infarction. *Stroke.* 1975;6:638–641.
116. Leopold NA, Hirsch LF, Ray T. Paroxysmal facial neuralgia secondary to a posterior communicating artery aneurysm. *Surg Neurol.* 1980;14:221–223.
117. Lesoin F, Rousseau M, Petit H, et al. Spontaneous

development of an intracavernous arterial aneurysm into a carotid-cavernous fistula: case report. *Acta Neurochir (Wien).* 1984;70:53–58.

118. Linskey ME, Sekhar LN, Hirsch W Jr, et al. Aneurysms of the intracavernous carotid artery: clinical presentation, radiographic features and pathogenesis. *Neurosurgery.* 1990;26:71–79.
119. Little JR, Blomquist GA, Ethier R. Intraventricular hemorrhage in adults. *Surg Neurol.* 1977;8:143–149.
120. Locksley HB. Report on cooperative study of intracranial aneurysms and subarachnoid hemorrhage, section V, I: natural history of subarachnoid hemorrhage, intracranial aneurysms and arteriovenous malformations. *J Neurosurg.* 1966;25:219–239.
121. Locksley HB. Report on cooperative study of intracranial aneurysms and subarachnoid hemorrhage, sectionV, II: natural history of subarachnoid hemorrhage, intracranial aneurysms and arteriovenous malformations based on 6838 cases in the cooperative study. *J Neurosurg.* 1966;25:321–368.
122. Lodge SD, Walker GF, Stewart MJ. Aneurysm of the left internal carotid artery simulating a pituitary tumor. *Br Med J.* 1927;2:1179–1180.
123. Lukin RR, Chambers AA, McLaurin R, et al. Thrombosed giant middle cerebral aneurysms. *Neuroradiology.* 1975;10:125–129.
124. Lustbader JM, Miller NR. Painless, pupil-sparing but otherwise complete oculomotor nerve paresis caused by a basilar artery aneurysm: case report. *Arch Ophthalmol.* 1988;106:583–584.
125. Madonick MJ, Savitsky N. Spinal fluid sugar in subarachnoid hemorrhage. *J Nerv Ment Dis.* 1948; 108:45–53.
126. Maiuri F, Gangemi M, Corriero G, et al. Anterior communicating artery presenting with sudden paraplegia. *Surgl Neurol.* 1986;25:397–398.
127. Marcus AO, Demakas JJ, Ross HA, et al. Optochiasmatic arachnoiditis with treatment by surgical lysis of adhesions, corticosteroids, and cyclophosphamide: report of a case. *Neurosurgery.* 1986;19:101–103.
128. Marion DW, Segal R, Thompson ME. Subarachnoid hemorrhage and the heart. *Neurosurgery.* 1986;18:101–106.
129. McFadzean RM, Hadley DM, McIlwaine GG. Optochiasmal arachnoiditis following muslin wrapping of ruptured anterior communicating artery aneurysms. *J Neurosurg.* 1991;75:393–396.
130. McMahon AJ. Diabetes insipidus after subarachnoid hemorrhage from an anterior communicating artery aneurysm. *Scott Med J.* 1988;33:208–209.
131. Merva W, Jamshidi S, Kurtzke J. Posterior communicating artery aneurysm as a cause of seizures. *Neurology.* 1985:35:620–622. Letter.
132. Michael WF. Posterior fossa aneurysms simulating tumors. *J Neurol, Neurosurg Psychiatry.* 1974;37: 218–223.
133. Mohr G, Ferguson G, Khan M, et al. Intraventricular hemorrhage from ruptured aneurysms: retrospective analysis of 91 cases. *J Neurosurg.* 1983: 58:482–487.
134. Mohr JP. *Manual of Clinical Problems in Neurology.* 2nd ed. Boston, Mass: Little Brown and Co.; 1989:4–184.
135. Morley TP, Barr HWK. Giant intracranial aneurysms: diagnosis, course, and management. *Clin Neurosurg.* 1969;16:73–94.
136. Morota N, Kobayashi S, Sugita K, et al. Giant aneurysms of the horizontal segment of the anterior cerebral artery: report of two cases. *Neurosurgery.* 1991;29:97–101.
137. Morota N, Ohtsuka A, Kameyama S, et al Obstructive hydrocephalus due to a giant aneurysm of the internal carotid artery bifurcation. *Surg Neurol.* 1988;29:227–231.
138. Nishimoto A, Fujimoto S, Tsuchimoto S, et al Anterior inferior cerebellar artery aneurysm: report of three cases. *J Neurosurg.* 1983;59:697–702.
139. Noms JW. Effects of cerebrovascular lesions in the heart. *Neurol Clin.* 1983;1:87–90.
140. Norlén G, Olivecrona H. The treatment of aneurysms of the circle of Willis. *J Neurosurg.* 1953; 10:404–415.
141. Norwood EG, Kline LB, Chandra-Sekar B, et al. Aneurysmal compression of the anterior visual pathways. *Neurology.* 1986;36:1035–1041.
142. O'Hare TH. Subarachnoid hemorrhage: a review. *J Emerg Med.* 1987;5:135–148.
143. Ohno K, Monma S, Suzuki R, et al. Saccular aneurysm of the distal anterior cerebral artery. *Neurosurgery.* 1990;27:907–913.
144. Ojemann RG, Crowell RM. *Surgical Management of Cerebrovascular Disease.* Baltimore, Md: Williams & Wilkins; 1983:127–265.
145. Okawara SH. Warning signs prior to rupture of an intracranial aneurysm. *J Neurosurg.* 1973;38:575–580.
146. Oppenheimer SM, Hachinski VC. The cardiac consequences of stroke. *Neurol Clin.* 1992; 10:167–176.
147. Ostergaard JR. Headache as a warning symptom of impending aneurysmal subarachnoid hemorrhage. *Cephalalgia.* 1991;11:53–55.
148. Ostergaard JR. Warning leak in subarachnoid hemorrhage. *Br Med J.* 1990; 301:190–191.
149. Papo I, Caruselli G, Salvolini U. Aneurysm of the superior cerebellar artery. *Surg Neurol.* 1977;7:15–17.
150. Pasqualin A, Bazzan A, Cavazzani P, et al Intracranial hematomas following aneurysmal rupture: experience with 309 cases. *Surg Neurol.* 1986;25: 6–17.
151. Pasquier F, Leys D, Vermersch P, et al Severe hypoglycorrhachia after subarachnoid hemorrhage: two cases with spontaneous recovery in adults. *Acta Neurol Belg.* 1987;87:76–79.
152. Perneczky A, Czech T. Prognosis of oculomotor palsy following subarachnoid hemorrhage due to aneurysms of the posterior communicating artery. *Zentralbl Neurochir.* 1984;45:189–195.
153. Perneczky A, Knosp E. Para- and infraclinoidal aneurysm: direct microsurgical repair. In: Proceedings of the International Symposium of Cavernous Sinus. Ljubljana, Yugoslavia; 1986:202–210.
154. Perria L, Rivano C, Rossi G, et al. Aneurysms of the bifurcation of the internal carotid artery. *Acta Neurochir (Wien).* 1968;19:51–68.
155. Pia HW, Fontana H. Aneurysms of the posterior cerebral artery. *Acta Neurochir (Wien).* 1977;38: 13–35.
156. Popovic E, Siu K. Ruptured intracranial aneurysms: a 12-month prospective study. *Med J Aust.* 1989;150:492–501.
157. Pritz MB. Evaluation and treatment of aneurysms of the vertebral artery: different strategies for different lesions. *Neurosurgery.* 1991; 29:247–256.
158. Reichenbach DD, Benditt EP. Catecholamines and

cardiomyopathy: the pathogenesis and potential importance of myofibrillar degeneration. *Hum Pathol.* 1970;1:125–150.
159. Rhoton AL, Day AL. Aneurysms and arteriovenous fistulate of the intracavernous carotid artery and its branches. In: Youmans JR, ed. *Neurological Surgery.* Philadelphia, Pa: WB Saunders; 1990;3: 1807–1830.
160. Ringel RA, Brick JF. Carotid-ophthalmic artery aneurysm masquerading as optic neuritis. *J Neurol Neurosurg Psychiatry.* 1986; 49:460. Letter.
161. Sahs AL, Nibblelink DW. *Aneurysmal Subarachnoid Hemorrhage: Report of Cooperative Study.* Baltimore, Md: Urban and Schwarzenberg; 1981:17.
162. Sahs AL, Perret GE, Nishiuka H, et al *Intracranial Aneurysms and Subarachnoid Hemorrhage: A Cooperative Study.* Philadelphia, Pa: Lippincott; 1969:296–308.
163. Sambrook MA, Hutchinson EC, Aber GM. Metabolic studies in subarachnoid hemorrhage and stroke, I: serial changes in acid-base values in blood and cerebrospinal fluid. *Brain.* 1973;96:171–190.
164. Sambrook MA, Hutchinson EC, Aber GM. Metabolic studies in subarachnoid hemorrhage and strokes, II: serial changes in cerebrospinal fluid and plasma urea electrolytes and osmolality. *Brain.* 1973;96:191–202.
165. Schisano G. Large anterior communicating artery aneurysm with temporal hemianopsia: case report. *J Neurosurg Sci.* 1985;29:267–271.
166. Scialfa G, Vaghi A, Valsecchi F, et al. Neuroradiological treatment of carotid and vertebral fistulas and intracavernous aneurysms. *Neuroradiology.* 1982;24:13–25.
167. Scott BA, Weinstein Z, Pulliam MW. Computer tomographic diagnosis of ruptured giant posterior cerebral aneurysms. *Neurosurgery.* 1988; 22:553–557.
168. Segal HD, McLaurin RL. Giant serpentine aneurysm: report of two cases. *J Neurosurg.* 1977;46: 115–120.
169. Sengupta RP, Gryspeerdt GL, Hankinson J. Carotid-ophthalmic aneurysms. *J Neur, Neurosurg, Psychiatry.* 1976;39:837–853.
170. Sengupta RP, Lassman LP, De Moraes AA, et al Treatment of internal carotid bifurcation aneurysms by direct surgery. *J Neurosurg.* 1975; 43:343–351.
171. Sherman DG, Salmon JH. Ocular bobbing with superior cerebellar artery aneurysm: case report. *J Neurosurg.* 1977;47:596–598.
172. Shimoda M, Yamada S, Yamamoto I, et al. Time course of CSF lactate level in subarachnoid hemorrhage: correlation with clinical grading and prognosis. *Acta Neurochir (Wien).* 1989;99:127–134.
173. Shintani A, Zervas NT. Consequence of ligation of the vertebral artery. *J Neurosurg.* 1972; 36:447–450.
174. Shoqeirat MA, Mayes A, MacDonald C, et al. Performance on tests sensitive to frontal lobe lesions by patients with organic amnesia: Leng and Parkin revisited. *Br J Clin Psychol.* 1990;29:401–408.
175. Silver AJ, Peterson ME Jr, Ganti SR, et al. CT of subarachnoid hemorrhage due to a ruptured aneurysm. *AJNR*. 1981;2:13–22.
176. Snyckers FD, Drake CG. Aneurysms of the distal anterior cerebral artery: a report on 24 verified cases. *S Afr Med J.* 1973; 47:1787–1791.
177. Solomon RA, Stein BM. Surgical approaches to aneurysms of the vertebral and basilar arteries. *Neurosurgery.* 1988;23:203–208.
178. Sørenson P, Lundorf E. Giant aneurysm of the vertebral artery simulating intracranial tumor at the foramen magnum. *Neuroradiology.* 1988; 30:359.
179. Soria E, Camell H, Dang H. Pupil-sparing oculomotor palsy caused by fusiform arteriosclerotic aneurysm of the basilar artery: case report. *Angiology.* 1989;40:921–927.
180. Stark RJ. Supranuclear ophthalmoplegia with basilar artery aneurysms. *Surg Neurol.* 1979; 12:447–452.
181. Stehbens WE. Pathology of intracranial arterial aneurysms and their complications. In: Fox JL ed. *Intracranial Aneurysms.* New York, NY: Springer-Verlag; 1983;1:272–357.
182. Steimle R, Jacquet G, Cotte-Rittaud M, et al. Volumineux anéurisme pseudo-tumoral partiellement thrombos é du territoire de la sylvienne. *Neurochir.* 1977; 23:73–80.
183. Steinberger A, Ganti SR, McMurtry JG III, et al Transient neurological deficits secondary to saccular vertebrobasilar aneurysms: report of two cases. *J Neurosurg.* 1984;60:410–413.
184. Stewart RM, Samson D, Diehl J, et al. Unruptured cerebral aneurysms presenting as recurrent, transient neurologic eeficits. *Neurology.* 1980;30:47–51.
185. Striph G, Slamovits JL, Burde RM. Visual recovery following prolonged amaurosis due to compressive optic neuropathy. *J Clin Neuro Ophthalmol.* 1984; 4:189–195.
186. Sugar O, Tinsley M. Aneurysm of terminal portion of anterior cerebral artery. *Arch Neurol Psychiatry.* 1948;60:81–85.
187. Sugita K, Kobayashi S, Takemae T, et al. Giant aneurysms of the vertebral artery: report of five cases. *J Neurosurg.* 1988;68:960–966.
188. Sugiura M, Yozawa Y, Kubo O, et al. Myocardial damage—myocytolysis caused by subarachnoid hemorrhage. [In Japanese.] *No To Shinkei..* 1985; 37:1155–1161. English abstract.
189. Suzuki H, Sato S, Suzuki Y, et al. Increased endolethin concentrations in CSF from patients with subarachnoid hemorrhage. *Acta Neurol Scand.* 1990;81:553–554.
190. Tabbaa MA, Ramirez-Lassepas M, Snyder BD. Aneurysmal subarachnoid hemorrhage presenting as cardiorespiratory arrest. *Arch Int Med.* 1987; 147: 1661–1662.
191. Takaku A, Fukawa O, Suzuki J. A case of priapism with a ruptured intracranial aneurysm. *J Neurol.* 1979;221:279–283.
192. Talman WT, Alonso DR, Reis DJ. Chronic lability of arterial pressure in the rat does not evolve into hypertension. *Clin Sci.* 1980;59(suppl):4055–4075.
193. Terao H, Muraoka I. Giant aneurysm of the middle cerebral artery containing an important blood channel: case report. *J Neurosurg.* 1972; 37:352–356.
194. Thurel C, Rey A, Thiébaut JB. Anéurysmes carotido-ophthalmiques. *Neurochir.* 1974;20: 25–39.
195. Tomasello F, Albanese V, Cioffi FA. Giant serpentine aneurysms: a separate entity. *Surg Neurol.* 1979;12:429–432.
196. Tomsak RL, Masaryk TJ, Bates JH. Magnetic resonance angiography (MRA) of an isolated aneurysmal third nerve palsy. *J Clin Neuro Ophthalmol.*

1991;11:16–18.
197. Torner JC, Kassell NF, Wallace RB, et al. Preoperative prognostic factors for rebleeding and survival in aneurysm patients receiving antifibrinolytic therapy: report of the cooperative aneurysm study. *Neurosurgery.* 1981;9:506–513.
198. Trobe JD, Glaser JS, Quencer RC. Isolated oculomotor paralysis: the product of saccular and fusiform aneurysms of the basilar artery. *Arch Ophthalmol.* 1978;96:1236–1240.
199. Troost BT, Walker JE, Cherington M. Hypoglycorrhachia associated with subarachnoid hemorrhage. *Arch Neurol.* 1968;19:438–442.
200. VanDellen JR. Intracavernous traumatic aneurysms. *Surg Neurol.* 1980;13:203–207.
201. Vermeulen M, Hasan D, Blijenberg BG. Xanthochromia after subarachnoid hemorrhage needs no revisitation. *J Neurol Neurosurg Psychiatry.* 1989;52:826–828.
202. Versavel M, Witmer JP, Matricali B. Giant aneurysm arising from the anterior cerebral artery and causing isolated homonymous hemianopsia. *Neurosurgery.* 1988;22:560–563.
203. Vincent FM. Hypoglycorrhachia after subarachnoid hemorrhage. *Neurosurgery.* 1981;8:7–9.
204. Vincent FM, Zimmerman JE. Superior cerebellar artery aneurysm presenting as an oculomotor nerve palsy in a child. *Neurosurgery.* 1980;6:661–664.
205. Viñuela F, Fox A, Chang JK, et al. Clinico-radiological spectrum of giant supraclinoid internal carotid artery aneurysms. *Neuroradiology.* 1984;26:93–99.
206. Volpe BT, Hirst W. Amnesia following the rupture and repair of an anterior communicating artery aneurysm. *J Neurol Neurosurg Psychiatry.* 1983;46:704–709.
207. Waga S, Fujimoto K, Morooka Y. Dissecting aneurysm of the vertebral artery. *Surg Neurol.* 1978;10:237–239.
208. Waga S, Ohtsubo K, Handa H. Warning signs in intracranial aneurysms. *Surg Neurol.* 1975;3:15–20.
209. Wallace M, Peerless S, Drake CG. Giant intracranial aneurysms. In: Youmans JR, ed. *Neurological Surgery.* Philadelphia, Pa: WB Saunders; 1990;3:1742–1762.
210. Walton JN. *Subarachnoid Hemorrhage.* Edinburgh, Scotland: Livingstone; 1956:287.
211. West P, Todman D. Chronic cluster headache associated with a vertebral artery aneurysm. *Headache.* 1991;31:210–212.
212. Wilkins RH, Rengachary SS. *Neurosurgery.* New York, NY: McGraw Hill; 1985;1:169–210.
213. Wilkins RH, Rengachary SS. *Neurosurgery.* New York, NY: McGraw Hill; 1985;2:1383–1500.
214. Wisoff JH, Flamm ES. Aneurysms of the distal anterior cerebral artery and associated vascular anomalies. *Neurosurgery.* 1987;20:735–741.
215. Wood JH. *Subarachnoid Hemorrhage: Neurobiology of Cerebrospinal Fluid.* New York, NY: Plenum; 1980;1:279–286.
216. Yamada K, Hayakawa T, Ushio Y, et al. Therapeutic occlusion of the vertebral artery for an unclippable vertebral artery aneurysm: relationship between site of occlusion and clinical outcome. *Neurosurgery.* 1984;15:834–838.
217. Yamanaka C, Hirohata T, Kiya K, et al. Basilar bifurcation aneurysm associated with bilateral internal carotid artery occlusions. *Neuroradiology.* 1987;29:84–88.
218. Yamaura A. Diagnosis and treatment of vertebral aneurysms. *J Neurosurg.* 1988;69:345–349.
219. Yasargil MG. *Surgery of Intracranial Aneurysms and Results: Carotid-Ophthalmic Aneurysms.* New York, NY: Georg Thieme Verlag; 1984:43–55.
220. Yasargil MG, Carter LP. Saccular aneurysms of the distal anterior cerebral artery. *J Neurosurg.* 1974;40:218–223.
221. Yasargil MG, Fox JL. Operative approach to aneurysm of the anterior communicating artery. In: Krayenb HLH ed. *Advanced and Technical Standards in Neurosurgery.* New York, NY: Springer-Verlag; 1975;2:115–128.
222. Yasargil MG, Smith RD. Middle cerebral artery aneurysms. In: Youmans JR ed. *Neurological Surgery.* 2nd ed. Philadelphia, Pa: WB Saunders; 1982;3:1663–1696.
223. Yock DH Jr, Larson DA. Computerized tomography of hemorrhage from anterior communicating artery aneurysms with angiographic correlation. *Radiology.* 1980;134:399–407.
224. Yoshimoto T, Uchida K, Suzuki J. Surgical treatment of distal anterior cerebral artery aneurysms. *J Neurosurg.* 1979;50:40–44.
225. Zager EL. Isolated trigeminal sensory loss secondary to a distal anterior inferior cerebellar artery aneurysm: case report. *Neurosurgery.* 1991;28:288–291.
226. Zlotnik EI, Sklyut JA, Smejanovich AF, et al. Saccular aneurysm of the anterior inferior cerebellar artery-internal auditory artery. *J Neurosurg.* 1982;57:829–832.

CHAPTER 3

# Imaging of Cerebral Aneurysms

John Perl II, MD, Thomas J. Masaryk, MD, and Issam A. Awad, MD, MSc, FACS

Approximately 28,000 intracranial aneurysms rupture each year in North America; half of these patients die within the first 30 days following rupture.[31] The prevalence of unruptured incidental aneurysms in autopsy series ranges from 1.3% to 7.9%.[55,71] A more recent angiographic study by Atkinson et al found a 1% prevalence of anterior circulation aneurysms.[7] The low prevalence of incidental aneurysms suggested by this study combined with the significant mortality and morbidity associated with ruptured aneurysms emphasizes the need for urgent evaluation of the symptomatic patients, and also the identification of asymptomatic patients at high risk for intracranial aneurysms.[7,86]

Intracranial aneurysms can be located intra- or extradurally. Extradural aneurysms involve the internal carotid arteries (ICAs) below the ophthalmic segment. Intradural aneurysms usually involve the distal ICAs, vessels of the circle of Willis, the bifurcation or trifurcation of the middle cerebral arteries (MCAs), and the vertebrobasilar trunk.[51] Aneurysms involving more peripheral cerebral vessels are less common and are usually due to inflammatory, infectious, traumatic, or tumoral etiology.[23,54,74,87] Posterior circulation aneurysms constitute 5% to 15% of cases.

Classification of aneurysms is often based on either the histologic and morphologic architecture or the etiology of the aneurysm. The morphologic appearance is commonly classified as saccular, or fusiform. The etiologies of aneurysms include congenital (berry), atherosclerotic, inflammatory, mycotic, dissecting, and neoplastic. The imaging evaluation of aneurysms includes demonstration of number, location, size, and morphologic appearance, as well as the location of the neck in the case of saccular aneurysms.[39] All of these factors play a vital role in the approach to therapy. In addition, it is imperative to define associated vascular variants or anomalies (such as hypoplastic/aplastic segments of the circle of Willis, carotid/basilar artery anastomosis, and supply or absence of vertebral or carotid arteries).[39]

The presence of subarachnoid and/or parenchymal clot, vasospasm, cerebral edema, infarction, or hydrocephalus are additional factors important to prognosis, medical management, and surgical planning.[39] Thus, the role of imaging is critical in the evaluation of the symptomatic patient, and is becoming better defined in evaluation of high-risk asymptomatic populations.

## Intracranial Berry Aneurysms

There exist certain patient populations with a high risk of harboring cerebral berry aneurysms: patients with polycystic kidney disease, cerebral arteriovenous malformations (AVMs), fibromuscular dysplasia, coarctation, and some connective tissue disorders.[5,62,81,88] In addition, there have been reports of families with a high incidence of intracranial aneurysms.[13,62,81,88,104]

The evaluation of asymptomatic cerebral aneurysms is evolving, with conventional catheter angiography remaining the gold standard. Invasive studies, however, are not typically performed in the asymptomatic patient unless another imaging modality is suggestive of an aneurysm. The less-invasive techniques that can be performed include computed tomography (CT), intravenous digital subtraction angiography (IVDSA), and magnetic resonance imaging (MRI) with magnetic resonance angiography (MRA).

Symptomatic patients can be divided into two groups: those that present with acute headaches/meningismus secondary to subarachnoid hemorrhage (SAH), and those that present with a focal mass effect such as a cranial nerve palsy. CT and catheter angiography currently remain the front-line diagnostic modalities in the clinical evaluation of acute SAH, although in certain circumstances, MRI and MRA play important roles, emerging, in the absence of SAH, as initial diagnostic regimens.

## *Computed Tomography*

CT can certainly detect intracranial aneurysms; however, the role in asymptomatic patients is unclear because of the variety of techniques employed in daily practice. The reports of CT-sensitivity to intracranial aneurysms have widely varied from 100% in one series to zero in another.[113,116] The most optimistic study was poorly controlled and the method of analysis was not revealed. The authors admit that both false positives and negatives may occur with relative frequency.[116] Other variables including system resolution, use and timing of contrast injection, and aneurysm size are all important in the reported detection rates.

Ruptured aneurysms are most frequently associated with SAH, less commonly with cerebral hematoma and/or intraventricular hemorrhage. Rarely, the rupture results in a subdural hematoma.[59] The etiology of the hemorrhage is often detected with noncontrast-enhanced CT, which provides a rapid assessment of the location and size of the hemorrhage. Prediction of the aneurysm location and evaluation of complications including infarction, mass effect, and hydrocephalus are also possible.[28,42,57,61,70] Contrast-enhanced CT in the setting of SAH occasionally can more accurately determine the location and etiology of the hemorrhage, but the additional contrast load may pose limitations if acute conventional angiography is planned.[42,61,68,88]

The hyperdensity of acute hemorrhage with respect to brain on a CT examination reflects primarily the hemoglobin and protein of blood.[75] In physiologic ranges, the hematocrit and hemoglobin have a linear relationship.[75] A patient that is significantly anemic could have a hemorrhage that is isodense to brain. Intracranial hematomas evolve over a time, becoming progressively lower in attenuation coefficient approaching isodensity to normal brain at approximately one week.[14,73]

Eighty to ninety percent of patients with SAH will have a positive CT examination (Figure 1).[3,67] This is important inasmuch as those patients with a classic clinical presentation and normal CT scan must have a spinal tap to fully exclude SAH. The blood in SAH evolves in a similar fashion to other intracranial hematomas on CT.[3] The location of the SAH can have predictive value of the location of the aneurysm rupture.[57,61,63,90] Moreover, some patterns of an SAH may imply nonaneurysmal or cryptogenic etiology,[4,96,108] and may be useful in directing subsequent angiographic evaluation. Di Lorenzo et al and Iwanaga et al have described scenarios in which the CT demonstrated SAH while the initial angiogram was negative, and followup angiography or surgery proved the presence of an aneurysm.[29,57] The many possible causes of negative angiography in acute SAH will be addressed later.

Silver et al described the pattern in 81 consecutive patients with SAH. The distribution

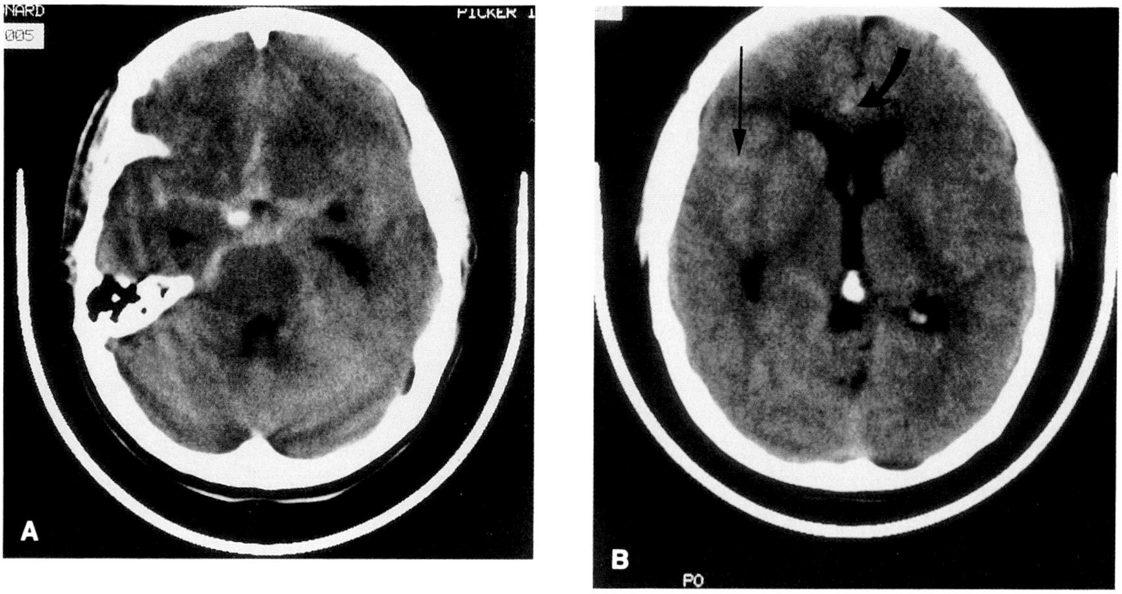


*Figure 1. SAH from an acute (< 1 hour) anterior communicating artery aneurysm. (A) Noncontrast-enhanced CT images demonstrate high attenuation in the suprasellar cistern extending to the prepontine cistern, anteriorly into the intrahemispheric cistern and the basal portions of the sylvian fissure. (B) Note subtle high attenuation identified in the mid-portion of the sylvian fissure (straight arrow) and subtle round small area of high attenuation in the interhemispheric fissure just anterior to the genu of the corpus callosum from the anterior communicating artery aneurysm (curved arrow). There is enlargement of the ventricles, especially the temporal horns due to early hydrocephalus.*

of the hemorrhage generally corresponds to the area of the aneurysm which has bled. The presence of parenchymal hemorrhage is more specific of an MCA or an anterior communicating artery aneurysm, while intraventricular hemorrhage is more prevalent with an anterior communicating artery, basilar summit, or posterior inferior cerebellar artery (PICA) aneurysm rupture.[61,96] Hemorrhage into the anterior portion of the pericallosal cistern is more suggestive of an anterior communicating artery or anterior cerebral artery (ACA) aneurysm rupture.[90] Interhemispheric hemorrhage is an otherwise nonspecific finding.[96] Hemorrhage within the sylvian fissure without pericallosal or interhemispheric blood suggests distal ICA, posterior communicating artery, or MCA aneurysm rupture.[96] Interparenchymal septal hematomas are only seen with anterior communicating artery aneurysm ruptures (Figure 2).[90] Inferior medial frontal hemorrhages occur in both anterior communicating artery and distal ICA aneurysm ruptures.[96] Corpus callosal hematomas are seen with rupture of pericallosal artery aneurysms. Hematomas in the deep frontal, lateral frontal, and temporal lobes may result from MCA, posterior communicating artery, and distal ICA aneurysm ruptures.[96] Exclusive temporal lobe hemorrhages are seen in ruptures of MCA and, rarely, posterior communicating artery aneurysms.[90,96]

Basal ganglionic hemorrhages are common in the setting of aneurysm rupture, and can be impossible to differentiate from primary hypertensive hemorrhages.[96] Perimesencephalic and interpeduncular hemorrhages extending into the lateral sylvian fissures are seen in basilar tip aneurysm ruptures.[96] Two studies evaluating perimesencephalic SAH with extension only to the ambient and basal portion of the sylvian fissure concluded this it is almost always nonaneurysmal in origin.[84,109] In both studies combined there were only two aneurysm ruptures out of 144 cases of perimesencephalic SAH, which had been inaccurately labeled as benign hemorrhages. Intraventricular hemorrhage or parenchymal

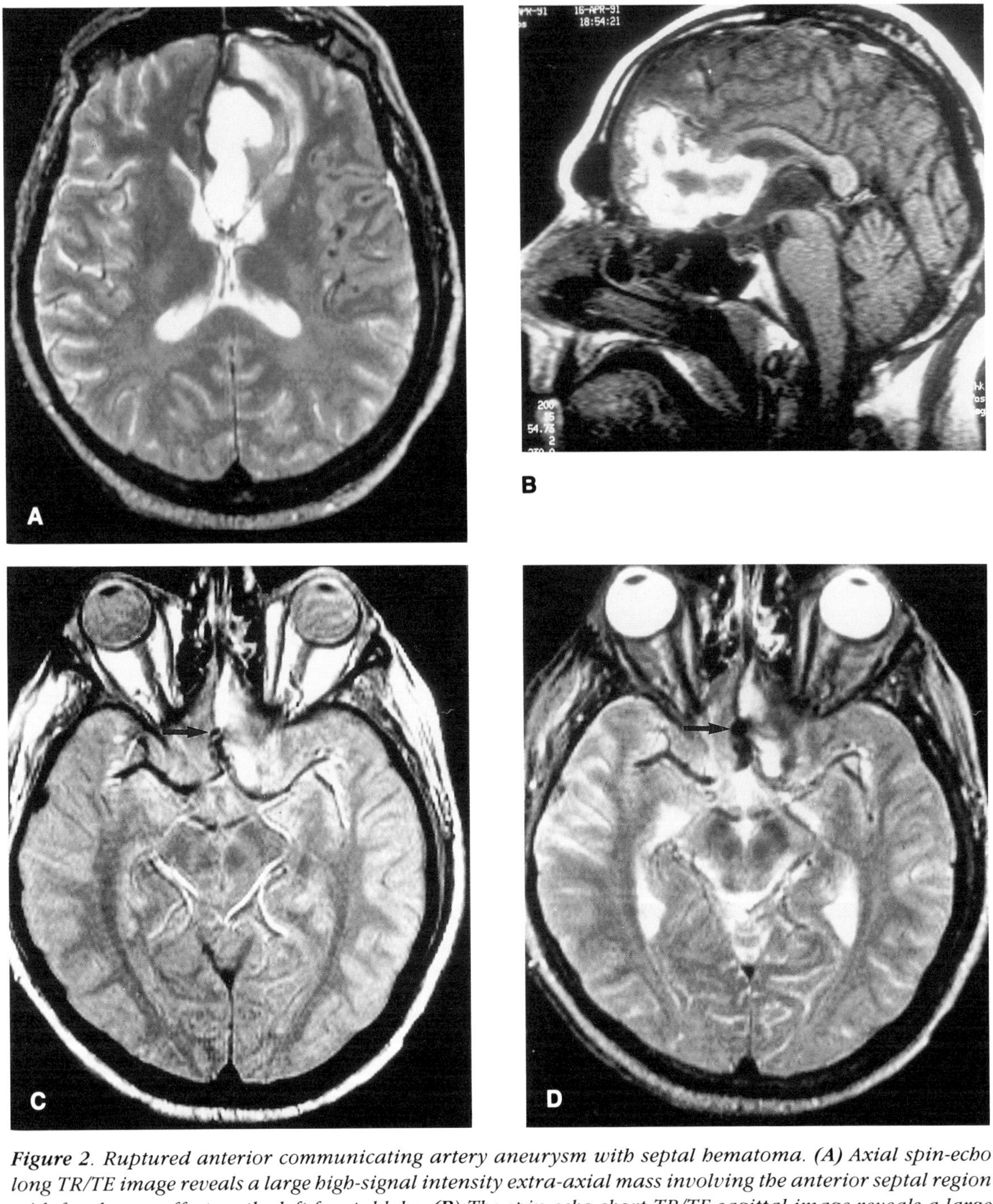


*Figure 2.* *Ruptured anterior communicating artery aneurysm with septal hematoma.* ***(A)*** *Axial spin-echo long TR/TE image reveals a large high-signal intensity extra-axial mass involving the anterior septal region with focal mass effect on the left frontal lobe.* ***(B)*** *The spin-echo short TR/TE sagittal image reveals a large high-signal mass with a low-signal central portion. This is due to hemorrhage in various stages of evolution. Note that there is as yet no hemosiderin rim.* ***(C,D)*** *Axial long TR/short TE and long TR/TE images. At the level of the anterior communicating artery there is high-signal intensity identified adjacent to the A1 segment of the left anterior cerebral artery extending anteriorly and medially. In the region of the anterior communicating artery, there is a bulbous rounded area which becomes more obvious on the long TE images (arrows), which more clearly demonstrate signal loss due to flow. This demonstrates the anterior communicating artery aneurysm.*

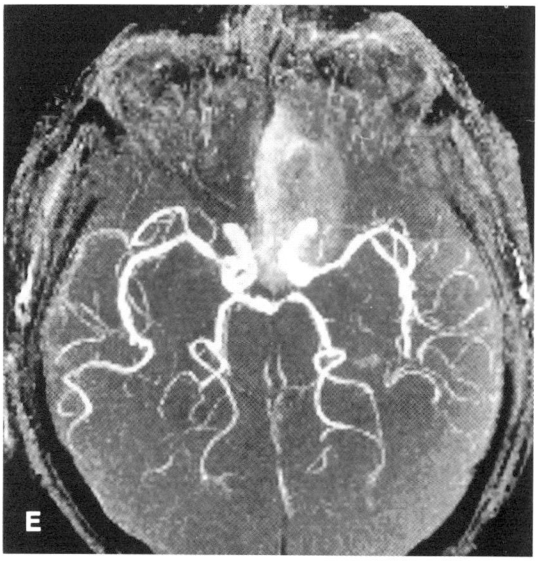


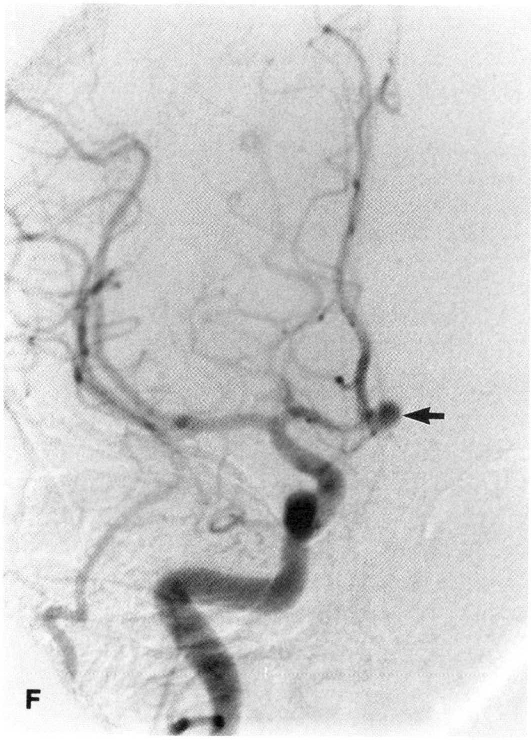


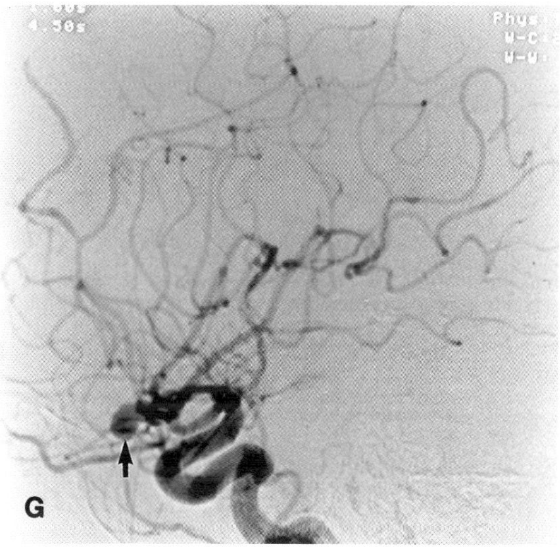


*Figure 2. (E) Three-dimensional time-of-flight (TOF) MRA does not demonstrate the aneurysm. Note the high signal intensity due to the hemoglobin from the septal hematoma. (F,G) Anterior and lateral IADSA images clearly demonstrate anterior communicating artery aneurysm (arrows) extending directly anteriorly. Note the subtle narrowing of the distal A1 segment possibly related to early vasospasm or focal mass effect from the hematoma.*

hemorrhage was never seen in cryptic nonaneurysmal hemorrhage.[84,109] The size and location of the subarachnoid hematoma in the basal cisterns are the most reliable ways to predict subsequent vasospasm.[4,28,35,58,80,96] Vasospasm occurred in 20 of 22 patients with large, thick hematomas, and in 5 of 19 patients with no blood or diffuse SAH on CT.[58] Black described a high association of both vasospasm (74%) and hydrocephalus (67%) with large SAHs.[16] Decreased attenuation on CT indicative of ischemia or infarction also has a strong correlation with vasospasm.[80,96] CT plays an additional vital role in the immediate postoperative management to evaluate forevacuation of hematomas, mass effect from edema, and intra-axial fluid or air collections, in addition to the previously mentioned complications of SAH in combination with aneurysm rupture.

Contrast-enhanced high-resolution CT (1.5-mm slice thickness) has been utilized for symptomatic and/or ruptured aneurysm detection in two studies, and has detected 5 of

5 aneurysms and 74 of 76 aneurysms, respectively.[77,89] With conventional CT imaging, the sensitivity of the technique was unacceptably low (18% to 64%).[6,42] A recent study by Teasdale et al evaluated thin-section (1.5-mm contiguous images) contrast-enhanced CT with multiple reformations in different planes in patients with oculomotor (III) palsies. In the patients without SAH, CT detected all posterior communicating artery aneurysms (all of which were greater than 7 mm in diameter). Other detected abnormalities, however, which were thought to represent additional aneurysms, actually represented vessel loops.[103] In patients with SAH and oculomotor palsies, all posterior communicating artery aneurysms were reliably detected, but an intracavernous aneurysm on the contralateral side was not identified.[103]

## *Magnetic Resonance Imaging*

The advantage of MRI in neuroimaging relates to superior contrast resolution between different tissues. Rapidly flowing blood is devoid of signal on the conventional spin-echo sequences used for brain imaging. Two components result in this signal loss: (1) fast flow (flight) of blood relative to the timing of the radiofrequency pulse sequence, and (2) motion in the presence and direction of the magnetic field gradients used to localize the signal within the magnet.[20,108,111] The rapid flow signal loss results from flowing protons that do not remain in the slice volume long enough to receive both the necessary 90° and 180° radiofrequency pulses. Additionally, fast flow creates increased random motion of protons in the presence of imaging gradients, resulting in the loss of proton-phase coherence and thus a decrease in signal intensity.[20] Consequently, nonthrombosed aneurysms often appear as areas of absent signal on conventional spin-echo MR scans (Figure 3).

There are also three circumstances that result in increased signal intensity from flowing blood: flow-related enhancement, even-echo rephasing, and diastolic pseudogating.[19,111,112] Flow-related enhancement is the most important, and is due to unsaturated, fully magnetized protons entering the excited image slice, thus emitting a strong (i.e. high) signal relative to the partially saturated protons in the adjacent tissues, which have not fully recovered from the previous excitation (Figure 4).[19] This is seen most prominently at the inflowing edge of the imaging volume.

Other nonvascular flow phenomena that may result in inappropriate diagnosis (of aneurysm) is that of cerebrospinal fluid (CSF) motion from adjacent transmitted vascular pulsations, which may give rise to areas of CSF hypointensity surrounding a vessel, thus simulating an aneurysm. This is due to signal mismappings from phase shift,[25] which are usually noted on long TR/short TE and long TR/TE images as hypodensities adjacent to vessels such as the basilar artery.[25] Another manifestation of the same phenomenon with both large and small vessels are motion artifacts, which are recognized as a series of alternating dark and light bands arising from the pulsating vessels due to spatial signal misregistration that is seen in the phase-encoding direction (Figure 5).

Another pitfall in MRI evaluation of aneurysms is the apparent flow void that can be seen in the paraclinoid region and may represent a pneumatized anterior clinoid process.[41] This mistake can be avoided if a gradient-echo flow-imaging protocol is utilized.[41] Small nonthrombotic aneurysms will usually demonstrate the signal characteristics of the supplying vessel, specifically the fast-flow-related enhancement, or flow void, depending on the pulse sequence selected.

The size of a nonthrombosed aneurysm on MRI correlates well with the angiographic size.[105] Both angiography and MRA underestimate the size of a partially thrombosed aneurysm. Compared to CT, MRI certainly provides much better delineation of the exact location and the relationship to the adjacent neural structures (Figures 4,5).[8,15,78,100] The artery from which the aneurysm arises usually is identified, but identifying the aneurysm neck is frequently not possible.[86] Analysis of

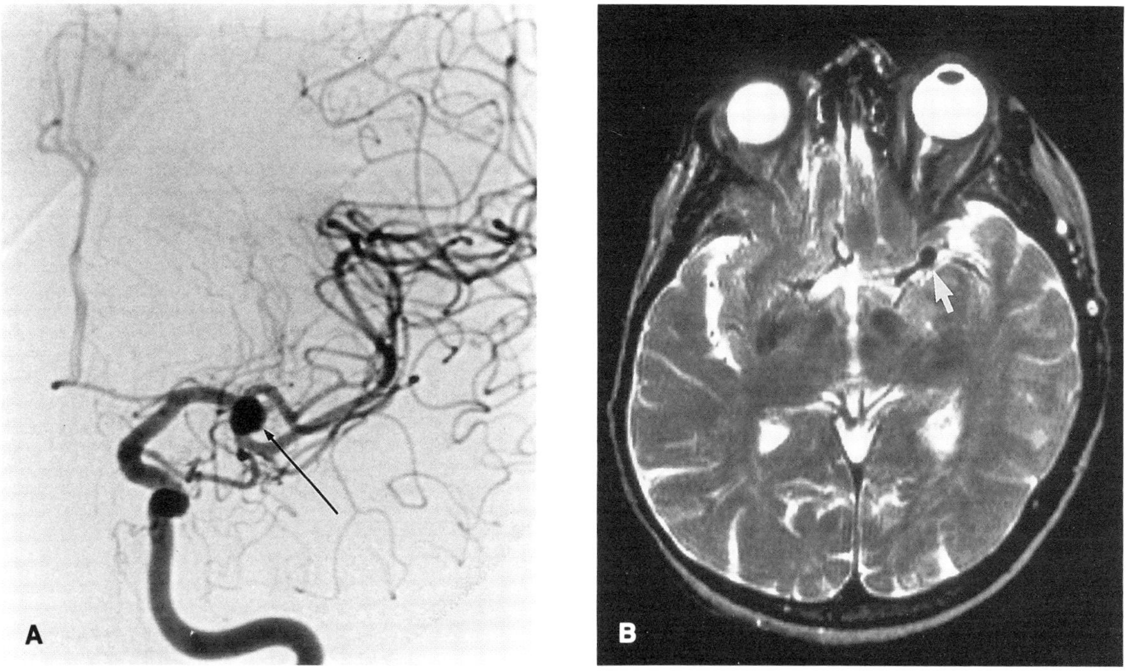


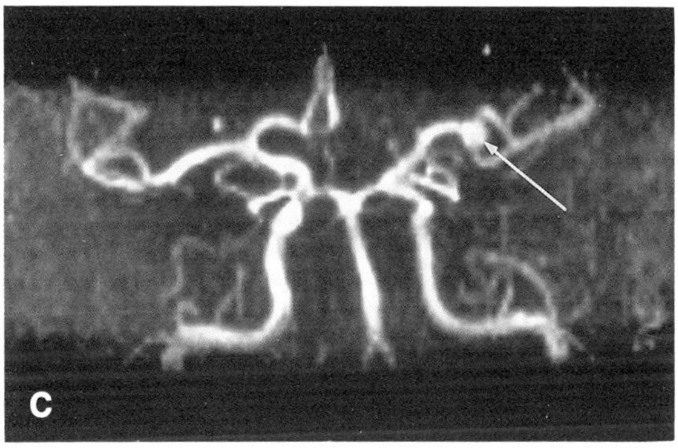


***Figure 3.*** *Asymptomatic right MCA aneurysm (arrows). **(A)** AP IADSA demonstrates an aneurysm arising off the left MCA bifurcation. **(B)** Axial spin-echo long TR/TE image reveals a rounded area of flow void clearly contiguous with the horizontal segment of the MCA. Note the striking tissue contrast between flowing blood and the adjacent brain and CSF. **(C)** MRA at the level of the circle of Willis clearly demonstrates the aneurysm arising from the MCA. The size of the aneurysm is equal on the spin-echo images and MRA because there is no thrombus narrowing the lumen.*

individual MRA partitions may allow better delineation of the aneurysm neck (Figure 4).

Many aneurysms less than 1 cm in size may not be demonstrated on spin-echo sequences. It is important to recognize that most spin-echo images have an interslice gap between-slices, and therefore small aneurysms could easily be missed, especially if the aneurysm is not located centrally within the voxel.[105] Using contiguous images almost always allows detection. An alternative way to address this problem is described by Ross et al using both spin-echo MRI and gradient-echo MRA together.[86]

### *Magnetic Resonance Imaging in Subarachnoid and Parenchymal Hemorrhage*

Acute SAH is difficult to detect by MRI. The signal emitted from blood is related to the oxidative state of hemoglobin and its breakdown products. The environment of CSF is quite different than that of brain parenchyma, which explains the striking contrast between intra- and extra-axial hemorrhages.[18] In acute SAH, there is very slight T1 shortening of CSF, which results in slight increases in signal

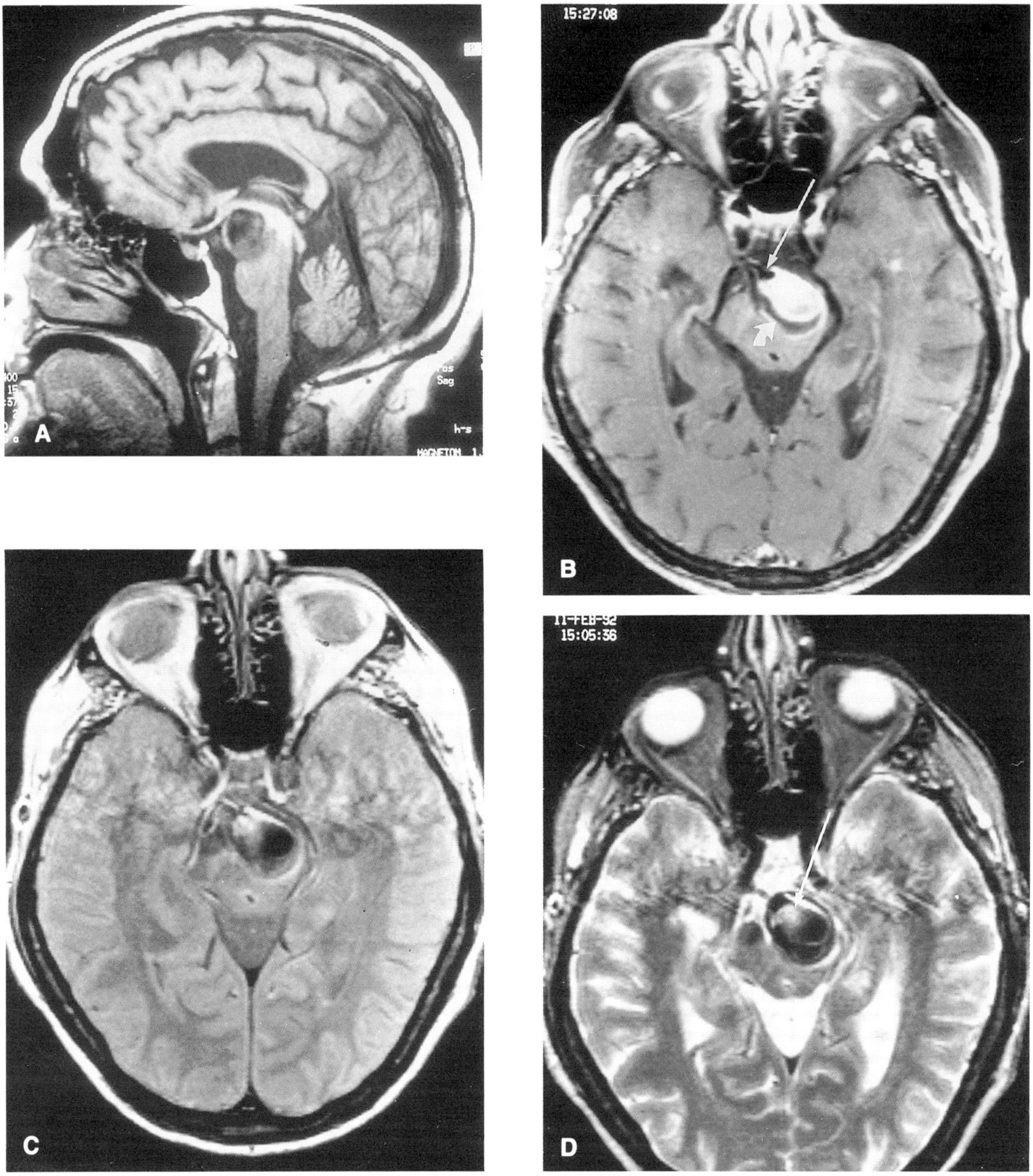


*Figure 4. Partially thrombotic giant basilar tip aneurysm. **(A)** A giant basilar tip aneurysm demonstrates signal void and compression of the brain stem on a short TR/TE image. **(B)** Axial image through the level of the aneurysm neck (arrow) demonstrating the flow void from the high-velocity blood on the short TR/TE image and the higher signal intensity from the slower-flowing blood within the central lumen of the aneurysm. Note the relatively hypointense rim due to the partially thrombosed wall (curved arrow). **(C,D)** The flow void on the longer TR images reveals the sensitivity of the T2-weighted sequences to slow-flowing blood. Notice the high signal intensity within the central portion, most prominent on the long TR/TE-weighted image, due to refocusing of slow flow by gradient-moment nulling (arrow).*

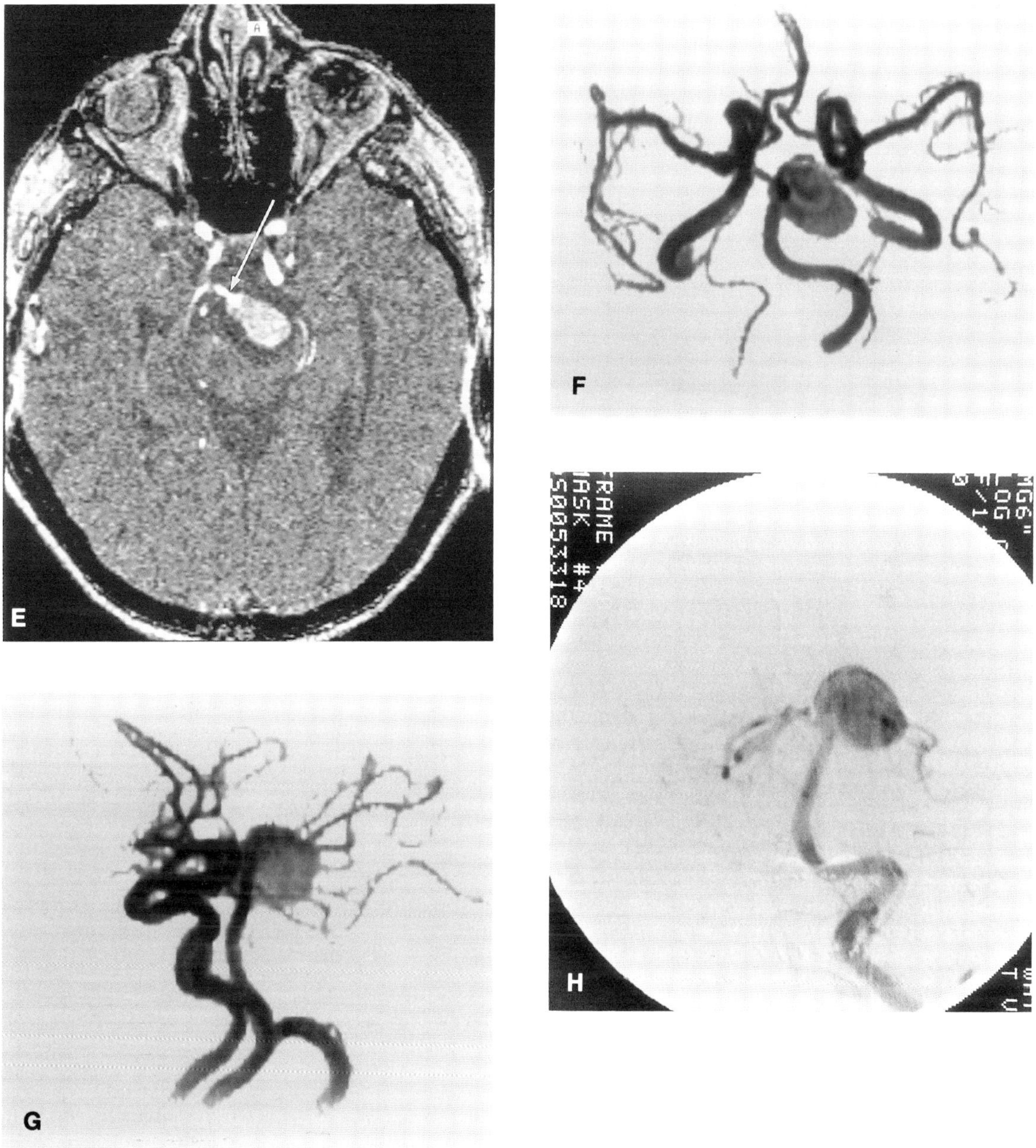


***Figure 4E–H.*** ***(E)*** *The axial slice from a three-dimensional TOF angiogram clearly separates flowing blood, which appears bright (arrow), from thrombus, which results in relatively decreased signal intensity in the aneurysm. The spin-echo sequences demonstrate the true size of the nonthrombosed portion of the aneurysm. The MRA slice also accurately delineates the width of the aneurysm neck (arrow) relative to the P1 segments.* ***(F,G)*** *The maximum intensity projection-processed MRA demonstrates the large aneurysm arising off the basilar tip with a patent posterior cerebral artery. Note the multiple projections obtainable from one sequence. This clearly demonstrates the relationship of the aneurysm to the adjacent vascular structures.* ***(H)*** *Townes, view DSA (see photos and legends for I and J on page 52).*

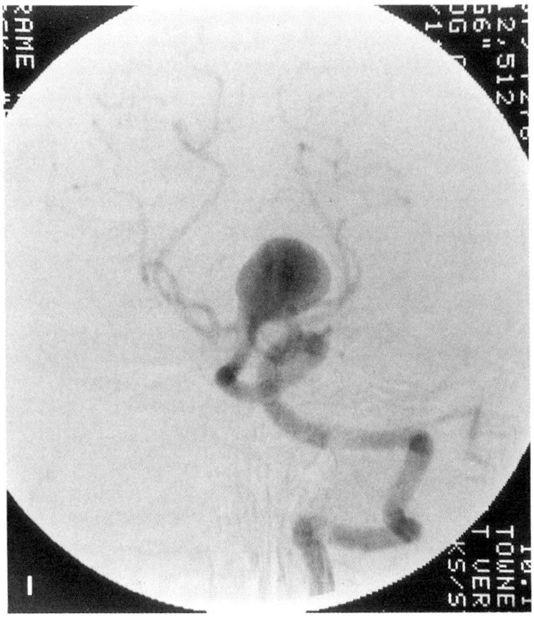


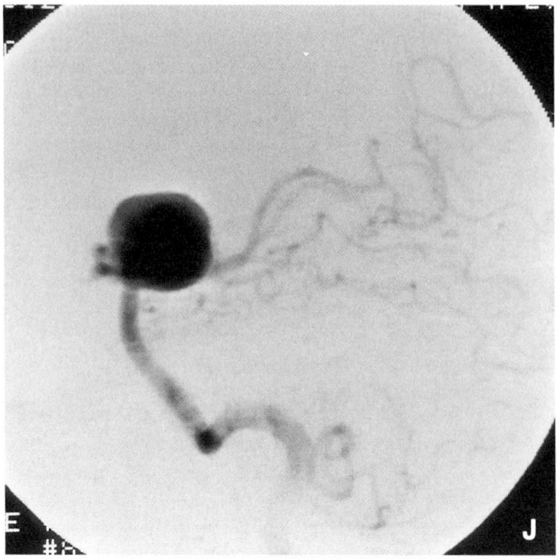


*Figure 4I,J. Waters, and lateral DSA. IADSA demonstrates the aneurysm located superiorly and to the left. The aneurysm is arising off the distal basilartip. The PCA is patent*

intensity on the short TR/TE images.[18] It takes several days for a significant amount of deoxyhemoglobin to convert to methemoglobin, resulting in obvious increased signal intensity in short TR/TE images. This is probably related to the high $O_2$ tension in CSF (as opposed to that of a typical intraparenchymal hematoma).[18] Since there is ongoing resorption of red blood cells (RBCs) from CSF, MR visualization of small SAHs may be impossible. Thus, CT remains the diagnostic test of choice in the setting of acute SAH.[18] MRI, however, can elegantly detect the complications of SAH, specifically ischemia and infarction, and hemosiderosis (Figure 6).

While MRI is not sensitive to acute small SAH, the tissue contrast in smaller parenchymal hematomas adjacent to an aneurysm and larger SAH allows detection. This may be important in the setting of a patient with multiple cerebral aneurysms in which one has ruptured,[50,99] especially in patients with no angiographic or CT findings to suggest the location of the rupture.

As discussed earlier, parenchymal hemorrhages evolve differently than blood in the CSF due to the local environment. Parenchymal hemorrhage maturation, from the hyperacute to the chronic stages, has been extensively described.[9,45] Acute hematomas (1–7 days) are isointense or slightly hypointense to gray matter and brain on short TR/TE (T1-weighted) spin-echo images, and are markedly hypointense centrally on long TR/TE (T2-weighted) spin-echo images. This is a result of preferential T2-proton relaxation enhancement by deoxyhemoglobin in the intact RBCs. Subacute hematomas (weeks–months) are hyperintense to brain on both short TR/TE and long TR/TE images as a result of the paramagnetic free intracellular methemoglobin (Figure 2).[47] In subacute and chronic hematomas there is a hypointense rim on short TR/TE-weighted images, which becomes markedly hypointense on long TR/TE weighted images. This is due to hemosiderin and ferritin deposition, which also demonstrates preferential T2-proton relaxation enhancement (Figure 6).[9,47] The preferential T2-relaxation enhancement in acute hematomas and in hemosiderin/ferritin is field dependent, and increases as the square of the magnetic field.[45–47] In addition, the susceptibility effect due to the hemosiderin/ferritin is directly related to the TE. Therefore, the hypointense rim thickens with longer TE-weighted images.[45] Gradient-echo MR imaging can detect both acute and chronic

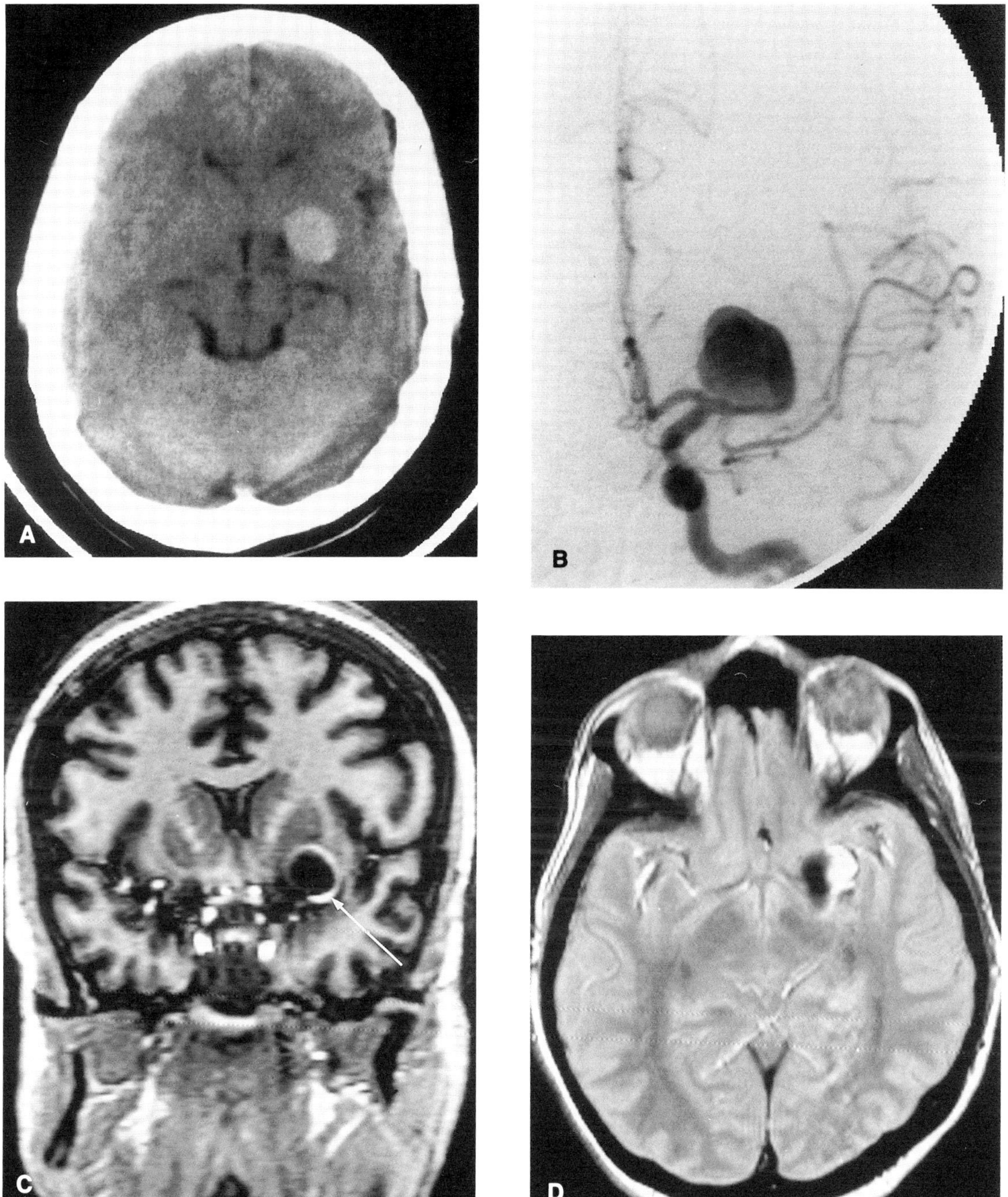


*Figure 5. Nonthrombotic giant middle cerebral aneurysm. **(A)** Axial noncontrast-enhanced CT demonstrates a hyperdense mass lesion in the suspected region of the MCA. The high attenuation is due to the fact that normal blood (hemoglobin 15g/dl) has an attenuation coefficient of approximately 52 Houndsfield units, approximately 10–20 units greater than the attenuation of gray and white matter, respectively.[77] **(B)** AP IADSA internal carotid angiogram demonstrates a giant aneurysm arising off the horizontal segment of the MCA with absence of flow to the lenticulostriates. **(C)** Low flip angle three-dimensional volume gradient-echo coronal image (MP RAGE). Flow-related enhancement is seen in fast-flowing blood on this sequence. The flow void centrally is indicative of slow-flowing blood in the aneurysm, and the hyperintense rim is due to the jet of fast-flowing blood (arrow). **(D)** The long TR images (long TR/short TE, long TR/TE axial images) demonstrate mixed signal intensity within the aneurysm due to turbulent flow.*

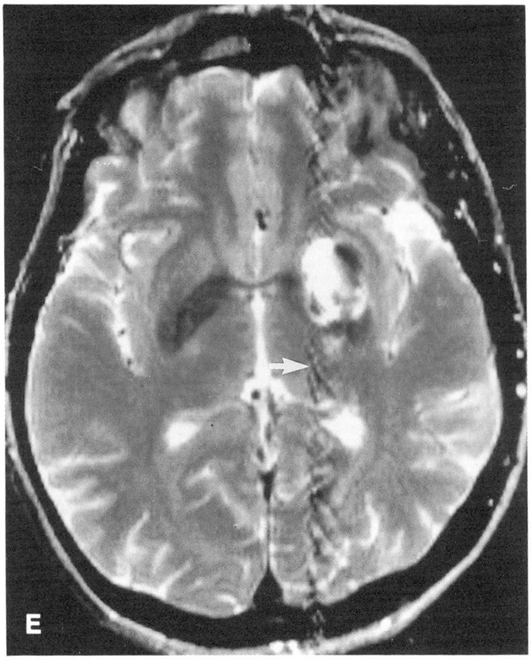


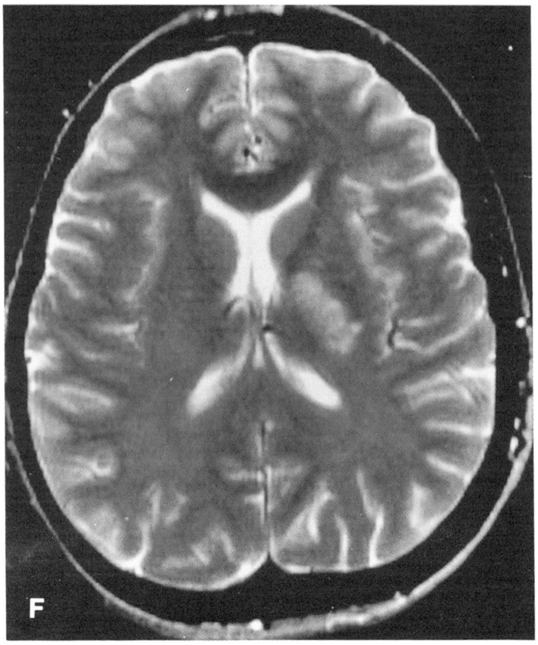


***Figure 5.*** *(E) The spatial misregistration ghosting artifact (arrow) is best appreciated on the long TR/TE images along the phase-encoding axis, proving the vascular origin of the mass. (F) The long TR/TE-weighted images demonstrate high-signal intensity within the posterior limb of the internal capsule due to compromise of the lenticulostriates. (G) three-dimensional TOF MIP angiogram demonstrates the aneurysm arising off the horizontal segment in the MCA. The distal segments of the MCA are patent.*

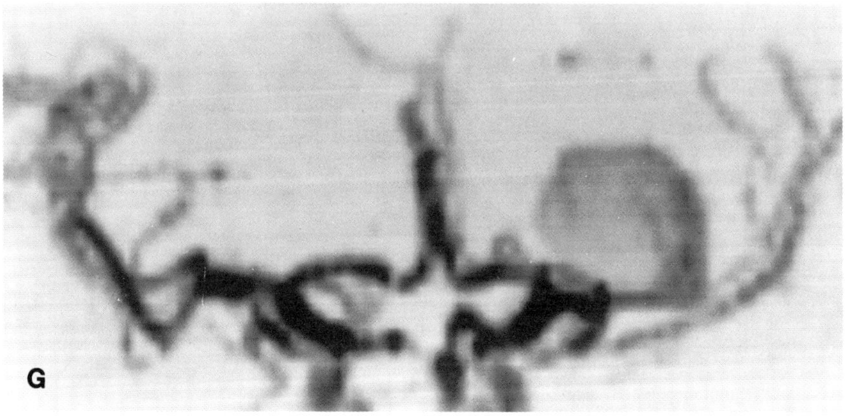


hemorrhage not seen on conventional spin-echo techniques. This is attributed to the greater sensitivity of the gradient-echo technique to magnetic field inhomogeneities resulting from imperfect signal refocusing.[9]

## *Magnetic Resonance Angiography*

MRA is a rapidly evolving technique which, when used with the combination of spin-echo technique, shows significant promise. In the retrospective study by Ross et al, conventional MRI and MRA complemented each other, resulting in a sensitivity of 95% and a specificity of 100% compared to intra-arterial DSA (IADSA).[86] At least 1 aneurysm in each of 19 patients with saccular or giant intracranial aneurysms proven by IADSA was detected by a three-dimensional time-of-flight (TOF) MRA in 28 controls not thought to have aneurysms. The MRA adequately demonstrated the circle of Willis and the MCA bifurcation/trifurcation. The carotid siphon proved problematic to fully characterize because of signal dropout from the uncompensated turbulent flow.

TOF MRA is created by flow-related enhancement in vessels using gradient-echo volume images, which provide vascular contrast. Projection angiograms are created using computerized reconstruction algorithms (Figure 3).[71] MRA has some pitfalls (Figure 4). If an aneurysm is partially thrombosed, MRA may underestimate the true size or miss the aneurysm analogous to conventional catheter angiography. Moreover, cranial hemorrhage may result in misleading images.[117] The high signal intensity from methemoglobin within a hemorrhage on the original images is picked up by a computerized reconstruction algorithm (usually a maximum intensity projection). This may obscure or simulate flow within an aneurysm (see Figure 2). Slow or turbulent flow in or around the vessels supplying the aneurysm may cause incomplete or suboptimal visualization due to decreased inflow of unsaturated protons that normally provide the high signal in TOF MRAs.[93] For these reasons MRA is not appropriate for patients suspected of acute SAH.

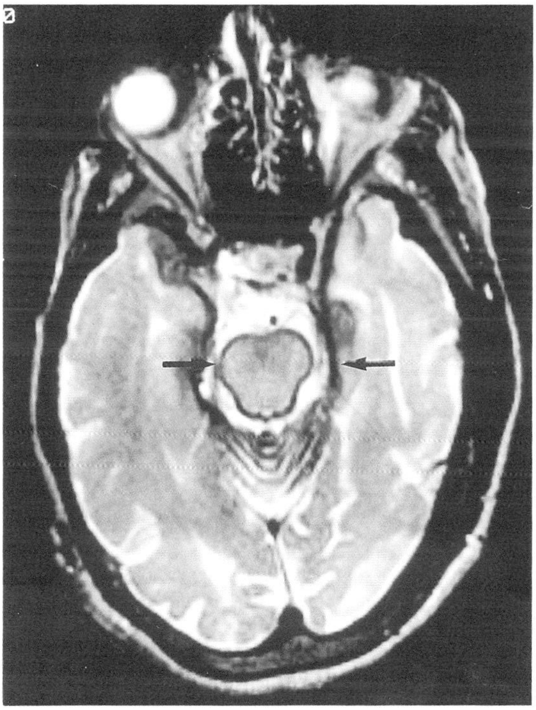

*Figure 6. Superficial hemosiderosis from an SAH. Spin-echo long TR/TE image. A rim of hypointensity is identified along the surfaces of the pons, the medial surfaces of the temporal lobe, and the cerebellar vermis. This is most obvious on the long TR/TE images as these are most prone to the susceptibility changes from the hemosiderin/ferritin deposition.*

MRI in combination with MRA holds promise for evaluation of unruptured aneurysms in both symptomatic and asymptomatic patients.[86] While the spatial resolution of MRA is certainly less than that of intra-arterial angiography, it is high enough to detect aneurysms as small as 2–3 mm. This has practical importance: both Locksley and McCormick et al found no SAHs from aneurysms smaller than 3 mm.[65,72] It was concluded by Levey et al in a rigorous decision analysis of polycystic kidney disease patients that intra-arterial angiography should not be performed on a routine basis in this population because its benefit is significant only if the prevalence of aneurysms exceeds 30%, the surgical complication rate is less than 1%, and the patient is under 25 years of age.[62] The current data suggests that MRI with MRA could provide a noninvasive test that has the sensitivity and specificity to significantly impact high-risk, asymptomatic populations.[86]

## *Angiography*

Conventional film screen and, now, IADSA are the diagnostic standards for the evaluations of intracranial aneurysms. Angiography provides the most accurate assessment of any diagnostic imaging study of the aneurysm location, size, shape, neck, relationship to the adjacent vessels, and potential multiplicity. Moreover, angiography can directly evaluate for the presence of vasospasm (Figure 7).

Aneurysm detection by cerebral angiography has been estimated to exceed 90%,[65] with recent angiographic techniques probably

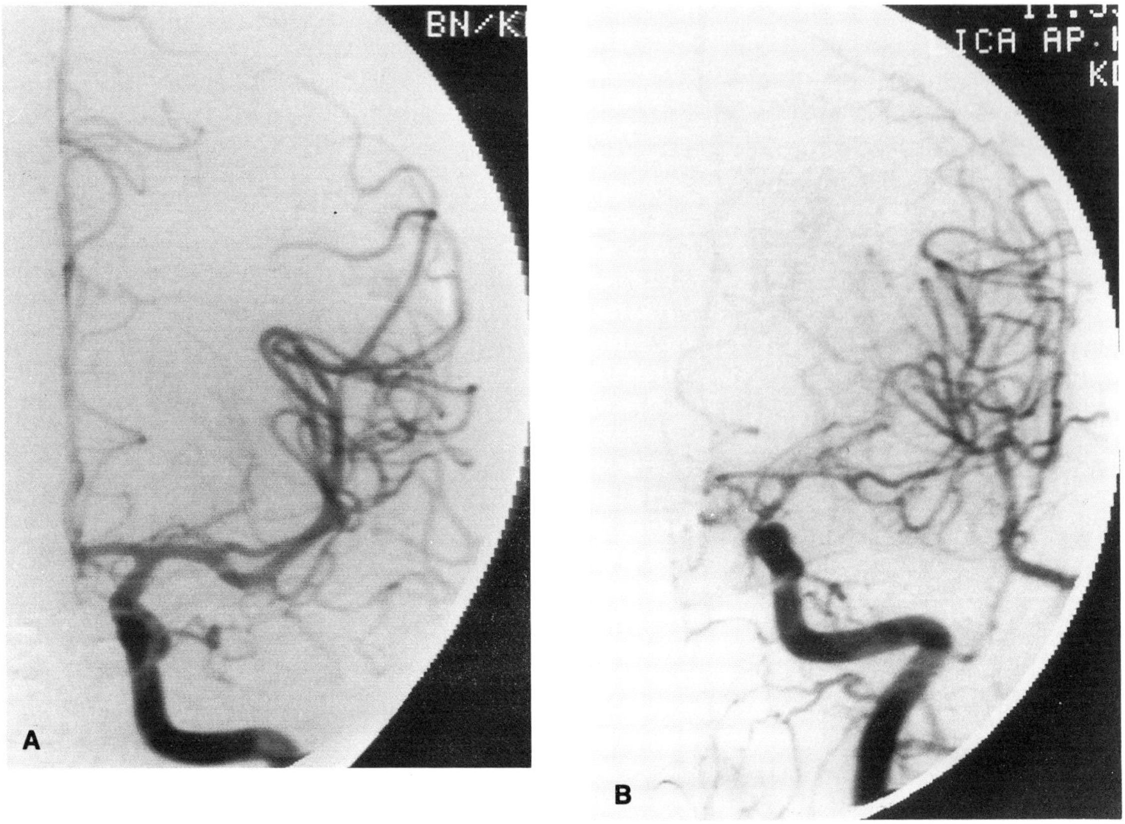


***Figure** 7. Vasospasm following SAH. **(A)** Initial anteroposterior (AP) angiogram demonstrating normal ACA and MCAs. **(B)** AP angiogram 3 days later (postclipping) demonstrating marked narrowing of the lumen of the distal ICA, ACA, and MCA. There is severe concentric narrowing subsequent to vasospasm. Note the near complete absence of flow through the ACA and the MCA. The lenticulostriates are barely visible.*

allowing even higher sensitivity. In the setting of acute SAH, more than 80% will be proven related to aneurysmal rupture. False negative rates on initial pancerebral angiography have varied widely from 2% to 23%, with more recent series estimating initial false negative rates in the order of 11.7% to 16%.[38,55,56] The proposed etiologies of false negative angiograms include vasospasm, peculiar flow patterns, thrombosis of the aneurysm, technically inadequate studies, and inaccurate interpretation.[17,29,38,43,95] These factors may be minimized but not totally eliminated by technical improvements. A second or third angiogram may visualize an aneurysm that was "missed" despite a technically satisfactory study.[17]

Initially, IADSA studies suffered from inadequate spatial resolution. With newer small focal spots and 1024 x 1024 matrix DSA suites, the diagnostic differences between the resolution of conventional film screen technique and digital angiography are insignificant. While the inherent spatial resolution of film screen angiography continues to be superior to digital angiography, the contrast resolution on the latter is greater. The net system resolution is probably close to the same. This has been supported clinically with intra-arterial digital subtraction studies acquired at lower spatial resolution (512 x 512 matrix).[106]

With respect to patient safety, a recent study (1990) demonstrated that persistent neurologic deficits occurred in approximately .09%, and transient deficits were observed in 0.45% of patients undergoing IADSA. The reduced complication rate in comparison with former studies seems to be related to the decreased examination time with DSA as well as the use of new iso-osmotic and nonionic contrast media.[48] Persistent neurologic deficits were defined as focal deficits that did not resolve within 24 hours. Transient neurologic deficits consisted of cortical blindness, paralysis, dysphasia, severe vertigo, double vision, and nystagmus, all of which lasted less than 24 hours.

Due to the high frequency of multiple aneurysms,[65,114] cerebral angiography in the setting of SAH is only complete if all the intracranial vessels are visualized. This approach should be followed only if no evidence of severe vasospasm is identified. At times specific angiographic techniques such as compression of the contralateral carotid artery to the side of carotid injection, or compression of the ipsilateral carotid artery to a vertebral injection to visualize the anterior communicating or posterior communicating arteries respectively should be employed.[5] If the initial angiogram is unrevealing and no other etiology for the hemorrhage is detected on MRI, a repeat angiogram is indicated,[55,56] although there are other authors who refute this assertion.[38,43] Iwanaga et al correlated findings of SAH on CT with negative initial catheter angiography. The following suggestions for followup angiography were made:

> If CT scans (within four days of SAH) show no detectable blood primarily in the perimesencephalic cisterns, further angiographic studies are probably not required. On the other hand if CT scans show a thin or thick subarachnoid blood, particularly with blood in the basal frontal interhemispheric fissure, angiographic studies should be repeated early and would be likely to uncover an initially cryptic aneurysm.[55]

Other studies support Iwanaga's observations of the benign prognosis of small perimesencephalic SAH.[84,109] If a repeat angiogram is to be performed, it is suggested that it be done in 10 to 14 days after the initial SAH.[5,95] SAH may also arise from the spine, which should also be considered in a negative workup of the intracranial contents.

In the setting of ruptured intracranial aneurysm in a patient with multiple aneurysms, certain findings on angiography may help determine the aneurysm responsible for SAH. These findings include: focal mass effect on the adjacent vessels, focal vasospasm, or a focal protrusion from the aneurysm dome, which is an indication of the bleeding defect in the aneurysm wall.[5] In addition, a multilobulated aneurysm is a less-reliable sign that may incriminate the ruptured aneurysm. Moreover, in patients with multiple aneurysms, an additional clue to determining which aneurysm has ruptured is provided by the size of the aneurysm. In a study by Wood of 105 patients with multiple aneurysms, the largest of the aneurysms had ruptured in 87%.[115] If there are several aneurysms identified on the same parent vessel, the more proximal aneurysm, unless thrombosed, ruptures most frequently.[27]

## *Intravenous Digital Subtraction Angiography (IVDSA)*

IVDSA alone is not considered adequate for evaluation of unruptured intracranial aneurysms. The spatial resolution is relatively poor, but of greater importance, the multiple overlapping vessels and limited number of views allow for an unacceptably high rate of both false positive and negative results.[37,104]

The role of IVDSA for acute SAH is not well established because of the early experience with limited spatial resolution, artifacts, and multiple overlapping vessels. With newer equipment, many of the technical problems have been addressed; however, there remains the persistence of overlapping vessels from the simultaneously opacified cerebral and craniofacial vascular supply.[26,34] In addition, there are a limited number of views that can be obtained per projection due to the large contrast bolus required for each projection. For these reasons IVDSA has fallen out of favor in the evaluation of aneurysms.

### *Transcranial Doppler*

Transcranial doppler (TCD) has emerged as an effective noninvasive technique to evaluate and monitor disturbances in cerebral hemodynamics due to vasospasm from SAH (Figure 8). [1,2,85,92] This technique only readily evaluates the proximal segments of the anterior cerebral artery, MCA, and occasionally the posterior cerebral arteries.[92] Vasospasm distal to these segments may not be accurately assessed.[2] The finding of vasospasm correlates reasonably well with the amount of SAH identified in the basal cisterns on CT.[91,92] With small amounts of SAH the increase in flow velocity is only mild to moderate.[93] Increasing flow velocities preceded both asymptomatic and symptomatic ischemia on CT.[91,92] TCD may also be utilized in the timing of surgical repair of aneurysms.[85] Some authors advocate early operation only if vasospasm is absent or mild, and judicious delay in the presence of fulminant major vessel spasm.

## Giant Intracranial Aneurysms

Approximately 2.5% to 7% of all intracranial aneurysms are classified as giant aneurysms[24,66] (greater than 25 mm in size), although some authors likewise regard aneurysms greater than 15 mm.[82,97] Giant aneurysms most frequently present with either a space occupying lesion, or compression of adjacent structures.[24,101,102,110] These aneurysms can be saccular or fusiform in morphology, which affects therapeutic decisions of either direct surgical clipping, endovascular therapy with or without preservation of the parent artery, or Hunterian (proximal) occlusion of the supplying artery.[102,110] Collateral flow in the circle of Willis also needs to be evaluated prior to parent artery occlusion,[110] as well as the patient's tolerance to temporary test-occlusion of the vessel.

### *Computed Tomography*

Three CT patterns have been described with giant aneurysms: completely thrombotic, partially thrombotic, and nonthrombotic.[83] Nonthrombotic thin-walled giant aneurysms appear the same size on arteriography and CT, and are slightly hyperdense to brain on noncontrast CT (Figure 5). As expected, all are markedly enhanced with contrast.[44,79,83] While the diagnosis is often clear-cut, the location and configuration of giant aneurysms can cause them to be confused with other extra-axial and occasionally intra-axial mass lesions such as meningioma, craniopharyngioma, or pituitary adenoma.[79,83]

The most specific CT pattern is seen in partially thrombotic giant aneurysms,[83] which demonstrate a rim of hyperdensity of variable thickness on noncontrast-enhanced CT. Many have a visible curvilinear peripheral calcification,[44,79,83] the relationship of which to the surgical neck is important and often best delineated on coronal images, as calcification at the surgical neck makes aneurysm clipping considerably more difficult.[30] Following contrast administration, central or peripheral enhancement is seen and the rim-enhancement is not seen angiographically.[79,83] There is often no correlation between the angiographic and CT sizes of the aneurysm as a result of the luminal thrombus. Thrombosed giant aneurysms demonstrate a ring-shaped hyperdense area with peripheral enhancement after contrast administration. No central or eccentric enhancement in the region of the expected lumen is identified.[83] Bony erosion and remodeling can be seen on both CT and plain films. With special dynamic contrast-enhanced CT, the ability to differentiate giant aneurysms from other extra-axial masses is improved by the differential in the amount and rate of contrast enhancement.[82]

### *Magnetic Resonance Imaging*

MRI of giant aneurysms is complementary to CT. It provides a much better delineation

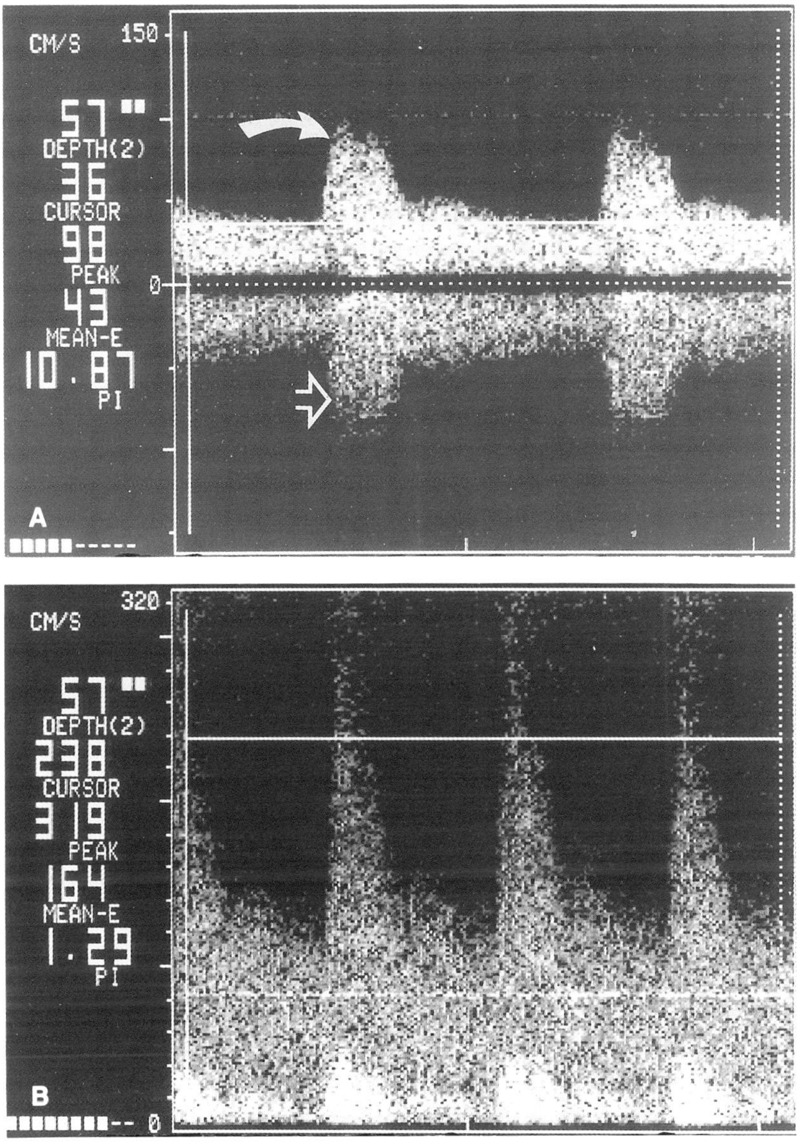


***Figure 8.*** *TCD ultrasound of vasospasm.* ***(A)*** *TCD velocity tracings from 3 days apart, both obtained at 57 mm from the skin surface of the right MCA and bifurcation. The superior waveform indicates flow towards the probe and represents the MCA (curved arrow). The inverted trace indicates flow away from the transducer and represents anterior cerebral artery flow (open arrow). The window of the transducer is approximately 1 cm, and therefore the simultaneous tracing localizes the sample to the ICA bifurcation. The normal mean velocity is 43 cm/sec, normal for the MCA. The anterior cerebral artery is often a mirror image but may demonstrate slightly less mean velocity. The relatively straight white line across the image is a cursor at the diastolic level.* ***(B)*** *The recording at 3 days later demonstrates a single waveform. In the interval, severe multivessel vasospasm has developed. Note that the mean velocity is now 164 cm/sec and is in the moderate to severe category (greater than 200 is severe). Images courtesy of Dr. R. Lorig, Cleveland Clinic Foundation.*

of the intra- or extra-axial location of masses, and in the case of giant aneurysms it can usually establish a diagnosis with certainty. Most giant aneurysms are nonthrombotic or partially thrombosed, and therefore MRI evidence of flow is depicted.[8,78] Commonly, there is signal void; however, high signal in slow-flowing vessels may be seen due to flow-related enhancement or even echo rephasing.[8,78] The signal intensity of thrombus on both short TR/TE and long TR/TE images demonstrates mixed signal intensity with a heterogeneous distribution on all spin-echo weighted sequences (Figure 4).[78,107] One series described a relatively specific appearance on MR, consisting of a laminated appearance of thrombus in different stages of evolution.[8] Concentric zones of various signal intensity surrounding free methemoglobin (hyperintense) with a patent lumen were identified on all spin-echo pulse sequences.[8] Centrally, all spin-echo sequences demonstrate high signal intensity immediately adjacent to the patent lumen (signal void), representing free methemoglobin.[8,78,107] In contrast with intracranial parenchymal hematomas in which the initial hyperintensity is peripheral, in giant aneurysm thrombus formation the initial hyperintensity is detected centrally.[8] Perianeurysmal hemorrhage may also be seen surrounding the brain parenchyma and will vary in appearance according to age.[8]

In contrast to CT, MRI does not readily detect calcifications or establish exact relationships to the paranasal sinuses and cortical bone as well as CT.[100] These relationships are important,[100] as proximity to the skull base may hinder satisfactory placement of aneurysm clips. On the other hand, MRI provides relatively good detail of the relationship of the parent artery to the aneurysm, but frequently not precisely enough to evaluate if the aneurysm is suitable for surgical clipping.[107] In giant aneurysms where the central flow void is not well depicted either due to thrombus or to slow flow, the use of slow-flow sequences may also be helpful[107] in both pre- and post-therapy assessment. One small series of six patients with giant aneurysms thrombosed by balloon embolization were followed with MRI. Of the aneurysms that were 100% occluded, all demonstrated a decrease in physical size on followup MRI. The one patient who had a 90% obliteration of the lumen demonstrated no change in the size of giant aneurysm over a 2-year followup.[100] Thrombus formation in an incompletely thrombosed giant aneurysm differs from organizing thrombus in a completely thrombosed aneurysm.[100] The thrombosis after occlusion is due to stasis, a mechanism analogous to venous (red) thrombosis rather than arterial (white) thrombosis.[60,100] This is reflected in the appearance on MRI. Iatrogenically induced thrombosis demonstrates an area of hyperintensity at 5–10 days on short TR/TE and long TR/short TE images. The long TR/TE images demonstrate hypointensity. At 4–6 weeks, induced thrombus was hyperintense on all spin-echo sequences where spontaneous hemorrhage still had areas of hypointensity, but these had increased in signal intensity from the subacute stage (5–10 days).[60,103]

## *Magnetic Resonance Angiography*

Careful selection of technique is important with MRA because lack of visualization suggesting complete thrombosis may be seen artifactually due to slow flow. Therefore, optimization of TOF MRA is important in slow-flowing lesions. The two-dimensional TOF MRA technique has the advantage over the three-dimensional TOF technique in providing strong flow-related enhancement even in the setting of slow flow.[57] However, both TOF techniques will incorporate material with high signal (such as red thrombus in giant aneurysms) into the maximum intensity projection image (Figure 2). Phase-contrast MRA techniques use a mask data set, which is subtracted from the flowing blood data set. High signal intensity on short TR/TE images such as methemoglobin do not simulate flowing blood as they are removed from the maximum intensity projection images analogous to the bony and soft tissue structures on DSA.

### *Angiography*

As with smaller aneurysms, angiographic evaluation typically defines the morphology and the width of the neck of the aneurysm. A morphologic and physiologic evaluation of the circle of Willis is also possible. The relationship of the surrounding vessels, and both the afferent and efferent arterial pedicles of the aneurysm may be identified.[110] A clear view of the neck of the aneurysm is often difficult to obtain, especially in region of the carotid, ophthalmic, and ICA bifurcation aneurysms.[110] Contralateral injection of the carotids as well as the vertebrobasilar system with compression of the ipsilateral carotid may be utilized to help visualize the collateral function of the circle of Willis.[110] Angiography best establishes the precise relationship of the aneurysm with the parent artery.[103] Thrombosed giant aneurysms will demonstrate a mass effect on the adjacent small vessels, stenosis, or occlusion of the parent vessel or its branches.

## Postoperative Imaging

### *CT and MRI*

Several studies suggest that postoperative MRI of patients with a successfully clipped aneurysm is safe and provides more useful information than does CT.[21,52] Regardless of the

TABLE 1
**Common Aneurysm Clips and MRI Compatibility***

| Aneurysm Clips | Deflection/ Movement | Highest Field Strength (T) | Reference |
|---|---|---|---|
| Drake (DR14, DR24) (Edward Weck, Triangle Park, NJ) | Yes | 1.44 | 12, 76 |
| Drake (DR16) (Edward Weck) | Yes | 0.147 | 76 |
| Drake (301 SS) (Edward Weck) | Yes | 1.5 | 12, 94 |
| Heifetz (17-7PH) (Edward Weck) | Yes | 1.89 | 22, 33 |
| Heifetz (Elgiloy) (Edward Weck) | No | 1.89 | 12, 22, 33 |
| Mayfield (301 SS) (Codman & Shurtleff, Randolph, MA) | Yes | 1.5 | 94 |
| Mayfield (304 SS) (Codman & Shurtleff) | Yes | 1.89 | 33 |
| McFadden (301 SS) (Codman & Shurtleff) | Yes | 1.5 | 12, 94 |
| Olivecrona | No | 1.44 | 76 |
| Pivot (17-7PH) (V. Mueller) | Yes | 1.89 | 33 |
| Scoville (EN58J) (Downs Surgical, Decatur, GA) | Yes | 1.89 | 12, 33 |
| Sugita (Elgiloy) (Downs Surgical) | No | 1.89 | 12, 33 |
| Sundt-Kees (301 SS) (Downs Surgical) | Yes | 1.5 | 12, 94 |
| Sundt-Kees Multi-Angle (17-7PH) (Downs Surgical) | Yes | 1.89 | 12, 33 |
| Vari-Angle (17-7PH) (Codman & Shurtleff) | Yes | 1.89 | 33 |
| Vari-Angle McFadden (MP35N) (Codman & Shurtleff) | No | 1.89 | 12, 33 |
| Vari-Angle Micro (17-7PM SS) (Codman & Shurtleff) | Yes | 0.15 | 10, 12 |
| Vari-Angle Spring (17-7PM SS) (Codman & Shurtleff) | Yes | 0.15 | 10, 12 |
| Yasargil (316 SS) (Aesculap) | No | 1.89 | 33 |
| Yasargil (Phynox) (Aesculap) | No | 1.89 | 33 |

* Modified with permission from Shellock FG, Curtis JS. MR imaging and biomedical implants, materials, and devices: an updated review. *Radiology*. 1991;180:541-550.[94]

chemical composition of the aneurysm clip, most CT images are markedly degraded by beam-hardening artifacts arising from the aneurysm clip.[21,52] With MRI there are also artifacts caused by paramagnetic properties of the alloys within the surgical clips resulting in local distortion and inhomogeneities of the magnetic field.[52] Both CT and MR images of the region immediately adjacent to the clip are severely degraded, rendering them uninterpretable.[52] The amount of artifact created on these imaging modalities relates to both the clip size and the alloy composition of the clip.[52]

Nonferromagnetic aneurysm clips (not deflected in a magnetic field) have been available for a number of years from several manufacturers. The difficulty arises in distinguishing the ferro- from the nonferromagnetic clips once they have been placed. This becomes especially important in imaging a patient in whom there is remote placement

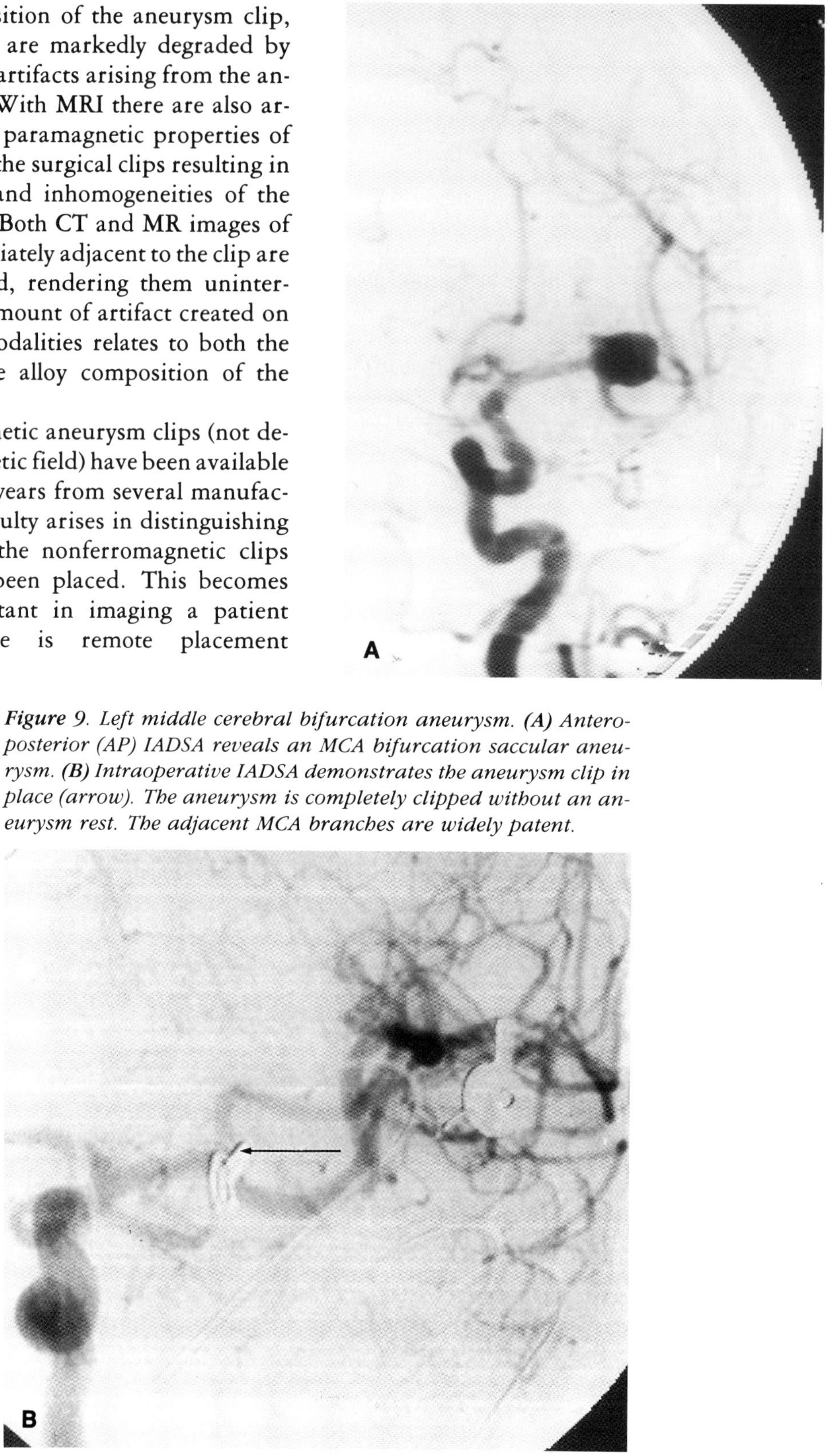


*Figure 9. Left middle cerebral bifurcation aneurysm. (A) Anteroposterior (AP) IADSA reveals an MCA bifurcation saccular aneurysm. (B) Intraoperative IADSA demonstrates the aneurysm clip in place (arrow). The aneurysm is completely clipped without an aneurysm rest. The adjacent MCA branches are widely patent.*

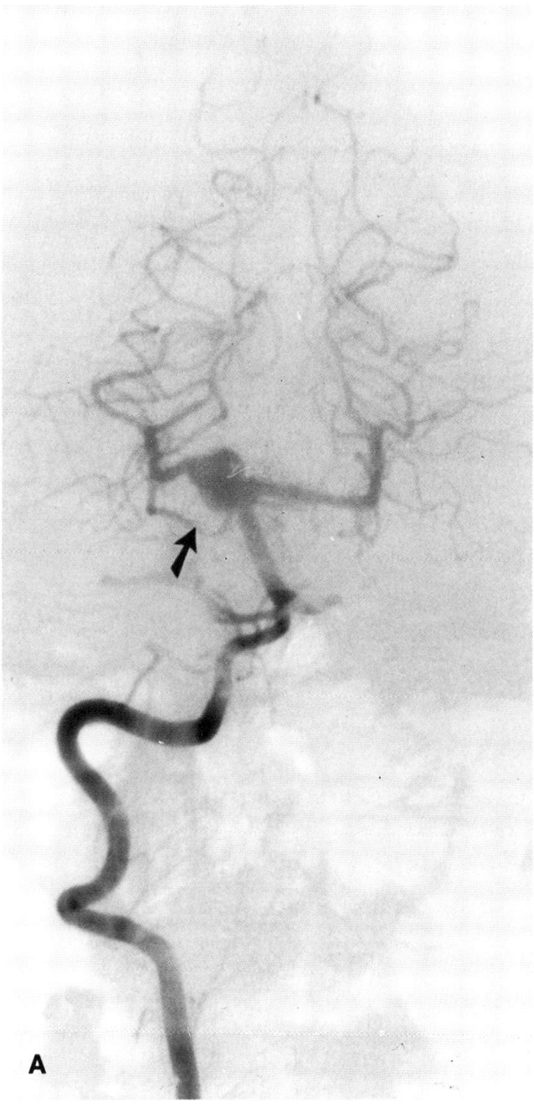


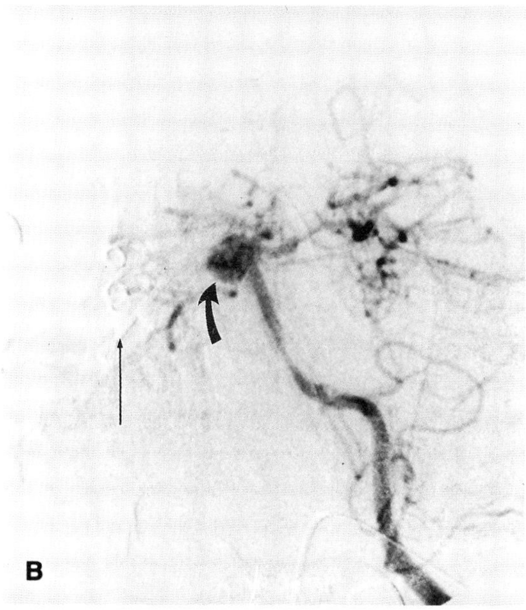


***Figure 10.*** *Right posterior cerebral artery aneurysm.* ***(A)*** *Anteroposterior (AP) IADSA reveals a saccular aneurysm arising off the P1 segment of the right posterior cerebral artery (arrow).* ***(B)*** *During surgery the aneurysm ruptured; profuse, nearly lethal bleeding was controlled with numerous clips. It appeared that the aneurysm was satisfactorily obliterated, but the view was obscured by numerous clips. The intraoperative oblique IADSA demonstrates the surgical clips (straight arrow) and the persistent aneurysm (curved arrow). The clips were carefully removed one by one, and the aneurysm was successfully obliterated following temporary clip application on the parent artery.*

of an aneurysm clip. Complete documentation of the brand and model of the clip should be specifically included in the patient record, thus allowing patients with nonferromagnetic clips to have access to MRI. Several authors have studied and compiled lists of aneurysm clips that have no deflection in magnetic fields and are therefore safe for magnetic imaging (Table 1). This safety does not imply that there will be no artifact, only that there will be no deflection, alleviating the risk of dislodging the aneurysm clip.[12,52,94]

## *Intraoperative and Postoperative Angiography*

Postoperative and, more recently, intraoperative angiography should be performed in all patients where placement of the aneurysm clip across the aneurysm neck cannot be completely visualized at surgery.[64] Postclipping angiography is the only way to ensure that the entire aneurysm is obliterated.[64] Opening of the aneurysm after clipping, a common practice at some institutions, does not prove that there is not a residual neck.[64] In the past, residual aneurysm necks or outpouchings at the site of the aneurysm clip have been thought to be inconsequential; however, it is now known that recurrent aneurysms from these sites are relatively common.[32,64] In the Feuerberg et al study, the incidence of rebleeding from an aneurysm rest was 0.38% to 0.79% per year during the 4- to 13-year observation period.[40] This is extremely important in younger patients.[40,64] In the 27 patients with aneurysm rests, incidence of rupture of the aneurysm rest was 3.8% over the 8 years of clinical followup.[40] Other authors' work support this data.[64]

An intraoperative IADSA achieves many of the same goals as a postoperative angiogram, and allows adjustment of the aneurysm clip to obliterate the entire neck of the aneurysm at the time of the initial surgery (Figure 9).[11,36,51] Intraoperative evaluation of the surgical repair prior to closure of the surgical wound allows recognition and correction of many technical defects, potentially reducing the operative complications and eliminating the need for reoperation (Figures 9–10).[11,51] Failure to recognize and correct a suboptimal anatomic repair can result in increased perioperative ischemic, delayed ischemic, and possibly hemorrhagic complications. This also allows for the intraoperative evaluation of the adjacent or parent vessels to ensure that they are not being compressed or occluded by the clip (Figures 11–12). Now that technologic advances are such that intraoperative

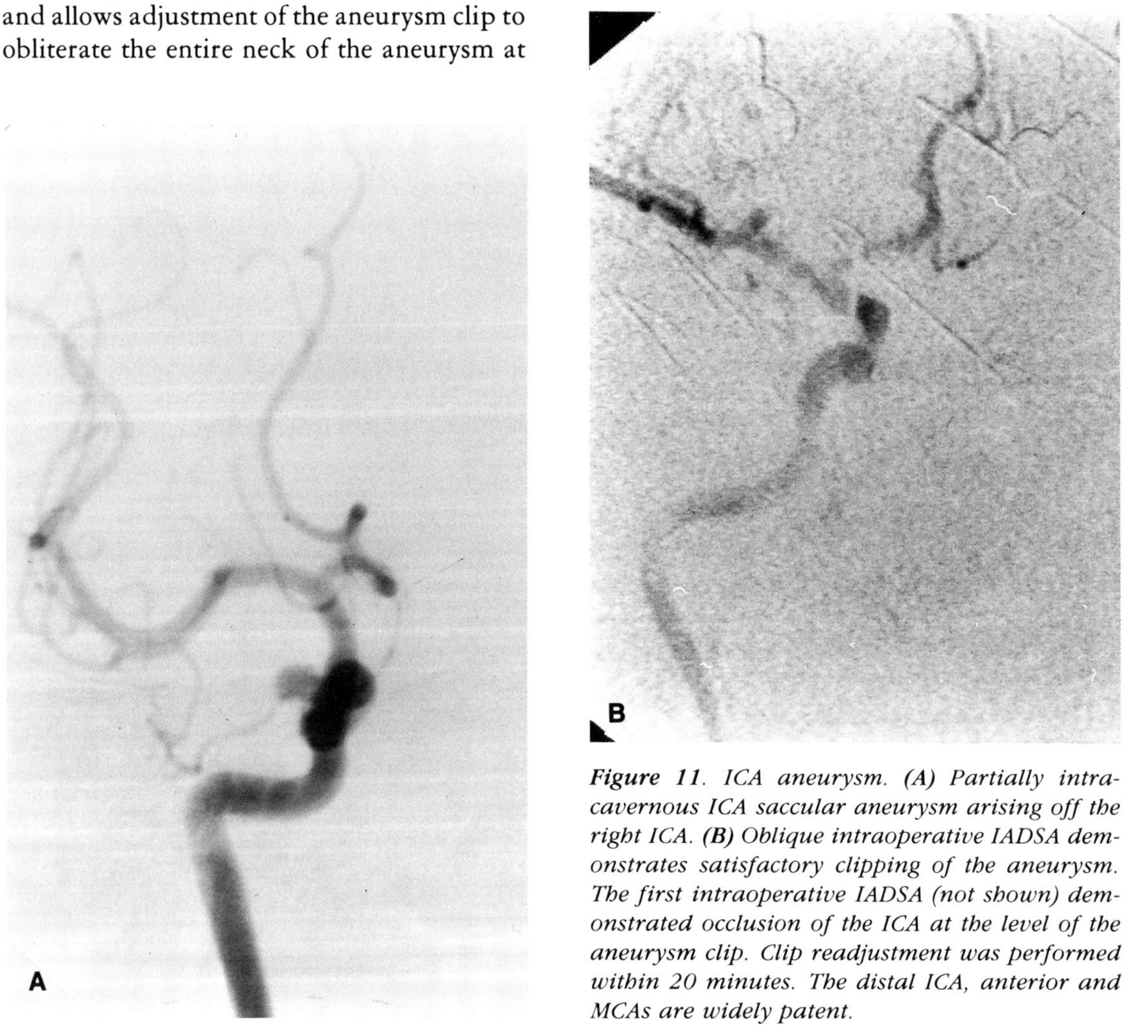


***Figure 11**. ICA aneurysm. **(A)** Partially intracavernous ICA saccular aneurysm arising off the right ICA. **(B)** Oblique intraoperative IADSA demonstrates satisfactory clipping of the aneurysm. The first intraoperative IADSA (not shown) demonstrated occlusion of the ICA at the level of the aneurysm clip. Clip readjustment was performed within 20 minutes. The distal ICA, anterior and MCAs are widely patent.*

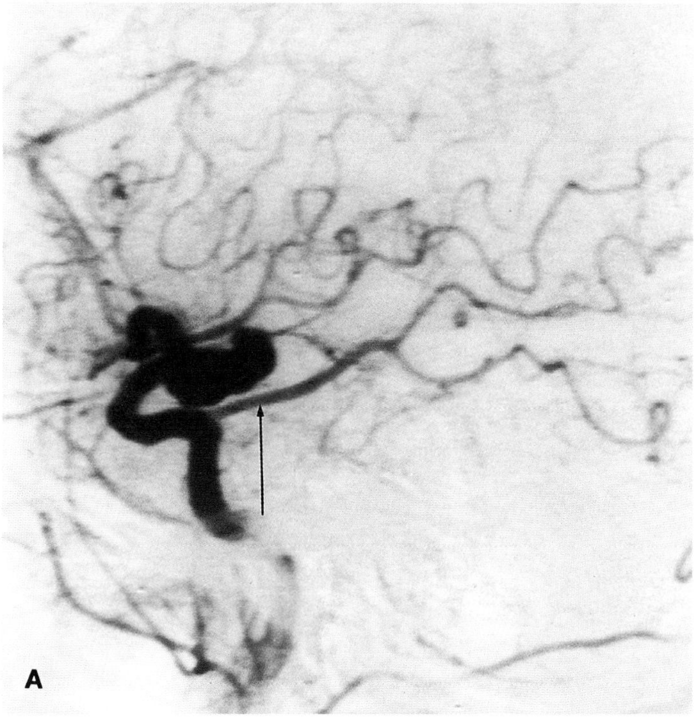


***Figure 12.*** *Posterior communicating artery aneurysm. (A) Lateral IADSA study reveals a lobulated giant aneurysm arising off the distal ICA. There is persistent fetal origin of the posterior cerebral artery (arrow). (B) Intraoperative lateral IADSA demonstrates satisfactory clipping of the aneurysm; however, the posterior cerebral artery is not identified. (C) With repositioning of the aneurysm clip, the aneurysm is still satisfactorily obliterated. The posterior cerebral artery again is opacified (arrow).*

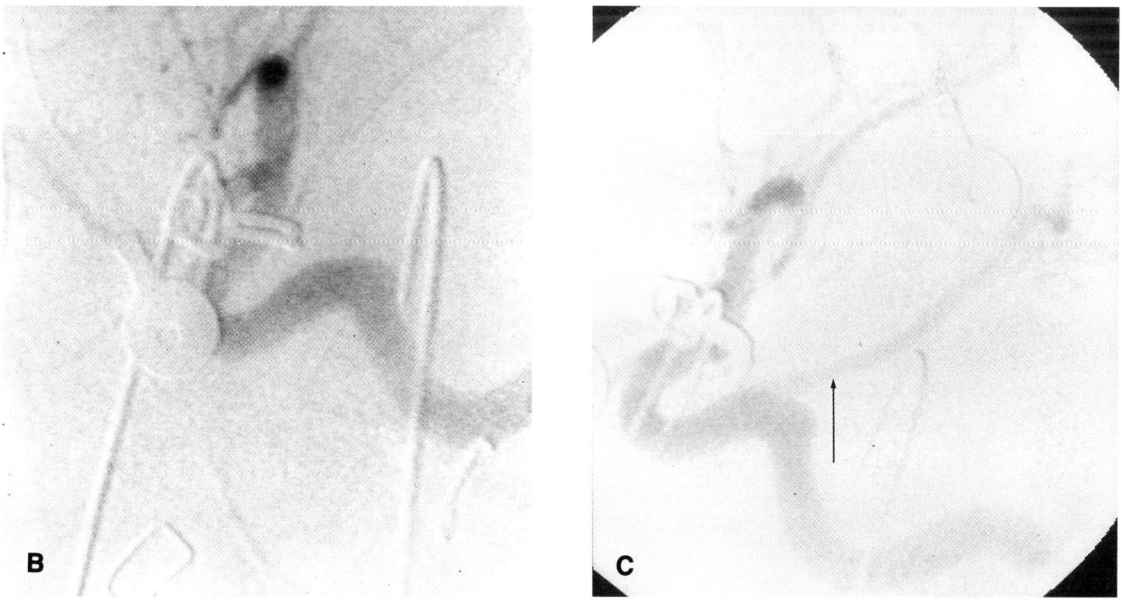

DSA is not only feasible but easily performed, it is more logical to immediately confirm the effectiveness of the surgical repair.

Perhaps the most important aspect of an intraoperative angiogram is presurgical planning of the intraoperative study. More specifically, patient preparation and positioning is of upmost importance to ensure safe and expeditious performance of the exam. The patient's upper head, neck, and chest must be free of any obscuring radiopaque material. The operating suite must be organized so that manipulation of the angiography unit will not contaminate the surgical field or limit motion of the angiographic unit (Figures 13–14). This is achieved with the patient in a supine position on a radiolucent operating table (Amsco Model Quantum 3080 RC). The scrub table is placed so the most cephalad extent of the table is approximately at the level of the patient's xyphoid process (Figure 14). The patient's head should be placed in a radiolucent head rest (Omni Medical 4-point fixation or Mayfield Radiolucent 3-point Head Rest A-1082). Access to the groin is unimpeded under the overhead scrub table holding the surgical instruments. (Figure 14).

The angiographic technique consists of placing a femoral sheath into the left common femoral artery after induction of general anesthesia. A 6 French sheath is used and infused with heparinized normal saline (1,000 units of heparin/250 ml of normal saline) at 20 ml/hr. At the time of angiography, the operating microscope is moved and the surgical field is protected with sterile drapes. In addition, the angiographic C-arm is covered with sterile bags (Figure 13). Angiography of the vessels is performed in a superselective fashion, with a 5 French catheter. Multiple angiographic projections are performed, including the angiographic projection that demonstrated the aneurysm neck at the best advantage preoperatively. All injections are performed by hand. The C-arm angiographic unit (Siemens Siremobil 2000) should perform digital subtraction and collect display angiographic studies in a dynamic and static mode. The length of time that intraoperative angiography adds to the procedure is approximately 15 to 30 minutes.

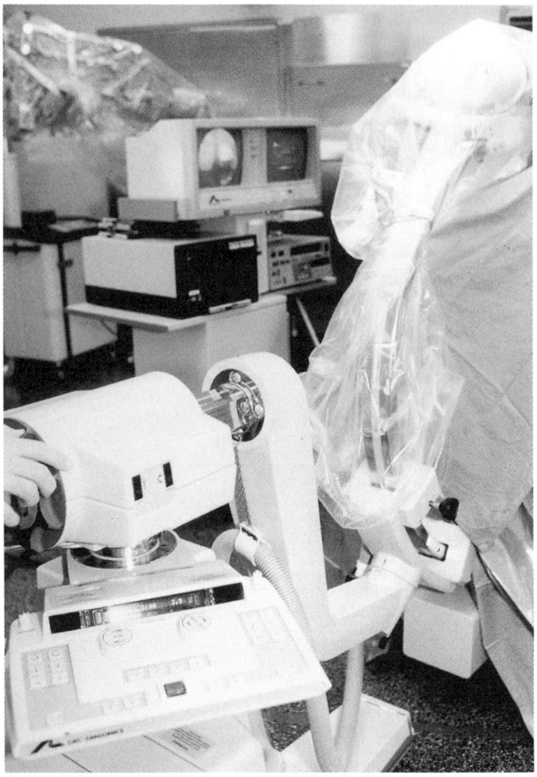

***Figure 13****. Intraoperative DSA. The operating microscope is removed, and the surgical field and the C-arm are draped. The digital subtraction unit is in place over the patient's head in this photograph. The operating microscope is seen in the background.*

The frequency of incomplete aneurysm clipping has been reported in two series ranging from 4% to 5%.[11] It has also been reported by Martin et al that false negative intraoperative angiograms may occur; however, since that series, there have been enough technical advances, especially in intraoperative equipment, that this would be expected to be less prevalent. Multiple projections also reduce false negative results. Intraoperative DSA is routinely used in aneurysm and other neurovascular surgical procedures at the authors' institution. If intraoperative angiography is not available, postoperative angiography is probably indicated.[64] In the cases

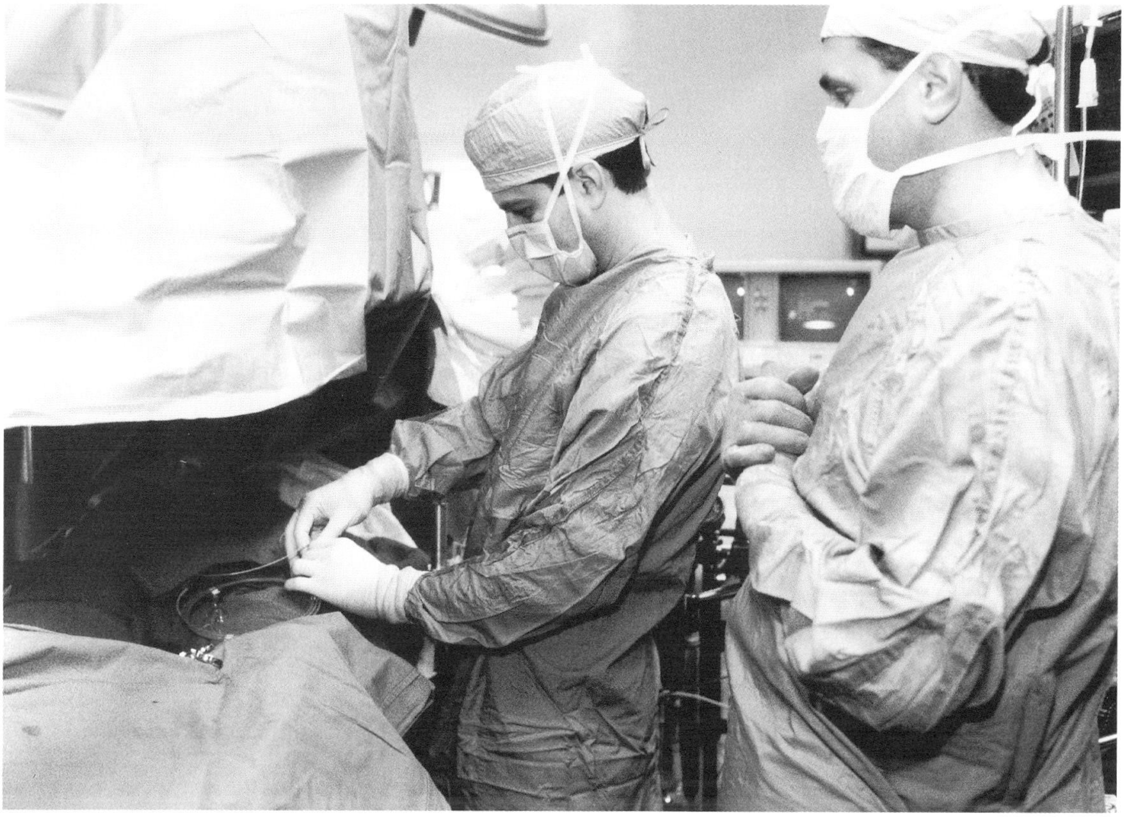

*Figure 14. Intraoperative angiography. The catheter is being placed through the femoral sheath, which had been introduced immediately after induction by anesthesia. The scrub table is above the patient with the most cephalad extent approximately at the level of the xyphoid process to allow the C-arm to visualize the arch for selection of the desired cerebral vessel.*

where a small residual aneurysm rest is present and immediate reoperation is not indicated, a followup angiogram in 3–5 years is probably in order.[66]

## References


1. Aaslid R, Huber P, Nornes H. Evaluation of cerebrovascular spasm with transcranial Doppler ultrasound. *J Neurosurg.* 1984;60:37–41.
2. Aaslid R, Markwalder T-M, Nornes H. Noninvasive transcranial Doppler ultrasound recording of flow velocity in basal cerebral arteries. *J Neurosurg.* 1982;57:769–774.
3. Adams HP Jr, Kassell NF, Torner JC, et al. CT and clinical correlations in recent aneurysmal subarachnoid hemorrhage: a preliminary report of the cooperative aneurysm study. *Neurology.* 1983;33: 981–988.
4. Alexander MSM, Dias PS, Uttley D. Spontaneous subarachnoid hemorrhage and negative cerebral panangiography. *J Neurosurg.* 1986;64:537–542.
5. Allcock JM. Aneurysms. In: Newton TH, Potts DG, eds. *Radiology of the Skull and Brain.* St. Louis, Mo: Mosby;1974;2:2435–2489.
6. Asari S, Satoh T, Sakurai M, et al. Delineation of unruptured cerebral aneurysms by computerized angiotomography. *J Neurosurg.* 1982;57:527 534.
7. Atkinson JLD, Sundt TM Jr, Houser OW, et al. Angiographic frequency of anterior circulation intracranial aneurysms. *J Neurosurg.* 1989;70: 551–555.
8. Atlas SW, Grossman RI, Goldberg HI, et al. Partially thrombosed giant intracranial aneurysms: correlation of MR and pathologic findings. *Radiology.* 1987;162:111–114.
9. Atlas SW, Mark AS, Grossman RI, et al. Intracranial hemorrhage: gradient-echo MR imaging at 1.5 T comparison with spin-echo imaging and clinical applications. *Radiology.* 1988;168:803–807.
10. Barrafato D, Henkelman RM. Magnetic resonance imaging and surgical clips. *Can J Surg.* 1984;27: 509–512.
11. Barrow DL, Boyer KL, Joseph GJ. Intraoperative angiography in the management of neurovascular disorders. *Neurosurgery.* 1992;30:153–159.
12. Becker RL, Norfray JF, Teitelbaum GP, et al. MR imaging in patients with intracranial aneurysm

clips. *AJNR.* 1988;9:885–889.

13. Belber CJ, Hoffman RB. The syndrome of intracranial aneurysm associated with fibromuscular hyperplasia of the renal arteries. *J Neurosurg.* 1968; 28:556–559.
14. Bergström M, Ericson K, Levander B, et al. Variation with time of the attenuation values of intracranial hematomas. *J Comput Assist Tomogr.* 1977; 1:57–63.
15. Biondi A, Scialfa G, Scotti G. Intracranial aneurysms: MR imaging. *Neuroradiology.* 1988; 30:214–218.
16. Black PM. Hydrocephalus and vasospasm after subarachnoid hemorrhage from ruptured intracranial aneurysms. *Neurosurgery.* 1986;18:12–16.
17. Bohmfalk GL, Story JL. Intermittent appearance of a ruptured cerebral aneurysm on sequential angiograms. *J Neurosurg.* 1980;52:263–265.
18. Bradley WG Jr, Schmidt PG. Effect of methemoglobin formation on the MR appearance of subarachnoid hemorrhage. *Radiology.* 1985;156:99–103.
19. Bradley WG Jr, Waluch V. Blood flow: magnetic resonance imaging. *Radiology.* 1985;154: 443–450.
20. Bradley WG Jr, Waluch V, Lai K-S, et al. The appearance of rapidly flowing blood on magnetic resonance images. *AJR.* 1984;143:1167–1174.
21. Brothers MF, Fox AJ, Lee DH, et al. MR imaging after surgery for vertebrobasilar aneurysm. *AJNR.* 1990;11:149–161.
22. Brown MA, Carden JA, Coleman RE, et al. Magnetic field effects on surgical ligation clips. *Magn Reson Imaging.* 1987;5:443–453.
23. Buckingham MJ, Crone KR, Ball WS, et al. Traumatic intracranial aneurysms in childhood: two cases and a review of the literature. *Neurosurgery.* 1988;22:398–408.
24. Bull J. Massive aneurysms at the base of the brain. *Brain.* 1969;92:535–570.
25. Burt TB. MR of CSF flow phenomenon mimicking basilar artery aneurysm. *AJNR.* 1987;8:55–58.
26. Carmody RF, Smith JRL, Seeger JF, et al. Intracranial applications of digital intravenous subtraction angiography. *Radiology.* 1982;144:529–534.
27. Crompton MR. Mechanism of growth and rupture in cerebral berry aneurysms. *BR Med J.* 1966;1: 1138–1142.
28. Davis JM, Davis KR, Crowell RM. Subarachnoid hemorrhage secondary to ruptured intracranial aneurysm: prognostic significance of cranial CT. *AJNR.* 1980;1:17–21.
29. Di Lorenzo N, Guidetti G. Anterior communicating aneurysm missed at angiography: report of two cases treated surgically. *Neurosurgery.* 1988; 23: 494–499.
30. Drake CG. Giant intracranial aneurysms: experience with surgical treatment in 174 patients. *Clin Neurosurg.* 1979;26:12–95.
31. Drake CG. Management of cerebral aneurysm. *Stroke.* 1981;12:273–283.
32. Drake CG, Friedman AH, Peerless SJ. Failed aneurysm surgery. Reoperation in 115 cases. *J Neurosurg.* 1984;61:848–856.
33. Dujovny M, Kossovsky N, Kossowsky R, et al. Aneurysm clip motion during magnetic resonance imaging: in vivo experimental study with metallurgical factor analysis. *Neurosurgery.* 1985;17:543–548.
34. Enzmann DR, Brody WR, Riederer G, et al. Intracranial intravenous digital subtraction angiography. *Neuroradiol.* 1982;23:241–251.
35. Fisher CM, Kistler JP, Davis JM. Relation of cerebral vasospasm to subarachnoid hemorrhage visualized by computerized tomographic scanning. *Neurosurgery.* 6:1–9.
36. Foley KT, Cahan LD, Hieshima GB. Intraoperative angiography using a portable digital subtraction unit. *J Neurosurg.* 1986;64:816–818.
37. Forbes GS, Earnest F IV, Kispert DB, et al. Digital angiography: Introducing digital techniques to clinical cerebral angiography practice. *Mayo Clin Proc.* 1982;57:683–693.
38. Forster DMC, Steiner L, Hakanson S, et al. The value of repeat panangiography in cases of unexplained subarachnoid hemorrhage. *J Neurosurg.* 1978;48:712–716.
39. Fox JL. Management of aneurysms of anterior circulation of intracranial procedures. In: Youmans JR, ed. *Neurological Surgery.* 3rd ed. Philadelphia, Pa: Saunders; 1990:1689–1732.
40. Feuerberg I, Lindquist C, Linqvist M, et al. Natural history of postoperative aneurysm rests. *J Neurosurg.* 1987;66:30–34.
41. Gean AD, Pile-Spellman J, Heros RC. A pneumatized anterior clinoid mimicking an aneurysm on MR imaging. Report of two cases. *J Neurosurg.* 1989;71:128–132.
42. Ghoshhajra K, Scotti L, Marasco J, et al. CT detection of intracranial aneurysms in subarachnoid hemorrhage. *AJR.* 1979;132:613–616.
43. Gilbert JW, Lee C, Young B. Repeat cerebral panangiography in subarachnoid hemorrhage of unknown etiology. *Surg Neurol.* 1990;33:19–21.
44. Golding R, Peatfield RC, Shawdon HH et al. Computer tomographic features of giant intracranial aneurysms. *Clin Rad.* 1980; 31:41–48.
45. Gomori JM, Grossman RI, Goldberg HI, et al. Intracranial hematomas: imaging by high-field MR. *Radiology.* 1985;157:87–93.
46. Gomori JM, Grossman RI, Goldberg HI, et al. Occult cerebral vascular malformations: high-field MR imaging. *Radiology.* 1986;158:707–713.
47. Gomori JM, Grossman RI, Hackney DB, et al. Variable appearances of subacute intracranial hematomas on high-field spin-echo MR. *AJNR.* 1987; 8:1019–1026.
48. Grzyska U, Freitag J, Zeumer H. Selective cerebral intraarterial DSA: complication rate and control of risk factors. *Neuroradiol.* 1990;32:296–299.
49. Hacker RJ, Krall JM, Fox JL. Data, I and II. In: Fox JL, ed. *Intracranial Aneurysms.* New York, NY: Springer Verlag; 1983;1: 19–117.
50. Hackney DB, Lesnick JE, Zimmerman RA, et al. MR identification of bleeding site in subarachnoid hemorrhage with multiple intracranial aneurysms. *J Comput Assist Tomogr.* 1986;10:878–880.
51. Hieshima GB, Reicher MA, Higashida RT, et al. Intraoperative digital subtraction neuroangiography: a diagnostic and therapeutic tool. *AJNR.* 1987;8: 759–767.
52. Holtås S, Olsson M, Romner B, et al. Comparison of MR imaging and CT in patients with intracranial aneurysm clips. *AJNR.* 1988;9:891–897.
53. Housepian EM, Pool JL. A systematic analysis of intracranial aneurysms from the autopsy file of the Presbyterian Hospital 1914 to 1956. *J Neuropathol Exp Neurol.* 1958;17:409–423.

54. Hove B, Andersen BB, Christiansen TM. Intracranial oncotic aneurysms from choriocarcinoma. case report and review of the literature: *Neuroradiol.* 1990;32:526–528.
55. Iwanaga H, Wakai S, Ochiai C, et al. Ruptured cerebral aneurysms missed by initial angiographic study. *Neurosurgery.* 1990;27:45–51.
56. Juul R, Fredriksen TA, Ringk R. Prognosis in subarachnoid hemorrhage of unknown etiology. *J Neurosurg.* 1986;64:359–362.
57. Keller PJ, Drayer BP, Fram EK, et al. MR angiography with two-dimensional acquisition and three-dimensional display. *Radiology.* 1989;173:527–532.
58. Kistler JP, Crowell RM, Davis KR, et al. The relation of cerebral vasospasm to the extent and location of subarachnoid blood visualized by CT scan: a prospective study. *Neurology.* 1983;33: 424–436.
59. Kondziolka D, Bernstein M, ter Brugge K, et al. Acute subdural hematoma from ruptured posterior communicating artery aneurysm. *Neurosurgery.* 1988;22:151–154.
60. Kwan ESK, Wolpert SM, Scott RM, et al. MR evaluation of neurovascular lesions after endovascular occlusion with detachable balloons. *AJNR.* 1988;9:523–531.
61. Laissy J-P, Normand G, Monroc M, et al. Spontaneous intracerebral hematomas from vascular causes: predictive value of CT compared with angiography. *Neuroradiol.* 1991;33:291–295.
62. Levey AS, Pauker SG, Kassirer JP. Occult intracranial aneurysm in polycystic kidney disease: when is cerebral arteriography indicated? *New Engl J Med.* 1983;308:986–994.
63. Liliequist B, Lindqvist M, Valdimarsson E. Computed tomography and subarachnoid hemorrhage. *Neuroradiology.* 1977;14:21–26.
64. Lin T, Fox AJ, Drake CG. Regrowth of aneurysm sacs from residual neck following aneurysm clipping. *J Neurosurg.* 1989;70:556–560.
65. Locksley HB. Report on the Cooperative Study of Intracranial Aneurysms and Subarachnoid Hemorrhage. Section V, I: natural history of subarachnoid hemorrhage, intracranial aneurysms and arteriovenous malformations based on 6368 cases in the cooperative study. *J Neurosurg.* 1966;25:219–239.
66. Locksley HB. Report on the Cooperative Study of Intracranial Aneurysms and Subarachnoid Hemorrhage. Section V, II: natural history of subarachnoid hemorrhage, intracranial aneurysms and arteriovenous malformations. Based on 6368 cases in the coopertaive study. *J Neurosurg.* 1966; 25:321–368.
67. MacDonald A, Mendelow AD. Xanthochromia revisited: a re-evaluation of lumbar puncture and CT scanning in the diagnosis of subarachnoid hemorrhage. *J Neurol, Neurosurg, Psychiatry.* 1988;51: 342–344.
68. Martin NA, Bentson J, Viñuela F, et al. Intraoperative digital subtraction angiography and the surgical treatment of intracranial aneurysms and vascular malformations. *J Neurosurg.* 1990;73: 526–533.
69. Masaryk TJ, Lewin JS, Laub G. Magnetic resonance angiography. In: Stark DD, Bradley WG, eds. *Magnetic Resonance Imaging.* St. Louis, Mo: Mosby Yearbook; 1991: 299–314.
70. McCormack J, Peyster RG, Brodner RA, et al. CT visualization of ruptured berry aneurysm within hematoma: the flip-flop sign. *J Comput Assist Tomogr.* 1986;10:28–31.
71. McCormick WF. Problems and pathogenesis of intracranial arterial aneurysms. In: Toole JF, Moosey J, Janeway R, eds. *Cerebrovascular disorders* 2nd edition. New York: Grune Straffon; 1971: 219–231.
72. McCormick WF, Acosta-Rua GJ. The size of intracranial saccular aneurysms. An autopsy study. *J Neurosurg.* 1970;33:422–427.
73. Messina AV, Chernik NL. Computed tomography: the "resolving" intracerebral hemorrhage. *Radiology.* 1975;118:609–613.
74. Nakstad P, Nornes H, Hauge HN. Traumatic aneurysms of the pericallosal arteries. *Neuroradiol.* 1986;28:335–338.
75. New PFJ, Aronow S. Attenuation measurements of whole blood and blood fractions in computed tomography. *Radiology.* 1976;121:635–640.
76. New PFJ, Rosen BR, Brady TJ, et al. Potential hazards and artifacts of ferromagnetic and nonferromagnetic surgical and dental materials and devices in nuclear magnetic resonance imaging. *Radiology.* 1983;147:139–148.
77. Newell DW, LeRoux PD, Dacey R Jr, et al. CT infusion scanning for the detection of cerebral aneurysms. *J Neurosurg.* 1989;71:175–179.
78. Olsen WL, Brant-Zawadzki M, Hodes J. Giant intracranial aneurysms: MR imaging. *Radiology.* 1987;163:431–435.
79. O'Neill M, Hope T, Thomson G. Giant intracranial aneurysms: diagnosis with special reference to computerized tomography. *Clin Radiol.* 1980;31: 27–39.
80. Pasqualin A, Rosta L, Da Pian R, et al. Role of computed tomography in the management of vasospasm after subarachnoid hemorrhage. *Neurosurgery.* 1984;15:344–353.
81. Perret G, Nishioka H. Report on the cooperative Study of Intracranial Aneurysms and Subarachnoid Hemorrhage, section VI: Arteriovenous malformations: an analysis of 545 cases of craniocerebral arteriovenous malformations and fistulae reported to the cooperative study. *J Neurosurg.* 1966;25:467.
82. Pinto RS, Cohen WA, Kricheff II, et al. Giant intracranial aneurysms: rapid sequential computed tomography. *AJNR.* 1982;3:495–499.
83. Pinto RS, Kricheff II, Butler AR, et al. Correlation of computed tomographic, angiographic, and neuropathological changes in giant cerebral aneurysms. *Radiology.* 1979;132:85–92.
84. Rinkel GJE, Wijdicks EFM, Vermeulen M, et al. Nonaneurysmal perimesencephalic subarachnoid hemorrhage: CT and MR patterns that differ from aneurysmal rupture. *AJNR.* 1991;12:829–834.
85. Romner B, Ljunggren B, Brandt L, et al. Correlation of transcranial Doppler sonography findings with timing of aneurysm surgery. *J Neurosurg.* 1990;73:72–76.
86. Ross JS, Masaryk TJ, Modic MT, et al. Intracranial aneurysms: evaluation by MR angiography. *AJNR.* 1990;11:449–456.
87. Rout D, Sharma A, Mohan PK, et al. Bacterial aneurysms of the intracavernous carotid artery. *J Neurosurg.* 1984;60:1236–1242.
88. Schievink WI, Limburg M, Dreissen JJR, et al. Screening for unruptured familial intracranial

aneurysms: subarachnoid hemorrhage 2 years after angiography negative for aneurysms. *Neurosurgery.* 1991;29:434–438.
89. Schmid UD, Steiger HJ, Huber P. Accuracy of high resolution computed tomography in direct diagnosis of cerebral aneurysms. *Neuroradiol.* 1987; 29: 152–159.
90. Scotti G, Ethier R, Melancon D, et al. Computed tomography in the evaluation of intracranial aneurysms and subarachnoid hemorrhage. *Radiology.* 1977;123:85–90.
91. Seiler RW, Grolimund P, Aaslid R, et al. Cerebral vasospasm evaluated by transcranial ultrasound correlated with clinical grade and CT-visualized subarachnoid hemorrhage. *J Neurosurg.* 1986;64: 594–600.
92. Sekhar LN, Wechsler LR, Yonas H, et al. Value of transcranial Doppler examination in the diagnosis of cerebral vasospasm after subarachnoid hemorrhage. *Neurosurgery.* 1988;22:813–821.
93. Sevick RJ, Tsuruda JS, Schmalbrock P. Three-dimensional time-of-flight MR angiography in the evaluation of cerebral aneurysms. *J Comp Assist Tomgr.* 1990;14:874–881.
94. Shellock FG, Curtis JS. MR imaging and biomedical implants, materials, and devices: an updated review. *Radiology.* 1991;180:541–550.
95. Shuaib A, Lee MA, Johns RD, et al. Subarachnoid hemorrhage and normal angiography: should the angiogram be reviewed by a second neuroradiologist? *Can J Neurol Sci.* 1988;15:413–416.
96. Silver AJ, Pederson ME Jr, Ganti SR, et al. CT of subarachnoid hemorrhage due to ruptured aneurysm. *AJNR.* 1981;2:13–22.
97. Sonntag VK, Yuan RH, Stein BM. Giant intracranial aneurysms: a review of 13 cases. *Surg Neurol.* 1977;8:81–84.
98. Steiner H, Lammer J, Kleinert R, et al. Dissecting aneurysm of cerebral arteries in congenital vascular deficiency. *Neuroradiology.* 1986;28:331–334.
99. Stone JL, Crowell RM, Gandhi YN, et al. Multiple intracranial aneurysms: magnetic resonance imaging for determination of the site of rupture. Report of a case. *Neurosurgery.* 1988; 23:97–100.
100. Strother CM, Eldevik P, Kikuchi Y, et al. Thrombus formation and structure and the evolution of mass effect in intracranial aneurysms treated by balloon embolization: emphasis on MR findings. *AJNR.* 1989;10:787–796.
101. Sundt TM Jr, Piepgras DG. Surgical approach to giant intracranial aneurysms: operative experience with 80 cases. *J Neurosurg.* 1979;51:731–742.
102. Symon L, Vajda J. Surgical experiences with giant intracranial aneurysms. *J Neurosurg.* 1984; 61:1009–1028.
103. Teasdale E, Statham P, Straiton J, et al. Non-invasive radiological investigation for oculomotor palsy. *J Neurol, Neurosurg, Psychiatry.* 1990; 53:549–553.
104. ter Berg JWM, Overtoom TMD, Ludwig JW, et al. Detection of unruptured familial intracranial aneurysms by intravenous digital subtraction angiography. *Neuroradiology.* 1987;29:272–276.
105. Teresi LM, Davis SJ. Cerebral vascular malformations. In: Stark DD, Bradley WG, eds. *Magnetic Resonance Imaging* St. Louis, Mo: Mosby Yearbook, 1991: 1.
106. Touho H, Karasawa J, Tazawa T, et al. Intraarterial digital subtraction angiography for definitive diagnosis of intracranial aneurysms. *AJNR.* 1988; 9:1157–1161.
107. Tsuruda JS, Halbach VV, Higashida RT, et al. MR evaluation of large intracranial aneurysms using cine low flip angle gradient-refocused imaging. *AJR.* 1988;151:153–162.
108. Valk PE, Hale JD, Crooks LE, et al. MRI of blood flow: correlation of image appearance with spin-echo phase shift and signal intensity. *AJR.* 1986; 146:931–939.
109. van Gijn J, van Dongen KJ, Vermeulen M, et al. Perimesencephalic hemorrhage: a nonaneurysmal and benign form of subarachnoid hemorrhage. *Neurology.* 1985;35:493–497.
110. Viñuela F, Fox A, Chang JK, et al. Clinico-radiological spectrum of giant supraclinoid internal carotid artery aneurysms: observations in 93 cases. *Neuroradiol.* 1984;26:93–99.
111. von Schulthess GK, Higgins CB. Blood flow imaging with MR: spin-phase phenomena. *Radiology.* 1985;157:687–695.
112. Waluch V, Bradley WG. NMR even echo rephasing in slow laminar flow. *J Comput Assist Tomogr.* 1984;8:594–598.
113. Weisberg L. Direct visualization of intracranial aneurysms by computed tomography. *Computerized Tomogr.* 1981;5:191–199.
114. Wilson FMA, Jaspan T, Holland IM. Multiple cerebral aneurysms: a reappraisal. *Neuroradiol.* 1989;31:232–236.
115. Wood EH. Angiographic identification of the ruptured lesion in patients with multiple cerebral aneurysms. *J Neurosurg.* 1964;21:182–198.
116. Yamamoto Y, Asari S, Sunami N, et al. Computed angiotomography of unruptured cerebral aneurysms. *J Comput Assist Tomogr.* 1986;10:21–27.
117. Yousem DM, Balakrihnan J, Debrun JM, et al. Hyperintense thrombus of GRASS MR images. Potential pitfall in flow evaluation. *AJNR.* 1990;11: 51–58.

# CHAPTER 4

# Perioperative Management of Ruptured Aneurysms

Gene H. Barnett, MD, and Donald M. Whiting, MD

In the hours and days following aneurysmal subarachnoid hemorrhage (SAH), the patient is subject to potential complications which may be neurologically devastating and even fatal. Attention to details of management may prevent many of these disorders, or at least allow their prompt recognition and treatment.

Early, aggressive management of SAH can substantially reduce the morbidity and mortality of the initial hemorrhage.[34] For this reason, a comprehensive, coordinated surgical/medical approach is taken by the Cerebrovascular Service and Neurosurgical Intensive Care Unit (NICU) at the Cleveland Clinic Foundation for such patients. Early efforts focus on stabilization and prevention of rehemorrhage until surgical obliteration of the source of bleeding can be effected. In the days following hemorrhage, cerebral vasospasm may develop, the treatment of which must be modified depending upon whether the aneurysm has been surgically repaired. Other complications, such as hydrocephalus or seizures, can arise at any time in the postoperative period and may lead to secondary brain injury or potentiate rehemorrhage.

The authors' approach to the medical management of these patients is outlined in Table 1. A thorough description of these techniques along with the rationale also are provided in Table 1 and in this chapter.

## Systemic Stabilization

Cardiac, pulmonary, or electrolyte abnormalities often follow SAH. These potentially fatal disturbances may delay surgery, or lead to secondary injury of the brain due to ischemia, hypoxia, or seizures. Clinical vigilance with appropriate therapy usually can avert these more serious consequences.

### *Cardiac Complications*

Electrocardiographic changes are common following SAH and include arrhythmias[19,31,49,77,78] and waveform changes consistent with ischemia[19,31,79] or infarction.[3] It is believed that most of these abnormalities are the result of a massive rise in circulating catecholamine levels occurring at the time of hemorrhage.[14,19,51,52] Although waveform changes were once considered to be a curiosity of cerebral injury, it is now recognized that these changes must be viewed as genuine evidence of cardiac dysfunction and treated accordingly. Early use of beta-adrenergic blockers has been shown to reduce catecholamine-mediated complications.[14,52] In addition to a 12-lead electrocardiogram (ECG), cardiac iso-enzymes should be obtained, and evidence of infarction treated appropriately.

Serious cardiac arrhythmias (atrioventric-

## TABLE 1
## Cleveland Clinic NICU Subarachnoid Hemorrhage Guidelines

**I. Prevent rehemorrhage.**

A. By limiting elevations of aneurysmal transmural pressure gradient.

1. Keep patient *flat* in a darkened, quiet room, and limit visitors. Begin stool softeners (pericolace 1 bid).
2. Beta adrenergic blockers (e.g. propranolol 10 mg p.o. qid, or 1 mg IV qid.) Dosage may be increased if necessary to reduce systolic arterial blood pressure to less than 120 mm Hg. Do not discontinue unless patient is profoundly bradycardic (< 45 beats/min), asthmatic, or hypotensive (systolic BP < 90 mm Hg). Taper if possible.
3. Sedate: Phenobarbital, 30–60 mg IV or p.o., tid. Use additional sedation as required (e.g. more phenobarbital, benzodiazepines, antipsychotics, anesthesia, and paralysis).
4. Antihypertensive drip at bedside (sodium nitroprusside 100 mg/250 ml 0.9% NaCl, or esmalol HCl 5 gm/500 ml 0.9% NaCl). Titrate to maintain systolic blood pressure less than120 mm Hg. (Consider raising BP limit to 150 mm Hg in chronic hypertensive patients.) Avoid excessive beta adrenergic blockade, especially in geriatric patients.
5. Treat seizures (phenytoin load 18 mg/kg, then 1.5 mg/kg q8h) for documented or suspected seizure only.
6. Prevent transient hypertension from uncomfortable procedures (such as suctioning) with medullary suppressant (lidocaine HCl 1–2 mg/kg IV bolus, or methohexital 0.5–1.5 mg/kg IV).

B. By preventing clot lysis.

1. If surgery is delayed or patient is at unusually high risk of rebleeding, consider antifibrinolytic therapy (aminocaproic acid load 4–5 gm/250 ml 0.9% NaCl over 1 hour, then 1–1.25 gm/hr IV) continuous infusion until surgery. Discontinue should patient develop thromboembolic complication or evidence of vasospasm.
2. No prostaglandin inhibitors (aspirin, nonsteroidal anti-inflammatory agents) until aneurysm is clipped.

**II. Avoid ischemic/hypoxic complications.**

A. Place pulmonary artery catheter after patient has been adequately sedated. Try to achieve pulmonary artery wedge pressure (PAWP) between 14–18 mm Hg (5% purified plasma protein fraction, 5% or 25% albumin, or blood as appropriate). Determine patient's optimum wedge pressure. Maintenance crystalloid infusion of 75 ml/hr of normal saline, total (adjust sodium dosage as necessary).

B. Maintain hematocrit (Hct) at 33% to 38% by volume expansion, transfusion, or phlebotomy (in this order).

C. Maintain arterial blood oxygen saturation 95% or greater.

D. Maintain blood glucose between 100–200 mg/dl. Obtain Accuchecks at least q4h or more frequently if required. Begin feeding 2–3 days posthemorrhage. Start gradually, and use parenteral feeding if obtunded or at risk for aspiration.

E. Do not allow patient to become volume-depleted from "salt wasting" or contrast-induced osmotic diuresis. Hydrate with 250 ml D5 NS prior to angiography, or D5 1.5 NS if the patient is hyponatremic.

F. Begin cerebroselective dihydropyridine (nimodipine 60 mg p.o./NG q4h).

**III. Monitor/treat complications of SAH.**

A. Any change in level of consciousness should be assessed by a CT scan (to check for hydrocephalus, rebleed, or infarction); arterial blood gas to check for hypoxia; serum chemistries and drug levels to check for metabolic or toxic effects; and TCD to assess vasospasm. If TCD shows vasospasm, or no other cause is apparent, refer to vasospasm guidelines.

B. If hydrocephalus, place ventricular catheter (or lumbar puncture [LP] drain if clearly communicating hydrocephalus). Drain if ICP ≥ 15 mm Hg. If frequent drainage required then drain continuously at this level. Overdrainage may precipitate hemorrhage.

C. If history or clinical evidence of aspiration, begin empiric antibiotic therapy (ticarcillin/clavulanate 3/0.1 gm q4–6 h. and tobramycin 1 mg/kg q8 h [adjust dosage in renal insufficiency]).

**IV. Vasospasm Guidelines:**

A. Optimize cardiac hemodynamics to maximize cerebral blood flow.

1. Patient should have a pulmonary artery catheter. Attempt to achieve PAWP of 14-18 mm Hg:
   Unclipped: 5% purified plasma protein fraction, 5% or 25% albumin or blood as appropriate.
   Clipped: Dextran 40, load with 80 ml over 1 hr, then 40 ml/hr.
2. Consider use of desmopressin (0.25–.5 ml IV bid) if unable to optimize PAWP due to brisk diuresis. Determine patient's optimum PWP by maximal cardiac output. (Revise with each change in PEEP or CPAP).
3. Increase systolic blood pressure:
   Unclipped: 140–160 mm Hg (max).
   Clipped: 210 mm Hg (max), maintain at lowest blood pressure that induces neurologic improvement.
   Dopamine (200 mg/250 ml D5 0.9% NaCl), dobutamine (250 mg/l D5 0.9% NaCl), or norepinephrine (4 mg/l D5 0.9% NaCl) with renal dose dopamine (1 mcg/kg/min) or phenylephrine (10 mg/250 ml D5 0.9% NaCl). Continue propranolol and sedation as this may prevent wide swings in pressure.
4. Discontinue antifibrinolytic agents.

B. Monitor severity of vasospasm.

1. TCD daily if clinical vasospasm, qod if subclinical vasospasm.
2. Angiography if TCD shows evidence of vasospasm immediately prior to surgery, or if vasospasm symptoms progress despite maximal medical therapy.

C. Endovascular therapy of vasospasm.

1. For cases with progressive cerebral vasospasm despite maximal medical therapy, *before* development of significant brain infarction.
2. Angiography with focal intra-arterial papaverine titrated to improvement of angiographic spasm.

ular dissociation, idioventricular rhythms, and ventricular tachycardia) occur in 20% to 40% of patients following SAH.[3,31,77] More benign rhythm disturbances, such as premature ventricular complexes, bradyarrhythmias, or supraventricular tachycardia occur in the majority of patients.[3,16,31,77] Cardiac arrhythmias occur most commonly in the first 2 days following SAH, perhaps associated with corrected Q-T intervals (QTC) prolongation, and may lead to sudden death.[3,18,31,77] Continuous cardiac monitoring should therefore be performed routinely.

As beta-adrenergic blocking agents provide substantial cardiac protection following SAH, they are only withheld for bradycardia (less than 45 beats per minute), with associated hypotension, heart block, heart failure, or specific contraindications to the use of beta blockers such as asthma or hypersensitivity. Bradyarrhythmias with hypotension may be treated with atropine (0.5–1.0 mg, intravenously).[78]

### *Pulmonary Complications*

The immediate time period following SAH may be complicated by pulmonary dysfunction secondary to aspiration pneumonia or neurogenic pulmonary edema. Screening tests, in addition to careful pulmonary examination on admission, include arterial blood gas and chest radiograph.

Witnessed or suspected aspiration should be treated empirically with a third-generation cephalosporin and aminoglycoside. If necessary, a sputum culture can be collected by nasotracheal or endotracheal suction; however, precipitation of rehemorrhage must be considered. In this setting, the patient's cough reflex may be blunted by the intravenous administration of methyl-hexitol (50–100 mg, intravenously)[59] or lidocaine (1.0–1.5 mg/kg, intravenously).[42,67]

Elevated cardiac filling pressures or capillary disruption due to elevated circulating catecholamines may lead to pulmonary edema.[42] The treatment of severe pulmonary edema with resultant oxygen desaturation includes use of a pulmonary artery catheter with measurement of the pulmonary artery occlusion pressure (PAOP) as a guideline for therapy. Elevated PAOP should be reduced to between 12–15 mm Hg using loop diuretics, after-load reducing agents, or a combination of the two.[63] Excessive hypovolemia must be avoided as it may lead to multiorgan dysfunction or potentiate clinical vasospasm.[36] Continuous positive airway pressure (CPAP) or positive end expiratory pressure (PEEP) are fundamental parts of the management of severe pulmonary edema. A CPAP mask and elevated $FiO_2$ may be sufficient to support a patient in mild pulmonary edema. Pulmonary support should be titrated to maintain an oxygen saturation of at least 93% so as to avoid a hypoxic insult to the brain. CPAP or PEEP may be used with relative impunity unless brain compliance is low with high intracranial pressure (ICP), as it may then result in further elevation of ICP.[23,42]

### *Hyponatremia*

Hyponatremia can occur in up to one third of patients following SAH. Impaired consciousness, seizures, and brain swelling may be promoted by low serum sodium concentration; therefore, early detection and treatment are required. Recent studies point toward cerebral salt wasting as being the primary cause of this disorder,[17,53,61] and not the syndrome of inappropriate anti-diuretic hormone secretion (SIADH). Such patients are typically hypovolemic, therefore fluid restriction is *not* an appropriate treatment to correct the low sodium. Rather, volume expansion with isotonic or hypertonic saline is very effective and has no untoward effect on vasospasm. Until hyponatremia is corrected, free water intake should be restricted, but not overall fluid intake.

## Neurologic Management

### *Prevention of Rehemorrhage*

Rehemorrhage following aneurysmal SAH is associated with a mortality rate of nearly

TABLE 2
**Commonly Used Clinical Grading Scales for Subarachnoid Hemorrhage**

**Hunt–Hess Scale**

| Grade | Neurologic Status |
|---|---|
| I | Asymptomatic or mild headache |
| II | Moderate to severe headache, nuchal rigidity, can have oculomotor palsy |
| III | Confusion, drowsiness, or mild focal signs |
| IV | Stupor or hemiparesis |
| V | Coma, moribund, and/or extensor posturing |

**Cooperative Aneurysm Study Scale**

| Grade | Neurologic Status |
|---|---|
| I | Free of symptoms |
| II | Mildly ill, alert and responsive, headache present |
| III | Moderately ill (lethargic, headache, no focal signs; or alert, focal signs present) |
| IV | Severely ill (stuporous, no focal signs; or drowsy, focal signs present) |

**World Federation of Neurological Surgeons**

| Grade | Neurologic Status |
|---|---|
| I | No focal signs; Glasgow Coma Scale Score 15 |
| II | No focal signs; Glasgow Coma Scale Score 13–14 |
| III | Focal signs; Glasgow Coma Scale Score 13-14 |
| IV | Glasgow Coma Scale Score 7–12; with or without focal signs |
| V | Glasgow Coma Scale Score 6 or less; with or without focal signs |

50%[48] and peaks in the first 48 hours of the ictus.[7,33,38] Clearly, reducing the likelihood of rehemorrhage would have a major impact on outcome. When possible, early surgery may virtually eliminate the risk of rebleeding,[29,46] reduce the incidence or severity of cerebral vasospasm by removing subarachnoid clots,[5,25,46,69–72] and allow induced hypertension as a means of treating cerebral vasospasm. Timing of surgery is a multifactorial decision based on the patient's general medical status, neurologic status (Table 2), and the aneurysm location.

Patients in good neurologic condition (Hunt–Hess Grade I or II), or those clinically deteriorating in association with an intracerebral hematoma, are usually treated with early surgery.* This may also be considered in Grade III, and even some Grade IV patients,[79] although surgery is typically delayed for most Grade III–V patients or those deemed medically unstable.

Prior to surgery, the patient remains at risk of rehemorrhage. A major focus of intensive care unit (ICU) treatment at this time is to minimize the risk of rebleeding. Efforts are directed at reducing the pressure gradient across the aneurysm wall (i.e. transmural pressure equals intracranial mean arterial pressure [MAP] minus ICP), and impairing dissolution of the clot that seals the site of previous rupture.

At hemorrhage, a marked increase in ICP occurs which may help to promote hemostasis.[28] For patients with normal ICP, keeping the patient flat in bed may reduce transmural pressure by maximizing ICP. If ICP is high and requires ventricular drainage, potential rebleeding secondary to overdrainage may be avoided by draining cautiously and judiciously, and only for pressures greater than 15 mm Hg.

Prevention of even brief periods of hypertension is paramount in preventing rehemorrhage[1,35,62] (Figure 1). Traditional measures focus on avoiding any stimulus potentially leading to agitation or excitement resulting in a rise in blood pressure.[13,34,54,60,68] Such patients are confined to bed in dimly-lit rooms with limited visitation and liberal use of sedation. Compared to unrestricted hospital activity, these measures can reduce the risk of rehemorrhage.[13,54] Autonomic suppressants such as lidocaine (1.0–1.5 mg/kg, intravenously) or methylhexatol (50–120 mg, intravenously)[59] are administered prior to procedures such as placement of invasive lines, intubation or suctioning. A potent hypotensive agent such as sodium nitroprusside or esmalol should be available premixed at the bedside to facilitate control of hypertension in these situations. General comfort measures

*References 4,6,24,32,34,46,47,65,66,68–70,72,80,81

also include mild sedation (phenobarbital 30–60 mg, qid),[13,34] dexamethasone (4 mg, qid)[13,34,60] which may minimize headache from chemical meningitis and brain edema, and liberal use of codeine or morphine for analgesia.

Appropriate blood pressure parameters following SAH remain controversial. In general, the systolic blood pressure should be maintained within approximately 5% of the patient's usual pressures.[13,35,60,62] In practice, we maintain the systolic blood pressure of nonhypertensive patients below 110 mm Hg, and hypertensive patients below 150 mm Hg.[13] Unless contraindicated, propranolol (10–20 mg, orally, tid, or 1 mg, intravenously, tid) is prescribed, as this agent is thought to have a "smoothing" effect on blood pressure, is cardioprotective, and may even have cerebral protective actions.[45,51,52]

Severe agitation in labile or refractory hypertension may require heavy sedation, or perhaps even anesthesia with paralysis and mechanical ventilation. Sedative agents thatmay be used in this setting include Versed, Proprofal, or benzodiazepines. Intravenous haloperidol (1–2 mg prn) may be particularly useful for episodes of psychosis.

Sedation may be temporarily withdrawn or tapered to validate the neurologic examination or obtain consent if the patient is otherwise stable. Even poor-grade patients are sedated as they respond to environmental stimuli with marked blood pressure fluctuations.

Rising blood pressure or the need for higher doses of antihypertensive agents may be due to increasing ICP (hydrocephalus or cerebral edema), cerebral vasospasm, or tachyphylaxis to or toxicity of the antihypertensive agent. When detected, these trends must be evaluated and appropriate action taken.

## *Hydrocephalus*

Obstruction of cerebrospinal fluid (CSF) outflow due to intraventricular clot may result in acute hydrocephalus in the hours or days following aneurysmal SAH. External or internal ventricular drainage is required; however

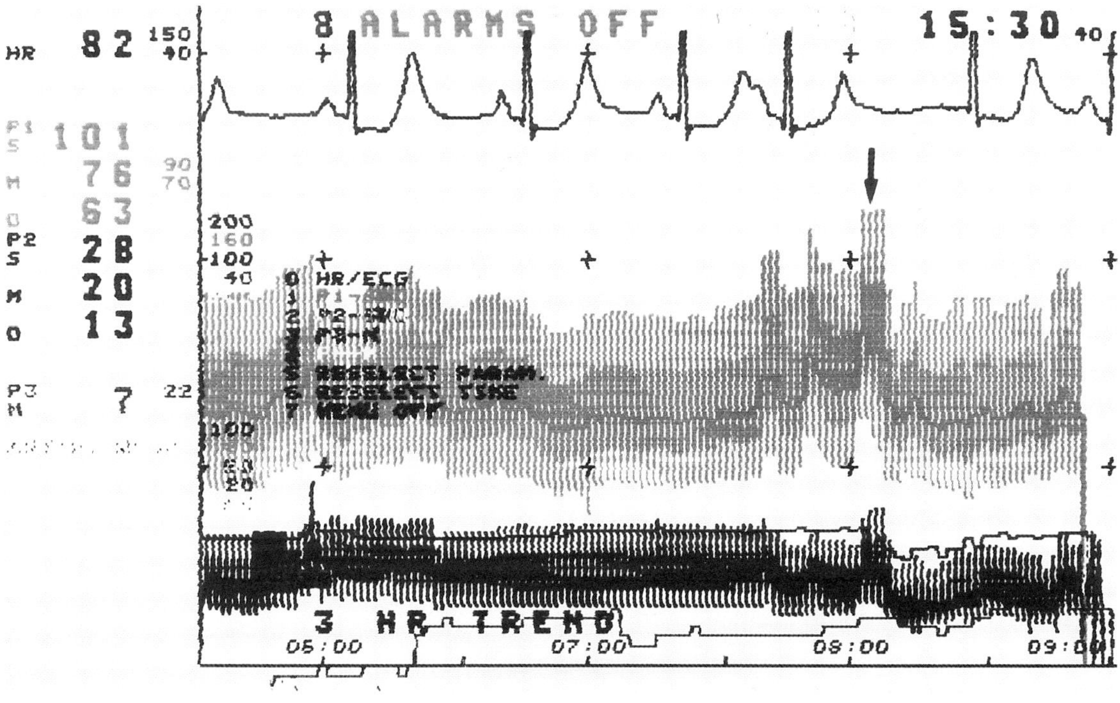


*Figure 1. Three-hour trend showing elevated systolic blood pressure (160 mm Hg) preceding aneurysm rerupture (arrow).*

catheter obstruction, requiring flushing or replacement of the device, occurs frequently. Use of thrombolytic agents to dissolve ventricular clots in this setting has been proposed but carries the potential for rehemorrhage.

Symptomatic communicating hydrocephalus may develop from days to months post-SAH. Early hydrocephalus may be treated with ventricular or lumbar drainage, often with ultimate resolution of ventricular enlargement. Late hydrocephalus, frequently associated with normal CSF pressures, usually requires placement of a shunt.

While the aneurysm remains unclipped, CSF drainage to treat hydrocephalus should be tempered by the risk of rehemorrhage secondary to elevation of the aneurysm transmural pressure.

## *Cerebral Vasospasm*

Angiographic vasospasm affects up to 70% of patients following SAH, but only about one third develop symptomatology attributable to this disorder. Clinical symptoms commonly begin a few days posthemorrhage, peaking by day seven and resolving over a period of weeks.[37,41] Symptoms include confusion, altered mental status, or new focal deficit unattributable to other identifiable causes such as hematoma, rehemorrhage, hydrocephalus, or metabolic imbalance.

Nimodipine prophylaxis (60 mg q4h, orally or by nasogastric tube) has been shown to decrease the incidence of symptomatic vasospasm and to improve overall outcome from ischemic complications following aneurysmal SAH.[2,6] Angiographic spasm does not appear to decrease significantly, however, and any benefit may be attributed to microcirculatory enhancement or direct cellular protection. Occasional pronounced hypotension or other potentially harmful side effects might outweigh the usefulness of nimodipine. Other calcium channel blockers for the prevention and treatment of vasospasm are currently under investigation. Early surgery may decrease the incidence of vasospasm by allowing more immediate clearance of spasmogenic substances from the cerebrospinal cisterns. Intracisternal therapy with thrombolytic agents or other pharmacologic manipulations might prove beneficial in the future at preventing or treating vasospasm.

Clinical deficits secondary to vasospasm can be ameliorated by improving cerebral blood flow.[84] Improvement of rheologic characteristics, oxygen delivery, and hemodynamic augmentation all have proven to be successful.[35,37,50,56,57] Early detection can allow prompt intervention which may minimize or prevent clinical deterioration. Transcranial Doppler (TCD) has proven to be a sensitive detector of vasospasm of major subarachnoid vessels. TCD is routinely performed on an every other day basis following SAH (Figure 2), with more frequent examinations performed in the event of clinical or angiographic vasospasm. Therapy is then continued until TCD hypervelocity has largely resolved.

## *Hemodynamic Measures*

Hypertensive therapy is the traditional approach to the management of cerebral vasospasm. While the aneurysm is unclipped, it must be understood that induced hypertension could lead to rehemorrhage. In this setting, the authors reduce the use of antihypertensives, allowing the blood pressure to rise by 20–30 mm Hg.[36] Since patients tend to become hypertensive in response to vasospasm, pressors therefore are rarely needed. If the patient has already had aneurysm obliteration, systolic blood pressures can safely be allowed to rise to 200 mm Hg or more.[26,36,44] Pressors such as dobutamine, phenylephrine, dopamine, or levo-ephedrine may be required to overcome spasm-induced ischemia.[26,36,44,58] When relatively pure alpha agonists are used to augment blood pressure, a renal dose (1–2 $\mu$g/kg/min) is added in an effort to protect the renal and splanchnic circulation.

Optimization of blood rheology and cardiac output has become better understood in recent years. The use of invasive cardiac monitoring such as the pulmonary artery catheter allows optimization of hemodynamics and,

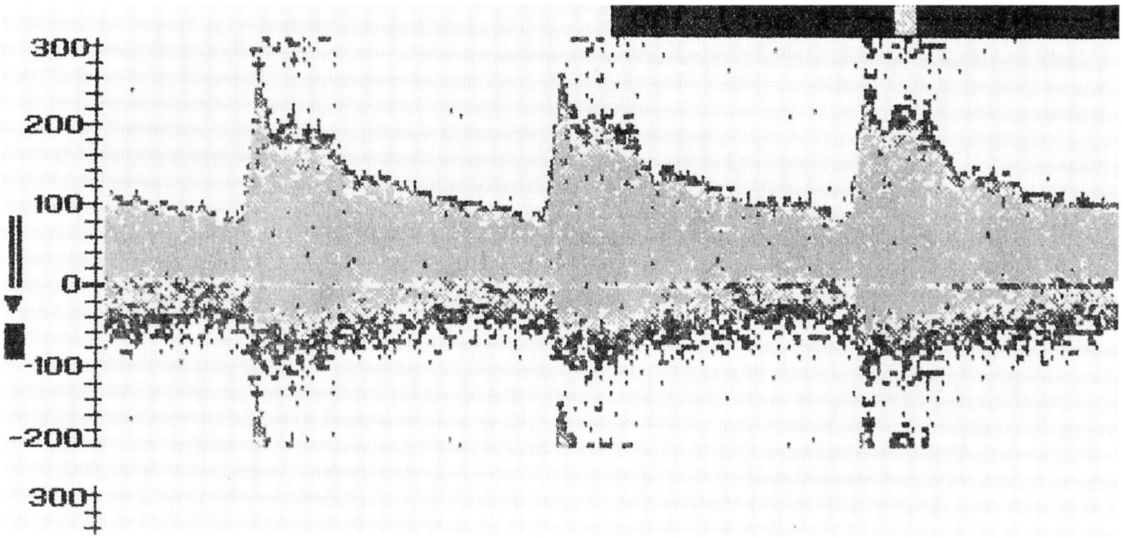


*Figure 2. TCD showing high velocity consistent with moderately severe vasospasm of the MCA.*

particularly, cardiac output. Following SAH, patients are typically hypovolemic,[2] a condition potentiating clinical vasospasm.[36,50,56] Returning the patient to a more euvolemic or slightly hypervolemic state (as determined by PAOP of 14–18 mm Hg) will result in improved cardiac output and cerebral blood flow,[36,57,76] possibly resulting in improvement of clinical deficits without artificially augmenting blood pressure.[36,37] Correction of hypovolemia may be achieved by the use of isotonic or hypertonic crystalloid solutions, colloid infusions, and/or packed red blood cells (RBCs) (if anemic), so as to optimize cardiac filling pressures and maintain hematocrit (Hct) at 33% to 37%, thereby optimizing blood viscosity.[29,50,75]

Balloon angioplasty has recently been used to mechanically overcome focal vessel spasm and improve distal perfusion (see Chapter 11 on endovascular techniques).[86] There is concern about reperfusion complications (i.e. hemorrhagic edema) with this technique, and also the risk of fatal vessel rupture by mechanical overdilation. Intra-arterial infusion of papaverine in the spasmed artery may be equally effective and much safer, but may require retreatment due to short-lived benefits. This modality currently is considered on our service for cases of progressive symptoms secondary to vasospasm despite the maximal medical measures outlined above.

## *Antifibrinolytic Therapy*

The CSF has potent fibrinolytic activity potentially leading to dissolution of the clot which seals the aneurysm. Therefore, another strategy to prevent rebleeding is pharmacologic blockade of fibrinolysis, such as aminocaproic acid (5 gm intravenous bolus, followed by 1.5 gm/hr infusion), which has been demonstrated to reduce the risk of rebleeding.[1,30,40] Unfortunately, this antifibrinolytic action may also potentiate the development of focal cerebral ischemia, hydrocephalus, thrombophlebitis, and pulmonary embolus.[7,11,39,40,68] As several studies have shown no overall difference in morbidity and mortality with the use of antifibrinolytics,[39,40,64] these agents are used infrequently, especially when the patient is treated with early surgery. Their use may still be considered with aneurysms that will require delayed surgery.

## *Seizures*

Seizure activity may occur in the immediate time period following SAH, potentially resulting in acute hypertension or mechanical stresses that may lead to rebleeding. For this reason, the authors favor use of prophylactic anticonvulsants,[10,68] such as phenytoin (18 mg/kg intravenous load, followed by 4–5 mg/kg/24 hours) or carbamazepine (200 mg, orally or p. r., tid), which should provide adequate prophylaxis in most cases.

Efforts to directly modify cerebral blood flow using pharmacologic agents have been largely unsuccessful.* Cerebroselective dihydropyridine calcium channel blockers, however, have proven to be effective in some animal and human clinical studies. Nimodipine is presently the only commercially available agent of this class. These agents are thought to provide leptomeningeal collateral artery dilation,[4,27] may improve RBC deformability, and have an antiplatelet aggregation effect.[4,15,27] The development of super-selective endovascular techniques is an interesting new approach to the mechanical dilation of cerebral arteries in spasm. At present, this approach is investigational, however, and not widely used.[86] Intra-arterial papaverine is currently being used on an investigational basis at several centers including The Cleveland Clinic Foundation, and the preliminary anecdotal experience has been encouraging.

An aggressive approach to the patient with symptomatic cerebrovasospasm usually results in minimal, if any, permanent neurologic sequelae, particularly if the aneurysm has been clipped, thereby allowing more aggressive hemodynamic hypertensive therapy.

## Conclusions

Optimal patient management following SAH involves close coordination of surgical and medical therapies. Recent advances in pharmacologic strategies having specific effects on the brain vasculature, and new developments in cerebral protective strategies should continue to improve the neurologic outcome of patients with this disorder.

*References 8,9,12,20–22,43,55,63,73,76,82,84,85

## References

1. Adams HP Jr, Nibbelink DW, Torner JC, et al. Antifibrinolytic therapy in patients with aneurysmal SAH. *Arch Neurol.* 1981;38:25–29.
2. Allen GS, Ahn HS, Preziosi TJ, et al. Cerebral arterial spasm: a controlled trial of nimodipine in patients with subarachnoid hemorrhage. *N Engl J Med.* 1983; 308:619–624.
3. Andreoli A, di Pasquale G, Pinelli G, et al. Subarachnoid hemorrhage: frequency and severity of cardiac arrhythmias: a survey of 70 cases studied in the acute phase. *Stroke.* 1987;18:558–564.
4. Auer LM. Pial arterial vasodilation by IV nimodipine in cats. *Drug Res.* 1981;31:1423–1425.
5. Auer LM. Acute surgery of cerebral aneurysms and prevention of symptomatic vasospasm. *Acta Neurochir (Wien).* 1983;69:273–281.
6. Auer LM. Preventive nimodipine and acute aneurysm surgery: heading for the control at complications after aneurysmal subarachnoid hemorrhage. *Neurochirurgia (Stuttg).* 1985;28:87–92.
7. Ausman JI, Diaz FG, Malik GM, et al. Current management of cerebral aneurysms: is it based on facts or myths? *Surg Neurol.* 1985;24:625–635.
8. Baskin DS, Kieck CF, Hosobuchi Y. Naloxone reversal and morphine exacerbation of neurologic deficits secondary to focal cerebral ischemia in baboons. *Brain Res.* 1984;290:289–296.
9. Bell BA, Miller JD, Neto NG, et al. Effect of naloxone on deficits after aneurysmal subarachnoid hemorrhage. *Neurosurgery.* 1985;16:498–501.
10. Biller J, Godersky JC, Adams HP Jr. Management of aneurysmal subarachnoid hemorrhage. *Curr Concepts Cerebrovasc Dis Stroke.* 1988;23:13–18.
11. Burchiel KJ, Hoffman JM, Bakay RA. Quantitative determination of plasma fibrinolytic activity in patients with ruptured intracranial aneurysms who are receiving Σ-aminocaproic acid: relationship of possible complications of therapy to the degree of fibrinolytic inhibition. *Neurosurgery.* 1984;14: 57–63.
12. Chyatte D, Sundt TM Jr. Response of chronic experimental cerebral vasospasm to methylprednisolone and dexamethasone. *J Neurosurg.* 1984;60: 923–926.
13. Crowell RM. Aneurysms and arteriovenous malformations. *Neurol Clin.* 1985;3:291–312.
14. Cruickshank JM, Neil-Dwyer G, Lane J. The effect of oral propranolol upon ECG changes occurring in SAH. *Cardiovasc Res.* 1975;9:236–245.
15. Dale J, Landmark KH, Myhre E. The effects of nifedipine, a calcium antagonist, on platelet function. *Am Heart J.* 1983;105:103–105.
16. Di Pasquale G, Lusa AM, Manini GL, et al. Cardiac arrhythmias associated with subarachnoid hemorrhage: prospective study with Holter electrocardiographic recording. [In Italian]. *G Ital Cardiol.* 1984; 14:323–329. English abstract.
17. Diringer M, Landenson PW, Stern BJ, et al. Plasma atrial natriuretic factor and subarachnoid hemorrhage. *Stroke.* 1988;19:1119–1124.
18. Estanol BV, Marin OS. Cardiac arrhythmias and sudden death in subarachnoid hemorrhage. *Stroke.* 1975;6:382–386.
19. Feibel JH, Campbell RG, Joynt RJ. Myocardial damage and cardiac arrhythmias in cerebral infarction and SAH: correlation with increased systemic cate-

cholamine output. *Trans Am Neurol Assoc.* 1976; 101:242–244.
20. Flamm ES, Kim J, Lin J, et al. Phosphodiesterase inhibitors and cerebral vasospasm. *Arch Neurol.* 1975;32:569–571.
21. Flamm ES, Yasargill MG, Ransohoff J. Control of cerebral vasospasm by parenteral phenoxybenzamine. *Stroke.* 1972;3:421–426.
22. Fleischer AS, Raggio JF, Tindall GT. Aminophylline and isoproterenol in the treatment of cerebral vasospasm. *Surg Neurol.* 1977;8:117–121.
23. Frost EA. Effects of P.E.E.P. on ICP and compliance in brain-injured patients. *J Neurosurg.* 1977; 47:195–200.
24. Fujiwara S, Matsubara T, Hachisuga S. Results of microsurgical management of ruptured intracranial aneurysms. *Acta Neurochir (Wien).* 1983;68: 227–237.
25. George B, Roux FX, Begue T, et al. Arguments in favor of early surgery for intracranial aneurysms. [In French]. *Neurochirurgie.* 1984;30:31–34. English abstract.
26. Giannotta SL, McGillicuddy JE, Kindt GW. Diagnosis and treatment of postoperative cerebral vasospasm. *Surg Neurol.* 1977;8:286–290.
27. Gioia AE, White RP, Bakhtian B, et al. Evaluation of the efficacy of intrathecal nimodipine in canine models of chronic cerebral vasospasm. *J Neurosurg.* 1985;62:721–728.
28. Grote E, Hassler W. The critical first minutes after subarachnoid hemorrhage. *Neurosurgery.* 1988;22: 654-661.
29. Grotta J, Ackerman R, Correia J, et al. Whole blood viscosity parameters and cerebral blood flow. *Stroke.* 1982;13:296–301.
30. Guidetti B, Spallone A. The role of antifibrinolytic therapy in the preoperative management of recently ruptured intracranial aneurysms. *Surg Neurol.* 1981; 15:239–248.
31. Hoff JT. Cerebral protection. *J Neurosurg.* 1986; 65:579–591.
32. Hunt WE, Kosnik EJ. Timing and perioperative care in intracranial aneurysm surgery. *Clin Neurosurg.* 1974;21:79–89.
33. Inagawa T, Kamiya K, Ogasawara H, et al. Rebleeding of ruptured intracranial aneurysms in the acute stage. *Surg Neurol.* 1987;28:93–99.
34. Kassell NF, Boarini DJ, Adams HP Jr, et al. Overall management of ruptured aneurysms: comparison of early and later operation. *Neurosurgery.* 1981;9: 120–128.
35. Kassell NF, Drake CG. Review of the management of saccular aneurysms. *Neurol Clin.* 1983;1:73–86.
36. Kassell NF, Peerless SJ, Durward QJ, et al. Treatment of ischemic deficits from vasospasm with intravascular volume expansion and induced arterial hypertension. *Neurosurgery.* 1982;11:337–343.
37. Kassell NF, Sasaki T, Colohan AR, et al. Cerebral vasospasm following aneurysmal subarachnoid hemorrhage. *Stroke.* 1985;16:562–572.
38. Kassell NF, Torner JC. Aneurysmal rebleeding: a preliminary report from the Cooperative Aneurysm Study. *Neurosurgery.* 1983;13:479–481.
39. Kassell NF, Torner JC, Adams HP. Antifibrinolytic agents do not alter mortality following aneurysmal SAH. *Stroke.* 1984;15:188. Abstract.
40. Kassell NF, Torner JC, Adams HP. Antifibrinolytic therapy in the acute period following aneurysmal SAH. *J Neurosurg.* 1984;61:225–230.
41. Kazner E, Sprung C, Adelt D, et al. Clinical experience with nimodipine in the prophylaxis of neurological deficits after subarachnoid hemorrhage. *Neurochirurgia (Stuttg).* 1985;28:110–113.
42. Kennedy SK. Airway management and respiratory support. In: Ropper AH, Kennedy SF, eds., *Neurological and Neurosurgical Intensive Care. 2nd ed.* Rockville, MD: Aspen Publishers; 1988:57–84.
43. Kistler JP, Lees RS, Candia G, et al. Intravenous nitroglycerin in experimental cerebral vasospasm: a preliminary report. *Stroke.* 1979;10:26–29.
44. Kosnik EJ, Hunt WE. Postoperative hypertension in the management of patients with intracranial arterial aneurysms. *J Neurosurg.* 1976;45:148–154.
45. Little JR, Latchaw JP Jr, Slugg RM, et al. Treatment of acute focal cerebral ischemia with propranolol. *Stroke.* 1982;13:302–307.
46. Ljunggren B, Brandt L, Kågström E, et al. Results of early operations for ruptured aneurysms. *J Neurosurg.* 1982;54:473–479.
47. Ljunggren B, Brandt L, Sundbärg G, et al. Early management of aneurysmal subarachnoid hemorrhage. *Neurosurgery.* 1982;11:412–418.
48. Locksley HB. Report on the Cooperative Study of Intracranial Aneurysms and SAH; section V. II: natural history of SAH, intracranial aneurysms and AVM based on 6368 cases in the cooperative study. *J Neurosurg.* 1966;25:321–368.
49. Mikolich JR, Jacobs WC, Fletcher GF. Cardiac arrhythmias in patients with acute cerebrovascular accidents. *JAMA.* 1981;246:1314–1317.
50. Muizelaar JP, Becker DP. Induced hypertension for the treatment of cerebral ischemia after SAH. *Surg Neurol.* 1986;25:317–325.
51. Neil-Dwyer G, Cruickshank J, Stratton C. Beta-blockers, plasma total creatine kinase and creatine kinase myocardial isoenzyme, and the prognosis of subarachnoid hemorrhage. *Surg Neurol.* 1986;25: 163–168.
52. Neil-Dwyer G, Walter P, Cruickshank JM. Beta-blockade benefits patients following a subarachnoid hemorrhage. *Eur J Clin Pharmacol.* 1985;28(suppl 1):25–29.
53. Nelson PB, Seif SM, Maroon JC, et al. Hyponatremia in intracranial disease; perhaps not the syndrome of inappropriate secretion of antidiuretic hormone (SIADH). *J Neurosurg.* 1981;55:938 941.
54. Nibbelink DW, Torner JC, Henderson WG. Intracranial aneurysms and SAH: report of a randomized treatment study, IV-A: regulated bed rest. *Stroke.* 1977;8:202–218.
55. Oba M, Mizoi K, Fujimoto S, et al. Effect of postischemic administration of mannitol, vit. E, dexamethasone and perfluro chemicals on cerebral ischemia. In: Setzler RF, Carter LP, Selman WR, et al, eds. *Cerebral Revascularization for Stroke.* New York, NY: Thieme Stratton; 1985: 267–274.
56. Pritz MB. Treatment of cerebral vasospasm. *Surg Neurol.* 1984;21:239–244.
57. Pritz MB, Giannotta SL, Kindt GW, et al. Treatment of patients with neurological deficits associated with cerebral vasospasm by intravascular volume expansion. *Neurosurgery.* 1978;3:364–368.
58. Ritchie WL, Weir B, Overton TR. Experimental SAH in cynomolgus monkey: evaluation of treatment with hypertension, volume expansion, and ventilation. *Neurosurgery.* 1980;6:57–62.
59. Ropper AH, Rockoff MA. Treatment of intractanial pressure. In: Ropper AH, Kennedy SF, eds. *Neuro-*

*logical and Neurosurgical Intensive Care, 2nd ed.* Rockville, Md., Aspen Publishers, 1988: 23–41.
60. Ropper AH, Zervas NT. Outcome one year after SAH from cerebral aneurysm. *J Neurosurg.* 1984; 60:909–915.
61. Rosenfeld JV, Barnett GH, Sila CA, et al. The effect of subarachnoid hemorrhage on blood and CSF atrial natriuretic factor. *J Neurosurg.* 1989;71:32–37.
62. Rosenwasser RH, Delgado TE, Buchheit WA, et al. Control of hypertension and prophylaxis against vasospasm in cases of subarachnoid hemorrhage: a preliminary report. *Neurosurgery.* 1983;12:658–661.
63. Rothberg CS, Weir B, Overton TR. Treatment of subarachnoid hemorrhage with sodium nitroprusside and phenylephrine: an experimental study. *Neurosurgery.* 1979;5:588–595.
64. Schisano G. The use of antifibrinolytic drugs in aneurysmal SAH. *Surg Neurol.* 1978;10:217–222.
65. Shephard RH. Ruptured cerebral aneurysms; early and late prognosis with surgical treatment: a personal series, 1958-1980. *J Neurosurg.* 1983;59:6–15.
66. Six EG, Clark JB, Early CB. Subarachnoid hemorrhage and intracranial aneurysms: a review of assessment and early management. *Milit Med.* 1983;148: 497–501.
67. Steinhaus JE, Gaskin L. A study of intravenous lidocaine as a suppressant of cough reflex. *Anesthesiology.* 1963;24:285–290.
68. Sundt TM J, Kobayashi S, Fode NC, et al. Results and complications of surgical management of 809 intracranial aneurysms in 722 cases. *J Neurosurg.* 1982; 56:753–765.
69. Suzuki J, Onuma T, Yoshimoto T. Results of early operations on cerebral aneurysms. *Surg Neurol.* 1979;11:407–412.
70. Takahashi S, Sonobe M, Nagamine Y. Early operations for ruptured intracranial aneurysms. *Acta Neurochir (Wien).* 1981;57:23–31.
71. Taneda M. Effect of early operation for ruptured aneurysms on prevention of delayed ischemic symptoms. *J Neurosurg.* 1982;57:622–628.
72. Taneda M. The significance of early operation in the management of ruptured intracranial aneurysms: an analysis of 251 cases hospitalized within 24 hours after subarachnoid hemorrhage. *Acta Neurochir (Wien).* 1982;63:201–208.
73. Tani E, Maeda Y, Fukumori T, et al. Effect of selective inhibitor of thromboxane $A^2$ synthetase on cerebral vasospasm after early surgery. *J Neurosurg.* 1984;61:24–29.
74. Thomas DJ, Marshall J, Russel RWR, et al. Effect of hematocrit on cerebral blood-flow in man. *Lancet.* 1977;2:941–943.
75. Tranmer BI, Gross CE, Kindt GW, et al. Pulsatile versus nonpulsatile blood flow in the treatment of acute cerebral ischemia. *Neurosurgery.* 1986;19: 724–731.
76. Varsos VG, Liszczak TM, Han DH, et al. Delayed cerebral vasospasm is not reversible by aminophylline, nifedipine, or papaverine in a "two-hemorrhage" canine model. *J Neurosurg.* 1983;58: 11–17.
77. Vidal BE, Dergal EB, Cesarman E, et al. Cardiac arrhythmias associated with subarachnoid hemorrhage: Prospective study. *Neurosurgery.* 1979; 5:675–680.
78. Weidler DJ. Myocardial damage and cardiac arrhythmias after intracranial hemorrhage: a critical review. *Stroke.* 1974;5:759–764.
79. Weir B, Aronyk K. Management mortality and the timing of surgery for supratentorial aneurysms. *J Neurosurg.* 1981;54:146–150.
80. Wheelock B, Weir B, Watts R, et al. Timing of surgery for intracerebral hematomas due to aneurysm rupture. *J Neurosurg.* 1983;58:476–481.
81. Whisnant JP, Phillips LH II, Sundt TM Jr. Aneurysmal subarachnoid hemorrhage: timing of surgery and mortality. *Mayo Clin Proc.* 1982;57:471–475.
82. White RP, Hagen AA, Robertson JT. Effects of nonsteroid anti-inflammatory drugs on subarachnoid hemorrhage in dogs. *J Neurosurg.* 1979;51:164–171.
83. Wilkins RH. Attempted prevention or treatment of intracranial arterial spasm: a survey. *Neurosurgery.* 1980;6:198–210.
84. Zervas NT, Hori H, Rosoff CB. Experimental inhibition of serotonin by antibiotic: prevention of cerebral vasospasm. *J Neurosurg.* 1974;41:59–62.
85. Zervas NT, Kuwayama A, Rosoff CB, et al. Cerebral arterial spasm: modification by inhibition of platelet function. *Arch Neurol.* 1973;28:400–404.
86. Zubkov YN, Nikiforov BM, Shustin VA. Balloon catheter technique for dilation of constricted cerebral arteries after aneurysmal SAH. *Acta Neurochir (Wien).* 1984;70:65–79.

# CHAPTER 5

# Anesthetic Management

Armin Schubert, MD

## The Neurosurgical/ Neuroanesthesia Relationship

In the early days of surgery, surgeons were solely responsible for their patients' anesthesia. Anesthetists, if present, were subordinate to the surgeon. As physicians developed an interest in anesthesia, the presence of anesthesiologists in the operating room became more prominent. Surgeons frequently resented this intrusion into their domain, however, and confrontations over optimal anesthetic management were common: when anesthesiologists, for example, began to introduce the use of endotracheal tubes, a good number of surgeons would proscribe their use.

While vestiges of animosity between surgeons and anesthesiologists persist to the present day, modern operative management has seen the development of a cooperative team approach in several specialized areas. Perhaps the most shining example is that encompassing the perioperative care of the neurologic surgical patient. Today, neurosurgeons have come to depend on the input and expertise of the neuroanesthesiologist to help manage patients both intraoperatively and postoperatively. Anesthesiologists specializing in this field have developed interest and expertise in the critical care of neurologic patients, frequently continuing their postoperative management. Neuroanesthesiologists and neurosurgeons are accustomed to maintaining a close level of communication regarding patient management, as well as collaboration in areas of mutual scientific interest and educational activities.

This special collaborative relationship began to develop with the need for operative management of intracranial aneurysms and arteriovenous malformations (AVMs).[108] Surgical success at treating cerebral aneurysms was made possible by modern microsurgical technique, but surgical advances in anesthetic management contributed significantly as well.[36,184] The close cooperation of neurosurgeons and anesthesiologists made possible the conditions of a relaxed, quiet brain for optimal exposure, as well as effective management of hemorrhage and ischemia. Further contributions came through the anesthesiologist's interest in neurophysiologic monitoring methods.

## The Preoperative Anesthetic Evaluation

In preparing a patient for anesthesia for aneurysm clipping, the anesthesiologist will focus on several points that become crucially important for anesthetic management. While a brief survey of concurrent medical problems is made, the main focus will be on assessing the severity of the intracranial bleed and associated cardiac abnormalities, particularly the possibility of concomitant myocardial injury. To properly tailor anesthetic intervention, one needs to know about the presence and degree of severity of cerebral vasospasm, hydrocephalus, and intracranial mass effect. To acquire an accurate picture of the patient's medical and neurologic status, it is necessary for surgeon and anesthesiologist to directly communicate their awareness of the latest diagnostic evaluations or changing neurologic conditions. Anesthesiologists must be aware of certain basic facts concerning intracranial aneurysms to appreciate issues in surgical management and to contribute meaningfully to perioperative care.

## *Evaluation of Neurologic Status*

### *Prevalence and Prognosis*

The prevalence of asymptomatic cerebral aneurysms by angiogram is 0.65%,[185] although autopsy estimates of asymptomatic cerebral aneurysm prevalence have ranged from 4% to 17%.[143] Drake reports that approximately 17% of asymptomatic cerebral aneurysms eventually rupture.[37] The incidence of cerebral aneurysm rupture is approximately 12 in 100,000.[125,130] Among neurosurgical lesions, cerebral aneurysms rank as a leading cause of morbidity and mortality. Peak age-related incidence is in the fourth and fifth decades (middle age), with women suffering about 60% of events.[143] Approximately 30,000 cases of ruptured cerebral aneurysm present annually in North America. Less than 30% recover without major disability, while about 50% of patients die from the first bleed or its complications; many ruptured aneurysms, however, go unrecognized. Only a little less than half are operated on. Overall surgical mortality is approximately 10%.

Conservative medical (i.e. nonsurgical) management of subarachnoid hemorrhage (SAH) results in a higher overall mortality (> 40%) within 6 months of the original hemorrhage.[115,152] Thereafter, the rate of rebleeding was 2.2% per year for 10 years, and then 0.86% a year for the next decade. Rebleeding carries a 78% mortality. These figures underscore the considerable risk associated with the nonsurgical conservative management of intracranial aneurysms.

### *Location of the Aneurysm*

Because the neuroanesthesiologist is concerned about both intraoperative and postoperative monitoring of neurologic status, he or she must have a working knowledge of anatomic relationships with regard to the intracranial vascular lesion. This will not only direct a screening physical examination, but also will help in planning intraoperative neurophysiologic monitoring.

Cerebral aneurysms usually arise at a cerebral vessel bifurcation. Most (88%) are supratentorial. They are believed to arise from anatomic defects in the vessel wall and are aggravated by hemodynamic stress. The most common sites[127] are the internal carotid/anterior cerebral artery (ACA) junction, internal carotid/posterior communicating artery (PCA) junction, anterior communicating artery/ACA junction, and middle cerebral artery (MCA).

Preoperatively, the neuroanesthesiologist will want to review the radiographic appearance of the lesion with the neurosurgeon and communicate any recommendations regarding perioperative neurophysiologic monitoring or the need for such special techniques, as cerebral protective therapy or rapid infusion devices.

### *Presentation and Severity Classification*

The most common presenting symptom is headache with or without loss of consciousness. Prodromal "sentinel leaks" occur in about 70% of patients who suffer a ruptured cerebral aneurysm,[37] and are frequently missed. Actual rupture of the aneurysm usually causes impressive symptoms (i.e. worst headache of the patient's life). Headache and associated neurologic deficit are caused by the increased intracranial pressure (ICP) that develops with rupture. In patients who survive the initial bleed, ICP normalizes as the aneurysm seals. However, damage from the first bleed may result in a spectrum of neurologic dysfunction. Hunt and Hess created a classification of cerebral aneurysms based on clinical signs and symptoms (Table 1)[57] that is useful as an indicator of overall prognosis as well as of surgical risk. Age, preoperative hypertension,[6,84] and preoperative neurologic condition (Hunt–Hess grade) correlate strongly with survival.[162] In addition, a higher severity grade alerts to the greater likelihood of concomitant intracranial hypertension,[168] vasospasm,[24] lower cerebral blood flow (CBF),[96] poor autoregulation,[159] and poor $CO_2$ reactivity.[97,169] Knowledge of a patient's neurologic grade is, therefore, invaluable to the anesthesiologist in devising a plan for optimal ventilatory and blood pressure management, as well as in assessing possible neurologic deterioration. Not infrequently, the anesthesiologist is the first person to provide a limited neurologic assessment on the day of surgery. Significant changes in neurologic status should be noted and communicated immediately to the operating surgeon. Deterioration may indicate rebleeding[167] or new onset of cerebral vasospasm, necessitating postponement of surgery. Furthermore, preoperative neurologic grading serves as a guide to postoperative evaluation of neurologic status, allowing the anesthesiologist to assess more accurately the need for interventions to distinguish between anesthetic and surgical causes of postoperative neurologic changes.

### *Recognition of Major Neurologic Threats*

Classically, anesthesiologists have been taught to think of candidates for aneurysm surgery as falling into one of two pathophysiologic patterns,[117] from which the priorities of perioperative anesthetic management flow.[143] In the so-called "ischemic-edematous pattern" of SAH (type I), an initial sharp rise of ICP above diastolic blood pressure is seen at the time of the hemorrhage.[116] ICP then promptly falls within minutes due to tamponading of the vessel and platelet plugging of the rupture site. Cerebral ischemia may initially produce seizures or a depressed level of consciousness, but neurologic function rapidly improves. In the first few days following SAH, the brain presents an "angry," swollen appearance in response to the limited fresh hemorrhage that, particularly in higher severity grades, is associated with cerebral edema. The latter may also be present if cerebral vasospasm has resulted in a large area of infarction. Priorities for anesthetic management are prevention of rebleeding, adequate brain volume control, and avoidance of conditions known to worsen ischemia.

The "hemorrhagic-compressive pattern" (type II SAH) is associated with a large initial hemorrhage that is not tamponaded locally. It then proceeds to intracerebral hemorrhage with clot formation, resulting in intracranial hypertension, frequently with midline shift. Cushing's response may be seen, and emer-

**TABLE 1**
**Hunt–Hess Grading of Subarachnoid Hemorrhage***

| Grade | Type | Perioperative Mortality (%) |
|---|---|---|
| I | Mild symptoms (e.g. slight headaches) | 0–5 |
| II | Severe headache, cranial nerve palsy | 2–10 |
| III | Drowsiness, mild focal neurologic deficit | 10–15 |
| IV | Stupor, severe hemiparesis | 60–70 |
| V | Coma, decerebrate posturing | 70–100 |

*Severe systemic disease (hypertension, diabetes, arteriosclerotic cardiovascular disease [ASCVD], chronic obstructive pulmonary disease [COPD] or arteriographic evidence of vasospasm places patient in the next less favorable category

gent evacuation of the hematoma, with or without clipping of the aneurysm, must be undertaken. The focus of anesthetic management shifts to immediate control of intracranial hypertension and maintenance of cerebral perfusion pressure (CPP).

Not all patients fit neatly into the above categories. It is important for the anesthesiologist to assess the contributing and complicating pathophysiology[167] of each case, as well as the patient's present condition, in order to prioritize management goals. In this context, one must bear in mind that, depending on the post-SAH time course, neurologic deterioration may occur secondary to rebleeding, vasospasm, edema, or hydrocephalus (see Table 2).

### Rebleeding

Recurrence of cerebral hemorrhage in the perioperative period carries a high morbidity and mortality rate.[9] Approximately two-thirds of patients whose aneurysms rebleed will die. The highest rate of rebleeding after SAH secondary to ruptured cerebral aneurysm occurs within 24 hours of the original hemorrhage.[58] The cumulative risk of rebleeding at 2 weeks post-SAH is 20%.[184] Prevention of recurrent SAH usually encompasses a regimen of bed rest, sedation, and rigorous control of blood pressure using oral or parenteral antihypertensive agents. Epsilon-aminocaproic acid was used extensively at one time to prevent clot lysis and subsequent recurrent hemorrhage. Clinical data, however, not only failed to demonstrate that antifibrinolytic therapy reduces mortality after SAH,[2] but also implicated it in increasing the risk of delayed cerebral ischemia.[54] Measures to prevent rebleeding of a ruptured cerebral aneurysm (i.e. blood pressure control, appropriate sedation, prevention of coughing) must be continued both in the immediate preanesthetic period and intraoperatively, prior to successful clipping.

TABLE 2
**Frequency of Major Perioperative Complications in Aneurysm Patients.[60]**

| | |
|---|---|
| Vasospasm | 27% |
| Brain swelling | 12% |
| Hydrocephalus | 12% |
| Rebleeding | 12% |
| Intracranial hematoma | 8% |

### Hydrocephalus

Arachnoid villi may become obstructed following SAH, which leads to hydrocephalus in 20% of patients, which is usually accompanied by a subacute deterioration in mental status and treated with ventriculostomy. The presence of preoperative unrelieved hydrocephalus signals a potential for development of intracranial hypertension during the early phase of general anesthesia, and is particularly worrisome with posterior fossa lesions. The anesthesiologist may well wish to inquire about the appropriateness of ventriculostomy placement prior to surgery. The presence of hydrocephalus or other evidence of intracranial hypertension should prompt meticulous adherence to measures designed to prevent intracranial hypertension during induction of anesthesia, endotracheal intubation, and positioning (Table 3).

### Vasospasm

The term "vasospasm" is probably a misnomer. Although the vessel initially will go into spasm as a result of contact with extravascular blood (thus contributing to its own sealing), the later "spasm" perhaps constitutes more of a structural change in the blood vessel (i.e. a vasculopathy exacerbated by fibrin deposition and wall thickening) than a readily reversible "vasoconstriction." Therefore, vasospasm is also referred to as "delayed cerebral ischemia." Because the presence of significant cerebral vasospasm requires certain adjustments in anesthetic management, it is important for the anesthesiologist to be aware of its presentation and treatment. It is also incumbent upon the surgeon to communicate the presence of significant spasm to the anes-

TABLE 3
**Strategies to Prevent Increases in Intracranial Pressure (ICP) During Endotracheal Intubation and Positioning**

**A. Anesthetic depth**
- Adequate depth of anesthesia
- Euvolemia allows tolerance of adequate depth
- Need for "preventive" top-up boluses of intravenous anesthetics
- Potent inhaled agents not useful beyond 1 MAC

**B. Neuromuscular blockade**
- Ablation of train-of-four
- Adequate top-up dosing with short-acting relaxants

**C. Blood pressure control**
- Cannot always be achieved with anesthetics alone
- Keep near low end of patient's preoperative range
- Assume CBF is pressure passive
- Stop laryngoscopy if blood pressure rises above 10 mm Hg
- Administer top-up dose prior to next attempt at laryngoscopy
- Use vasodepressors that do not dilate cerebral vessels (esmolol, labetalol)

**D. Ventilation**
- Adequate hypocarbia ($PaCO_2$: 27–33 mm Hg)
- End-tidal $PCO_2$ can severely underestimate $PaCO_2$
- Confirm $PaCO_2$ by blood gas analysis
- Avoid hypoxia-related cerebral vasodilation

thesiologist so that appropriate hemodynamic and ventilatory care can be planned.

Typically, vasospasm presents as a subacute deterioration in the patient's mental status, with or without neurologic deficit. It is seen in approximately 30% to 40% of patients admitted with SAH;[54,62] usually, it begins 24–72 hours post-SAH, peaks on days 6–8, and resolves by about the 12th day.[173] Vasospasm is probably due to breakdown of erythrocytes in the subarachnoid space with release of vasoactive substances such as serotonin, prostaglandins, catecholamines, and breakdown products of hemoglobin. It is radiographically identifiable, with the most prominentspasm occurring in the larger cerebral vessels. Grubb and colleagues[50] found significantly decreased CBF and cerebral metabolic rate of oxygen ($CMRO_2$) in patients with SAH, although cerebral blood volume (CBV) was significantly increased. These results imply that cerebral vasospasm occurs mainly in the large, radiographically visible extraparenchymal vessels, accompanied by compensatory vasodilation of intraparenchymal vessels. It is estimated that up to 80% of patients suffering an SAH will demonstrate angiographic evidence of vasospasm.[60] Only 17% to 30% develop ischemic neurologic deficits attributable to the vasospasm, however, since critical CBF reduction may not occur despite arteriographic changes.

The treatment of cerebral vasospasm currently involves administration of calcium channel blockers specific for cerebral vessels hypervolemic, hemodilutive, hypertensive therapy, in addition to general supportive intensive care measures. Each modality has implications for anesthetic management of patients undergoing aneurysm clipping. As reviewed by Wilkins,[182] many agents have been administered in an attempt to both prevent and attenuate cerebral vasospasm, but to date, the only drugs showing promise are centrally active calcium entry blockers. Nimodipine and nicardipine cross the blood-brain barrier and block influx of extracellular calcium, a primary source of calcium ions for cerebral arteries. In the study by Allen et al,[5] 10 of 60 patients without nimodipine treatment developed neurologic deficit, versus 5 of 56 patients treated with nimodipine, and only 1 of those patients developed a "severe" deficit. Their conclusion was that nimodipine prevents the occurrence of severe vasospasm, rather than attenuating the severity of vasospasm. Furthermore, Ljunggren et al[83] treated 60 patients suffering from SAH secondary to ruptured cerebral aneurysm with early surgery (less than 72 hours) plus postoperative intravenous nimodipine, and reported a 3% incidence of postoperative fixed neurologic deficit, compared to a 13% incidence of postoperative fixed neurologic deficit in patients treated with early surgery but no nimodipine. Interestingly, the incidence of angiographically identifiable vasospasm was similar in both groups, implying that nimodipine may exert its effects primarily on the smaller cerebral vessels. Pial vessel dilatation is frequently observed at operation in patients treated with nimodipine.[151]

The effects of nimodipine on intraoperative hemodynamics and anesthetic requirements consist of a minimal decrease in the systolic blood pressure postintubation and prior to incision.[150,151] There was no difference in overall volatile anesthetic requirement between patients who had received nimodipine and those who had not. The cardiovascular effects of nimodipine and nicardipine consist primarily of a modest reduction in blood pressure (by 10% to 20%), an important decrease (50%) in systemic vascular resistance, and a corresponding increase in cardiac output. Warner et al[171] reported no major untoward effects during the intraoperative management of 13 patients treated with nicardipine. However, nicardipine-treated patients required more fluids and less supplemental isoflurane.

Several studies have shown that induced hypervolemia and hypertension may reverse neurologic deficit caused by vasospasm-induced cerebral ischemia. Kassell, Peerless, et al[61] expanded intravascular volume with whole blood or packed red cells to raise the pulmonary capillary wedge pressure to 18–20 mm Hg. If no improvement was noted, a vasopressor or an inotrope (norepinephrine, dopamine, or dobutamine) was added and titrated against neurologic condition with a maximal systolic arterial pressure to 240 mm Hg (mean arterial pressure [MAP] 150), or a maximal systolic pressure of 160 mm Hg if the aneurysm was not obliterated. Of 58 patients, 43 improved, 9 were unchanged, and 6 deteriorated. Other investigators also observed a salutary neurologic response to hypervolemic hemodilution and hypertension in patients with cerebral vasospasm[8] and even used hypervolemia prophylactically after aneurysm clipping with encouraging results.[146]

The anesthesiologist may care for patients treated with this so-called "triple H" therapy (hypertension, hemodilution, and hypervolemia) and therefore needs to be familiar with possible resultant complications. In the face of impaired autoregulation (cerebral vasomotor paralysis), hypertension may produce vasogenic edema,[25] intracranial hypertension, and hemorrhagic cerebral infarct. Rebleeding from an unclipped cerebral aneurysm may also occur. While these problems exist theoretically, hypervolemic hypertensive therapy is widely utilized after aneurysm clipping, and has been shown to result in a sustained elevation of CBF.[122] Some patients will be able to tolerate the increase in ICP if hypervolemic and/or hypertensive therapy is utilized, while others with diminished intracranial compliance from brain swelling and/or cerebral edema may not. Because this mode of therapy is frequently associated with fluid overload and high-pressure pulmonary edema, especially in patients with limited myocardial reserve, close monitoring of cardiac performance is advisable, such as the monitoring of pulmonary artery occlusion pressure and cardiac output.

### *Timing of Surgical Intervention*

The two most feared complications of ruptured cerebral aneurysm are rebleeding from the aneurysm and cerebral vasospasm. Conservative management is not generally a viable option, so that timing of surgery becomes crucial. Surgical strategy has evolved to optimize the time of aneurysm clipping in an effort to minimize either complication. Definitive surgery has been proposed both "early" (up to 72 hours post-SAH) and "late" (greater than 10 days post-SAH), after resolution of vasospasm. Whether the anesthesiologist practices with surgeons who operate "early" or "late," understanding the advantages and drawbacks of each approach will optimize surgical operating conditions and patient safety.

Advantages of early surgery include decreased probability of rebleeding with an associated 70% to 80% fatality rate, reduced severity of vasospasm secondary to intraoperative removal of subarachnoid blood and breakdown products felt to cause vasospasm, and the relative safety of treating vasospasm with postoperative blood pressure elevation without concern for rerupture. A major disadvantage is the presence of a red, swollen brain, which makes surgical exposure and aneurysm clipping technically difficult. Late surgery affords better surgical conditions, but rebleeding and vasospasm are more likely to occur in the interim. Furthermore, conservative therapy includes bed rest, sedation, antihypertensive therapy, and antifibrinolytic therapy, all of which can be associated with further complications (fluid depletion, deep vein thrombosis, drug interactions, epsilon aminocaproic acid-exacerbated vasospasm).

Management mortality includes preoperative as well as postoperative mortality. Patients in Hunt–Hess Grades I and II have essentially the same mortality regardless of the time of operation. For patients in Grades III and IV, operative mortality decreases with time, while management mortality rises dramatically, implying that, as time progresses, patients in Grades III and IV die before surgery, presumably due to rebleeding and vasospasm. A review of the literature shows that many studies are flawed either because patients who are "too sick" for surgery are excluded, or because those who die preoperatively are not counted in the mortality statistics. It appears that while postoperative mortality may be somewhat reduced by operating "late," management mortality rises sharply during the preoperative period.[120] The anesthesiologist can therefore expect to encounter surgical practices which choose early intervention, as well as those in which late surgery is performed. It is the intent of this chapter to provide guidance in both situations.

## *Evaluation of Coexisting Medical Conditions*

### *Respiratory Status*

SAH can be associated with respiratory abnormalities from a variety of causes. The patient may have aspirated gastric contents during the initial ictus, and therefore present with hypoxemia and pneumonitis. Acute respiratory failure may result from aspiration and, in rare cases, from neurogenic pulmonary edema.[174] Assessment will include, at a minimum, determination of arterial blood gases and a chest radiograph. The severity of pulmonary dysfunction should be evaluated in an intensive care environment. Depending on severity, treatment may require supplemental oxygen and mechanical ventilatory support. Because of the importance of avoiding "secondary injury," such as may be caused by hypoxemia, hypercarbia, and the hemodynamic consequences of respiratory failure, early recognition and treatment of respiratory failure are imperative. When preoperative endotracheal intubation is deemed necessary (Table 4), the neuroanesthesiologist can provide valuable input and prevent dangerous hemodynamic fluctuations associated with laryngoscopy.

The preoperative anesthetic evaluation of the patient's respiratory status should include a directed physical examination, review of pulmonary history, and chest radiograph. If the patient is receiving ventilatory support, the ventilator settings should be noted. Special arrangements may be necessary to provide the same level of ventilatory support in the operating room (OR), as many OR ventilators cannot effectively ventilate patients who require high inflation pressure or minute volume, as may be needed in acute respiratory failure or sepsis.

TABLE 4

**Indications for Endotracheal Intubation Following SAH**

- Obtundation, with poor airway reflexes
- Intermittent upper airway obstruction
- Minute ventilation > 10 liters per minute
- Evolving aspiration syndrome
- $PaO_2 < 60$ mm Hg on $FIO_2 > 0.50$
- $PaCO_2 > 45$ mm Hg (acutely, unsedated)
- Need for ICP control

### *Electrolyte and Metabolic Abnormalities*

SAH can be associated with electrolyte abnormalities. Hyponatremia is present in 35% of patients following SAH,[180] and may represent either a fluid-deficient or a fluid–overloaded state. The now defunct method of "drying out" patients with SAH frequently resulted in a state of chronic hypovolemia, prompting appropriate secretion of antidiuretic hormone (ADH) with resultant water retention despite salt loss caused by diuretics. All too commonly, however, this hyponatremia was diagnosed as SIADH (syndrome of inappropriate ADH secretion) and treated with further fluid restriction.

During recent years, the concept of cerebral salt wasting has been described. Although its etiology is still debated, the concomitant secretion of atrial natriuretic factor (ANF) in many patients with SAH is notable. Unfortunately, the degree of hyponatremia does not correlate well with plasma levels of ANF,[34,136,] and a causative role has yet to be proven. Nevertheless, preoperative anesthetic evaluation should take into account the possibility of ongoing sodium loss and resultant relative hypovolemia, exacerbated by bed rest and diuretics.

Diuretic use may also result in hypokalemia, which should be corrected slowly if thought to be acute. Chronic hypokalemia due to long-term diuretic therapy requires large amounts of potassium because total body potassium stores are low. Unless digitalis is used concomitantly, chronically reduced serum potassium of as low as 3.0 meq/l has not been associated with a higher incidence of intraoperative arrhythmias.[166] When atrial or ventricular dysrhythmias are evident, however, serum potassium should be normalized preoperatively.

Inasmuch as glucose has been implicated in exacerbating central nervous system (CNS) ischemia,[75,132-134] one should endeavor to correct significant hyperglycemia ($>$ 200 mg/dl) prior to the operation. For this reason, anesthesiologists prefer not to administer glucose perioperatively, except to treat hypoglycemia. This practice, to which the author subscribes, necessitates frequent checks of serum glucose concentration.

Patients who come to surgery more than a few days post-SAH may be in a catabolic state with acetonuria and mild metabolic acidosis. Hypoproteinemia may result in diminished protein binding of anesthetics, thus requiring a downward dose adjustment. Alternatively, parenteral hyperalimentation may have been instituted. Preoperative evaluation should note type and condition of venous access. Recent subclavian venipuncture requires consideration of and evaluation for delayed appearance of pneumothorax. The presence of metabolic or electrolyte abnormalities referable to hyperalimentation should be determined, and appropriate plans for continuation or possible unintended discontinuation of hyperalimentation solutions should be made. In this context, it is again imperative to check the serum glucose level periodically and to have substituting solutions (10% dextrose) available for intravenous infusion.

### *Abnormal ECG, Acute Myocardial Infarct, and SAH*

Preoperative electrocardiogram (ECG) changes are present in 40% to 100% of patients with SAH.[91,149,172] They consist predominantly of prolongations in QT interval, ST-segment depression, changes in T-wave morphology, and prominent U waves.[33] Atrial and ventricular dysrhythmias are common, but pathologic Q waves are rarely observed. Patients with more severe neurologic impairment have a higher incidence of ECG changes.[91] During the same study, the incidence of intraoperative ECG changes was 35%, leading to a postoperative 65% prevalence of abnormal ECGs. Unless ECG changes fluctuated, they were not a predictor of outcome. Elevation in cardiac enzyme activity was not indicative of myocardial infarction (MI). It is noteworthy that in this study of 270 patients, no evidence of MI was documented despite the high incidence of perioperative ECG changes.

Because patients succumbing to SAH have been found on autopsy to have subendocardial hemorrhage, myocytolysis, and other cardiac muscle abnormalities, preoperative ECG abnormalities have given anesthesiologists cause for concern. Whether or not the ECG changes have pathophysiologic significance remains questionable. ECG changes, however, are not a good indicator of myocardial function. Yet, in an evaluation of concomitant electrocardiographic and echocardiographic monitoring, myocardial wall motion abnormalities appeared more frequently in neurologically sicker patients.[31] ECG changes accompanied echocardiographic abnormalities. Therefore, poor-grade patients with ECG abnormalities may be considered at highest risk for myocardial dysfunction. The possibility of acute MI developing in tandem with the progression of SAH exists, but it is very rare when measured against the high prevalence of ECG abnormalities in this condition.

When ECG changes occur in a nonspecific fashion post-SAH (i. e. are present diffusely in all leads), and are not associated with symptoms of coronary ischemia or hemodynamic instability, they can be considered insignificant. Surgery should proceed as planned. The vast majority of SAH-associated ECG changes appear to be benign and do not warrant postponement of surgery.[139] The postmortem histopathologic findings in SAH patients showing areas of focal myocardial necrosis reminiscent of "norepinephrine myocarditis"[172] may be associated with intense central sympathetic outflow that results from SAH-induced vasospasm to autonomic control centers such as the hypothalamus. Provided there are no contraindications, prophylactic administration of $\beta$-adrenergic blocking agents may not only be beneficial in preventing subendocardial damage following SAH,[112] but also may help control systemic hypertension and dysrhythmias.

The surgical team occasionally faces a dilemma in the patient who is scheduled for urgent aneurysm clipping but has a distinctly abnormal preoperative ECG. When the ECG shows changes suspicious for acute MI (principally due to the appearance of new and significant Q waves), further workup will be necessary.[179] Prolongation of the Q-T interval may predispose to development of malignant ventricular dysrhythmias secondary to subendocardial damage of the conducting system.[92] If a fresh MI is suspected on the basis of enzyme analysis or nuclear cardiology scanning techniques, it is prudent to wait as long as justifiable from the neurosurgical standpoint because the risk of myocardial rupture and malignant ventricular dysrhythmias is particularly high during the first 2 weeks post-MI. All possible steps to protect vulnerable myocardium should be taken if a patient with recent MI should, nevertheless, urgently require surgery. This may include a continuous assessment of pulmonary artery (PA) pressure, ventricular wall motion by transesophageal echo, and multi-lead ECG ST-segment analysis. In patients with an irritable ventricle, noninvasive methods to assess cardiac performance may be preferred, as PA catheterization can result in malignant ventricular dysrhythmias. Myocardial work should be minimized and nitroglycerin or other coronary dilators given prophylactically. Deliberate hypotensive techniques are contraindicated in this situation.

### *When Is an "Anesthesia Consultation" Appropriate?*

In certain instances, it is imperative that the anesthesiologist be consulted early to help determine optimal preoperative patient preparation (Table 5). Frequently, the "window of opportunity" for early surgery (i. e. time to development of vasospasm) is short, and efforts to optimally prepare the patient for surgery must be coordinated as expeditiously as possible. When the diagnosis of significant associated medical conditions is unclear (e. g. ventricular dysrhythmias, respiratory failure, hepatic dysfunction, new onset renal failure, MI, or unstable angina), the anesthesiologist and surgeon should work together to obtain a

TABLE 5
**Reasons for Obtaining Early Anesthesia Consultation in the Patient with SAH.**

1. **Severity of associated medical disease**
   - Unstable angina
   - Recent MI
   - Malignant dysrhythmia
   - History of recent congestive heart failure (CHF)
   - Severe bronchospastic disease
   - Bullous emphysema
   - $CO_2$ retention; severe COPD
2. **Uncertain diagnosis**
   - Dyspnea
   - Chest pain
   - Markedly elevated hepatic enzymes
3. **Unusual diseases with anesthetic implications**
   - Malignant hyperthermia
   - Porphyria
   - Depressive illness treated with monoamine-oxidase (MAO) inhibitors
4. **Unusual airway considerations**
   - Known difficult airway
   - Past airway-deforming surgery

satisfactory diagnosis and begin appropriate treatment. When the airway is in question (such as in patients with obvious airway deformities, prior airway-deforming surgery, or acute airway infection), the anesthesiologist should be consulted immediately since special procedures may be needed to prepare the patient and obtain airway control. Other conditions prompting consultation are a history or family history of malignant hyperthermia, porphyria, psychiatric disease treated with monoamine-oxidase inhibitors, severe hypertension (diastolic pressure ≥ 110 mm Hg), chronic obstructive airway disease, and significant impairment in myocardial function with poor exercise tolerance.

# Intraoperative Management

## *Semiurgent Early Aneurysm Clipping*

There is no evidence that any one anesthetic improves surgical outcome. Regardless of the particular anesthetic employed, there are a few important considerations to remember. These are:

1. prevention of rebleeding (minimize transmural aneurysm pressure);
2. facilitation of adequate surgical exposure;
3. preparation for intraoperative rupture; and
4. management of temporary ischemia.

Transmural aneurysm pressure, a variable equal to MAP minus ICP, is thought to determine the likelihood of rebleeding. In a patient with a ruptured cerebral aneurysm who presents for elective aneurysm clipping, the aneurysm may rebleed due to either an abrupt increase in arterial pressure or a sudden decrease in ICP. Theoretically, either mechanism could result in displacement of the clot that is plugging the aneurysm. Thus, it is of utmost importance for anesthesiologists and surgeons alike to avoid increases in the patient's transmural aneurysm pressure.

Arterial hypertension must be prevented during both the preinduction phase and the induction of anesthesia. This is done with the use of vasodilators (frequently, patients have been started on sodium nitroprusside [SNP], hydralazine, etc. in the intensive care unit). If mental status and airway are clear, adequate sedation is also indicated to avoid anxiety-related hypertension. Especially during the transfer to the OR and preinduction placement of invasive monitoring lines, blood pressure can quickly get out of control. Small increments of midazolam (0.5–1.0 mg) and fentanyl (25–50 μg) or sufentanil (5.0–7.5 μg) in conjunction with vasodepressors (esmolol, nitroglycerin, SNP) are appropriate treatment here. It should be noted that excessive sedation can result in hypoventilation and hypoxemia; supplemental oxygen should always be administered. Sedative premedications should be avoided in patients with severe neurologic grades (III and above) because of the increased likelihood of intracranial hypertension. Patients undergoing intracranial aneurysm surgery require direct arterial blood pressure monitoring to afford a continuingestimate of transmural aneurysm pressure. A central venous catheter is usually inserted to allow maintenance of euvolemia, especially when induced hypotension is contemplated. When computed tomography (CT) scan shows evidence of thick, subarachnoid blood collections, pointing to a high likelihood of postoperative vasospasm and ischemic sequelae,[2] placement of a PA catheter is warranted for optimal hypervolemic therapy.

Induction of anesthesia can be accomplished in many ways. After prehydration (Ringer's lactate, 6–8 ml/kg) and preoxygenation, the combination of sufentanil (1–1.5 μg/kg), thiopental (2–3 mg/kg), and vecuronium (0.1 mg/kg) generally allows intubation of the trachea without hypertensive responses. The author frequently administers these anesthetics by titration to blood pressure and heart rate, dividing the dose into several incrementally injected portions. Sufentanil can be replaced by fentanyl, 10–15 μg/kg. It is the author's clinical impression that sufentanil affords superior control of blood pressure. However, there exists a lingering controversy about its effects on CBF stemming from the observation that it increases CBF in dogs.[102] In situations where increased ICP is suspected (brain fullness frequently complicates early aneurysm surgery), the concentration of potent inhaled anesthetics (isoflurane, enflurane, halothane, and desflurane) should be minimized to less than 1 minimum alveolar concentration (MAC). When using such an anesthetic, isoflurane is preferred because of its salutary effects on cerebrospinal fluid (CSF) dynamics, lesser cerebrovasodilatory properties, fast emergence, and reputed capacity to act as a cerebral protectant. When elevated ICP is of concern, some would also advocate the elimination of nitrous oxide, a potential cerebrovasodilator. During the early part of the case, anesthetic management requires anticipation and prevention of hemodynamic stimulation accompanying endotracheal intubation, skeletal fixation, and periosteal retraction, all of which can markedly elevate blood pressure.

It is, likewise, important to avoid immediate precipitous hypocarbia. During induction, the patient should *not* be aggressively hyperventilated, because sudden hypocarbia may reduce ICP (and thus transmural aneurysm pressure) sufficiently to allow clot separation, thereby potentially causing recurrent hemorrhage. During positioning and the initial phase of the operation, "low normotension" is maintained, and a moderate level of hypocarbia is achieved ***gradually***. Precipitous hypocarbia is particularly hazardous when combined with systemic hypertension. Applicationof the head-pin holder is also associated with marked elevation in blood pressure. Various measures have been proposed to ablate this hemodynamic response. Although additional anesthetic in the form of thiopental, 2 mg/kg, or sufentanil, 0.3–0.5 μg/kg, may blunt the response, application of local anesthetic to the potential pin site is far more effective.[26,76]

Most aneurysm surgery is performed in the supine, lateral, or semilateral positions. Standard precautions for neurosurgical positioning are taken, including padding of bony prominences, assurance of adequate respiratory movements and avoidance of excessive head rotation and flexion. The endotracheal tube and anesthetic tubing is securely taped and routed to avoid unintentional dislodgment. When intraoperative cerebral angiography is planned, the anesthesiologist must be cognizant of the requirements for a sterile arterial connection site (usually femoral) and the work-space requirements of the neuroradiologist.

For maintenance of anesthesia, a continuous infusion of sufentanil (150 μg in 150 ml normal saline) at a rate of 0.20–0.5 μg/kg/hr, along with nitrous oxide (60%), oxygen, and low-dose isoflurane (< 0.5 MAC) is utilized frequently at the author's institution. However, fentanyl or even alfentanil may be substituted. When an opioid infusion is used, the infusion rate should be matched to the level of surgical stimulation. In particular, after dural incision, the infused amount should be titrated to the lowest feasible level to avoid large cumulative opioid doses. A recent evaluation of these three synthetic narcotics during craniotomy revealed no differences with respect to brain relaxation and time to awakening.[47]

Patients receiving alfentanil, however, required more vasopressor to maintain blood pressure prior to intubation. The rationale for opioid supplementation is a reduction in the requirements for inhalation anesthesia, better operating conditions,[16] and facilitation of emergence.[109] After dural incision, ICP is near-atmospheric and may be further reduced by use of a lumbar drain, which is placed by the neurosurgeon or anesthesiologist after induction of anesthesia and initially clamped. Drainage of CSF is begun only after removal of the cranial flap. Hyperventilation can now proceed aggressively to a $PaCO_2$ between 23–28 mm Hg, along with the administration of mannitol, 0.5–1.0 gm/kg. Mannitol has been implicated in promoting aneurysm rupture by transiently increasing CBV,[137] and should be used with caution prior to dural opening (i.e. administered slowly over 15–20 minutes). Despite these theoretic considerations, facilitation of surgical exposure through brain shrinkage (via mannitol, hypocapnia) is extremely important, as the risk of tissue injury from excessive retractor pressure or uncontrolled aneurysmal hemorrhage is prohibitive.[4] If the patient has residual vasospasm or other evidence of ongoing cerebral ischemia, hyperventilation should be more restrained ($PaCO_2$ of 30–32 mm Hg) to avoid adversely affecting collateral blood flow.

Cerebral autoregulation and $CO_2$ reactivity are impaired for at least 7 days following SAH.[32,159] It is therefore reasonable to expect a diminished brain reductive effect of hyperventilation in patients undergoing early aneurysm clipping. Similarly, CBF may not be well autoregulated, further emphasizing the need for tight control of blood pressure to avoid cerebral ischemia or overperfusion.

### *Induced Hypotension versus Cerebral Protection*

In recent years, there has been a tendency to manage aneurysm clipping without deep induced hypotension. There is no clear-cut evidence that hypotension prevents rupture;[30] yet there are indications that patients who are managed with hypotension experience a poorer neurologic outcome.[49]

Techniques used in place of hypotension include simple tamponade as well as temporary clipping of the feeder artery. When temporary clipping is planned, one depends on collateral circulation to prevent ischemia. Therefore, blood pressure is normalized and oxygen delivery maximized (normovolemia, hematocrit (Hct) = 32–35, $PaO_2 > 100$ mm Hg). If temporary occlusion is likely to extend beyond 5–1 0 minutes, protection with barbiturate (sodium thiopental [STP]) is a reasonable approach.[93] It is in the situation of temporary, reversible focal cerebral ischemia that barbiturates have been shown to possess protective properties,[111] even when administered as late as 1 hour following the insult.[142] Generally, 3–5 mg/kg STP is needed to induce electroencephalogram (EEG) burst suppression. As other anesthetics are reduced or eliminated, STP is titrated in small doses to avoid systemic hypotension. Burst suppression will last for 5–10 minutes. If possible, the temporary clip should be released after 10 minutes, additional barbiturate administered, and the clip reapplied. Continuous EEG monitoring is helpful to determine the endpoint for drug therapy. Because hypotension is due mostly to inadequate vascular filling, information from a PA catheter can be invaluable for maintaining favorable hemodynamics. Therefore, the author often elects to insert it at the beginning of the case if the likelihood of barbiturate therapy is substantial. An important principle to remember here is not to sacrifice blood pressure for barbiturate therapy, i.e. ***an adequate CPP must be maintained!*** Because of its lesser tendency than barbiturates to decrease blood pressure, etomidate has been used in this situation as well.[10] This agent produces cerebral metabolic and EEG effects similar to those produced by thiopental sodium. However, the experimental evidence for cerebral protection with etomidate is less secure when compared with barbiturates.

If barbiturate protection is needed for a longer period of time, a full loading dose of

STP, 30–35 mg/kg, is necessary (administered over 30–60 minutes), followed by an infusion of 1–3 mg/kg/hr, again titrated to EEG burst suppression. If less than 20 mg/kg of STP have been administered during the case, it is generally possible to awaken the patient at the end of the procedure.

## *Delayed Aneurysm Clipping*

Although there is a trend toward early surgical intervention in good-grade aneurysms, many centers still adopt the conservative approach of operating late, i. e. after the time expected for remission of cerebral vasospasm (10–14 days). Preoperative evaluation of these patients must take into consideration the following factors:

1. Patients may be more severely impaired neurologically, either because of permanent damage from intense vasospasm or because of an initial presentation in a poor Hunt–Hess severity grade. Conditions influencing the anesthesiologist's management include hemiparesis (avoidance of succinylcholine to prevent hyperkalemia; and attention to the site of neuromuscular blockade monitoring), and cranial nerve deficits (need for postoperative intubation or tracheostomy to protect the airway). Furthermore, patients may be fluid depleted because of prolonged bed rest, diuretic and steroid therapy, as well as poor oral fluid intake. The anesthesiologist may need to take steps to optimize preinduction fluid balance and adjust doses and types of peri-induction drugs. Prolonged bed rest and treatment with antifibronolytic agents predisposes to respiratory complications and deep vein thrombosis, partially prevented by pneumatic compression stockings. An inferior vena cava filter may have been placed. Pulmonary compromise may be present and should be evaluated adequately prior to surgery.
2. Patients may have developed secondary complications from SAH such as hydrocephalus, residual cerebral vasospasm, pulmonary aspiration, and ventilatory insufficiency requiring high-pressure mechanical ventilatory support (see earlier sections). When a ventricular catheter or other ICP measurement device is present, surgeon and anesthesiologist must be in agreement with regard to the perioperative management of these devices. The dedicated neuroanesthesiologist has a working knowledge of the benefits and shortcomings of the major ICP monitoring modalities, knows the pitfalls and complications that can arise from each, and is able to interpret ICP waveforms accurately. It is imperative that the neurosurgeon communicates his concerns regarding such devices to the anesthesiologist in situations other than routine.
3. In an attempt to treat cerebral vasospasm, the patient's cardiac status may have been compromised through fluid overload or myocardial ischemia. Hypervolemic hypertensive hemodilution therapy is associated with a 7% to 17% incidence of pulmonary edema.[8,61] The preoperative evaluation should carefully address these issues, as the risk of anesthesia increases dramatically in patients with ongoing congestive heart failure, coronary ischemia, or recent MI. If any of these conditions are suspected, a cardiology consultation should be obtained, and preoperative monitoring of PA pressure, use of nitrates, afterload reduction, or inotropic therapy considered. In the rare case, postponement of aneurysm clipping can be justified on cardiac grounds. The rationale is to bridge the period of high risk for malignant dysrhythmias and myocardial rupture (2 weeks) post-MI and to decrease the risk of reinfarction (at least 6 weeks for all MIs, longer for nontransmural MI).[43] The mortality of patients suffering a postoperative MI exceeds

50%. Assessment of cardiac risk by nuclear cardiology imaging studies (dipyridamole thallium) or coronary angiography will be helpful in defining the risk-benefit relationship of proceeding with surgery. As much as 50% of vascular surgery patients with thallium redistribution (indicative of ongoing myocardial ischemia) suffered perioperative ischemic cardiac complications.[13]

When considered for delayed aneurysm surgery, patients ordinarily would not be expected to have residual vasospasm. Therefore, the need for a PA catheter to adjust cardiac filling pressure for vasospasm therapy may be needed only occasionally. Its use is still recommended in the patient whose myocardial function is more than minimally compromised. In the absence of cerebral vasospasm, induced hypotension is considered acceptable, although the surgeon may still opt for temporary occlusion of feeder vessels. The considerations for electrophysiologic monitoring of cerebral ischemic events and cerebral protection will also apply in delayed aneurysm clipping (see discussions in this chapter).

## *Emergent Evacuation of Intracerebral Hematoma After Subarachnoid Hemorrhage*

The patient who must undergo emergent evacuation of an intracerebral hematoma caused by aneurysmal rupture presents different management problems than the patient scheduled for elective aneurysm clipping. The overriding consideration here is ***increased ICP*** due to mass effect from the hematoma. Minimally acceptable preparation for anesthesia includes initial stabilization of airway and circulation, hemogram, electrolytes, coagulation profile, and cross-matching of blood for transfusion, as well as insertion of adequate intravenous and arterial cannulas. Some issues regarding cardiac and respiratory status may remain unresolved, but expectant anesthetic management usually suffices. Because of the emergent nature of the surgical procedure and the presence of intracranial hypertension, these patients are considered to have full stomachs and are therefore at risk for aspiration of gastric contents.

The patient is usually obtunded. There is evidence of mass effect on CT or magnetic resonance imaging (MRI) scans (midline shift, ventricular effacement, compressed basilar cisterns, etc). Cushing's reflex may be present (hypertension with bradycardia; sometimes hypertension alone) and may include respiratory arrest requiring immediate airway control. Efforts should be focused on permitting adequate CPP through reduction of ICP and avoidance of hypotension. Aggressive treatment of high blood pressure in the face of increased ICP may lead to further neurologic deterioration.[18] However, extreme hypertension may also contribute to further enlargement of the hematoma and reduced perfusion.

Timely airway control and mechanical ventilation may be life saving. Induction of anesthesia often is rapid, utilizing a combination of thiopental sodium, 2–5 mg/kg, opioids, and a larger dose of nondepolarizing neuromuscular relaxant (vecuronium, 0.25 mg/kg), while pressure on the cricoid cartilage is maintained to compress the esophagus, thus avoiding passive gastric reflux. Hyperventilation, mannitol, use of narcotics and barbiturates to reduce $CMRO_2$, and avoidance of volatile anesthetics are generally desirable. Cerebral perfusion must be maintained, and nonenthusiastic efforts to eliminate the patient's hypertension may actually reduce cerebral perfusion to critical levels. Depending on the location of the aneurysm, the surgeon may attempt to clip it at the same time as the hematoma is removed.[177] Massive blood loss can result from uncontrolled rebleeding of the aneurysm once the tamponading effect of the hematoma has been removed. Needless to say, these patients present difficult management problems for surgeon and anesthesiologist alike, and their prognosis is generally poor.

# Emergence and Early Postoperative Care

## *Selection of Anesthetic Technique That Allows Prompt Emergence*

The goal of the operative team is to allow the patient to emerge from anesthesia in such a way that neurologic status can be assessed immediately upon completion of the procedure. This is important for the timely diagnosis of neurologic problems requiring prompt intervention, such as clip malposition, intracranial hematoma, or vasospasm,[161] and surgeons and anesthesiologists must work together to achieve this goal. While the anesthesiologist selects a technique that allows smooth and timely emergence from anesthesia (see Table 6), the surgeon also contributes by providing updated estimates of the time required to complete the operation. This allows the anesthesiologist to tailor the administration of opioids, inhalation anesthetics, and muscle relaxants to the surgical requirements. Furthermore, the surgeon assists by avoiding excessive head motion and traction on the endotracheal tube during removal of the headpin holder and application of the surgical dressing. Care taken during these maneuvers can prevent stimulating a coughing spell, which would require administration of additional intravenous barbiturate or lidocaine, both of which can prolong emergence. The anesthesiologist's efforts to awaken patients promptly consist primarily of allowing sufficient time to eliminate volatile anesthetics and to reduce plasma concentrations of intravenous anesthetics so that the patient can awaken rapidly. This task is frequently complicated by relatively intense surgical stimuli towards the end of the case (i. e. galeal closure, head wrap), which require substantial anesthetic depth. A new, potent inhaled anesthetic may aid significantly in this respect: desflurane, a highly fluorinated methylethyl-ether related closely to isoflurane, has recently been released in the USA for clinical use. By virtue of its low blood gas solubility, it is rapidly eliminated at a rate matched presently only by nitrous oxide. It offers the potential for rapid and precise titration to even intense surgical stimuli occurring at the end of procedures such as craniotomy for aneurysm clipping. Yet it provides for rapid wake-up time with less postoperative sedation than seen with conventional anesthetic regimes.[44]

TABLE 6
**Components of Anesthetic Technique Facilitating Rapid Emergence**

1. **Choice of Anesthetics**
   - Avoidance of high doses of potent inhaled anesthetics
   - Dose limits on intravenous anesthetics
   - Termination of opioid infusions 45–60 minutes prior to end of case
   - No long-acting agents (e.g., droperidol) or opioids within 60 minutes of end of case
   - Use of short-acting anesthetics or those with high rates of elimination
2. **Adjunctive Measures**
   - Avoidance of long-acting premedication
   - Reduction of anesthetic dose for age and MAC-reducing drugs
   - Monitoring of exhaled anesthetic concentration
   - Matching of anesthetic level to surgical stimulus

## *When To Extubate and When Not To*

If the patient's preoperative status is stable and the surgical procedure has been uneventful, extubation at the end of the case is expected. Preoperative obtundation usually indicates continued postoperative endotracheal intubation for airway protection. Likewise, if the surgical procedure has been long and difficult (>12 hours) or if the surgeon encounters an unacceptable degree of brain swelling, many elect to leave the patient intubated and ventilated in an intensive care setting. Furthermore, during surgery in the posterior fossa, postoperative intubation may need to be continued if damage to the glossopharyngeal (IX), vagus (X), or hypoglossal (XII) nerves or their nuclei is suspected. Premature extubation following extensive brain stem surgery may result in airway obstruction or inability to protect the lower airways from aspiration. Postoperative mechanical ventilation does not preclude assessment of neurologic status. Appropriate sedation with short-acting agents such as propofol administered by infusion (25–100 μg/kg/min allows patients to tolerate the endotracheal tube. By terminating the infusion, the patient's underlying neurologic status should be evident within 10–15 minutes.

## *Hemodynamic Management*

During the application of the head dressing and during endotracheal extubation, maximal sympathetic activation may occur due to the relatively light level of anesthesia. Systemic hypertension can also be seen as a result of the activation of catecholamine and renin-angiotensin systems in the aftermath of induced hypotension. This hypertensive response is undesirable in patients with recent intracranial surgery and can be catastrophic if unclipped aneurysms are still present. Short-acting agents such as esmolol, and NTG, as well as the longer-acting combined alpha and beta blocker labetalol, can be used effectively to keep blood pressure and heart rate under control during this period.[110] The use of labetalol reduces SNP requirements dramatically following cerebrovascular surgery without apparent side effects.[123] However, approximately 10% of patients may show persistent hypertension despite treatment with labetalol and require additional therapy with hydralazine or SNP. Blood pressure should be monitored continuously in the postoperative period. This includes transport to the recovery area and diagnostic imaging facilities. Even if the procedure has been uneventful, postoperative vasospasm, cerebral edema, brain swelling, or hematoma formation may occur. For these reasons, most patients are monitored in an intensive care setting for 48 to 72 hours postoperatively. Intraoperative diuretic therapy and radiographic contrast material contribute to ongoing urinary fluid losses in the early postoperative period. Fluid therapy aims to expand the patient's circulating volume with crystalloid, colloid, or blood in an attempt to prevent postoperative vasospasm. Blood pressure is maintained at normal to slightly elevated levels. Nimodipine has become an important postoperative strategy for vasospasm prevention.

## *Emergent Return to the Operating Room*

Unexpected, new neurologic deficits in the immediate postoperative period require aggressive work-up, including cerebral angiography and CT scanning. Malposition of an aneurysm clip or significant intracranial hemorrhage can require urgent return to the OR. The latter indication may be encountered more frequently if immediate postoperative intrathecal injection of tissue plasminogen activation for prevention of vasospasm enjoys more widespread use.[40] It is imperative that surgeons and anesthesiologists communicate well during this period so that the anesthetic management can be adjusted to the pathophysiologic process at hand (temporary ischemia vs. ICP).

Despite the need for urgent control of the airway, one should resist the temptation to secure the airway without adequate pharmacologic preparation, thus avoiding detrimental hemodynamic intracranial consequences. Choice of anesthetics should take into account the virtual certainty of pneumocephalus (avoidance of $N_2O$) and the prolonged action of succinylcholine after recent administration of acetylcholinesterase inhibitors. Further consideration should be given to continued availability of blood products and the need for cerebral protective measures if clip-related ischemia is suspected. The need for postoperative mechanical ventilation after a repeat intracranial procedure also increases, and appropriate plans should be made to accommodate this.

## Special Topics

### *Intraoperative Aneurysm Rupture and Massive Blood Loss*

#### *Risk and Incidence*

The incidence of intraoperative cerebral aneurysm rupture varies from 5% to 20%. While bleeding can occur during any intracranial aneurysm clipping, certain factors make the occurrence of major hemorrhage more likely. Giant aneurysms (>2.5 cm diameter) are more likely to bleed, as are aneurysms located in the basilar artery (BA) territory and at the anterior communicating artery.[3,49] Quality of surgical exposure seems to be an important factor, therefore it is important that anesthetic management provides for optimal intracranial conditions that allow good surgical exposure.

Another important aspect of intraoperative aneurysm rupture and bleeding is timing. Batjer and Samson[9] reported on intraoperative aneurysmal rupture and found 3 likely times for rupture. Rupture of the aneurysm prior to adequate surgical exposure occurs only rarely (1% of all cases), but is associated with a high mortality (75%). When aneurysm rupture occurs during induction of anesthesia or endotracheal intubation, continuation of the procedure and emergent or "rescue" clipping are indicated.[163] Rupture in this setting is probably related to increased transmural aneurysm pressure either as a result of increased MAP or rapid reductions in ICP during induction or surgical opening. In Batjer and Samson's study, rupture occurred almost as frequently during clipping (8%) as it did during dissection (9%). During clip application, rupture and bleeding can be severe, as large rents may result from improper clip application. Neurologic outcome was better when rupture occurred with adequate exposure and during sharp versus blunt dissection. A favorable neurologic outcome after intraoperative aneurysm rupture is still only expected in 50% of cases. Overall, intraoperative rupture led to a 38% incidence of "poor outcome," compared to a 12% incidence in patients who did not have intraoperative rupture.

If the aneurysm is ruptured during the approach to the vessel, another technique that may be employed includes manual compression of the ipsilateral carotid artery. Indeed, the surgeon may include the ipsilateral neck into the sterile field for compression or ligation of the carotid artery to allow proximal control, depending on the perceived likelihood for aneurysmal rupture. For that reason, the anesthesiologist and neurosurgeon should agree preoperatively on an appropriate site for preoperative insertion of the central catheter.

#### *Preparation*

The amount and rate of blood lost during intraoperative aneurysm rupture can be impressive, approaching 1 liter per minute. Because of this, the operative team must be prepared to deal with abrupt and major bleeding in any case of intracranial aneurysm clipping. As it is imperative that one be prepared for rapid transfusion at all times, certain basic precautions are necessary. Preoperatively, blood should be typed and a cross-match obtained for a minimum of four units for the average adult patient, with additional blood held in reserve. Prior to induction of anesthesia, the anesthesiologist should ensure availability of blood in close proximity to the OR. When the surgical dissection approaches the aneurysm proper, many prefer to have the blood in the OR and cross-checked against the patient's identification bracelet so that it is ready to infuse instantly. Large bore intravenous access should be secured (in the author's practice, this includes two 14–16-gauge, short peripheral intravenous cannulas, as well as central intravenous access). Pressure infusion and fluid-warming devices, as well as appropriate resuscitation fluids and drugs should be immediately at hand. Appropriate fluids include isotonic nonglucose-containing crystalloid solutions, 5% or 25% albumin, 6% hetastarch, blood, platelets, and fresh-frozen plasma. It should be mentioned in this context that 25% albumin provides the largest amount of intravascular fluid expansion for actual volume infused. In a situation where intravenous access is tenuous and other fluid therapy is clearly inadequate for the amount of bleeding, 25% albumin is the author's choice until further intravenous access can be attained.

When faced with aneurysms at higher risk for intraoperative rupture, the author also keeps a rapid infusion device (RID) on standby. This roller-pump–driven infusion device is generally capable of infusing up to 1.5 liters/minute. It requires sheath introducer (at least #7 French) access to the circulation and must be operated by trained personnel to avoid mechanical breakdown or complications such as air embolization. To minimize cost, the disposable tubing for the RID is not opened until significant bleeding has occurred. The set-up time should not exceed 5 minutes in the hands of trained personnel.

### *Measures to Facilitate Control of Bleeding*

When surgical control of the bleeding site has been lost, deep hypotension (MAP 40–45 mm Hg) is induced emergently. The rationale is that a brief period of drastically reduced blood flow will allow the surgeon to regain control. While the effectiveness of hypotension to prevent aneurysm rupture has been questioned,[30] it is all too frequently the only choice once uncontrolled bleeding occurs. When emergently inducing hypotension in this situation, bear in mind that it is not the time to worry about possible contraindications. Even if the patient has ischemic coronary vascular disease, one may start emergency hypotension as a life-saving measure. If bleeding is not controlled, the patient will exsanguinate. Also, although deep hypotension is desirable to regain control of bleeding, it may considerably compromise organ function. This effect is compounded if a shock state contributes to systemic hypotension. It is, therefore, imperative to fluid resuscitate aggressively at the same time. In this situation, the ability to determine cardiac filling (such as with the use of a PA catheter) is a welcome asset. Hypotension can be achieved with either nitroprusside or isoflurane. Newman, Gelb, and Lam[114] studied the use of isoflurane for profound hypotension and found that the global cerebral oxygen supply-demand balance was favorably influenced with this agent. CBF is also maintained during nitroprusside-induced hypotension, but nitroprusside does not decrease $CMRO_2$.

In addition to or in place of inducing systemic hypotension, one can also attempt to cause "local" hypotension by obtaining proximal control. This may take the form of externally accomplished temporary carotid artery compression or temporary surgical ligation. While this may be effective in the anterior cerebral circulation, brisk collateral flow through the circle of Willis frequently can render the effort futile. Posterior circulation bleeding is not amenable to this maneuver. During the last decade, better surgical exposure and understanding of cerebral tolerance to ischemia have led to the practice of temporary clipping of accessible feeder vessels (see discussion under "Cerebral Protection").

### *Circulatory Arrest*

In some institutions, giant and poorly accessible aneurysms are repaired under deep hypothermic circulatory arrest.[145,147,148] This approach is ineffective in an emergency situation involving torrential bleeding. However, when planned in advance, the technique allows the surgeon up to 60 minutes of operating time without concern for hemostatic control. The technique is expensive and requires two surgical teams. Unfortunately, the side effects of extracorporeal circulation (heparinization) and rewarming frequently negate the salutary attributes of this technique. It is not clear that circulatory arrest actually improves outcome for these patients.[12] The anesthetic techniques for managing deliberate circulatory arrest for the neurosurgical patient have been described.[160]

### *Fluids for Resuscitation*

Blood loss may be replaced initially with dextrose-free, full strength crystalloid (preferably normal saline, as Ringer's lactate contains approximately 10% free water). Although hemodilution with crystalloid was shown not to increase brain water in either the normal[189] or freeze-lesioned brain,[188] it is the clinical impression of many that brain edema is worsened postoperatively following large-scale crystalloid resuscitation. The author, therefore, initially uses a limited amount of Ringer's lactate or normal saline ($\leq$ 3 liters) and continues with colloid or blood as appropriate.

The use of hypertonic saline for resuscitation from shock has resulted in less brain edema and lower ICP in an animal model of intracranial mass lesion[181] and in closed head injury.[41] In a group of pediatric patients with closed head trauma, treatment with hypertonic saline lowered ICP for at least 2 hours. The short-term effects on human ICP following hypertonic saline may thus be beneficial in volume resuscitation for intraoperative hemorrhage, since brain swelling can be exacerbated by large-scale fluid resuscitation. Despite its theoretic advantage, hypertonic saline is not in routine clinical use even under the circumstances discussed here.

When colloid is used, 6% hetastarch is appropriate but must be limited to no more than 20 ml/kg lean body weight. At higher doses, a coagulopathy may result. During the initial phases of fluid resuscitation, when blood loss exceeds the rate of possible fluid replacement, 25% albumin may be pushed by syringe in the hope of recruiting up to four times the administered volume into the vascular space from interstitial fluid.

During massive hemorrhage, blood should be administered either as whole blood or in component form. While existing data on large blood loss situations during battle trauma in healthy, young adults suggest the need for platelet and coagulation factor therapy following one exchange transfusion, clinically diffuse oozing is often seen at an earlier stage. It is the consensus among neuroanesthesiologists and neurosurgeons at the author's institution that traditional recommendations regarding blood component therapy may need to be modified for intracranial surgery, and earlier administration of components such as fresh frozen plasma and platelets can be indicated. Nevertheless, the operative team must utilize blood products responsibly to minimize waste and exposure to blood-borne pathogens.

## *Neurophysiologic Monitoring During Aneurysm Surgery*

Successful intracranial aneurysm clipping occasionally requires temporary occlusion of feeding vessels. This may lead to cerebral ischemia and permanent damage when collateral circulation is inadequate. It has been suggested that electrophysiologic monitoring of neurologic function may allow adjustments in surgical and anesthetic technique to minimize ischemic conditions. When such monitoring is used intraoperatively, the anesthesiologist should be considered a part of the monitoring team, as the selection of anesthetics and acute physiologic management of the patient may directly impact on the quality of obtainable neurophysiologic information.

### *Surface Electroencephalogram*

The difficulty with this monitoring modality lies in its inability to reliably monitor the area at risk for ischemia. Frequently, when a full array of surface electrodes is placed preoperatively, a number are lost in the area of the surgical site. Brain decompressive measures introduce air between the inner table of the skull and the brain surface, attenuating the surface EEG signal and leading to preferential acquisition of signals originating in areas of distant cortex (which is apposed more closely to the inner table of the skull). Most importantly, the surface EEG cannot effectively monitor subcortical ischemia, such as occurs when lenticulostriate-perforating vessels may be included in the aneurysm clip, resulting in ischemia to the internal capsule.

### Cortical EEG

Because of the disadvantages of the surface EEG, limited direct corticography using subdural strip electrodes has been employed.[187] During pterional craniotomy for anterior circulation aneurysms, single-column subdural electrode strips are advanced under the edge of the craniotomy and placed in proximity to the motor strip.

### Evoked Potentials

Symon et al[157] popularized the use of somatosensory evoked potentials (SSEPs) to monitor for brain ischemia with aneurysm clip placement. These investigators monitored median nerve SSEPs during aneurysm surgery for carotid and MCA lesions. They reported an association between transient postoperative neurologic deficit and prolongation of central conduction time (CCT) greater than 10 msec, and used CCT to adjust placement of aneurysm clips. Further observations from this group[156] indicate that temporary occlusion appears safe for 12 minutes or less provided there are no appreciable changes in CCT. The rate at which the primary cortical SSEP waveform disappears was noted to correlate directly with the severity of postoperative deficits. Landi et al[73] believed that persistent prolongation of CCT beyond 9.5 msec for more than 10 minutes is associated with neurologic damage. Buchthal et al[19] observed that neurologic complications were not seen unless the SSEP was lost during the case. However, once SSEP loss was evident, there seemed to be little tolerance for further ischemia, and patients developed either transient or longer-lasting neurologic impairment if temporary occlusion persisted more than 2 minutes following loss of SSEP.

SSEPs are more likely to detect subcortical ischemia (such as that caused by occlusion of perforating vessels) than surface EEG. They also represent a measure of cortical blood flow. Evoked responses recorded from the cerebral cortex have been used as an index of CBF in animals.[67,158] During induced hypotension, the amplitude of the SSEP decreased progressively with blood pressure below 60 mm Hg, suggesting that such electrophysiologic changes were related to CBF.[38] A further series by Carter et al[21] confirms the association of prolonged CCT with low CBF and poor neurologic outcome. Although SSEPs may indicate the likelihood of postoperative neurologic deficit, their utility will not be accepted until it can be demonstrated that interventions in response to SSEP changes are possible and effective. Schramm et al[140] addressed this issue by using SSEPs to guide surgical technique by adjusting retractors, removing temporary clips, and repositioning aneurysm clips. Likewise, Friedman et al[46] report data that are suggestive of improved outcome as a result of interventions prompted by intraoperative SSEP changes. When SSEP changes occur, the anesthesiologist can also intervene by optimizing cerebral oxygen delivery through manipulations of blood volume, cardiac output, perfusion pressure, and blood gas tensions.

Surgery for clipping of posterior circulation aneurysms may be complicated by brain stem ischemia. Brain stem auditory-evoked potentials (BAEPs) have been used to monitor brain stem function in this situation. Neurologic outcome is predicted reasonably well by BAEP behavior with intraoperative manipulation.[72,82] Friedman et al reports a disappearance of the BAEP components beyond wave I to correlate with poor neurologic outcome. Additionally, delays of wave I-V and III by 1.9 and 2.0 msec, respectively, were associated with postoperative brain stem dysfunction. BAEPs are more sensitive to brain stem ischemia during BA clipping than SSEPs, presumably because of the remote anatomic neural pathway taken by the latter. BAEPs and the ECG as monitoring modalities for brain stem integrity have largely supplanted the practice of observing spontaneous respiratory activity,[99] although some groups have renewed interest in and report benefits from this practice.[90] Monitoring for respiration during posterior circulation aneurysm surgery is cumbersome and may compromise the operative field due to brain swelling from hypercarbia. Spontaneous ventilation also increases the risk of venous air embolism.

Anesthetics affect both EEG and evoked potentials. The goal of anesthetic management is to minimize such influences and to provide a stable environment facilitating the acquisition of neurophysiologic data (Table 6). When monitoring EEG for brain ischemia, a relatively light anesthetic regimen consisting of low-dose isoflurane ($\leq$ 0.5 MAC) and nitrous oxide ($\leq$ 60%) supplemented by opioids and muscle relaxants is satisfactory. Bolus doses of thiopental and other intravenous anesthetics, as well as abrupt changes in ventilation and blood pressure, should be avoided during such critical monitoring periods as application of temporary clips. Higher levels of isoflurane anesthesia, with its profound EEG depressant action (burst suppression at clinically relevant doses), may obscure ischemic changes.

SSEPs are more sensitive to anesthetics than BAEPs. With SSEPs, similar precautions must be taken for anesthetic management as are necessary for EEG monitoring. The cortical component of the SSEP is reduced in a dose-dependent fashion by potent inhaled anesthetics (e.g. isoflurane) as well as by nitrous oxide. Therefore, the concentrations of these agents are limited to $\leq$ 0.5 MAC and $\leq$ 50%, respectively. The use of relaxants and opioids is recommended, as it frequently eliminates the need for bolus injections at critical times.

When the neurophysiologic signal deteriorates, the anesthesiologist participates in eliminating confounding causes of such a change by assessing potential contributory systemic factors (see Table 7). These include hypoxemia, hypercarbia, anesthetic overdose, and hemodynamic deterioration. He or she may also be able to assist the electrophysiologist in assessing effective stimulus delivery by checking lead placement, neuromuscular block, and extremity position. The occurrence of an EEG or SSEP change suspected to represent ischemia should prompt immediate action consisting of improvement in blood pressure and oxygen delivery, clip repositioning, or interruption of temporary clipping.

### *Motor-Evoked Potentials*

Motor cortex stimulation by either electric or magnetic means evokes an electrophysiologic response that can be recorded at the level of the spinal cord, peripheral nerve, and muscle (EMG). Recordings from the latter two appear to be most sensitive to the effects of CNS injury. Levy found a reasonable correlation of neurosurgical interventions and motor-evoked potential (MEP) changes, especially during operation on the brain stem and spinal cord.[78] MEP monitoring is attractive because it may yield functional information about specific motor pathways, rather than compelling the observer to make inferences about motor function from sensory pathway data, as is the case for SSEPs. Problems with MEPs include the potential for triggering seizures, extreme sensitivity to anesthetics (EMG amplitude reduction of $\geq$ 90% with volatile anesthetics reported by Haghighi et al),[51] difficulty with specificity of cortical stimulation, and the need to maintain only very light levels of neuromuscular blockade. Currently, MEPs remain an experimental procedure.

### *Cerebral Blood Flow*

Intraoperative cortical CBF measurements have been used to predict the safe period of temporary clipping. If blood flow is high, as much as 15 minutes of temporary clipping may be safe.[119,121] This technique is complicated by technical difficulties as well as the possibility of undetected subcortical ischemia induced by occlusion of perforating branches. Because of the potentially high risk for ischemic complications during aneurysm clipping, monitoring of cerebral function by electrophysiologic means should be strongly considered in all but the most routine cases. The cerebral territory at risk should dictate the type of monitoring (e.g. median nerve SSEPs for MCA aneurysms because the MCA supplies somatosensory cortex of the hand area; lower extremity SSEPs for lesions putting the anterior cerebral artery territory at risk). When such monitoring is employed, the operative team must communicate well to allow accurate interpretation of electrophysiologic events. For the anesthesiologist this means selection of a technique which interferes least with EEG or evoked potentials (see Table 7), refraining from making sudden changes in the anesthetic regimen during critical monitoring periods, and being aware of the differential diagnosis of EEG and evoked potential changes (see Table 8).

## *Induced Hypotension*

### *Changing Surgical Requirements for Induced Hypotension*

Until recently, neurosurgeons required deep levels of induced hypotension (MAP = 50 mm Hg) for substantial periods of time prior to and during the clipping of intracranial aneurysms. With the advent of more sophisticated microsurgical techniques, and the recognition that temporary focal ischemia may be tolerated when adequate protective and countervailing measures are undertaken, the technique of deep induced hypotension has given way to temporary exclusion clipping of the aneurysm. During the initial surgical approach, blood pressure is kept in the low normal range. During exclusion clipping, in direct contrast to induced hypotensive technique, blood pressure is normalized and even slightly elevated to improve collateral circulation. At the same time, the anesthesiologist seeks to provide optimal cerebral oxygen delivery by maintaining good oxygenation (usually $PO_2 > 100$), blood rheology (Hct = 33–35), and only mild hypocapnia ($PCO_2 = 30 \pm 3$). Although many recommend normocapneic ventilatory management during potential cerebral ischemia (i.e. dur-

TABLE 7
**Anesthetic Techniques for EEG/SSEP Monitoring**

| | |
|---|---|
| **A. Premedication** | Low doses of:<br>• Opioid<br>• Benzodiazepine<br>• Neuroleptanalgesic |
| **B. Induction of anesthesia** | Avoid large doses of:<br>• Barbiturate<br>• Benzodiazepine |
| **C. Maintenance** | • Isoflurane ≤ 0.5 MAC (with $N_2O$ 50%)<br>• Isoflurane ≤ 1.0 MAC (alone)<br><br>Infusions:<br>• Fentanyl 1–3 μg/kg/hr<br>• Sufentanil 0.15–0.5 μg/kg/hr<br>• Alfentanil 0.75–1.5 μg/kg/min<br>• Adequate neuromuscular blockade to reduce muscle artifact |
| **D. Critical monitoring period** | • Avoid bolus-dosing of IV anesthetics<br>• Avoid change in volatile agent concentration |
| **E. In case of poor baseline SSEP morphology:** | • Eliminate $N_2O$<br>• Substitute etomidate (infusion of 10–20 μg/kg/min)<br>• Steroid supplement needed with etomidate |

TABLE 8
**Differential Diagnosis of EEG and Evoked Potential Changes**

| | |
|---|---|
| **A. Technical factors** | • Electrode impedance<br>• Circuit integrity<br>• Stimulus delivery<br>• Radiofrequency interference |
| **B. Systemic factors** | • Hypotension<br>• Hypoxemia<br>• Hypercarbia<br>• Anesthetics<br>• Hypothermia |
| **C. Neurologic factors** | • CNS ischemia<br>• Pneumocephalus<br>• Peripheral nerve ischemia/compression |

ing carotid endarterectomy),[88] the disadvantage of completely normalizing $PCO_2$ (i. e. deteriorating surgical exposure) outweighs the theoretic advantage of normocapnia. There is evidence that responsiveness of the cerebral circulation to carbon dioxide is at least partially preserved during induced hypotension.[138]

There are, however, situations that still require substantial reductions in blood pressure either on an elective or emergent basis. The neuroanesthesiologist should therefore be quite familiar with hypotensive techniques and be prepared to induce hypotension safely, effectively, and reversibly.

### *Safety and Contraindications*

The safety of induced hypotension is probably greater[56] than the overall morbidity and mortality rate of 3.2% indicated in early studies.[52] The principal components of such morbidity related to organ ischemia and late bleeding. Coronary, cerebral, and retinal artery thrombosis were reported in addition to renal insufficiency.[79] However, improvements in monitoring, drugs, and postoperative care are felt to result in a lower complication rate today.[104] Ischemic organ disease, be it cardiac, cerebrovascular, renal, or hepatic, is an important, yet still relative, contraindication to the use of *elective* hypotensive technique. Other obvious contraindications to elective induced hypotension include concomitant intracranial hypertension, significant cerebral vasospasm, and recent MI or stroke. On the other hand, the anesthesiologist must be prepared to induce hypotension *emergently* should the surgeon lose control of the circulation during catastrophic aneurysm rupture. Induced hypotension with simultaneous aggressive fluid resuscitation will then be the patient's only chance for survival, as the surgeon must be able to regain control of the bleeding site. Pre-existing hypertension does not represent an absolute contraindication to induced hypotension. However, the anesthesiologist and neurosurgeon should agree on a target level of blood pressure reduction based on the severity of the patient's hypertensive state prior to the surgical procedure. Under these circumstances, a blood pressure reduction of 30% from the preoperative baseline state is generally considered safe.[12] During deep induced hypotension, ventilation should be adjusted to approach normocarbia, as hypocarbia combined with hypotension may potentiate ischemic risks.[53]

### *Techniques for Induced Hypotension*

A multitude of techniques for inducing elective hypotension has been reported in the literature. More important than any specific technique should be the realization that appropriately induced hypotension is achieved through vasodilation of the periphery with maintenance of filling pressure, intravascular volume, and cardiac output, which usually increases. In no case should hypotension be brought about by hypovolemia or measures that resemble a shock state. In practice, there are a few techniques that are commonly used for the purpose of inducing hypotension during aneurysm clippings.

Lam and Gelb[71] studied the use of intermediate levels of isoflurane anesthesia (up to 2-MAC isoflurane-inspired concentration). Under these conditions, isoflurane provides a stable, easily reversed state of induced hypotension that is characterized by EEG burst suppression with depressed $CMRO_2$ and a reduction or maintenance of baseline CBF.[86] At the same time, it provides clinically excellent operative conditions without brain swelling.[71] Cardiac output remains unchanged while systemic vascular resistance decreases at stable filling pressures. In primates, isoflurane causes a dose-dependent abolition of CBF autoregulation, which persists up to 100 minutes following discontinuation.[165] Although a very controversial issue,[170] protective effects of isoflurane are felt by some to result from its cerebral metabolic suppressant effects.

Another widely used technique for induced hypotension consists of the administration of SNP by continuous infusion. SNP-induced hypotension activates the sympathetic and renin-angiotensin systems.[65] This technique frequently requires supplementation by either preoperative (propranolol, 20–60 mg, PO q 6 hs), intraoperative beta adrenergic blockade,[64] or preoperative therapy with an angiotensin-converting enzyme (ACE) inhibitor such as captopril, 3 mg/kg, PO.[186] Beta blockade and ACE inhibition also help prevent the rebound hypertension associated with termination of SNP therapy, since they reduce renin-angiotensin system output.[105] When not otherwise contraindicated, propranolol also can be titrated intraoperatively to a heart rate of 60–80 beats per minute. In cardiovascularly robust individuals, the initial dose can be 1 mg, repeated up to 0.1 mg/kg. Dose should be halved for older or debilitated patients. Beta blockade is contraindicated in patients with poor myocardial function and bronchospastic disease. The advantages of this technique are the potency and reliability of SNP in reducing blood pressure, its short half-life and easy reversibility, the large clinical experience accumulated with this agent, and the lack of cardiovascular depressant effect. Potential disadvantages include the possibility of adverse blood flow redistribution in the myocardium resulting in subendocardial ischemia,[45] as well as shunting of blood flow in the pulmonary circulation with resultant increases in shunt fraction. Furthermore, reflex tachycardia, insidious vasodilation and swelling of the cerebral vasculature,[164] rebound hypertension,[28] and extreme sensitivity to the agent in hypovolemic states may also occur. In patients with significant coronary ischemic disease, the sole use of SNP is less than ideal. In this situation the author prefers to use nitroglycerin supplemented with beta blocker therapy and isoflurane. Prolonged administration of high doses of SNP ($> 8$ mg/kg/min) can result in toxic blood levels of cyanide ($> 100$ mg/dl) and thiocyanate ($> 10$ mg/dl). The hallmark of cyanide toxicity is the inability of tissues to utilize oxygen. It is recognized by increasing tachyphylaxis and metabolic lactic acidosis with high central venous $PO_2$. Treatment with intravenous thiosulfate (150 mg/kg) and/or sodium nitrate (5 mg/kg) must be undertaken expeditiously, except in renal insufficiency where hydroxocobalamin is preferred.

Although intravenous nitroglycerin has been used to achieve induced hypotension, a subpopulation of neurosurgical patients is resistant to the action of this drug.[89] Adjunctive agents (beta blockers, labetalol, captopril) and measures such as deepening the level of anesthesia are usually necessary to achieve reliably the desired level of hypotension. Intravenous nitroglycerin may increase ICP by causing cerebral vasodilatation and brain swelling,[27,29] but it is not associated with the adverse distribution of blood flow in the myocardium. Except at very high doses, toxicity related to nitroglycerin is virtually unprecedented. Methemoglobinemia may occur theoretically, but is almost never seen.[22]

Esmolol, a short-acting beta blocker with minimal effect on the cerebral circulation, has been used for induction of neurosurgical hypotension in doses of approximately 200 μg/kg/min. When compared to SNP, there is less rebound hypertension and reflex tachycardia.[124] Esmolol can also be employed to decrease the dosing requirements for SNP.

Trimethaphan, a ganglionic blocker, has been used for induced hypotension in neurosurgery. It affects ICP less than SNP,[164] but may still cause intracranial hypertension.[59] This agent is no longer widely popular because of its side effects (histamine release, tachyphylaxis, pupillary dilation), possible adverse cerebral energy balance and oxygen availability at low mean arterial pressures,[87,101] and failure to maintain regional CBF.[1]

A relatively new hypotensive agent is adenosine, a short-acting nucleotide which leaves CBF unaffected, but reduces $CMRO_2$ approximately 15% when used to induce hypotension to a MAP of 45 mm Hg. It has no adverse effects on cerebral energy balance.[69] Its theoretic advantage is some degree of metabolic depression and less potential for vasomotor paralysis.[70] However, CBF behaves similarly with SNP-induced hypotension,[131] and a clear clinical benefit of adenosine remains to be demonstrated.

While infusions of short-acting drugs to induce hypotension are preferable because of their easy reversibility, agents with longer half-lives also play a role. Hydralazine, labetalol, alpha-methyldopa, and ACE inhibitors have all been used to either induce or facilitate the induction of hypotension during neurosurgical procedures. Except for the alpha- and beta-blocking agents, all vasodilators (including calcium channel blockers) can dilate the cerebral vasculature and may result in brain swelling. Although the anesthesiologist should be familiar with these drugs, no clear benefits are associated with longer-acting agents. The operative management of induced hypotension should employ a technique with which the anesthesiologist, the surgeon, and the intensivist providing the postoperative care are familiar.

### *Reversal of Hypotension*

Once the aneurysm has been successfully clipped, induced hypotension is usually swiftly reversed with an eye to avoiding rebound hypertension. Following nitroprusside and other vasodilator-induced hypotension, rebound hypertension is frequently seen[63] as a result of sympathetic activity in response to generalized vasodilation, activating the renin-angiotensin system. Plasma concentrations of catecholamines and renin-angiotensin are markedly elevated during induced hypotension.[65] Rebound hypertension can be prevented by beta adrenergic blockade or ACE inhibition.[186] It is treated with short-acting vasodilators, beta adrenergic blockade, and a moderate increase in the depth of anesthesia. When allowing blood pressure to normalize, the anesthesiologist and surgeon observe the patient's response, specifically looking for bleeding, brain swelling, and rebound hypertension. Bleeding points unrecognized during hypotension frequently appear and require careful attention to bring about hemostasis. Likewise, the surgeon may request a modest level of induced hypertension to test the integrity of the vascular clip or repair. To achieve this, the anesthesiologist carefully uses a vasopressor (phenylephrine 20–30 μg intravenous and/or ephedrine 5 mg) if blood pressure does not spontaneously reach the desired level (systolic blood pressure, 140–160 mm Hg). At this point, it is imperative to avoid precipitous administration of larger vasopressor doses, as this can lead to undesirable hypertension.

## *Cerebral Protection*

In the perioperative management of the patient with an intracranial aneurysm, the possibility of encountering cerebral ischemia exists because of the possible pre-existence of vasospasm, as well as the need for temporary clipping. The anesthesiologist, therefore, must be familiar with current strategies to facilitate protection from cerebral ischemia. Cerebral protection refers to an intervention initiated prior to the occurrence of brain ischemia. The concept is based on the premise that certain prophylactic measures can interfere with the cascade of events triggered by the injury. There are several mechanisms through which such a salutary effect may be achieved.

### *Reducing Demand for Energy*

Average brain oxygen consumption (i.e. $O_2$ extraction, $CMRO_2$) is, with the exception of myocardial tissue, higher than oxygen consumption in other body tissues and averages approximately 3.5 ml/100g/min. Total $CMRO_2$ consists of demand for energy by cellular "housekeeping" functions (membrane transport, mitochondrial function, etc.) and by neuronal electrical activity. Despite its high energy demand, the brain cannot store energy very well. In the face of complete ischemia, cerebral energy stores only sustain brain tissue for several minutes before irreversible injury, resulting from metabolic failure begins at the cellular level.[17] In some experimental situations, however, complete ischemia may be tolerated as long as 17 minutes.[75]

Cerebral protection through reduction of $CMRO_2$ must be achieved either by reduction of neuronal function (e.g. by the use of barbiturates and similar substances that reduce or eliminate spontaneous brain electrical activity) or by nonspecific slowing of all neuronal cellular processes (e.g. through hypothermia). It stands to reason that reduction of neuronal function will only be effective if the injury preserves some residual level of electrical (EEG) activity. Thus, it is not surprising that barbiturates have not been found effective in situations of experimental complete global ischemia or, clinically, in cardiac arrest. These insults are too severe to permit significant levels of neuronal electrical activity.

### *Blocking Mediators of Ischemic Injury*

Brain ischemia on a cellular level leads to depletion of high-energy phosphates necessary to maintain ionic gradients. Potassium leaves the cell, and sodium and calcium enter it. High intracellular levels of calcium activate phospholipases, which in turn produce free fatty acids from lipid membranes. Intracellular acidosis develops because of anaerobic metabolism and is worsened by the production of free fatty acids, which give rise to a variety of toxic metabolites including thromboxane, leukotriene, prostaglandin, etc. Lipid peroxidation is enhanced in the presence of iron complexes, free radicals are generated (a process that is intensified during reperfusion), and excitatory amino acids (glutamate, aspartate) are produced. These compounds have been implicated in potentiating the original ischemic injury (e.g. arachidonic acid metabolites by mediating postischemic hypoperfusion; excitatory amino acids by causing ischemia-induced seizure activity), and may have a direct toxic effect on neuronal cells.

### *Anesthetics as Cerebral Protectants*

An extensive array of pharmacologic agents have been studied for their potential to provide brain protection from ischemic/hypoxic insults. The following discussion is merely meant to highlight the major groups of drugs.

#### Barbiturates

The primary rationale for the use of barbiturates in protection against ischemic brain injury is the reduction of brain tissue energy demand resulting from cellular electrical functions. At a time when supply of nutrients may be critically low, energy demand would likewise be reduced, allowing tissue to survive at a lower level of nutrient delivery. Protective effects of barbiturates may also include prevention of lipid peroxidation,[42] reduction of cerebral edema,[135] and favorable redistribution of CBF, also referred to as "inverse steal."[15] However, one of the major benefits of barbiturate therapy is gained from its effectiveness in reducing ICP by affecting cerebral metabolism and, secondarily, CBF and volume. Since brain electric activity usually persists in patients with intracranial hypertension, barbiturate therapy would be expected to reduce $CMRO_2$, which "protects" brain tissue both by limiting cell energy demand at a time when blood flow may be compromised, and by improving perfusion pressure through reduction in ICP (CPP = MAP-ICP). In the treatment of intracranial hypertension, high-dose barbiturate therapy is generally reserved for the patient who fails other routine measures (hyperventilation, diuretics, CSF drainage, etc).

Barbiturates appear to be only effective at brain protection when ischemia is incomplete, (i.e. there is still some EEG activity). Experimental evidence is solid in demonstrating the protective effect of barbiturates in focal cerebral ischemia.[98] In focal ischemia, synaptic electrical activity is partially preserved, so that barbiturate therapy should reduce $CMRO_2$, improve the balance between energy demand and supply, and therefore be effective. Likewise, in the situation of open-chamber cardiac surgery, ischemia is incomplete and, in many instances, focal (i.e. emboli). The landmark study of Nussmeier et al[118] points towards effectiveness of barbiturates in this situation.

By contrast, in experimental global ischemia, barbiturates are ineffective at improving neurologic outcome and overall mortality. A large multicenter clinical trial of thiopental following cardiac arrest also failed to demonstrate a beneficial effect.[14] The following offers an explanation for the apparent discrepancy of barbiturate action in global versus focal ischemia. Barbiturates depress $CMRO_2$ only to the extent they depress cerebral electrical activity. In global ischemia (especially cardiac arrest), cerebral electrical synaptic activity is already depressed, so that significant further reduction in $CMRO_2$ by barbiturates would not be expected, thus accounting for the ineffectiveness of barbiturate resuscitation.

### Timing of Barbiturate Therapy

Presumably through one of the mechanisms described above, barbiturate therapy appears to provide some benefit, even if administered *after* a focal ischemic insult. Thus, barbiturates have been shown to diminish infarct size when administered following focal ischemia.[15] A beneficial effect was seen in primates when barbiturates were given up to 120 minutes after MCA occlusion.[142] Clinically, one may administer barbiturates even after the occurrence of cerebral ischemia (i.e. temporary aneurysm clip during uncontrolled hemorrhage), allowing first for hemodynamic stabilization to occur.

**Pentobarbital** is most commonly used for elective induction of barbiturate coma. It is more effective at lower doses than thiopental and has a serum half-life (elimination) of approximately 30 hours.[135] It is administered by loading dose (3–10 mg/kg) at 1 mg/kg/min, followed by continuous infusion at 1–2 mg/kg/hr. The use of blood levels (in the 25–40 mg/ml range) is not essential to therapy, but may prevent excessive recovery times from barbiturate coma. The therapeutic endpoint sought should be EEG evidence of near-abolition of cortical electrical activity in the form of burst suppression (4–8 EEG bursts/minute).

**Thiopental** is a rapidly acting barbiturate that is often used if the desired effect is necessary immediately (i.e. intraoperative). In this context, intravenous doses of 3–5 mg/kg will produce transient (< 10 minute) burst suppression and blood thiopental levels of 10–30 $\mu g/ml$.[106] There appears to be no advantage to longer-term use, as its elimination half-life is then comparable to that of pentobarbital. The cerebral protective effect of thiopental sodium has recently been demonstrated in the clinical situation of open-chamber cardiac surgery. In the absence of hypothermia and arterial inflow filtering, Nussmeier et al[118] demonstrated a clear reduction in major post-cardiopulmonary bypass neurologic deficits using high doses of thiopental (about 35 mg/kg) titrated to EEG evidence of burst suppression. Such high doses are not always necessary for temporary EEG suppression when brain protection is sought against surgically induced, reversible focal ischemia (e.g. intracranial aneurysms, extracranial-intracranial bypass, possibly carotid surgery). When temporary ischemia is produced during cerebral aneurysm clipping, intermittent doses of STP can be administered at the rate of 3–5 mg/kg every 5–10 minutes titrated to burst suppression. Provided the patient is normovolemic and administration is gradual, cardiovascular tolerance is surprisingly good. Most temporary ischemia can be handled with doses up to 20–25 mg/kg of thiopental. However, if requirements for protection continue, a continuous intravenous infusion must be started. Hourly dose requirement may initially be high (10–15 mg/kg/hr) to maintain the desired level of burst suppression, but soon can be tapered to approximately 2–5 mg/kg/hr.

**Methohexital** may afford a quicker recovery because of its somewhat shorter elimination half-life. In practice, however, it is less frequently used because of the possibility of exacerbation of seizure disorders.

**Etomidate**, an imidazole compound used for induction of general anesthesia, has cerebrovascular and metabolic effects not unlike those of barbiturates, and should therefore be similarly effective. Some, but less extensive, clinical experience exists with this agent in the area of brain protection and treatment of intracranial hypertension. One potential advantage of etomidate is its lesser myocardial depressive action. When etomidate was titrated to EEG burst suppression, up to 60 minutes of internal carotid temporary occlusion were well tolerated.[10] The dose of etomidate is approximately 0.4–0.5 mg/kg followed by increments of 0.1 mg/kg to achieve adequate EEG suppression. However, especially when administered by infusion, concerns about suppression of the adrenal-pituitary axis, EEG excitation, and a higher incidence of vomiting may outweigh the otherwise beneficial properties of etomidate.

**Propofol** is a sterically hindered phenol that can induce EEG burst suppression at clinically useful doses not associated with delayed emergence. While this drug does not result in parallel reductions in $CMRO_2$ and CBF,[55] $CMRO_2$ appears to remain coupled to CBF within reasonable tolerance limits. Despite some encouraging evidence that was reported recently,[66] at present there is insufficient experience to warrant recommending this agent for cerebral protection.

Complications of barbiturate therapy include depression of cardiac output, CPP, and even frank cardiovascular collapse in poorly hydrated patients. It is therefore often necessary to reverse hypovolemia and provide pharmacologic inotropic support. In most instances, this necessitates invasive cardiovascular monitoring, including the use of PA catheters. The profound respiratory depressant effect of barbiturates makes controlled mechanical ventilation mandatory, with all the potential risks and complications thereof. Longer-term barbiturate therapy (i.e. days) is associated with hypothermia, depression of immune responses, and subsequent risk, primarily, of pulmonary infectious complications.[11] It is evident that barbiturate coma should not be instituted lightly. A sophisticated intensive care setting is needed to support patients who are going to benefit from this mode of therapy. Neurologic evaluation of the patient in barbiturate coma is difficult. The use of ICP monitoring devices and electrophysiologic monitoring (e.g. evoked potentials, which can be monitored even when the EEG is isoelectric), coupled with early CT scan, MRI, or angiography can help identify adverse developments in a timely fashion.

**Isoflurane** suppresses brain electrical activity to the point of isoelectricity at clinically useful concentrations (1.5–2.0 MAC). Cerebral energy stores are well maintained with a degree of metabolic depression similar to that achievable with barbiturates.[113] Both laboratory and clinical studies have suggested a cerebral protective effect of isoflurane. In carotid endarterectomy patients, Messick et al[95] found that the regional CBF at which EEG evidence of ischemia appeared (the so-called "ischemic threshold") was significantly lower (i.e. 8–10 ml/100g/min) than had previously been observed with halothane (i.e. 18–20 ml/100g/min). Furthermore, Michenfelder et al[100] retrospectively reported a lower total incidence of EEG ischemia in carotid endarterectomy during isoflurane anesthesia when compared to other anesthetics. Although its efficacy as a cerebral protectant is still under debate, it has been used during temporary vessel occlusion for aneurysm surgery.[98] The anesthetic is titrated to EEG burst suppression and requires concomitant pharmacologic support of the circulation. However, the effect of isoflurane "protection" on neurologic outcome in focal ischemia is far from clear. Michenfelder's[100] retrospective data show *no difference in neurologic outcome* with either anesthetic regimen. Nehls, Todd, et al[111] demonstrated a protective effect for barbiturates, but not for isoflurane, in a baboon MCA occlusion model. By contrast, Milde et al[103] showed that if blood pressure was equal in both isoflurane- and barbiturate-treated primates, no difference in neurologic outcome could be demonstrated, possibly indicating an equivalent degree of protection from either drug. The issue of isoflurane protection in focal cerebral ischemia must therefore still be regarded as highly controversial. It is conceivable that isoflurane fails to exert a protective effect in focal ischemia because its cerebrovasodilatory properties induce a cerebral steal, shunting blood away from the ischemic focus. Barbiturates have been observed to cause a "reverse steal" (or "Robin Hood" effect), enhancing blood flow in the ischemic region.[15]

### *Nonanesthetic Protection*

**Nimodipine** improves neurologic outcome in patients recovering from aneurysmal SAH[5,129] and has become a standard prophylactic agent in such patients. It is presumed that this effect is mediated by nimodipine's action on small vessel cerebral vasospasm. When administered prior to experimental global ischemia, the drug also results in better neurologic outcome.[98] Nimodipine has shown promise when used to treat existing ischemia.

Elevated intracellular **glucose** concentration at the time of a cerebral ischemic insult may result in increased cellular lactic acidosis, thus worsening ischemic injury.[176] This effect has been observed both in focal[134] and global cerebral ischemia.[75] In the clinical setting, hyperglycemic stroke patients made a worse neurologic recovery than patients who were not hyperglycemic at the time of the stroke.[133] Likewise, blood glucose levels were significantly higher in cardiac arrest patients who did not awaken postoperatively than in those who did, and correlated with outcome in patients with closed head injury.[132]

While these clinical series may not prove that hypoglycemia caused the adverse outcome, available evidence strongly implicates the presence of excess glucose in the aggravation of ischemic injury. It is important to realize that even modest amounts of glucose (the equivalent of 1,000 ml 5% dextrose-containing intravenous fluid in humans), if administered before the global ischemic insult, augmented neurologic deficits significantly, despite blood glucose measurements below 200 mg/dl.[75] It is currently recommended that glucose-containing solutions be avoided in the management of operative patients at risk for neurologic injury. How tightly blood glucose needs to be controlled to obtain optimal effect is unclear. A clinical trial investigating the efficacy of steroids in head injury found the outcome to be worse in the steroid-treated group if ICP was elevated.[48] This result may be explained on the basis of mildly, but consistently, higher blood glucose levels in the steroid-treated patients (145 vs. 118 mg/dl). The implication of such observations may be that glucose needs to be tightly controlled in patients at risk for neurologic injury, although reduction of blood glucose to subnormal levels has not been found to be beneficial.[144]

### Mannitol

Ischemia may result in tissue swelling and secondary obstruction of brain tissue capillaries,[81] thus worsening the initial ischemic insult.[153] Breakdown of the blood brain barrier and onset of ischemic symptoms after feline MCA occlusion were delayed by administration of mannitol.[80] To improve microcirculatory flow during potential ischemic episodes, mannitol has been clinically employed prior to temporary clipping. It is noteworthy that these protective regimens incorporated other substances such as the antioxidant alpha-tocopherol (Vitamin E) and perfluorochemicals as well.[154,155]

### Hypothermia

Reduction of body temperature decreases oxygen consumption by 5% to 7% for every degree centigrade, so that $CMRO_2$ could be reduced by as much as 50% at a temperature of 27° C. Because hypothermia affects all cellular processes, it is a more efficient and powerful metabolic depressant tool than agents that affect $CMRO_2$ by merely depressing electrical activity. When electrical activity persists, barbiturates potentiate the cerebral metabolic depressant effect of hypothermia. Currently, with the exception of hypothermic cardiac arrest performed at some centers for certain giant aneurysms,[148] deep hypothermia is not practical for most neurosurgical interventions (carotid endarterectomy, routine cerebral aneurysm clipping, other temporary cerebrovascular occlusion). Anesthetic management for aneurysm clipping under hypothermic circulatory arrest has been described.[160] The technique involves monitoring with a PA catheter, slight head-up tilt to facilitate venous cerebral drainage during circulatory arrest, and frequent barbiturate loading to aid in cerebral protection. Complications may include coagulation defects on rewarming with resultant delayed intracerebral hemorrhage. Acidosis, cardiovascular instability, and pulmonary emboli have also been reported. Some centers are beginning to use mild hypothermia (34° to 35°C) routinely in cerebrovascular surgery where the risk of ischemic CNS injury is substantial. For a temperature reduction of 3°C, one may gain as much as a 20% reduction in $CMRO_2$, which may or may not be important as a protective mechanism. Mild hypothermia could also have important protective effects by slowing the release of excitatory neurotransmitters as well.[20] Not totally innocuous, mild hypothermia can slow metabolism of anesthetics and muscle relaxants, and lead to postoperative shivering and discomfort.[141] It is not associated with the more serious problems caused by deep hypothermia such as arrhythmias, coagulation defects, etc.

### Antagonists to Excitatory Neurotransmitters

Excitatory neurotransmitters such as glutamate and aspartate have been implicated as contributors to ischemic CNS injury. Excitatory amino acid receptors (especially N-methyl-D-aspartate or NMDA) are distributed in brain regions that are selectively vulnerable to ischemia, result in burst firing when activated, and could be responsible for postischemic seizure activity. The prophylactic administration of NMDA-antagonists MK801 and ketamine in a rat model of incomplete forebrain ischemia showed promise.[23] When given after the ischemic insult, however, MK801 failed to affect neurologic outcome in dogs and primates.[74,128] There is no basis at present to use ketamine clinically as a brain protective or resuscitative agent.

## *Practical Application of Protective Techniques*

Current recommendations for brain protection are apt to be vague. The most valid indication for utilizing pharmacologic brain protection is to buy time (i.e. rest the brain) while a temporary, and ultimately reversible, regional disruption in nutrient flow is expected to occur. Despite the recent interest in newer protective agents, the use of barbiturate protection is still valid and preferred in such clinical situations. Thus, barbiturate protection is reasonable during carotid endarterectomy if electrophysiologic or clinical evidence of ischemia does not resolve with conventional therapy (i.e. increase in circulating volume and blood pressure, insertion of shunt). In this situation one assumes that barbiturates will increase the brain's tolerance to ischemia, as other measures are taken to improve blood flow and lessen the vascular obstruction. Likewise, it has been said that barbiturates would be reasonable if a shunt is not used and EEG is not available for ischemia monitoring. Following cerebrovascular surgery, if an ischemic deficit is suspected to be surgically correctable (intimal flap, thrombus, or malpositioned aneurysm clip), one may choose to temporarily "rest" the brain with barbiturates while preparations are made to reoperate.

During cerebral aneurysm surgery, temporary clamping of feeder vessels may become necessary to control bleeding. If such clamping lasts more than 10 minutes, barbiturate protection is reasonable.[161] Induced hypotension during cerebral aneurysm surgery also may bring up the question of protective anesthetics. There is no evidence that isoflurane would specifically protect better than other reasonable anesthetics in this situation,[85] although its use represents an effective alternative to other methods of inducing hypotension. To add barbiturates during hypotension induced to control bleeding is fraught with the danger of cardiovascular collapse. However, once hemodynamic stability has been approached, careful loading with barbiturates is feasible, especially if the ischemic insult is expected to continue for some time before it can be corrected surgically. Mild hypothermia is also now occasionally used in anticipation of temporary cerebral ischemia during aneurysm clipping.

## *Pregnancy and Anesthetic Management for Cerebral Aneurysm Surgery*

SAH is the most common cerebrovascular complication during pregnancy and can be an important cause of maternal mortality.[94] The incidence is low (1 in 3,000–8,000 pregnancies) but rises as the pregnancy progresses. Pregnancy may be associated with a progression of aneurysm disease.[175] This is possibly related to the increasingly hyperdynamic cardiovascular state of the gravid patient. If the SAH is due to a ruptured cerebral aneurysm, neurosurgical management is indicated because of the high risk of rebleeding. It is generally agreed that both mother and fetus tolerate neurosurgical intervention, provided the appropriate precautions are taken. Cesarean section (C-section) is indicated only for obstetric complications, when the mother is clearly not salvageable, or when the hemorrhage occurs during labor, which is rare.

Prior to embarking on a neurosurgical procedure in a pregnant patient, it is important that the obstetrician, neurosurgeon, and anesthesiologist interact and agree on a well-planned course of action. Fetal monitoring via continuous abdominal Doppler and left uterine displacement should be maintained during the perioperative period. Immediate obstetric consultation should be available during the perioperative period.

Although many of the medications and techniques needed during surgical clipping of intracerebral aneurysms are known to have adverse effects on the uteroplacental unit and fetus (see Table 9), they have been used with relative impunity in practice. Anesthetic management of the pregnant patient involves premedication with an antacid or $H_2$ blocker to reduce gastric volume. Induction of anesthesia and endotracheal intubation should be managed rapidly to prevent aspiration, with cricoid pressure applied on induction. Continuous monitoring of arterial pressure and rigid control thereof are essential. The prophylactic administration of vasodilators is advisable in anticipation of major stimuli, such as intubation and incision. Depending on the stage of pregnancy, the safety of different anesthetics for the fetus must be considered. During the early stages of pregnancy, it is prudent to utilize agents that have a long record of safety (thiopental, morphine, curare, succinylcholine—potent inhaled anesthetics). The use of nitrous oxide is still considered somewhat controversial.[183] Light anesthesia and surgical stress may be associated with spontaneous uterine contractions and reduction in uterine blood flow. Phenylephrine, but not ephedrine, reduces uterine blood flow. The latter should therefore be used to elevate blood pressure pharmacologically, if needed.

If simultaneous C-section and aneurysm clipping are contemplated, the effect on neonatal responses of anesthetics administered prior to delivery should be considered. Narcotics are generally avoided to prevent neonatal depression.[178] Likewise, the concentrations of volatile agents and nitrous oxide are limited to prevent fetal hypoxia and excessive uterine bleeding. If hemodynamic activation cannot be reliably prevented without opioids, preparations to support neonatal ventilation by mechanical means should be made.

Controlled hyperventilation is necessary to obtain satisfactory operative conditions and allow safe exposure and clipping of the aneu-

TABLE 9
**Adverse Uteroplacental Drug Effects***

| Drug | Adverse Effects |
|---|---|
| Phenytoin | Minimal |
| Thiopental | Neonatal depression (> 8 mg/kg; human). Worsening of pre-existing fetal distress due to maternal hemodynamic effects |
| Lidocaine | Uterine hypertonus and vasoconstriction with fetal distress (toxic doses; sheep). Worsening of pre-existing fetal distress |
| Mannitol | Oligohydramnios with fetal hypo-osmolarity, hypernatremia, dehydration, cyanosis, and bradycardia (12.5 g/kg; rabbit). Fetal hyperosmolarity in humans 1 h after 200 g |
| Furosemide | Possibly dilation of ductus arteriosus. Electrolyte abnormalities |
| Nitroprusside | Decreased UVR.** Lethal fetal cyanide levels with onset of maternal tachyphylaxis (sheep). No fetal compromise in humans[184] |
| Nitroglycerin | Decreased UVR** (sheep) |
| Hydralazine | Decreased UVR** (sheep) |
| Propranolol | Decreased umbilical blood flow (sheep). Premature labor, worsening of pre-existing fetal distress. Neonatal acidosis, bradycardia, hypoglycemia, apnea[39] |
| Trimethaphan camsylate | Unstudied |
| Oxytocin | Possible mild hypotension, but used clinically without problems[178] |
| Hypothermia | Decreased uterine blood flow, but fetus also metabolically protected |
| Moderate Hyperventilation | Increased UVR; fetal metabolic acidosis only at maternal $PaCO_2 \leq 20$ |

*Adapted from Kofke et al [68]
**Uterine vascular resistance

rysm. Yet, alkalosis may reduce fetal oxygenation by reducing umbilical blood flow and shifting the hemoglobin dissociation curve to the left. Although investigations have yielded controversial results,[77,107,126] case reports of aneurysm clipping with hyperventilation during pregnancy suggest relative fetal safety unless there are complicating conditions such as uteroplacental insufficiency.

Induced hypothermia is likewise well tolerated in gravid animals[7] and patients.[35] Fetal mortality was generally associated only in the presence of exacerbating conditions such as uterine hypertonus, acidosis, and hypoxia. Induced hypotension has been safely managed with nitroglycerin and nitroprusside[68,183] despite initial concerns over the latter drug.

## References


1. Abe K, Demizu A, Kamada K, et al. Local cerebral blood flow with prostaglandin $E_1$ or trimethaphan during cerebral aneurysm clip ligation. *Can J Anaesth.* 1991;38:831–836.
2. Adams HP Jr, Kassell NF, Torner JC, et al. Predicting cerebral ischemia after aneurysmal subarachnoid hemorrhage: influences of clinical condition, CT results, and antifibrinolytic therapy: a report of the Cooperative Aneurysm Study. *Neurology* 1987;37:1586–1591.
3. Ades PE, Graftieaux JP. Ruptures anévrysmales per-opératoires: place et conséquence des clampages temporaires. *Agressologie.* 1990;31:351–356. English abstract.
4. Albin MS, Bunegin L, Dujovny M, et al. Brain retraction pressure during intracranial procedures. *Surg Forum.* 1975;25:499–500.
5. Allen GS, Ahn HS, Preziosi TJ, et al. Cerebral arterial spasm: a controlled trial of nimodipine in patients with subarachnoid hemorrhage. *N Engl J Med.* 1983;308:619–624.
6. Artiola i Fortuny L, Adams CBT, Briggs M. Surgical mortality in an aneurysm population: effects of age, blood pressure, and preoperative neurological state. *J Neurol Neurosurg Psychiatry* 1980; 43:879–882.
7. Assali NS, Westin B. Effects of hypothermia on uterine circulation and on the fetus. *Proc Soc Exp Biol Med.* 1962;109:485–488.
8. Awad IA, Carter P, Spetzler RF, et al. Clinical vasospasm after subarachnoid hemorrhage: response to hypervolemic hemodilution and arterial hypertension. *Stroke.* 1987;18:365–372.
9. Batjer H, Samson D. Intraoperative aneurysmal rupture: incidence, outcome, and suggestions for surgical management. *Neurosurgery.* 1986;18:701–707.
10. Batjer HH, Frankfurt AI, Purdy PD, et al. Use of etomidate, temporary arterial occlusion, and intraoperative angiography in surgical treatment of large and giant cerebral aneurysms. *J Neurosurg.* 1988; 68:234–240.
11. Belopavlovic M, Buchthal A. Barbiturate therapy in the management of cerebral ischaemia. *Anaesthesia.* 1980;35:271–278.
12. Black S. Cerebral aneurysm and arteriovenous malformation. In: Cucchiari RF, Michenfelder JD, eds, *Clinical Neuroanesthesia.* New York, NY: Churchill Livingstone; 1990:223–254.
13. Boucher CA, Brewster DC, Darling RC, et al. Determination of cardiac risk by dipyridomate-thallium imaging before peripheral vascular surgery. *N Engl J Med.* 1985;312:389–394.
14. Brain Resuscitation Clinical Trial I Study Group. Randomized clinical study of thiopental loading in comatose survivors of cardiac arrest. *N Engl J Med.* 1986;314:397–403.
15. Branston NM, Hope DT, Symon L. Barbiturates in focal ischemia of primate cortex: effects on blood flow distribution, evoked potential and extracellular potassium. *Stroke.* 1979;10:647–653.
16. Bristow A, Shalev D, Rice B, et al. Low-dose synthetic narcotic infusions for cerebral relaxation during craniotomies. *Anesth Analg.* 1987;66: 413–416.
17. Brockman SK, Jude JR. The tolerance of the dog brain to total arrest of circulation. *Bull Johns Hopkins Hosp.* 1960;106:74–80.
18. Brown MF, Benzel EC. Morbidity and mortality associated with rapid control of systemic hypertension in patients with intracranial hemorrhages. *J Neurosurg Anesth.* 1990;2:53–55.
19. Buchthal A, Belopavlovic M, Mooij JJ. Evoked potential monitoring and temporary clipping in cerebral aneurysm surgery. *Acta Neurochir (Wien).* 1988;93:28–36.
20. Busto R, Globus MY-T, Dietrich WD, et al. Effect of mild hypothermia on ischemia-induced release of neurotransmitters and free fatty acids in rat brain. *Stroke.* 1989;20:904–910.
21. Carter LP, Raudzens PA, Gaines C, et al. Somatosensory evoked potentials and cortical blood flow during craniotomy for vascular disease. *Neurosurgery.* 1984;15:22–28.
22. Chestnut JS, Albin MS, Gonzalez-Abola E, et al. Clinical evaluation of intravenous nitroglycerin for neurosurgery. *J Neurosurg.* 1978;48:704–711.
23. Church J, Zeman S, Lodge D. The neuroprotective action of ketamine and MK-801 after transient cerebral ischemia in rats. *Anesthesiology.* 1988; 69:702–709.
24. Chyatte D, Sundt TM Jr. Cerebral vasospasm after subarachnoid hemorrhage. *Mayo Clin Proc.* 1984; 59:498–505.
25. Cole DJ, Schell RM, Drummond JC, et al. Focal cerebral ischemia in rats: effect of phenylephrine-induced hypertension during reperfusion. *J Neurosurg Anesth.* 1992;4:78–84.
26. Colley PS, Dunn R. Prevention of blood pressure response to skull-pin head holder by local anesthesia. *Anesth Analg.* 1979;58:241–243.
27. Cottrell JE, Gupta B, Rappaport H, et al. Intracranial pressure during nitroglycerin-induced hypotension. *J Neurosurg.* 1980;53:309–311.
28. Cottrell JE, Illner P, Kittay MJ, et al. Rebound hypertension after sodium nitroprusside-induced hypotension. *Clin Pharmacol Ther.* 1980;27:32–36.
29. Dahl A, Russell D, Nyberg-Hansen R, et al. Effect of nitroglycerin on cerebral circulation measured by

transcranial Doppler and SPECT. *Stroke.* 1989; 20:1733–1736.
30. Dahlgren BE, Gordon E, Steiner L. Evaluation of controlled hypotension during surgery for intracranial aneurysms. *Excepta Medica.* International Congress Series. 1968;200:1232–1238.
31. Davies KR, Gelb AW, Manninen PH, et al. Cardiac function in aneurysmal subarachnoid hemorrhage: a study of electrocardiographic and echocardiographic abnormalities. *Br J Anaesth.* 1991;67:58–63.
32. Dernbach PD, Little JR, Jones SC, et al. Altered cerebral autoregulation and $CO_2$ reactivity after aneurysmal subarachnoid hemorrhage. *Neurosurgery.* 1988;22:822–826.
33. Di Pasquale G, Pinelli G, Andreoli A, et al. Holter detection of cardiac arrhythmias in intracranial subarachnoid hemorrhage. *Am J Cardiol.* 1987; 59:596–600.
34. Diringer MN, Lim JS, Kirsch JR, et al. Elevated plasma atrial natriuretic factor following subarachnoid hemorrhage: relationship to intraventricular and suprasellar blood. *Crit Care Med.* 1991; 19(suppl):S27. Abstract.
35. Donaldson JO. *Neurology of Pregnancy.* Philadelphia, PA: WB Saunders; 1978:124–128.
36. Drake CG. Aneurysm surgery: past, present and future. *Anesthesiol Clin.* Summer,1982;20:1–9.
37. Drake CG. Management of cerebral aneurysm. *Stroke.* 1981;12:273–283.
38. Eisenberg HM, Turner JW, Teasdale G, et al. Monitoring of cortical excitability during induced hypotension in aneurysm operations. *J Neurosurg.* 1979;50:595–602.
39. Ellis C, Fidler J. Drugs in pregnancy: adverse reactions. *Br J Hosp Med.* 1982;28:575–584.
40. Findlay JM, Weir BK, Kassell NF, et al. Intracisternal recombinant tissue plasminogen activator after aneurysmal hemorrhage. *J Neurosurg.* 1991; 75:181–188.
41. Fisher B, Thomas D, Peterson B. Hypotonic saline lowers raised intracranial pressure in children after head trauma. *J Neurosurg Anesth.* 1992;4:4–10.
42. Flamm ES, Demoupoulos HB, Seligman ML, et al. Possible molecular mechanisms of barbiturate-mediated protection in regional cerebral ischemia. *Acta Neurol Scand Suppl.* 1977;56:150–151.
43. Fleisher LA, Barash PG. Preoperative cardiac evaluation for noncardiac surgery: a functional approach. *Anesth Analg.* 1992;74:586–598.
44. Fletcher JE, Sebel PS, Murphy MR, et al. Psychomotor performance after desflurane anesthesia: a comparison with isoflurane. *Anesth Analg.* 1991; 73:260–265.
45. Fremes SE, Weisel RD, Mickle DAG, et al. A comparison of nitroglycerin and nitroprusside: I:Treatment of postoperative hypertension. *Ann Thor Surg.* 1985;39:53–59.
46. Friedman WA, Chadwick GM, Verhoeven FJ, et al. Monitoring of somatosensory evoked potentials during surgery for middle cerebral artery aneurysms. *Neurosurgery.* 1991;29:83–88.
47. From RP, Warner DS, Todd MM, et al. Anesthesia for craniotomy: a double blind comparison of alfentanil, fentanyl, and sufentanil. *Anesthesiology.* 1990;73:896–904.
48. Gelpke GJ, Braakman R, Habbema JDF, et al. Comparison of outcome in two series of patients with severe head injuries. *J Neurosurg.* 1983; 59:745–750.
49. Giannotta SL, Oppenheimer JH, Levy ML, et al. Management of intraoperative rupture of aneurysm without hypotension. *Neurosurgery.* 1991;28:531–536.
50. Grubb RL Jr, Raichle ME, Eichling JO, et al. Effects of subarachnoid hemorrhage on cerebral blood volume, blood flow, and oxygen utilization in humans. *J Neurosurg.* 1977;46:446–453.
51. Haghighi SS, Madsen R, Green KD, et al. Suppression of motor evoked potentials by inhalation anesthetics. *J Neurosurg Anesth.* 1990;2:73–78.
52. Hampton LJ, Little DM Jr, Rodabaugh GS, et al. Studies concerning prolongation of activity of succinylcholine. *Anesthesiology.* 1955;16:67–72.
53. Harp JR, Wollman H. Cerebral metabolic effects of hyperventilation and deliberate hypotension. *Br J Anaesth.* 1973;45:256–262.
54. Hijdra A, van Gijn J, Nagelkerke NJ, et al. Prediction of delayed cerebral ischemia, rebleeding, and outcome after aneurysmal subarachnoid hemorrhage. *Stroke.* 1988;19:1250–1256.
55. Hoffman WE, Kochs E. Propofol: an intravenous anesthetic for neuroanesthetic practice? *J Neurosurg Anesth.* 1992; 4:75–77.
56. Hugosson R, Högström S. Factors disposing to morbidity in surgery of intracranial aneurysms with special regard to sleep controlled hypotension. *J Neurosurg.* 1973;38:561–567.
57. Hunt WE, Hess RM. Surgical risk as related to time of intervention in the repair of intracranial aneurysms. *J Neurosurg.* 1968;28:14–20.
58. Jane JA, Kassell NF, Torner JC, et al. The natural history of aneurysms and arteriovenous malformations. *J Neurosurg.* 1985;62:321–323.
59. Karlin A, Hartung J, Cottrell JE. Rate of induction of hypotension with trimethaphan modifies the intracranial pressure response in cats. *Br J Anaesth.* 1988;60:161–166.
60. Kassell NF, Boarinin DJ. Perioperative care of the aneurysm patient. *Contemporary Neurosurg.* 1984; 6:1–6.
61. Kassell NF, Peerless SJ, Durward QJ, et al. Treatment of ischemic deficits from vasospasm with intravascular volume expansion and induced arterial hypertension. *Neurosurgery.* 1982;11:337–343.
62. Kassell NF, Sasaki T, Colohan ART, et al. Cerebral vasospasm following aneurysmal subarachnoid hemorrhage. *Stroke.* 1985;16:562–572.
63. Khambatta HJ, Stone JG, Khan E. Hypertension during anethesia on discontinuation of sodium nitroprusside-induced hypotension. *Anesthesiology.* 1979;51:127–130.
64. Khambatta HJ, Stone JG, Khan E. Propranolol alters renin release during nitroprusside-induced hypotension and prevents hypertension on discontinuation of nitroprusside. *Anesth Analg* 1981;60:569–573.
65. Knight PR, Lane GA, Hensiger RN, et al. Catecholamine and renin-angiotensin response during hypotensive anesthesia induced by sodium nitroprusside or trimethaphan camsylate. *Anesthesiology.* 1983;59:248–253.
66. Kochs E, Hoffman WE, Werner C, et al. The effects of propofol on brain electrical activity, neurologic outcome, and neuronal damage following incomplete ischemia in rats. *Anesthesiology.* 1992;

76:245–252.

67. Kochs E, Schulte am Esch J. Relationship between cerebral blood flow and somatosensory evoked potentials during graded incomplete ischemia in goats under general anesthesia. *Anesthesiology.* 1987; 67(suppl):A403. Abstract.
68. Kofke WA, Wuest HP, McGinnis LA. Cesarean section following ruptured cerebral aneurysm and neuroresuscitation. *Anesthesiology.* 1984;60:242–245.
69. Lagerkranser M, Bergstrand G, Gordon E, et al. Cerebral blood flow and metabolism during adenosine-induced hypotension in patients undergoing cerebral aneurysm surgery. *Acta Anaesthesiol Scand.* 1989;33:15–20.
70. Lam AM, Artru AA. Auto regulation of cerebral blood flow in response to adenosine-induced hypotension in dogs. *J Neurosurg Anesth* 1992;4:120–127.
71. Lam AM, Gelb AW. Cardiovascular effects of isoflurane-induced hypotension for cerebral aneurysm surgery. *Anesth Analg* 1983;62:742–748.
72. Lam AM, Manninen PH, Keane JF. Brain stem auditory evoked potential monitoring during vertebrobasilar occlusion therapy for posterior fossa aneurysms. *Anesthesiology.* 1984;61(suppl):A347. Abstract.
73. Landi A, Demo P, Carraro JR, et al. Intra-operative monitoring by means of somatosensory evoked potentials during aneurysm surgery. *Agressologie.* 1990;31:363–366.
74. Lanier WL, Perkins WJ, Ruud B, et al: Effect of the excitatory amino acid antagonist MK-801 on neurologic function following complete cerebral ischemia in primates. *Anesthesiology.* 1988;69 (suppl):A846. Abstract.
75. Lanier WL, Stangland KJ, Scheithauer BW, et al. The effects of dextrose infusion and head position on neurologic outcome after complete cerebral ischemia in primates: examination of a model. *Anesthesiology.* 1987;66:39–48.
76. Levin R, Hesselvik JF, Kourtopoulos H, et al. Local anesthesia prevents hypertension following application of the Mayfield skull-pin head holder. *Acta Anaesthesiol Scand.* 1989;33:277–279.
77. Levinson G, Shnider SM, de Lorimier AA. Effects of maternal hyperventilation on uterine blood flow and fetal oxygenation and acid-base status. *Anesthesiology.* 1974;40:340–347.
78. Levy WJ Jr. Clinical experience with motor and cerebellar evoked potential monitoring. *Neurosurgery.* 1987;20:169–182.
79. Lindop MJ. Complications and morbidity of controlled hypotension. *Br J Anaesth.* 1975;47:799–803.
80. Little JR. Modification of acute focal ischemia by treatment with mannitol and high-dose dexamethasone. *J Neurosurg.* 1978;49:517–524.
81. Little JR. Morphological changes in acute focal ischemia: response to osmotherapy. *Adv Neurol.* 1980;28:443–457.
82. Little JR, Lesser RP, Lueders H, et al. Brain stem auditory evoked potentials in posterior circulation surgery. *Neurosurgery* 1983:12:496–502.
83. Ljunggren B, Brandt L, Säveland H, et al. Outcome in 60 consecutive patients treated with early aneurysm operation and intravenous nimodipine. *J Neurosurg.* 1984;61:864–873.
84. Ljunggren B, Säveland H, Brandt L. Causes of unfavorable outcome after early aneurysm operation. *Neurosurgery.* 1983;13:629–633.
85. MacNab MS, Manninen PH, Lam AM, et al. The stress response to induced hypotension for cerebral aneurysm surgery: a comparison of two hypotensive techniques. *Can J Anaesth.* 1988;35:111–115.
86. Madsen JB, Cold GE, Hansen ES, et al. Cerebral blood flow and metabolism during isoflurane-induced hypotension in patients subjected to surgery for cerebral aneurysms. *Br J Anaesth.* 1987;59: 1204–1207.
87. Maekawa T, McDowall DG, Okuda Y. Brain-surface oxygen tension and cerebral cortical blood flow during hemorrhagic and drug-induced hypotension in the cat. *Anesthesiology.* 1979;51:313–320.
88. Mahla ME. Carotid artery surgery: anesthesia and monitoring. *Refresher Courses Anesth.* 1991;271:1–7.
89. Maktabi M, Warner D, Sokoll M, et al. Comparison of nitroprusside, nitroglycerin and deep isoflurane anesthesia for induced hypotension. *Neurosurgery.* 1986;19:350–355.
90. Manninen PH, Cuillerier DJ, Gelb AW, et al. Monitoring of brain stem function during posterior fossa surgery. *Can J Anaesth.* 1990;37(suppl):S23.
91. Manninen PH, Gelb AW, Lam AM, et al. Perioperative monitoring of the electrocardiogram during cerebral aneurysm surgery. *J Neurosurg Anesth.* 1990;2:16–22.
92. Marion DW, Segal R, Thompson ME. Subarachnoid hemorrhage and the heart. *Neurosurgery.* 1986;18:101–106.
93. McDermott MW, Durity FA, Borozny M, et al. Temporary vessel occlusion and barbiturate protection in cerebral aneurysm surgery. *Neurosurgery.* 1989;25:54–62.
94. Meincke DL, Hurt WG, Young HF. Ruptured intracranial aneurysms in pregnancy. *V Med.* 1976; 103:878–881.
95. Messick JM Jr, Casement B, Sharbrough FW, et al. Correlation of regional cerebral blood flow (rCBF) with EEG changes during isoflurane anesthesia for carotid endarterectomy: critical rCBF. *Anesthesiology.* 1987;66:344–349.
96. Meyer CH, Lowe D, Meyer M, et al. Progressive change in cerebral blood flow during the first three weeks after subarachnoid hemorrhage. *Neurosurgery.* 1983;12:58–76.
97. Meyer FB, Muzzi DA. Cerebral protection during aneurysm surgery with isoflurane anesthesia. *J Neurosurg.* 1992;76:541–543.
98. Michenfelder JD. Current status of brain protection. *Refresher Courses Anesth.* 1987;15:125–137.
99. Michenfelder JD, Gronert GE, Rehder K. Neuroanesthesia. *Anesthesiology.* 1969;30:65–100.
100. Michenfelder JD, Sundt TM, Fode N, et al. Isoflurane when compared to enflurane and halothane decreases the frequency of cerebral ischemia during carotid endarterectomy. *Anesthesiology.* 1987;67:336–340.
101. Michenfelder JD, Theye RA. Canine systemic and cerebral effects of hypotension induced by hemorrhage, trimethaphan, halothane, or nitroprusside. *Anesthesiology.* 1977;46:188–195.
102. Milde LN, Milde JH. The cerebral hemodynamic and metabolic effects of sufentanil in dogs. *Anesthesiology.* 1987;67(suppl):A570. Abstract.

103. Milde LN, Milde JH, Lanier WL, et al. Comparison of the effects of isoflurane and thiopental on neurologic outcome and neuropathology after temporary focal ischemia in recovery after cardiac arrest. *Ann Neurol.* 1984;15:59–63.
104. Miller E. Deliberate hypotension. In: Miller Rd, ed. *Anesthesia.* New York, NY: Churchill Livingstone; 1986:1949–1970.
105. Miller ED Jr, Ackerly JA, Vaughan ED Jr, et al. The renin-angiotensin system during controlled hypotension with sodium nitroprusside. *Anesthesiology.* 1977;47:257–262.
106. Moffat JA, McDougall MJ, Brunet D, et al. Thiopental bolus during carotid endarterectomy-rational drug therapy? *Can Anaesth Soc J.* 1983;30:615–622.
107. Motoyama EK, Rivard G, Acheson F, et al. Adverse effect of maternal hyperventilation on the fetus. *Lancet.* 1966;1:286–288.
108. Murtagh F, Smith DS. Reflections on the anesthesia-neurosurgical alliance. *J Neurosurg Anesth.* 1990;2:182–188.
109. Mutch WA, Ringaert KR, Ewert FJ, et al. Continuous opioid infusions for neurosurgical procedures: a double blind comparison of alfentanil and fentanyl. *Can J Anaesth.* 1991;38:710–716.
110. Muzzi DA, Black S, Losasso TJ, et al. Labetalol and esmolol in the control of hypertension after intracranial surgery. *Anesth Analg.* 1990;70:68–71.
111. Nehls DG, Todd MM, Spetzler RF, et al. A comparison of the cerebral protective effects of isoflurane and barbiturates during temporary focal ischemia in primates. *Anesthesiology.* 1987; 66:453–464.
112. Neil-Dwyer G, Walter P, Cruickshank JM, et al. Effect of propranolol and phentolamine on myocardial necrosis after subarachnoid hemorrhage. *Br Med J.* 1978;2:990–992.
113. Newberg LA, Milde JH, Michenfelder JD. The cerebral metabolic effects of isoflurane at and above concentrations that suppress cortical electrical activity. *Anesthesiology.* 1983;59:23–28.
114. Newman B, Gelb AW, Lam AM. The effect of isoflurane-induced hypotension on cerebral blood flow and cerebral metabolic rate for oxygen in humans. *Anesthesiology.* 1986;64:307–310.
115. Nishioka H, Torner JC, Graf CJ, et al. Cooperative study of intracranial aneurysms and subarachnoid hemorrhage: a long-term prognostic study, II: ruptured intracranial aneurysms managed conservatively. *Arch Neurol.* 1984;41:1142–1146.
116. Nornes H. The role of intracranial pressure in the arrest of hemorrhage in patients with ruptured intracranial aneurysm. *J Neurosurg.* 1973;39:226–234.
117. Nornes H, Magnaes B. Intracranial pressure in patients with ruptured saccular aneurysm. *J Neurosurg.* 1972;36:537–547.
118. Nussmeier NA, Arlund C, Slogoff S: Neuropsychiatric complications after cardiopulmonary bypass: cerebral protection by a barbiturate. *Anesthesiology.* 1986;64:165–170.
119. Ogawa A, Sato H, Sakurai Y, et al. Limitation of temporary vascular occlusion during aneurysm surgery: study by intraoperative monitoring of cortical blood flow. *Surg Neurol.* 1991;36:453–457.
120. Öhman J, Heiskanen O. Timing of operation for ruptured supratentorial aneurysms: a prospective randomized study. *J Neurosurg.* 1989;70:55–60.
121. Ohmoto T, Nagao S, Mino S, et al. Monitoring of cortical blood flow during temporary arterial occlusion in aneurysm surgery by the thermal diffusion method. *Neurosurgery.* 1991;28:49–54.
122. Origitano TC, Wascher TM, Reichman OH, et al. Sustained increased cerebral blood flow with prophylactic hypertensive hypervolemic hemodilution ("triple H" therapy) after subarachnoid hemorrhage. *Neurosurgery.* 1990;27:729–739.
123. Orlowski JP, Shiesley D, Vitd DG, et al. Labetalol to control blood pressure after cerebrovascular surgery. *Crit Care Med.* 1988;16:765–768.
124. Ornstein E, Matteo RS, Weinstein JA, et al. A controlled trial of esmolol for the induction of deliberate hypotension. *J Clin Anesth.* 1988;1:31–35.
125. Pakarinen S. Incidence, aetiology, and prognosis of primary subarachnoid hemorrhage: a study based on 589 cases diagnosed in a defined urban population during a defined period. *Acta Neurol Scand suppl.* 1967;29:1–28.
126. Parer JT, Eng E, Aoba H, et al. Uterine blood flow and oxygen uptake during maternal hyperventilation in monkeys at cesarean section. *Anesthesiology.* 1970;32:130–135.
127. Peerless SJ. Intracranial aneurysms. In: Newfield P, Cottrell JE, eds. *Handbook of Neuroanesthesia.* Boston, Mass: Little Brown & Co; 1983:173–206.
128. Perkins WJ, Lanier WL, Scheithauer BW, et al. Effect of an excitatory amino acid antagonist (MK-801) on neurologic outcome in a canine model of complete cerebral ischemia. *Anesthesiology.* 1988; 69(suppl):A582. Abstract.
129. Petruk KC, West M, Mohr G, et al. Nimodipine treatment in poor-grade aneurysm patients: results of a multicenter double-blind placebo-controlled trial. *J Neurosurg.* 1988;68:505–517.
130. Phillips LH II, Whisnant JP, O'Fallon WM, et al. The unchanging pattern of subarachnoid hemorrhage in a community. *Neurology.* 1980;30:1034–1040.
131. Pinaud M, Souron R, Lelausque J-N, et al. Cerebral blood flow and cerebral oxygen consumption during nitroprusside-induced hypotension to less than 50 mmHg. *Anesthesiology.* 1989;70:255–260.
132. Prough DS, Coker LH, Lee S, et al. Hyperglycemia and neurologic outcome in patients with closed head injury. *Anesthesiology.* 1988;69(suppl): A584. Abstract.
133. Pulsinelli WA, Levy DE, Sigsbee B, et al. Increased damage after ischemic stroke in patients with hyperglycemia with or without established diabetes mellitus. *Am J Med.* 1983;74:540–544.
134. Pulsinelli WA, Waldman S, Rawlinson D, et al. Moderate hyperglycemia augments ischemic brain damage: a neuropathologic study in the rat. *Neurology.* 1982;32:1239–1246.
135. Ropper AH, Kennedy SF. *Neurological and Neurosurgical Intensive Care.* 2nd edition. Rockville, Md: Aspen Publishers; 1988.
136. Rosenfeld JV, Barnett GH, Sila CA, et al. The effect of subarachnoid hemorrhage on blood and CSF atrial natriuretic factor. *J Neurosurg.* 1989;71:32–37.
137. Rosenørn J, Westergaard L, Hansen PH. Mannitol-induced rebleeding from intracranial aneurysm. *J Neurosurg.* 1983;59:529–530.
138. Roth S, Jones SC, Ebrahim ZY, et al. Local cortical blood flow and oxygen consumption during isoflurane-inducing hypotension: results in patients

undergoing intracranial aneurysm clipping. *Cleve Clin J Med.* 1989;56:766–770.

139. Samra SK, Kroll DA. Subarachnoid hemorrhage and intraoperative electrocardiographic changes simulating myocardial ischemia: anesthesiologist's dilemma. *Anesth Analg.* 1985;64:86–89.
140. Schramm J, Koht A, Schmidt G, et al. Surgical and electrophysiological observations during clipping of 134 aneurysms with evoked potential monitoring. *Neurosurgery.* 1990;26:61–70.
141. Schubert A. Should mild hypothermia be routinely used for human cerebral protection? The flip side. *J Neurosurg Anes.* 1992;4:216–220.
142. Selman WR, Spetzler RF, Roski RA, et al. Barbiturate coma in focal cerebral ischemia: relationship of protection to timing of therapy. *J Neurosurg.* 1982;56:685–690.
143. Shapiro HM. Physiology and pharmacology of the perioperative management of patients with intracranial aneurysms. *Refresher Courses Anesth.* 1982; 10:201–212.
144. Siemkowicz E, Hansen AJ. Clinical restitution following cerebral ischemia in hypo-, normo-, and hyperglycemic rats. *Acta Neurol Scand.* 1978;58:1–8.
145. Silverberg GD, Reitz BA, Ream AK. Hypothermia and cardiac arrest in the treatment of giant aneurysms of the cerebral circulation and hemangioblastoma of the medulla. *J Neurosurg.* 1981; 55:337–346.
146. Solomon RA, Fink ME, Lennihan L. Early aneurysm surgery and prophylactic hypervolemic hypertensive therapy for the treatment of aneurysmal subarachnoid hemorrhage. *Neurosurgery.* 1988; 23:699–704.
147. Solomon RA, Smith CR, Raps EC, et al. Deep hypothermic circulatory arrest for the management of complex anterior and posterior circulation aneurysms. *Neurosurgery.* 1991;29:732–737.
148. Spetzler RF, Hadley MN, Ragamonti D, et al. Aneurysms of the basilar artery treated with circulatory arrest, hypothermia, and barbiturate cerebral protection. *J Neurosurg.* 1988;68:868–879.
149. Stober T, Kunze K. Electrocardiographic alterations in subarachnoid haemorrhage: correlation between spasm of the arteries of the left side of the brain and T inversion and QT prolongation. *J Neurol.* 1982;227:99–113.
150. Stullken EH Jr, Balestrieri FJ, Prough DS, et al. The hemodynamic effects of nimodipine in patients anesthetized for cerebral aneurysm clipping. *Anesthesiology.* 1985;62:346–348.
151. Stullken EH Jr, Johnston WE Jr, Prough DS, et al. Implications of nimodipine prophylaxis of cerebral vasospasm on anesthetic management during intracranial aneurysm clipping. *J Neurosurg.* 1985; 62:200–205.
152. Sundt TM Jr, Whisnant JP. Subarachnoid hemorrhage from intracranial aneurysms: surgical management and natural history of disease. *N Engl J Med.* 1978;299:116–122.
153. Suzuki J, Tanaka S, Yoshimoto T. Recirculation in the acute period of cerebral infarction: brain swelling and its suppression using mannitol. *Surg Neurol.* 1980;14:467–472.
154. Suzuki J, Yoshimoto T, Kayama T. Surgical treatment of middle cerebral artery aneurysms. *J Neurosurg.* 1984;61:17–23.
155. Suzuki J, Yoshimoto T, Kodama N, et al. A new therapeutic method for acute brain infarction: revascularization following the administration of mannitol and perfluorochemicals: a preliminary report. *Surg Neurol.* 1981;17:325–332.
156. Symon L, Momma F, Murota T. Assessment of reversible cerebral ischemia in man: intraoperative monitoring of the somatosensory evoked response. *Acta Neurochir Suppl (Wien).* 1988;42:3–7.
157. Symon L, Wang AD, Costa E, et al. Perioperative use of somatosensory evoked responses in aneurysm surgery. *J Neurosurg.* 1984;60:269–275.
158. Teasdale G, Rowan JO, Turner J, et al. Cerebral perfusion failure and cortical activity. In: Ingvar DH, Lassen NA, eds. *Cerebral Function, Metabolism and Circulation.* Copenhagen: Munksgaard; 1977:23.14-23.25.
159. Tenjin H, Hirakawa K, Mizukawa N, et al. Dysautoregulation in patients with ruptured aneurysms: cerebral blood flow measurements obtained during surgery by a temperature-controlled thermoelectrical method. *Neurosurgery.* 1988; 23:705–709.
160. Thomas AN, Anderton JM, Harper NJN. Anaesthesia for the treatment of a giant cerebral aneurysm under hypothermic circulatory arrest. *Anaesthesia.* 1990;45:383–385.
161. Todd MM, Warner DS. Perioperative management of the patient with an intracranial aneurysm. *Refresher Courses Anesth.* 1989;17:227–242.
162. Torner JC, Kassell NF, Wallace RB, et al. Preoperative prognostic factors for rebleeding and survival in aneurysm patients receiving antifibrinolytic therapy: report of the Cooperative Aneurysm Study. *Neurosurgery.* 1981;9:506–513.
163. Tsementzis SA, Hitchcock ER. Outcome from "rescue clipping" of ruptured intracranial aneurysms during induction anaesthesia and endotracheal intubation. *J Neurol Neurosurg Psych.* 1985;48:160–163.
164. Turner JM, Powell D, Gibson RM, et al. Intracranial pressure changes in neurosurgical patients during hypotension induced with sodium nitroprusside or trimetaphan. *Br J Anaesth.* 1977;49:419–425.
165. Van Aken H, Fitch W, Graham DI, et al. Cardiovascular and cerebrovascular effects of isoflurane-induced hypotension in the baboon. *Anesth Analg.* 1986;65:565–574.
166. Vermeulen M, van Gijn J, Hijdra A, et al. Causes of acute deterioration in patients with a ruptured intracranial aneurysm. *J Neurosurg.* 1984;60:935–939.
167. Vitez TS, Soper LE, Wong KC, et al. Chronic hypokalemeia and intraoperative dysrhythmias. *Anesthesiology.* 1985;63:130–133.
168. Voldby B, Enevoldsen EM. Intracranial pressure changes following aneurysm rupture, I: clinical and angiographic correlations. *J Neurosurg.* 1982; 56:186–196.
169. Voldby B, Enevoldsen EM, Jensen FT. Cerebrovascular reactivity in patients with ruptured intracranial aneurysms. *J Neurosurg.* 1985;62:59–67.
170. Warner DS. Isoflurane: more than an anesthetic. *J Neurosurg Anesth.* 1990;2:319–321.
171. Warner DS, Sokoll MD, Maktabi M, et al. Nicardipine HCl: clinical experience in patients undergoing anaesthesia for intracranial aneurysm clipping. *Can J Anaesth.* 1989;36:219–223.
172. Weintraub BM, McHenry LC Jr. Cardiac abnormalities in subarachnoid hemorrhage: a resumé. *Stroke.* 1974;5:384–392.

173. Weir B, Grace M, Hansen J, et al. Time course of vasospasm in man. *J Neurosurg.* 1978;48:173–178.
174. Weir BK. Pulmonary edema following fatal aneurysm rupture. *J Neurosurg.* 1978;49:502–507.
175. Weir BK, Drake CG. Rapid growth of residual aneurysmal neck during pregnancy. *J Neurosurg.* 1991;75:780–782.
176. Welsh FA, Ginsberg MD, Rieder W, et al. Deleterious effect of glucose pretreatment on recovery from diffuse cerebral ischemia in the cat, II: Regional metabolite levels. *Stroke.* 1980;11:355–363.
177. Wheelock B, Weir B, Watts R, et al. Timing of surgery for intracerebral hematomas due to aneurysm rupture. *J Neurosurg.* 1983;58:476–481.
178. Whitburn RH, Laishley RS, Jewkes DA. Anaesthesia for simultaneous Caesarean section and clipping of intracerebral aneurysm. *Br J Anaesth.* 1990;64:642–645.
179. White JC, Parker SD, Rogers MC. Preanesthetic evaluation of a patient with pathologic Q waves following subarachnoid hemorrhage. *Anesthesiology.* 1985;62:351–354.
180. Whiting DM, Barnett GH, Little JR. Management of subarachnoid hemorrhage in the critical care unit. *Cleve Clin Med.* 1989;56:775–785.
181. Whitley JM, Prough DS, DeWitt DS. Shock plus an intracranial mass in dogs: cerebrovascular effects of resuscitation fluid choices. *Anesth Analg.* 1988;67(suppl):S259. Abstract.
182. Wilkins RH. Attempted prevention or treatment of intracranial arterial spasm: a survey. *Neurosurgery.* 1980;6:198–210.
183. Willoughby JS. Sodium nitroprusside, pregnancy and multiple intracranial aneurysms. *Anaesth Intensive Care.* 1984;12:358–360.
184. Wilson CB, Spetzler RF. Factors responsible for improved results in the surgical management of intracranial aneurysms and vascular malformations. *Am J Surg.* 1977;134:33–37.
185. Winn HR, Taylor J, Kaiser DL. Prevalence of asymptomatic incidental aneurysms: review of 4,568 arteriograms. *Stroke.* 1983;14:121. Abstract.
186. Woodside J Jr, Garner L, Bedford RF, et al. Captopril reduces the dose requirement for sodium nitroprusside induced hypotension. *Anesthesiology.* 1984;60:413–417.
187. Young WL, Solomon RA, Pedley TA, et al. Direct cortical EEG monitoring during temporary vascular occlusion for cerebral aneurysm surgery. *Anesthesiology.* 1989;71:794–799.
188. Zornow MH, Scheller MS, Todd MM, et al. Acute cerebral effects of isotonic crystalloid and colloid solutions following cryogenic brain injury in the rabbit. *Anesthesiology.* 1988;69:180–184.
189. Zornow MH, Todd MM, Moore SS. The acute cerebral effects of changes in plasma of osmolality and oncotic pressure. *Anesthesiology.* 1987;67:936–941.

# CHAPTER 6

# Early Versus Delayed Surgery for Ruptured Aneurysms

Mark E. Shaffrey, MD, Christopher I. Shaffrey, MD, and Neal F. Kassell, MD

The timing of aneurysm surgery has been a topic of major neurosurgical controversy. Optimal timing of surgery following aneurysmal subarachnoid hemorrhage (SAH) is a crucial management variable that not only can be reliably manipulated by the neurosurgeon but may significantly affect the outcome of the patient. Although the majority of an estimated 28,000 North Americans that suffer from ruptured intracranial aneurysms will survive the initial ictus in good health, only about 1 in 3 will recover to the fullest extent.[17] Thus, the medical and surgical management of aneurysmal SAH is still far from optimal.

Outcome following aneurysm rupture is influenced by many interrelated factors, including the severity of the initial hemorrhage, rebleeding, the timing and technical success of surgical management, and the prevention and treatment of complications.[35] Morbidity and mortality following SAH primarily result from effects of the initial hemorrhage, vasospasm, and rebleeding, in descending order of frequency.[22] The primary objective of aneurysm surgery is prevention of rebleeding through obliteration of the sac. Early surgical intervention, however, also affords the opportunity to influence the development or treatment of vasospasm.

Traditionally, the timing of aneurysm surgery has balanced the technical considerations of surgery with the risk of morbidity and mortality occurring during the interval between SAH and clipping. These considerations have resulted in two schools of thought. "Early" aneurysm surgery is typically considered to be from 0–3 days postictus, while "delayed" surgery generally is more than 7 days following initial SAH. Although in the past most surgical decisions have been influenced by anecdotal accounts of experience with each "school," the controversy has resulted in completion of a prospective, observational, nonrandomized evaluation of this problem—the International Cooperative Study on Timing of Aneurysm Surgery.

## History of Early Versus Delayed Aneurysm Surgery

Soon after Walter Dandy's earliest attempt to cure an aneurysm of the circle of Willis by direct obliteration of the aneurysmal sac in 1937, the appropriate timing of aneurysm surgery became a continuing topic of debate.[3] When intracranial operations for ruptured aneurysms became more prevalent in the late 1940s and early 1950s, early surgery was performed, usually on an urgent basis.[19] At this time, however, unacceptably high operative mortality rates were encountered primarily due to limitations in visualization, instrumentation, and neuroanesthesia.[19]

In 1953 Norlēn and Olivecrona published a pivotal paper reporting a 3% operative mortality rate for patients operated upon 3 weeks or more following aneurysmal SAH.[27] This was in stark contrast to those patients that underwent "acute" surgery (defined at that time as a few hours to 3 weeks following hemorrhage) who had a 53% mortality rate.[27] For the next 2 decades this paper greatly influenced the timing of surgical management of aneurysmal SAH, and has served as a cornerstone in the argument for the delayed surgical approach.[19]

In the early 1960s, Pool and Hunt remained proponents of early surgery for patients in good neurologic condition; however, delayed surgery was generally practiced.[13,31] In 1965, Norlēn published results which advocated surgery within the first 2 days following SAH to prevent the disastrous effects of rebleeding.[26] From the mid-1960s until the mid-1970s, the hazards of rebleeding and cerebral vasospasm became more clearly defined.[7,37] Death and disability due to these processes gave rise to further attempts at early surgery, but most reports continued to describe significantly increased operative morbidity and mortality with early surgical approaches.[11,12,20]

## The Influence of Technology on the Timing of Aneurysm Surgery

Over the past 25 years, reductions in surgical morbidity and mortality have paralleled technical advances, playing a major role in the relatively recent resurgence of early aneurysm surgery following aneurysmal SAH. In 1966, Pool and Colton reported the use of the dissecting microscope for aneurysm surgery,[32] and since that time, the operating microscope has become almost universal in the surgical treatment of intracranial aneurysms. Advantages arising from the use of the microscope include: improved visualization of complex or partially-obscured structures through magnification and illumination; more accurate ligation of the aneurysm neck while reducing the inadvertant occlusion of small perforators; removal of fresh clot from the basal cisterns, possibly reducing the risk of vasospasm; and the development of complex operative approaches to such regions as the cavernous sinus, the basilar trunk, and the distal vertebral arteries.[35]

Closely linked to the development of the operative microscope is the evolution of new generations of microinstruments. These include a wide range of microsurgical dissectors, forceps, scissors, knives, clip appliers, and needle holders that, in conjunction with the microscope, allow a more precise approach to the aneurysmal sac. Many advances also have occurred in the technology of aneurysm clips. Since the early hemostatic clips first used by Cushing, "cross-legged" clips have been developed which permit multiple applications and removals but which close with sufficient force to prevent dislodging by pulsatile arterial blood flow.[35] Other advances in clip technology include bayonet clips which improve visualization during clip application, fenestrated clips which allow ligation of the aneurysm neck with preservation of adjacent vessels, and "booster" clips which provide additional closing force for atherosclerotic and/or calcified aneurysm necks.[35,38,41]

The ability to operate on tight, swollen brain in the acute stage post-SAH is greatly aided by developments in neuroanesthesia. Brain relaxation may be approached by several means including controlled hypotensive anesthesia with isoflurane, hyperventilation, and mannitol. The neuroanesthesiologist plays a critical role in the use of hypothermic techniques. Moderate hypothermia is especially attractive in complex cases when there is increased risk of cerebral ischemia, thus making a reduction in the neuronal metabolic rate advantageous.[36]

The emergence of neurovascular surgery as a distinct subspecialty has provided well-trained and experienced surgeons who continually seek to improve upon the surgical results of the preceding generations. It is only in light of the advances in technology, anesthesia, and expertise that an enlightened comparison between early and delayed surgical management of aneurysmal SAH is possible. The most crucial areas for comparison include the effects of the timing of aneurysm surgery on rebleeding, vasospasm, operative morbidity and mortality, and overall management.

## Comparison of Early Versus Delayed Aneurysm Surgery

### *Rebleeding*

Aneurysmal rebleeding is the most cataclysmic and disabling event following initial SAH. The mortality rates from rebleeding have been cited between 70% to 90%.[33] The highest incidence of rebleeding is within the initial 24–48 hours and, in the absence of surgical treatment, there is a 20% to 30% incidence of rebleeding within 2 weeks of the initial ictus.[15,21,24,35] It has been estimated that 1 in 6 patients suffering aneurysmal SAH will die or become severely disabled from rebleeding.[17] Thus, early surgical obliteration of the aneurysm eliminates the potential for rebleeding during the highest risk period.

While awaiting a delayed surgical approach, there is theoretically significant advantage to impeding the lysis of the blood clot that seals the site of initial aneurysm rupture. The two most commonly prescribed antifibrinolytic drugs are the synthetic amino carboxylic acid derivatives, epsilon-aminocaproic acid (EACA) and tranexamic acid (AMCA), which effect antifibrinolytic activity by competitive inhibition of plasminogen activation.[9] From a clinical standpoint, however, while antifibrinolytic agents reduce rebleeding rates by almost 50%, there is a concurrent increase in ischemic neurologic deficits.[18] Therefore, rebleeding rates are diminished at the expense of increasing ischemic neurologic complications. The reason for this is unclear. Theories include: the possibility of increased propensity for cerebrovascular thrombotic events related to these medications; potential reduced clearing of the subarachnoid clot, prolonging the influence of the factors that cause vasospasm; or, it may be that the incidence of ischemia is not increased per se, but that drug-reduced mortality related to rebleeding results in more patients surviving to suffer the ischemic complications of vasospasm.[9,10,16,34]

Regardless of the etiology of the complications, there appears to be no well-defined role for antifibrinolytic therapy if surgical treatment is anticipated within the first 24–48 hours following SAH.[19] If surgery is to be delayed more than 2 days after admission, however, it may be considered reasonable to employ these agents, acknowledging the potential to develop or aggravate focal ischemic neurologic deficits.[35]

### *Vasospasm*

Although aneurysmal rebleeding is the most dramatic complication following initial rupture, cerebral vasospasm is the leading treatable cause of morbidity and mortality in tertiary care centers.[22] The occurrence rate of angiographic vasospasm has been estimated to be as high as 70% to 90% in the first 2 weeks following SAH.[1,14,19,40] The ischemic neurologic deficits resulting from vasospasm may occur in as many as half of patients demonstrating angiographic vasospasm.[20] It is encouraging, however, that clinical vasospasm appears to be waning, with attributed mortality rates decreasing from over 40% in the 1960s to 15% in the early 1980s to currently less than 8%.[20]

Early aneurysm clipping (prior to the onset of vasospasm) provides the opportunity for removal of subarachnoid clot and the irrigation of spasmogenic substances from the subarachnoid spaces. Predictably, mechanical clot removal results in only partial clearing of the subarachnoid hematoma, while incurring a significant risk of bruising pial banks and injuring small vessels.[35] Despite successful studies in the primate model, recent clinical studies cast doubt on the importance of mechanical clot removal in the deterrence of vasospasm.[14,28]

Another approach to the removal of subarachnoid clot is via thrombolytic therapy. This entails the irrigation of the subarachnoid space with recombinant tissue plasminogen activator (rTPA) or urokinase at the time of surgery and/or in the postoperative period. Preclinical data have demonstrated substantial clearing of large subarachnoid hematomas, and have suggested the prevention of arterial vasospasm and ischemic neurologic deficits.[5,6] The major concern of thrombolytic therapy is the risk of intracranial bleeding; therefore, more rigorous clinical trials are necessary to document safety and effectiveness.

A further potential benefit of early surgery is the more aggressive treatment of reversible ischemic deficits secondary to vasospasm, theoretically accomplished through optimization of the patient's hemodynamic and rheologic status. This is often referred to as hypervolemic, hypertensive hemodilution or "triple H" therapy.

Although "triple H" therapy is a poor alternative to definitive measures for preventing or reversing arterial narrowing, it will be an essential component in the treatment of cerebral vasospasm for the near future. Increasing arterial pressure, however, can result in rebleeding of previously unruptured aneurysms, and new bleeding from incidental but unsecured aneurysms.[20,30] Thus, the delay of surgical treatment may put the patient at risk for rebleeding if "triple H" therapy is necessary and the aneurysm is not obliterated.

## *Operative Morbidity and Mortality*

Prior to the early 1970s most reports indicated that there was a higher incidence of operative morbidity and mortality associated with early aneurysm surgery. The decision to delay surgery was appropriate based on superior operative results. Since that time, advances in expertise, technology, and neuroanesthesia have caused surgeons to reevaluate these results for both approaches. Most current anecdotal series find that operative mortalities in experienced hands are comparable with early or delayed strategies.[2,4,25,29,39]

Included as part of the Cooperative Study on the Timing of Aneurysm Surgery was a subjective evaluation by neurosurgeons of the relative "tightness" of the brain at the time of surgery. In nearly half of the patients operated upon on day 0 or 1, surgeons noted that the brains were tight.[25] In contrast, tight brains were noted in approximately 20% of patients who had surgery on day 10 or later.[23] However, despite a greater percentage of cases with the brain being "tighter" in early surgery, it was not associated with an increased operative morbidity in the form of brain contusions, lacerations, or the requirement for significant brain resection.[23]

## *Management Results*

Despite the advances in treatment of patients with aneurysmal SAH, at least half will die or become disabled. The final common denominator in treatment of ruptured intracranial aneurysms, and the ultimate comparison for early and delayed surgical approaches, is the total morbidity and mortality resulting from a particular course of treatment—the overall management results.

Delayed surgery was the standard for many years because resultant postoperative complications were few. With delayed surgery, however, many patients died or were severely disabled as a result of rebleeding or vasospasm during the interval between SAH and surgery. Milhorat and Krautheim reported a 0% operative mortality in delayed surgery patients, with the overall mortality rate being 65%.[25] The combined results of the International Cooperative Study on the Timing of Aneurysm Surgery revealed that management morbidity and mortality were equivalent in both early and late surgery groups.[22] The most favorable outcomes and lowest mortality rates were among alert patients for whom surgery was planned on days 0–3 and 11–14.[22] The group of patients who had surgery planned for days 7 through 10 had the least favorable outcome and the highest mortality rate.[22] It was found that the results of surgery were generally superior when the operation was performed subsequent to day 10 post-SAH but that the operative results were counterbalanced by the increased rate of complications occurring during the delay.[22]

Recently, patient data from North American centers in the International Cooperative Study on the Timing of Aneurysm Surgery (772 patients, 22% of the total study population) have undergone analysis for management results.[8] The overall outcome at 6 months in patients with surgery planned for days 0–3 and 11–32 were equivalent with regard to mortality, but the early patients had significantly improved rates of good recovery as compared with the delayed patients (71% versus 62%, $p < 0.01$).[8] In addition, since the data collection, reports by experienced aneurysm surgeons describe improved management morbidity and mortality with the initiation of a policy of early definitive aneurysm operations.[4,29]

## Conclusion

It is the authors' belief that initiation of a policy of early operation at centers with experienced surgeons and committed operative facilities will result in a superior overall outcome. As the incidence of vasospasm decreases with prophylactic therapy, and more effective methods of treatment for vasospasm continue to be developed, management results with early surgery should even further improve as compared to delayed surgery. However, instances for delaying surgery are still indicated and include: patients who present with severe vasospasm following SAH, those in poor medical condition at the time of presentation, and situations where full resources for early surgery may not be available.

## References


1. Adams HP Jr. Calcium antagonists in the management of patients with aneurysmal subarachnoid hemorrhage: a review. *Angiology.* 1990;41:1010–1016.
2. Chyatte D, Fode NC, Sundt TM Jr. Early versus late intracranial aneurysm surgery in subarachnoid hemorrhage. *J Neurosurg.* 1988;69:326–331.
3. Dandy WE. Intracranial aneurysm of the internal carotid artery: cured by operation. *Ann Surg.* 1938; 107:654–659.
4. Disney L, Weir B, Petruk K. Effect on management mortality of a deliberate policy of early operation on supratentorial aneurysms. *Neurosurgery.* 1987; 20:695–701.
5. Findlay JM, Weir BKA, Kanamaru K, et al. The effect of timing of intrathecal fibrinolytic therapy on cerebral vasospasm in a primate model of subarachnoid hemorrhage. *Neurosurgery.* 1990;26:201–206.
6. Findlay JM, Weir BKA, Kanamaru K, et al. Intrathecal fibrinolytic therapy after subarachnoid hemorrhage: dosage study in a primate model and review of the literature. *Can J Neurol Sci.* 1989;16:28–40.
7. Gibbs JR, O'Gorman P. Fibrinolysis in subarachnoid hemorrhage. *Postgrad Med J.* 1967;43: 779–784.
8. Haley EC Jr, Kassell NF, Torner JC. The International Cooperative Study on the Timing of Aneurysm Surgery: the North American experience. *Stroke.* 1992;23:205–214.
9. Haley EC Jr, Torner JC, Kassell NF. Antifibrinolytic therapy and cerebral vasospasm. *Neurosurg Clin N Am.* 1990;1:349–356.
10. Hoffman EP, Koo AH. Cerebral thrombosis associated with Amicar therapy. *Radiology.* 1979; 131:687–689.
11. Hunt WE, Hess RM. Surgical risk as related to time of intervention in the repair of intracranial aneurysms. *J Neurosurg.* 1968;28:14–20.
12. Hunt WE, Kosnick EJ. Timing and perioperative care in intracranial aneurysm surgery. *Clin Neurosurg.* 1974;21:79–89.
13. Hunt WE, Meagher JN, Barnes JE. The management of intracranial aneurysm. *J Neurosurg.* 1962;19:34–40.
14. Inagawa T. Effect of early operation on cerebral vasospasm. *Surg Neurol.* 1990;33:239–246.
15. Jane JA, Winn HR, Richardson AE. The natural history of intracranial aneurysms: rebleeding rates during the acute and long term period and implication for surgical management. *Clin Neurosurg.* 1977;24: 176–184.
16. Kangston E, Palma L. Influence of antifibrinolytic treatment on the morbidity in patients with subarachnoid hemorrhage. *Acta Neurol Scand.* 1972;48:257–258.
17. Kassell NF, Drake CG. Timing of aneurysm surgery. *Neurosurgery.* 1982;10:514–519.
18. Kassell NF, Haley EC, Torner JC. Antifibrinolytic therapy in the treatment of aneurysmal subarachnoid hemorrhage. *Clin Neurosurg.* 1986;33:137–145.
19. Kassell NF, Shaffrey CI, Shaffrey ME. Timing of aneurysm surgery. In: Wilkins RH, Rengachary SS, eds. *Neurosurgery Update* Vol 2. New York, NY: McGraw-Hill; 1990;2:95–99.
20. Kassell NF, Shaffrey ME, Shaffrey CI. Cerebral vasospasm following aneurysmal subarachnoid hemorrhage. In: Apuzzo MLJ, ed. *Brain Surgery: Complication Avoidance and Management.* New York, NY: Churchill Livingstone; 1992.
21. Kassell NF, Torner JC. Aneurysmal rebleeding: a preliminary report from the Cooperative Aneurysm Study. *Neurosurgery.* 1983;13:479–481.

22. Kassell NF, Torner JC, Haley EC Jr, et al. The International Cooperative Study on the Timing of Aneurysm Surgery. I: overall management results. *J Neurosurg.* 1990;73:18–36.
23. Kassell NF, Torner JC, Haley EC Jr, et al. The International Cooperative Study on the Timing of Aneurysm Surgery. II: surgical results. *J Neurosurg.* 1990;73:37–47.
24. McKissock W, Richardson A, Walsh L. Middle-cerebral aneurysms: further results in the controlled trial of conservative and surgical treatment of ruptured intracranial aneurysms. *Lancet.* 1962;2:417–421.
25. Milhorat TH, Krautheim M. Results of early and delayed operations for ruptured intracranial aneurysms in two series of 100 consecutive patients. *Surg Neurol.* 1986;26:123–128.
26. Norlén G. Some aspects of the surgical treatment of intracranial aneurysms. *Clin Neurosurg.* 1963; 9:214–222.
27. Norlén G, Olivecrona H. The treatment of aneurysms of the circle of Willis. *J Neurosurg.* 1953;10: 404–415.
28. Nosko M, Weir BKA, Lunt A, et al. Effect of clot removal at 24 hours on chronic vasospasm after SAH in the primate model. *J Neurosurg.* 1987;66:416–422.
29. Öhman J, Heiskanen O. Timing of operation for ruptured supratentorial aneurysms: a prospective randomized study. *J Neurosurg.* 1989;70:55–60.
30. Origitano TC, Wascher TM, Reichman OH, et al. Sustained increased cerebral blood flow with prophylactic hypertensive hypervolemic hemodilution ("Triple-H" therapy) after subarachnoid hemorrhage. *Neurosurgery.* 1990;27:729–740.
31. Pool JL. Timing and techniques in the intracranial surgery of ruptured aneurysms of the anterior communicating artery. *J Neurosurg.* 1962;19:378–388.
32. Pool JL, Colton RP. The dissecting microscope for intracranial vascular surgery. *J Neurosurg.* 1966; 25:315–318.
33. Rosenørn J, Eskesen V, Schmidt K, et al. The risk of rebleeding from ruptured intracranial aneurysms. *J Neurosurg.* 1987;67:329–332.
34. Rydin E, Lundberg PO. Tranexamic acid and intracranial thrombosis. *Lancet.* 1976;2:49. Letter.
35. Shaffrey ME, Shaffrey CI, Kassell NF. Surgical management of ruptured intracranial aneurysms. In: Adams HP, ed. *Handbook of Cerebrovascular Diseases.* New York, NY: Decker: 1993;509–518.
36. Stone DJ. Anesthesia for intracranial vascular surgery. In: Sperry RJ, Stirt JA, Stone DJ, eds. *Manual of Neuroanesthesia.* Philadelphia, Pa: BC Decker; 1989:131–142.
37. Stornelli SA, French JD. Subarachnoid hemorrhage: factors in prognosis and management. *J Neurosurg.* 1964;21:769–780.
38. Sugita K, Hirota T, Iguchi I. Comparative study of the pressure of various aneurysm clips. *J Neurosurg.* 1976;44:723–727.
39. Suzuki J, Yoshimoto T. Early operation for the ruptured intracranial aneurysm—especially the cases operated within 48 hours after the last subarachnoid hemorrhage. *Neurol Surg (Tokyo).* 1976;4:135–141.
40. Tettenborn D, Dycka J. Prevention and treatment of delayed ischemic dysfunction in patients with aneurysmal subarachnoid hemorrhage. *Stroke.* 1990; 21(suppl IV):85–89.
41. Weir B. *Aneurysms Affecting the Nervous System.* Baltimore, Md.: Williams & Wilkins, 1987;88–93, 429–432, 625–629.

# CHAPTER 7

# Surgical Treatment of Anterior Circulation Aneurysms

Robert A. Solomon, MD

This chapter focuses on the technical aspects of surgical treatment of anterior circulation berry aneurysms. No attempt is made to discuss the management of subarachnoid hemorrhage (SAH) , giant aneurysms, posterior circulation aneurysms, or cavernous sinus aneurysms. These subjects are addressed in other chapters.

## History

The surgical management of intracranial aneurysms dates back nearly 200 years when the first cases of cervical carotid ligation were performed for patients with intracranial hemorrhage. Some of these cases were undoubtedly aneurysms, but the first confirmed intracranial aneurysm treated by carotid ligation was reported by Sir Victor Horsley in 1885.[13] Carotid ligation went on to become the standard neurosurgical treatment for cerebral aneurysms until the middle of the 20th Century.

The first reported attempt at direct ligation of an intracranial aneurysm was by Zeller in 1911.[26] An intraoperative rupture led to the patient's death. A successful intracranial aneurysm operation was first performed by Norman Dott in Great Britain in 1931.[5] A small ruptured carotid artery bifurcation aneurysm was directly wrapped with muscle and the patient made an excellent recovery. The first successful clipping of an intracranial aneurysm was done in 1937 by Walter Dandy using a silver vascular clip. The patient made a complete recovery following clipping of the posterior communicating artery aneurysm, and the modern era of aneurysm surgery was launched.[2]

The 1940s and 1950s saw a great expansion in both the number of neurosurgeons and their capabilities. During this time neurosurgeons became well acquainted with the techniques necessary to approach intracranial aneurysms at any location and to mechanically obliterate the aneurysm neck.[6,14,15,19,20] Sophisticated instrumentation and vascular clips were developed by numerous surgeons and manufacturers to facilitate clipping of intracranial aneurysms. With the advent of the operating microscope in neurosurgery in the 1960s, aneurysm surgery again took a leap forward.

Although a number of surgeons used the microscope to operate on intracranial aneurysms, most of the credit for the modern microsurgical approach to anterior circulation aneurysms must go to Yasargil, who popularized the pterional craniotomy for anterior circulation aneurysms.[33] He emphasized the importance of the modern neurosurgeon being facile with microsurgical techniques, stressed the advantages of minimizing brain retraction by complete removal of the sphenoid wing, and detailed the cisternal ap-

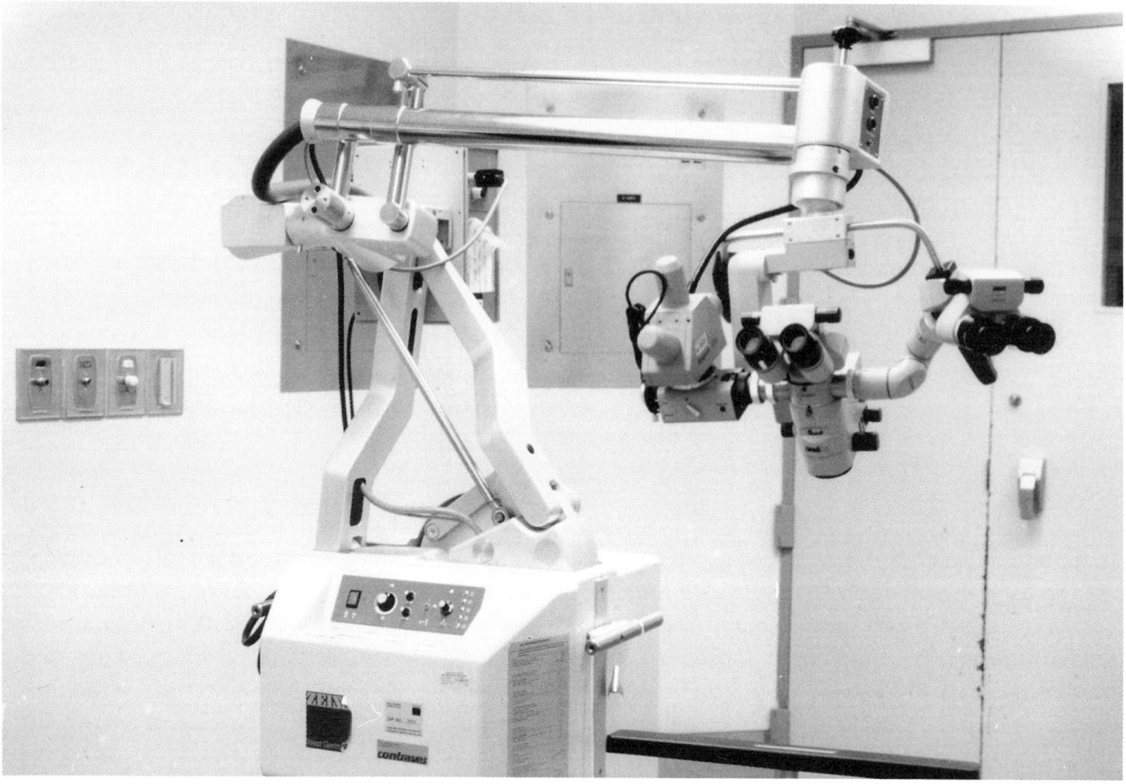

*Figure 1. The Zeiss operating microscope with the Contraves stand is the standard for microneurosurgical procedures.*

proaches necessary to arrive at anterior circulation aneurysms in any location with minimal brain retraction and trauma.[31,32]

## Equipment and Instrumentation

Proper equipment and operating room instrumentation are critical to the success of neurosurgical procedures. Nowhere are these factors more important than in aneurysm surgery. The operating microscope allows neurosurgeons to work through very narrow openings in the skull, mandating long, delicate instruments to work at the depths of the operative field. Each surgeon develops a personal preference of dissection instruments, suction tips, clip appliers, and aneurysm clips. There is no specified list of equipment that every microneurosurgeon must have, but each surgeon must develop a repertoire of a variety microsurgical instruments capable of performing multiple technical maneuvers. The surgeon must feel comfortable and have practice in using the equipment.

The Zeiss operating microscope with the Contraves stand has become the standard instrument for microsurgical procedures (Figure 1). This microscope, with its excellent optics and coaxial illumination, can be positioned with ease to accommodate any desired angle of vision through the operative opening.

Suction tips form one of the most critical pieces of microsurgical instrumentation. Having a straight suction tube connected to the wall suction reduces the efficacy and potential utilization of the suction tip in microneurosurgery. Microsuction tips designed by Fukushima are particularly useful. These suction tips come in various lengths and diameters, with a continuously tapered shaft that prevents clogging of the suction tip lumen. A thumb hole allows for continuous absolute

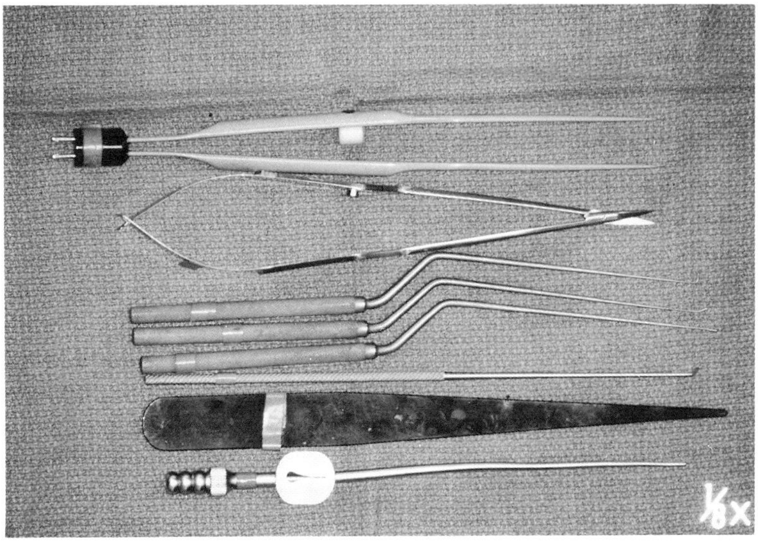


*Figure 2. A sampling of the types of instruments required for microneurosurgery. From top to bottom, they are: (1) insulated Rhoton bipolar forceps with 3 mm tips; (2) bayonetted pinch scissors; (3) bayonetted and straight distractors with tips of various shapes and sizes; (4) tapered retractor; and, (5) Fukushima microsuction device.*

control of suction pressure from zero suction to full force suction, allowing the surgeon to use the tip both as a dissector and as a well-controlled device to remove unwanted fluids and tissue fragments.

An array of dissectors with various tips of different size and angulation are mandatory for aneurysm dissection (Figure 2). Sharp dissection is often preferable to blunt dissection around an aneurysm since the sharp dissection avoids traction on a precarious aneurysm dome. A disposable blade such as the Beaver eye blade makes an excellent cutting instrument with a reliably sharp tip.

The clip applier is critically important and perhaps even of greater importance than the aneurysm clip. A variety of clip appliers are offered by various instrument manufacturers and all of them have specific advantages and disadvantages. The Fukushima clip appliers allow clip application at any angle while maintaining a very low profile of the tip of the clip applier.[22] This factor becomes critical when applying clips into deep exposures and when navigating around critical structures that must be preserved (Figure 3).

## Pterional Craniotomy

Except in rare circumstances, all anterior circulation aneurysms and aneurysms around the basilar apex can be accessed by the pterional craniotomy. This approach is designed to take advantage of naturally occurring planes and spaces that can be used to expose the base of the brain without significant brain retraction. The orbital roof and sphenoid wing occupy a space under the frontal lobe and between the frontal and temporal lobes. Removal of the sphenoid wing and flattening of the orbital roof opens a pathway that requires only minimal enlargement with frontal lobe retraction to provide operative exposure to the parasellar region. Dissection and opening of the sylvian fissure also allows for widened exposure of this space, increasing access to the prepontine cisterns and middle cerebral artery.

### *Patient Positioning*

Positioning is critical to increasing the positive contribution of gravity and decreasing

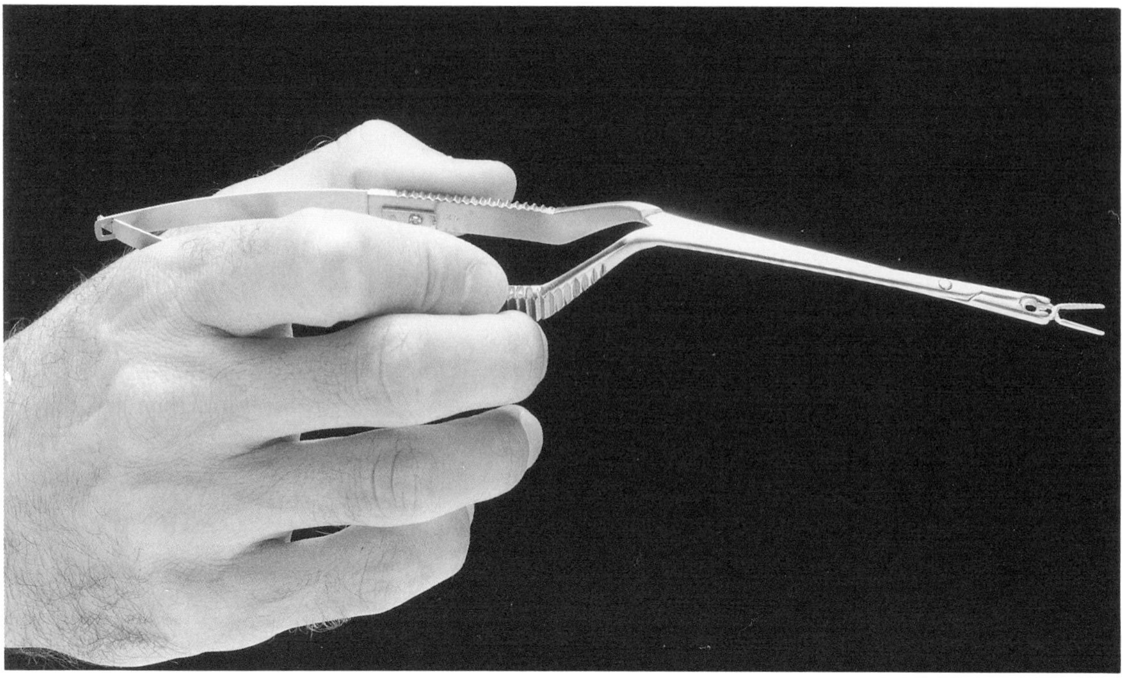

*Figure 3.* *Solomon/Fukushima clip applier holding a straight Yasargil clip.*

the negative contributions of venous engorgement. The patient is positioned supine with the head of the bed elevated about 10° to 15° to ensure that final position of the head is above the level of the heart. The neck is maximally extended (Figure 4). The head is elevated slightly and then rotated between 20° to 45° away from the side of the craniotomy (Figure 5).

For carotid aneurysms, the amount of rotation should be about 45°, but for midline aneurysms of the anterior communicating artery and basilar apex, the rotation is minimized to only 15° to 20°. Such positioning will minimize venous pressure and allow gravity to enhance the relaxation of the frontal lobes away from the orbital roof. The head should always be held in a rigid three-point fixation device such as the Mayfield-Kees head holder.

## Soft Tissue Dissection

The incision begins 1 cm anterior to the external auditory meatus and extends from the zygoma, following the hairline anteriorly to the midline. This incision is cosmetically invisible since hair will hide the scar. An inci-

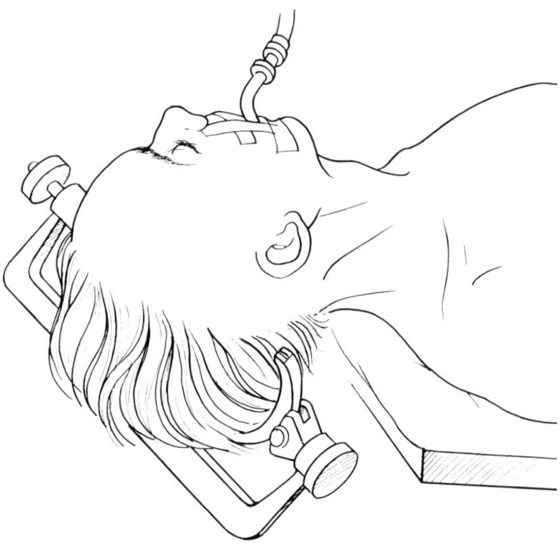

***Figure 4.*** *Drawing of the patient's head position. The head of the bed is elevated about 10° to 15°. The neck is maximally extended and the skull is held in rigid pin fixation with the Mayfield-Kees holder.*

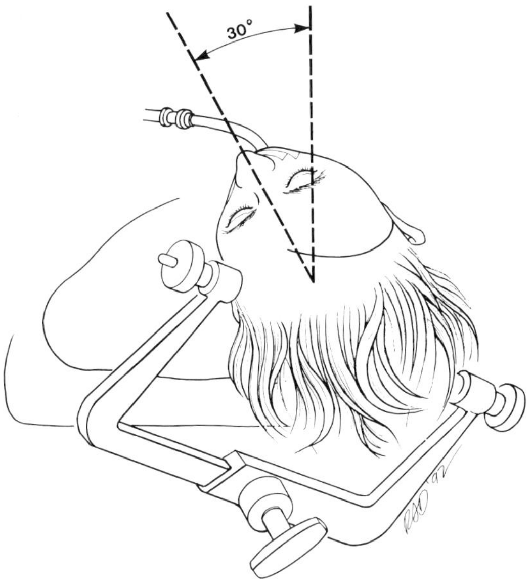


*Figure 5. Another view of the patient's head position, showing 30° angulation of the head away from the side of the intended craniotomy.*

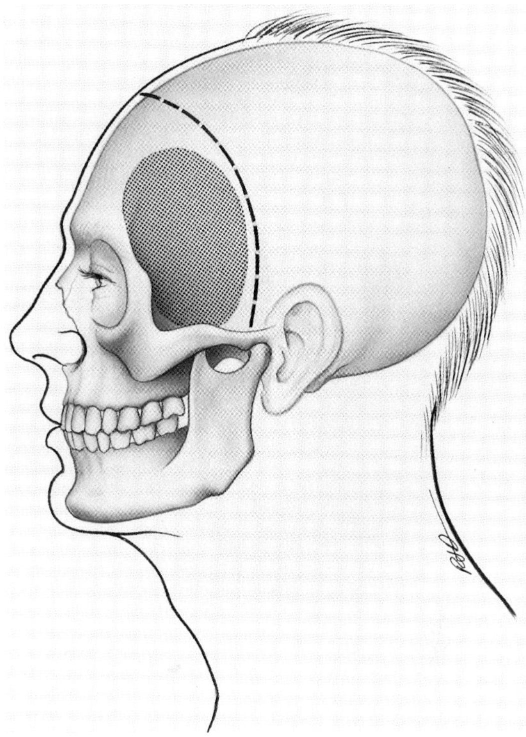

*Figure 6. Drawing of the skull shows the location of the scalp incision and the shaded area indicating the approximate location of the pterional craniotomy.*

sion in the posterior aspect of the temporalis muscle allows the muscle and the scalp flap to be elevated anteriorly as a single layer. This method of anterior elevation of the muscle, as opposed to the interfascial temporalis flap described by Yasargil,[31] minimizes the potential risk to the frontalis branch of the facial nerve. During elevation of the muscle flap from its insertion on the superior temporal line, it is usually advisable to leave a small cuff of the fascia attached to the frontal bone: when the muscle is repaired at the end of the case, the muscle can then be reattached to its proper bony insertion.[25]

## *Craniotomy*

The bone flap can be turned either with a craniotome or using multiple burr holes and Gigli saws (Figure 6). A single burr hole can best be placed in the temporal squamosa underneath the temporalis muscle in the posterior aspect of the bony exposure. Using the craniotome inserted into the bony opening on the temporal squamosa, the bone cut starts superiorly along the posterior border of the bony exposure, extending across the linea temporalis, then curving gradually anteriorly to a point above the orbital rim and about 3–4 cm medial to the orbital attachment of the zygoma. The cut then turns inferiorally, following the orbital ridge crossing the linea temporalis as far anterior as possible so that the cut corresponds to the position of the frontal fossa floor. At this point, the sphenoid wing is encountered and further inferior cutting with the craniotome is blocked. A second cut is made inferiorly and anteriorly from the burr hole to the inferior edge of the sphenoid wing.

The bone flap can then be fractured across the sphenoid wing and gentle epidural dissection will free the bone flap from its dural attachments. The dura is freed in an epidural fashion away from the orbital roof and the sphenoid wing. Using a high-speed drill with a cutting burr, the orbital roof is flattened, removing major bumps, and making the bony opening flush with the frontal fossa floor. The lateral part of the sphenoid wing is removed with the drill or small rongeurs as indicated by the individual anatomy in each case. It is best to remove the sphenoid all the way down to the superior orbital fissure, thereby ensuring the maximum amount of bony removal possible to enlarge the opening down to the parasellar region.

### *Dural Opening*

The dura is opened in a semilunar fashion, creating a flap that can be retracted anteriorly. The incision is started at the most superior and anterior aspect of the bony opening, then extended across the frontal lobe, across the sylvian fissure, and then across the temporal lobe, arching back anteriorly to the most inferior and anterior aspect of the bony opening. When this incision is flapped anteriorly and secured with sutures, the epidural space around the sphenoid can be effectively closed off from the operative field so that oozing during the microsurgical aspects of the operation will be minimized. Through this incision in conjunction with a proper bony opening, satisfactory brain dehydration, and cerebrospinal fluid (CSF) removal, the frontal lobe is generally relaxed sufficiently so that a view down to the optic nerve is possible without brain retraction. At this point in the operation, the operating microscope is brought into the field and the rest of the operation utilizes microsurgical techniques. Further steps vary depending on the location and size of the aneurysm, and these issues will be discussed individually in subsequent sections.

## Brain Relaxation Techniques

Satisfactory brain relaxation is critical to a successful aneurysm operation. This factor is most compelling during the treatment of recently ruptured aneurysms where intracranial pressure (ICP) can reach as high as several hundred millimeters of water. Such intracranial hypertension in the setting of extensive SAH has been called red angry swollen brain, a condition presumed to obstruct the technical process of early aneurysm surgery.[7] However, following the rupture of an aneurysm, the elevated intracranial pressure is not actually due to brain parenchymal swelling but to obstructed CSF flow and blood clots in the basal cisterns. Therefore, with extensive CSF drainage, adequate brain relaxation can be achieved in all patients in Grades I–III and most patients in Grades IV and V.[23]

The CSF must be drained prior to the dural opening to reduce ICP to near normal. In most instances, the insertion of an intraoperative spinal drainage catheter in the lumbar thecal sac is the preferred method. In cases with obvious hydrocephalus on preoperative computed tomography (CT) scans, however, a ventriculostomy can effect significant decompression and usually provides adequate relaxation.

The author uses spinal drainage in all patients who are within 2 weeks of an SAH at the time of surgery. Following the induction of general anesthesia, the patient is turned in the lateral decubitus position and, using a 14-gauge Tuey needle, a spinal puncture is performed in the lumbar region. A small ureteral catheter is then passed into the thecal sac and the metallic needle removed. This catheter can then be manipulated by the anesthesiologist to withdraw CSF based on the observations of the surgeon. Usually, between 60 and 100 ml of fluid are removed to provide adequate relaxation during acute aneurysm surgery.

The second most useful technique for brain relaxation is the use of intravenous mannitol. The bolus administration of between 1–2 grams per kilogram of body weight, delivered at about the time of the skin incision, will produce relaxation by brain dehydration. Mannitol also offers some protection from cerebral ischemia and is therefore especially useful in cases where temporary clip application is anticipated. Mannitol is used in all aneurysm operations, regardless of whether the aneurysm is ruptured or unruptured at the time of surgery.

Patient positioning, as mentioned in the previous section, is also critical so as not to unnecessarily increase ICP secondary to poor venous drainage. Therefore, it is important to ensure that the patient's head is positioned above the heart (1) so that venous pressure will be below zero, and (2) so that the neck is not excessively turned, which can kink the jugular veins and increase the venous tension in the head.

The patient should be mildly hyperventilated with $PCO_2$ between 25–30 torr. Currently available anesthetic gases such as isoflurane have minimal contributions to ICP elevation, and therefore are preferable to the previously used agents such as halothane.

## Supraclinoid Carotid Aneurysms

### *Anatomy of the Internal Carotid Artery*

The internal carotid artery (ICA) passes through the petrous bone in the carotid canal and then passes upward, forward, and medially over the foramen lacerum to reach the inferior and posterior aspect of the cavernous sinus. Within the cavernous sinus the carotid artery passes the posterior lateral aspect of the sella turcica and then curves anteriorly, continuing along the lateral aspect of the sella. As it approaches the anterior portion of the sella, the artery loops upward and medially to the top of the cavernous sinus, completing the siphon portion of the carotid artery.

The most important branch of the intracavernous portion of the ICA is the meningohypophyseal trunk. This vessel arises from the lower portion of the siphon and projects posteriorly branching into three main units: the tentorial artery, the dorsal meningeal artery, and the inferior hypophyseal artery. Two other relatively common branches arise from this segment of the carotid artery. These are the artery of the inferior cavernous sinus and the capsular artery of McConnel.

The carotid artery emerges from the cavernous sinus inferior and medial to the anterior clinoid process. The artery is enveloped in a fold of dura which forms the carotid cave. This section of the carotid artery has been termed the clinoidal segment, and is not truly in the subarachnoid space.[3] While still inferior to the anterior clinoid process, the carotid artery then enters the carotid cistern and thus the subarachnoid space. The cisternal compartmentalization of the subarachnoid space is somewhat variable but has been very well described by Yasargil.[31]

The branches of the ICA above the cavernous sinus include the ophthalmic artery, one or more superior hypophyseal arteries, the posterior communicating artery, the anterior choroidal, and the terminal branches of the ICA—the anterior and middle cerebral arteries. On rare occasions, the ophthalmic artery and the superior hypophyseal arteries can arise within the cavernous sinus. The ophthalmic artery is the first major branch and is directed anteriorly and medially to follow the optic nerve back into the orbit. The superior hypophyseal artery is inferiorally and medially directed to supply the pituitary stalk, tuber cinereum, anterior lobe of the pituitary, and the inferior surface of the optic nerves.

Usually the largest branch of the ICA before its termination is the posterior communicating artery, which arises inferolaterally from the carotid artery and courses posteriorly and medially to connect with the proximal portion of the posterior cerebral artery (PCA) in the posterior fossa. Numerous important perforating branches arise from the posterior communicating artery and supply the inferior optic chiasm, optic tract, and portions of the medial hypothalamus and inferior thalamus.[10]

The anterior choroidal artery, which is occasionally duplicated, arises just distally to the posterior communicating artery, usually on the inferolateral aspect of the internal carotid

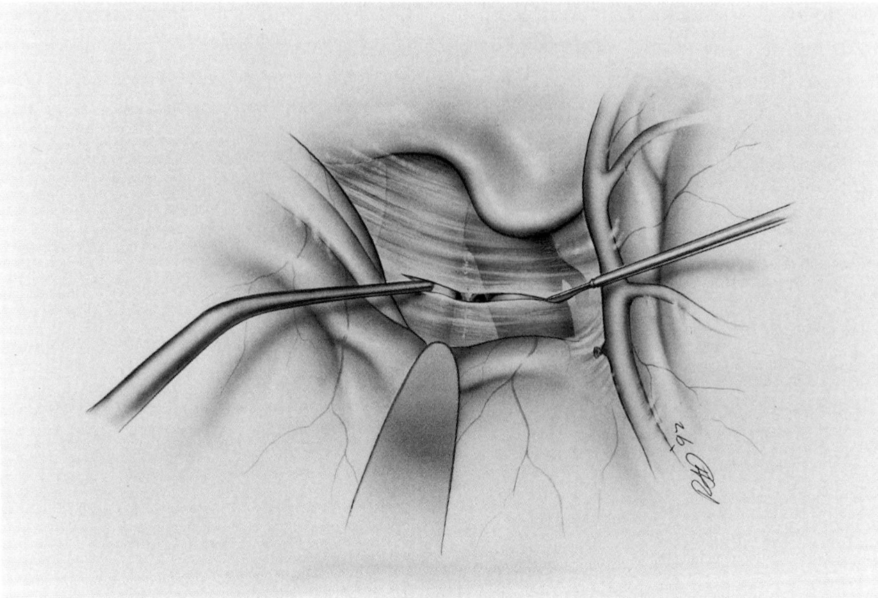

*Figure 7. Drawing of the initial brain retraction of the frontal lobe, exposing the right carotid-ophthalmic cisterns. Note the optic nerve on the left and the carotid artery on the right. The temporal lobe is unretracted to the right of the drawing. A microsuction device is in the surgeon's left hand and an arachnoid knife is being used in the right hand to open the cistern over the carotid artery.*

artery. The anterior choroidal artery passes posteromedially to enter the crural cistern. The artery usually gives off an uncal branch to supply the cortex of the uncus, the posteromedial amygdala, the anterior hippocampus,the dentate gyrus, and the tail of the caudate nucleus. The other major branch supplies the optic chiasm, the posterior two thirds of the optic tract, the medial part of the globus pallidus, the genu of the internal capsule, and portions of the thalamus and midbrain.

Perforators from the ICA are highly variable and some of the perforators that normally arise from the major named branches of the ICA can arise directly from the artery itself. For example, neural structures usually supplied by the anterior choroidal artery may be supplied by small perforators arising directly off the ICA. These perforators are usually important when aneurysms of the carotid bifurcation are considered. A complete description of the variability and destination of these perforators has been presented by Gibo et al.[10]

## *Initial Brain Retraction*

Following completion of the pterional craniotomy and the dural opening, a retractor is placed on the inferior surface of the frontal lobe to enlarge the tunnel of vision from the surface of the brain down to the paraclinoid region. The initial retractor should be placed so that the optic nerve is clearly visualized. The optic cistern, which encases the optic nerve, is stretched and thereby prepared for the initial arachnoid dissection (Figure 7). Once the optic nerve has been identified and the arachnoid has been stretched, it is time to introduce the microscope to the operative field and the remainder of the surgery is conducted under magnification and coaxial illumination.

## *Sylvian Fissure Splitting*

Splitting of the sylvian fissure is not mandatory for most aneurysms of the ICA at the posterior communicating origin and the anterior choroidal origin. Smaller aneurysms in these locations generally can be adequately exposed with frontal lobe retraction alone, when the brain has been properly relaxed. Therefore, sylvian fissure dissection is not routinely performed with most carotid aneurysms.

Opening the sylvian fissure does, however, enhance the exposure of the carotid artery and ICA aneurysms. A sylvian fissure split should be considered for all aneurysms that are more than 2 cm in size as well as for any aneurysm that has an angiographic configuration indicating that the surgery might be unusually challenging from a technical standpoint. There is very little downside to opening the sylvian fissure in any aneurysm operation; this maneuver has been proposed by Yasargil to be a standard component of aneurysm surgery in the anterior circulation.[31,32] In the author's experience, sylvian fissure dissection is required only with aneurysms of the middle cerebral artery (MCA) and the carotid bifurcation, but is advantageous for giant aneurysms and complex aneurysms in any location in the anterior circulation.

Sharp dissection is necessary to commence the sylvian fissure dissection. The sylvian fissure dissection is usually started at a point on the surface of the brain where the frontal operculum and the temporal lobe are in apposition. The exact point of entry into the sylvian fissure is not critical; the most advantageous spot is usually where transparent arachnoid is present. The venous anatomy on the surface of the sylvian fissure is highly variable. Multiple large veins often follow the course of the sylvian fissure to drain into the sphenoparietal or cavernous sinuses. These veins are generally associated with the temporal lobe on the temporal side of the sylvian fissure. Therefore, it is almost always advisable to enter the fissure on the frontal side of these veins. When there are no large veins on the surface, the arachnoid dissection is facilitated.

Once the cistern of the sylvian fissure has been entered, the dissection proceeds by gently spreading the lips of the fissure from the inside and progressing proximally while applying pressure on both walls of the fissure, the overlying bridging tissues are stretched, facilitating sharp dissection of these bridging fibers. Once the sylvian fissure has been definitively entered, subsequent dissection is carried on from "inside out." This maneuver assures that the pial surfaces of the frontal operculum and the temporal lobe are not violated. The goal, which is sometimes impossible to achieve, is to keep both pial surfaces completely intact and to separate the two lobes in the subarachnoid space.

The sylvian fissure dissection begins distally and proceeds proximally until all of the bridging arachnoid fibers between the frontal and temporal lobes have been divided, especially those that cover the carotid cistern. Occasionally, there may be bridging veins from the frontal to the temporal lobes and these may have to be divided to facilitate complete separation of the two lobes. It is not possible that arterial structures irrigate both frontal and temporal lobes. Therefore, when an artery has been definitely established to provide penetrating vessels into one of the two lobes, the dissection can be carried forth on the side of the vessel away from the penetrating branches. This concept is important when the two pial surfaces are densely adherent.

Occasionally the orbital frontal gyrus may indent into the temporal lobe, obscuring the CSF cistern. There is then no choice but to pursue a subpial dissection through the adherent portion of the fissure. The only true landmarks for location of the fissure in these cases are the distal branches of the middle cerebral artery, which travel in the sylvian fissure.

## *Opening the Basal Cisterns*

Arachnoid dissection with sequential opening of the basal cisterns is the key to exposure of all intracranial aneurysms. Opening the cisterns allows for CSF drainage and removal of tethers from the inferior surface of the brain to the skull base. These maneuvers create brain relaxation, ease retraction, and widen the tunnel of vision down to the skull base.

The first step with carotid aneurysms is to open the optic cistern encasing the ipsilateral optic nerve (Figure 7). The cistern is best opened by using sharp dissection with a microknife blade. A disposable Beaver eyeblade is preferred for this dissection. The goal is to free the optic nerve totally from attachments to the frontal lobe to improve exposure of the entire carotid artery. The carotid cistern is incised separately, starting from the proximal portion just lateral to the optic nerve, adjacent to the anterior clinoid process. The cistern is opened over the carotid artery, but the dissection is limited to the diameter of the artery and is not extended laterally. This precaution is especially important with recently ruptured aneurysms because of the risk of traumatizing the aneurysm dome before complete dissection of the neck has been undertaken. The carotid cistern is opened far enough at first only to visualize the most proximal portion of the carotid artery and prepare that segment of the carotid artery for temporary clipping, if necessary.

Following this initial exposure, increased frontal lobe retraction is usually required to visualize more distal portions of the carotid artery. The cistern is then opened distally along the main trunk of the carotid artery. With posterior communicating artery aneurysms, the dissection needs to extend only to a point just distal to the aneurysm neck so that enough room is created to place temporary clips both proximally and distally to the aneurysm. In this fashion, if an intraoperative rupture were to occur during the dissection of the neck, temporary clips could be applied to the carotid artery.

For carotid bifurcation aneurysms, the entire carotid cistern must be opened, as well as the cisterns surrounding the proximal A1 and M1 arteries. Visualization of all three arterial components of the carotid bifurcation is mandatory to provide satisfactory control in the event of aneurysm rupture or if temporary clipping is otherwise required.

## *Dissection of the Aneurysm Neck*

A critical aspect of aneurysm surgery is avoidance of intraoperative rupture. Handling intraoperative rupture is discussed in detail in a subsequent section. The most important way to avoid intraoperative rupture is to leave the dome of the aneurysm undisturbed. This point is critical when dealing with recently ruptured aneurysms and less important, although certainly good practice, when dealing with unruptured aneurysms.

Posterior communicating and anterior choroidal aneurysms generally project posteriorly and laterally, often under the petroclinoid ligament and into the oculomotor (III) nerve. These domes can occasionally be attached to the petroclinoid ligament or project directly above the petroclinoid ligament into the medial aspect of the temporal lobe. A recently ruptured aneurysm will generally be tethered by one of these structures; therefore, retraction on the carotid artery can potentiate intraoperative rupture. For all of these reasons, the initial dissection of any aneurysm should be limited to the neck of the aneurysm. The neck is the only critical part of the aneurysm anatomy that needs to be established prior to definitive clipping (Figure 8).

With posterior communicating artery aneurysms, the origin of the posterior commu-

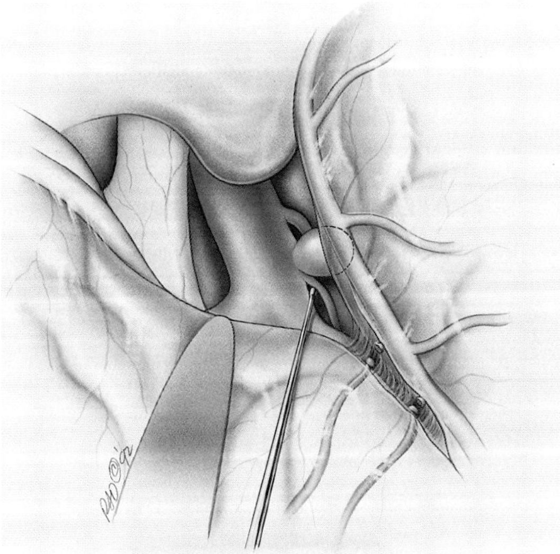

***Figure 8.*** *Drawing of the exposure of an anterior choroidal aneurysm. Note the sylvian fissure has been largely undisturbed and the temporal lobe is not retracted off the dome of the aneurysm. The anterior choroidal artery is clearly identified prior to clip application.*

nicating artery should be isolated and separated from the aneurysm so that clipping can proceed without compromising the artery. Except in cases of persistent fetal origin of the posterior cerebral artery, compromise of the carotid end of the posterior communicating artery is generally not a critical problem. Although important perforators originate from the posterior communicating artery, the artery is bilaterally supplied and generally will fill from either the posterior circulation or the carotid artery. If it is impossible to easily delineate the origin of the posterior communicating artery without disrupting the dome of the aneurysm, it is better to place the initial clip across the aneurysm neck, including the posterior communicating artery, than to risk an intraoperative rupture. In some instances, the posterior communicating artery arises directly on the opposite side of the aneurysm neck and is therefore not able to be visualized until the aneurysm is clipped.

Compromise of a direct origin of the posterior cerebral artery off the carotid can lead to a major and possibly devastating stroke. In these cases, if the origin of the artery cannot be appreciated prior to clipping the aneurysm, temporary clips may be advisable so that the aneurysm dome can be retracted and the origin of the vessel clearly seen prior to placement of the initial clip.

The aneurysm neck is best delineated with a blunt microprobe which is first passed proximal to the aneurysm along the neck at its point adjacent to the carotid artery. After the probe has been placed well past the presumed neck of the aneurysm, the same maneuver is carried forth on the distal side of the aneurysm neck. After dissection proximally and distally, it is advantageous to feel the back side of the aneurysm neck. Although this part of the neck cannot be visualized, palpating underneath the aneurysm neck with curved or angled microdissectors holds several advantages: (1) this kind of dissection ensures that there is not an unseen component of the aneurysm bulging posteriorly that might be punctured by improper clip placement; and, (2) dissection around the posterior aspect of the aneurysm neck gives some indication of the width of the neck and thereby the length of clip required.

Clipping of anterior choroidal aneurysms requires a slightly different consideration because the preservation of the anterior choroidal artery is a critical component of the operation (Figure 9). If the anterior choroidal artery cannot be visualized because the aneurysm neck is overlying the origin of the artery, it is advisable to place temporary clips on the carotid artery and retract the dome of the aneurysm so that the anterior choroidal artery can be definitively identified prior to clip placement. This artery is small, easily injured, and does not tolerate temporary clipping. Even with posterior communicating artery aneurysms, it is good practice to clearly identify the anterior choroidal artery prior to the placement of any clips so that it is not possible to accidentally include the anterior choroidal artery in the clip.

A wide enough passageway must be dissected on either side of the aneurysm neck to allow unobstructed passage of the aneurysm clip. Blunt tools are usually sufficient for the final dissection of the neck region of the aneurysm, but if there are arachnoid bands from the carotid artery to the dome of the aneurysm it is wise to cut these bands sharply, using microscissors so as to avoid excessive traction on either the carotid artery or the aneurysm dome. Manipulation of these structures can lead to an intraoperative rupture.

Numerous important perforators are often hidden behind the dome of aneurysms at the carotid bifurcation. Perforators going up to the anterior perforated substance and the anterior choroidal artery are in proximity to the posterior aspect of bifurcation aneurysms. Care must be exercised during neck dissection to make sure that the perforators are swept off the aneurysms and that a proper depth for clip placement is determined.

## *Clip Placement*

Although exposure of posterior communicating artery aneurysms is the simplest of the intracranial aneurysm procedures, the clip-

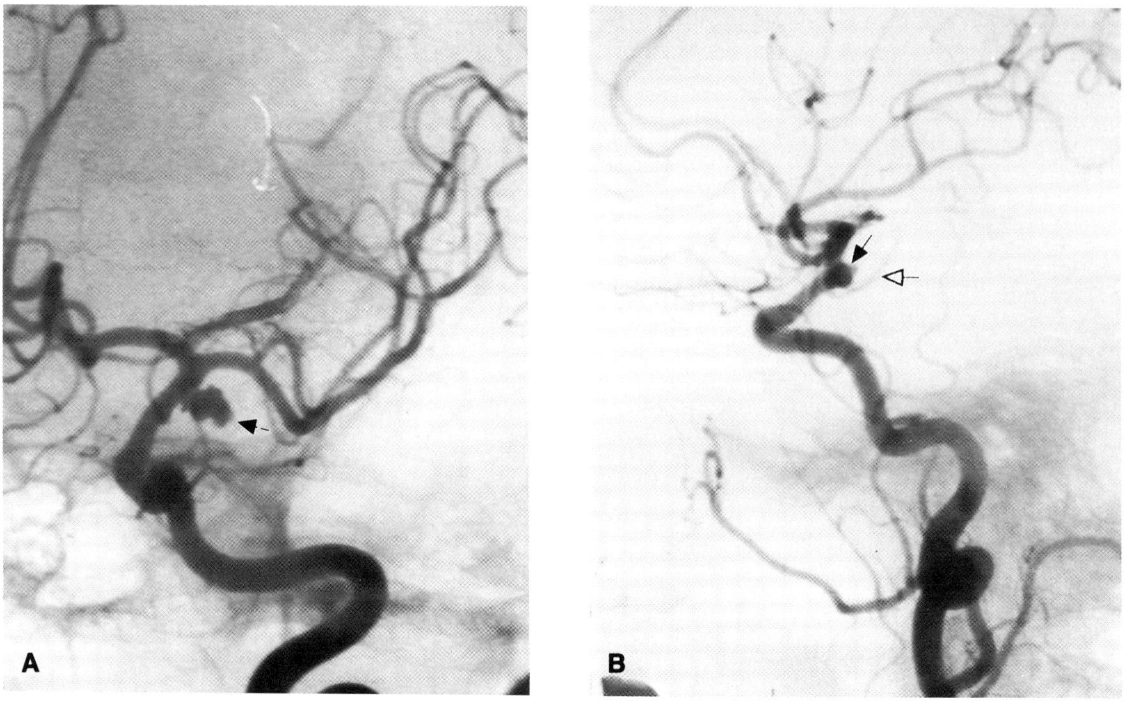


*Figures 9A,B. Anteroposterior (AP) (A) and lateral (B) angiogram depicts a carotid aneurysm and the origin of the anterior choroidal artery. The closed arrows point to the aneurysm and the open arrow on the lateral angiogram points to the anterior choroidal artery.*

ping of these aneurysms may be extremely difficult. Often the anterior clinoid process or the proximal portion of the petroclinoid ligament can interfere with visualization or clipping of the proximal side of the neck of the aneurysm. In some instances, it is necessary to cut the attachment of the petroclinoid ligament from the clinoid, or even to drill off the anterior clinoid process just to gain access to the proximal side of the neck of a posterior communicating aneurysm.

The other complicating factor in clip placement is that posterior communicating aneurysms often project almost directly posteriorly from the carotid artery instead of manifesting the more common lateral projection. In these instances, only a part of the dome and neck of the aneurysm is visualized. If a straight clip is used to clip the aneurysm, the clip blades may travel along the dome of the aneurysm and not truly across its neck. Closure of the clip blades on the dome can precipitate devastating rupture of the aneurysm since the aneurysm could be torn in an area that is not easily visualized. It is critical, therefore, to ensure that the clip passes only across the neck region of the aneurysm (see Figure 21).

If a straight clip has to angle underneath the carotid artery, sometimes there is not enough room up against the temporal lobe to angle the clip applier. In such instances, a curved clip is advantageous in clipping aneurysms that are underneath the carotid artery as viewed by the surgeon. However, the curved clips carry the increased danger of catching unseen perforators on the posterior aspect of the carotid artery.

Curved clips must be used with great care, and generally only in cases where sacrifice of the posterior communicating artery is permissible by angiographic criteria (Figure 10). A curved clip is very hazardous to use with anterior choroidal artery aneurysms: even if the primary anterior choroidal artery is well seen, supernumerary anterior choroidal arteries or perforators can be easily included in a curved

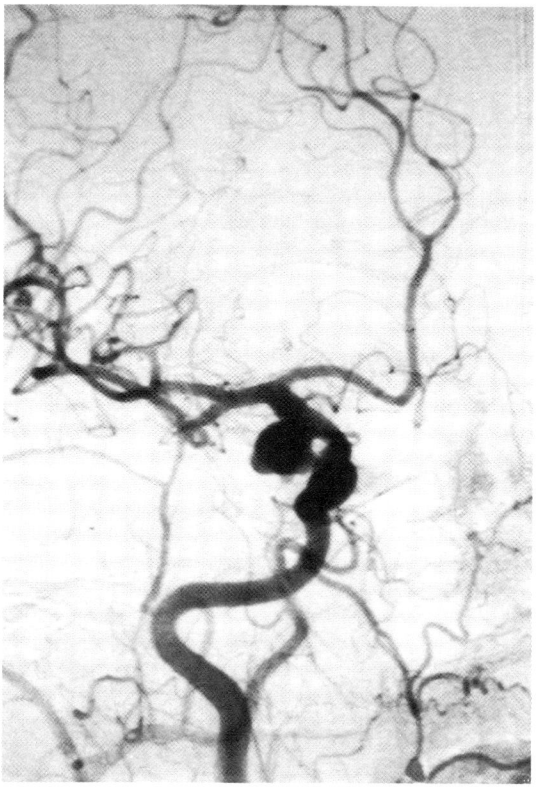

*Figure 10A. Preoperative anteroposterior angiogram shows a large irregular, recently ruptured, posterior communicating aneurysm.*

clip. Viewing the neck of the aneurysm from the medial side of the carotid artery helps insure that the clip can pass all the way across the carotid without compromising posteriorly projecting perforating vessels.

Protection of perforators behind the aneurysm dome is critical with carotid bifurcation aneurysms (Figure 11). Perforator damage in these cases is usually attributable to using a longer aneurysm clip that allows the distal part of the blades to catch deep perforators.

## *Clip Inspection*

Following placement of the aneurysm clip, the clip must be completely inspected to insure that the clip blades have traversed the width of the neck of the aneurysm and that the parent vessel or perforators are not compromised. If problems are identified by clip inspection, the clip should be moved into a more satisfactory orientation. Almost all neurologic complications of aneurysm surgery can be traced to faulty clip placement.

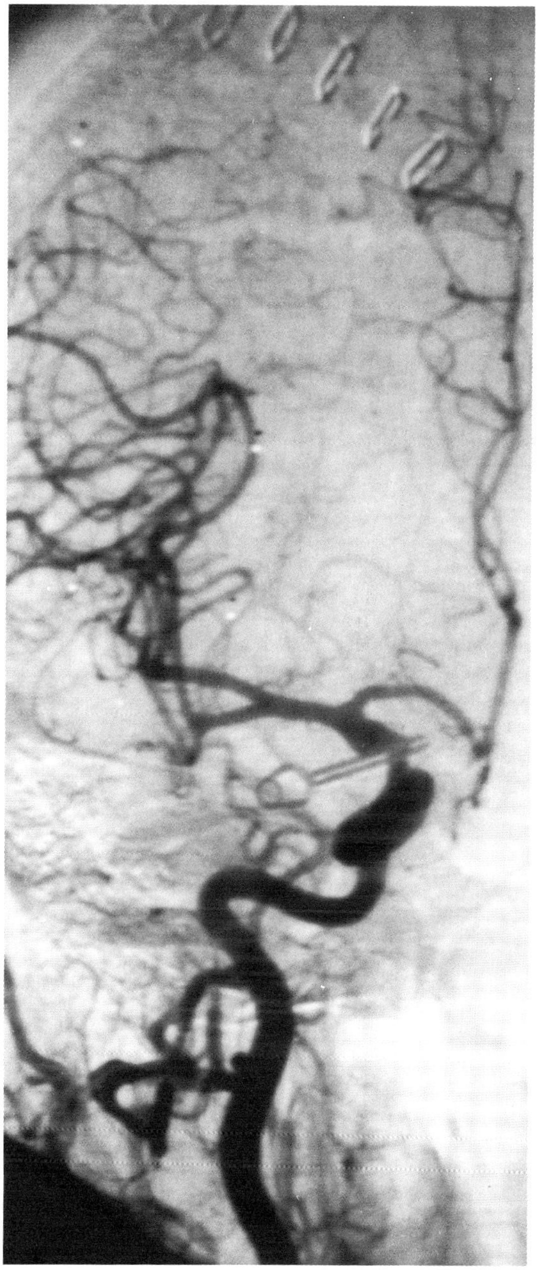

*Figure 10B. Postoperative angiogram shows a successfully clipped aneurysm, using a Yasargil clip that passes from the lateral to the medial side of the carotid artery. This clip position would be unacceptable in patients with persistent fetal circulation.*

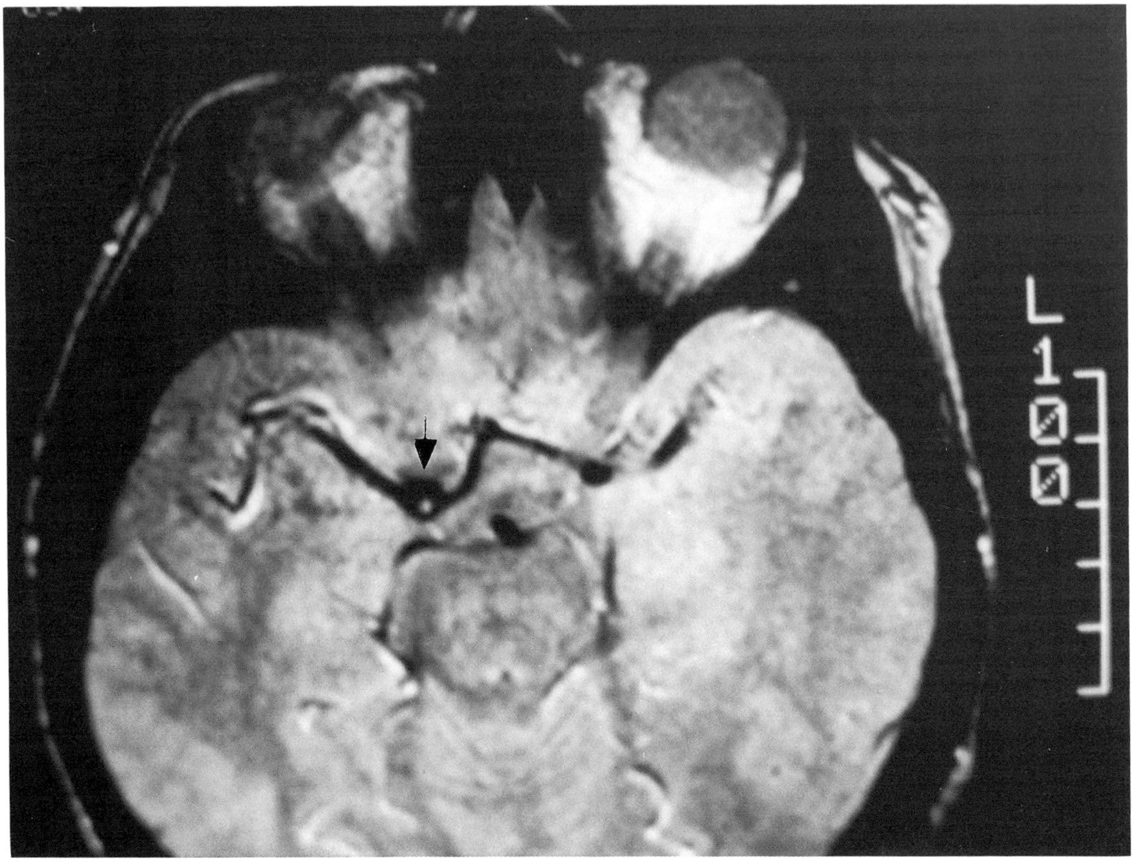


*Figure 11A. Preoperative magnetic resonance image (MRI) of a patient with a 1 cm right carotid bifurcation aneurysm. The arrow points to the aneurysm which separates the anterior and middle cerebral arteries.*

When moving an aneurysm clip, it is best to place a clip on the dome of the aneurysm, distal to the initial clip, allowing space for the first clip to be adjusted to its proper location. The distal clipping will maintain the aneurysm in a contracted state, easing the reapplication of the primary clip and preventing hemorrhage.

The final maneuver after aneurysm clipping and before closure is to puncture the aneurysm dome. This is the only true test to determine that the aneurysm has been obliterated. If there continues to be arterial flow in the aneurysm, back-up clips will must be applied or the primary clip changed to a better location. Failure to needle an aneurysm dome is equivalent to an ostrich putting its head in the sand. It is always better to know at this point in the operation that the aneurysm has not been improperly clipped, than to get a telephone call at 2:00 AM informing you that the patient has suffered a devastating postoperative rupture.

## Paraclinoid Aneurysms

### *Anatomy and Terminology*

The neurosurgical literature is replete with a confusing array of nomenclature to describe carotid aneurysms that arise adjacent to the anterior clinoid process. In the author's experience, paraclinoid aneurysms can conveniently be classified into three categories: (1) aneurysms that arise within the *cavernous sinus* with or without projections into the subarachnoid space; (2) ophthalmic aneurysms that arise in association with the ophthalmic

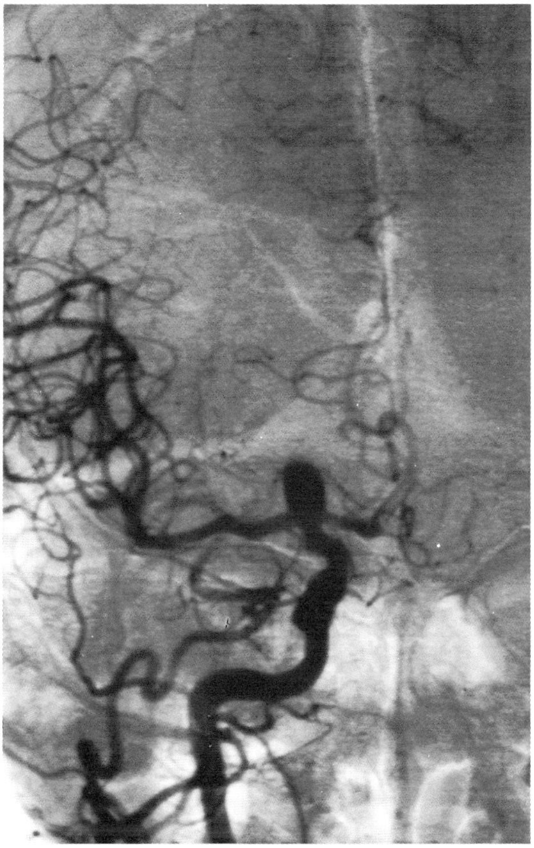

*Figure 11B. Anteroposterior angiogram shows the carotid bifurcation aneurysm. Note the small perforators in proximity to the dome of the aneurysm.*

artery and project superiorly; (3) and ***superior hypophyseal*** aneurysms that project medially and posteriorly toward the optic chiasm.[3]

This classification scheme has relevance to surgical anatomy and operative approach. With ophthalmic aneurysms, the surgical view of the carotid artery is generally obstructed by the dome of the aneurysm that overlies the parent vessel. These aneurysms project directly into the optic nerve or displace the nerve medially, kinking the nerve at the proximal opening of the optic canal. The superior hypophyseal aneurysms project away from the carotid artery, and the carotid artery is usually lateral or even overlying the dome of the aneurysm. The aneurysms project back into the optic chiasm and suprasellar region.

Cavernous sinus aneurysms require that the cavernous sinus be opened in order to expose the aneurysm and gain proximal control of the aneurysm neck. Often aneurysms that lie completely or mostly within the cavernous sinus cannot be clipped and require endovascular treatment, proximal carotid occlusion, or trapping. The dural carotid ring marks the beginning of the so-called supraclinoid portion of the ICA.

Aneurysms that arise below the ring usually remain totally extradural in location and therefore are not particularly dangerous lesions in terms of intracranial hemorrhage. These lesions reside mostly in the cavernous sinus, but may extend into the carotid cave between the cavernous sinus and the subarachnoid space.

Some aneurysms arising below the dural carotid ring can expand the ring and project superiorly into the subarachnoid space. These lesions usually have an investment of dura around the base of the subarachnoid projection, which often forms a waist around the aneurysm that may be visualized on angiography. Operative intervention for intracavernous aneurysms and aneurysms that arise partially within the cavernous sinus require mastery of the anatomy around the cavernous sinus and experience with specialized extradural approaches necessary to deal with vascular lesions in this location.[4]

## *Removal of the Anterior Clinoid Process*

The key to successful surgery of ophthalmic aneurysms, superior hypophyseal aneurysms, or aneurysms within the cavernous sinus, is removal of the anterior clinoid process and the roof of the optic foramen. The extent of bony removal depends in large part on the configuration and exact type of aneurysm being approached. For aneurysms that involve the cavernous sinus, an extensive extradural resection of the roof of the orbit, the optic foramen, the anterior clinoid process, and parts of the sphenoid bone surrounding the superior orbital fissure is necessary to ex-

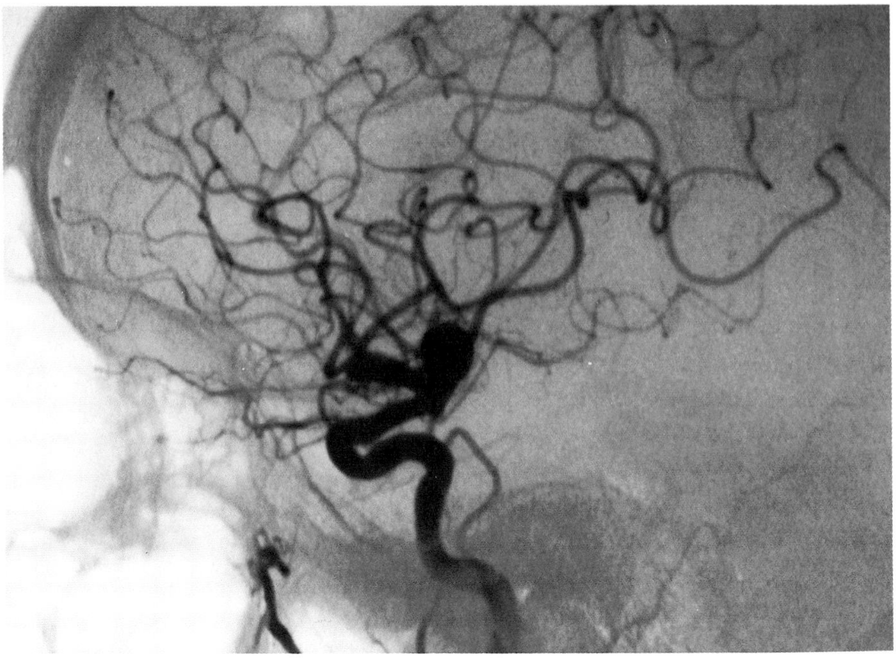

*Figure 11C. Lateral angiogram demonstrates the upward projection of the carotid bifurcation aneurysm into the right hemisphere.*

pose the soft-tissue regions of the anterior aspect of the cavernous sinus and the proximal carotid artery. Although this extensive bony resection is not usually required for aneurysms arising at the ophthalmic artery and superior hypophyseal artery, the extradural approach facilitates subsequent intradural aspects of the operative procedure and eliminates the requirement of using a high-speed air drill adjacent to the dome of an intracranial aneurysm.

The negative aspect of extradural bony removal is the removal of bone prior to visualization of the aneurysm and the distal carotid artery. Aneurysms of the superior portions of the cavernous sinus can severely erode the clinoid process inferiorally, and during bony removal the aneurysm or proximal portions of the ICA are subject to traumatic injury. Meticulous technique and awareness of these possibilities can reduce the hazards of the extradural approach. If problems arise or the anterior clinoid process is noted to have osseous attachments in addition to those to the superior orbital fissure and the inferior strut of the optic foramen, it is best to open the dura and obtain control of the ICA prior to final removal of the anterior clinoid process.

The author prefers the extradural approach to all complex and giant aneurysms of the paraclinoid region. This approach guarantees maximum removal of bony structures prior to dissection of the aneurysm. With small aneurysms of the ophthalmic and superior hypophyseal regions, intradural drilling of the medial aspect of anterior clinoid process and the proximal portion of the optic foramen usually provides sufficient visualization of the neck of the aneurysm and allows for controlled clipping (see Figure 12).

Prior to drilling the anterior clinoid process, it is advisable to establish proximal and distal control of the internal carotid artery in case there is rupture of the aneurysm. Usually it is necessary to cut down in the cervical region and expose the proximal ICA, holding a vascular ligature available for emergency

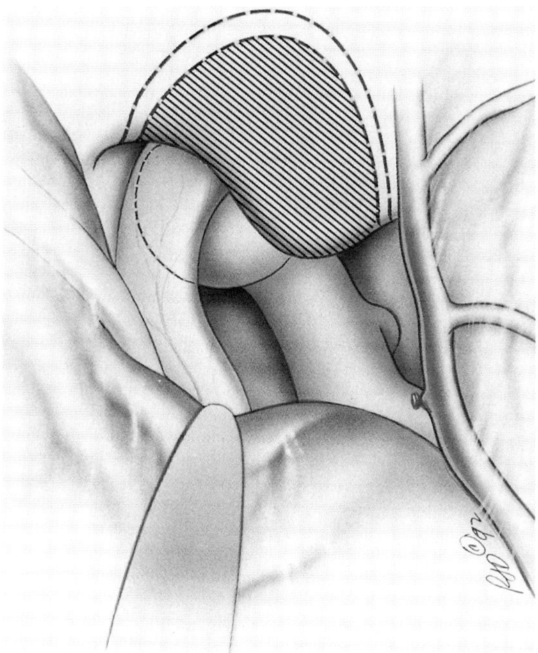

*Figure 12A. Drawing of the initial exposure of a carotid ophthalmic aneurysm. The right optic nerve is stretched over the dome of a 1 cm ophthalmic aneurysm. The superior-most dotted line indicates the location of the dural incision for creating the semilunar flap used to expose the bone over the optic foramen and anterior clinoid process. The bone removed by drilling is represented by the cross-hatched area.*

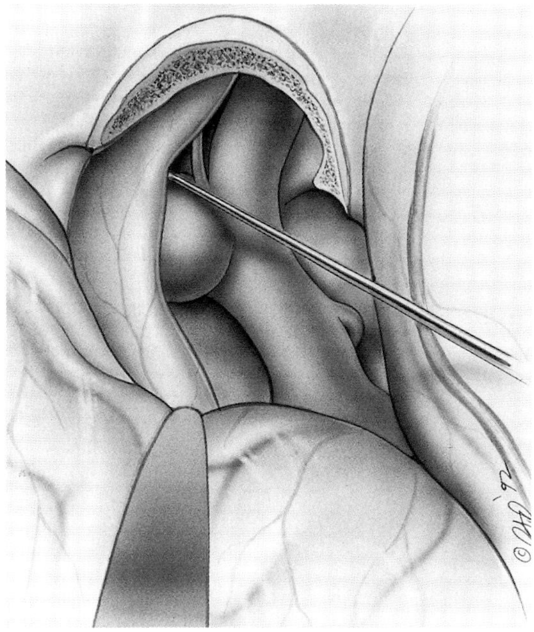

*Figure 12B. Representation of the view after drilling of the anterior clinoid process and opening of the optic foramen. Note all of the dura has been removed and visualization of the proximal carotid artery in the clinoidal space allows easy access to both sides of the aneurysm.*

occlusion. The supraclinoid carotid artery distal to the aneurysm is also dissected and prepared for temporary clipping, if the need should arise.

Following the establishment of proximal and distal control, a semilunar flap of dura is opened over the anterior clinoid process and the optic foramen. The flap extends from the medial side of the optic foramen to the lateral side of anterior clinoid process. This flap, when reflected inferiorly, serves as a buffer covering the ICA, the aneurysm, and the optic nerve. Drilling of the optic foramen and anterior clinoid process can usually be accomplished using a high-speed diamond burr without major risk to the neurovascular structures.

After drilling, the dura is completely removed over the optic nerve and the proximal internal carotid artery usually as far down as the dural ring. This approach exposes enough of the proximal portion of the internal carotid artery to allow clipping of the aneurysm, but usually does not expose enough proximal artery to obtain intracranial proximal and distal control. A cut-down in the neck should always accompany this type of aneurysm exposure.

The unroofing of the optic foramen and opening of the falciform ligament overlying the optic nerve is critical to decompressing the optic nerve This allows superior elevation of the nerve for complete exposure of the medial side of paraclinoid aneurysms. The optic nerve is frequently angulated around the medial side of the aneurysm or stretched directly over the dome of the aneurysm. The tether at the proximal portion of the optic foramen often provides a site for injury to the optic nerve. Opening of the optic foramen is beneficial and increases the safety of optic nerve manipulation during clipping of these aneurysms.

### *Clip Placement*

Ophthalmic aneurysms are generally amenable to clipping with a straight clip. The clip is best oriented along the axis of the internal carotid artery, minimizing the risk of deformation of the parent artery. This type of clip placement is very difficult to achieve due to the confines of the exposure. The clip can be oriented perpendicular to the axis of the internal carotid artery, especially with small ophthalmic artery aneurysms, as long as care is taken not to distort the lumen of the parent vessel (see Figure 13). Such distortion is usually not a problem with aneurysms less than 2 cm in size. The distortion of the carotid artery can be a major problem with giant aneurysms in this location, especially when calcification is present in the neck of the aneurysm. Great care must be taken to insure that sufficient lumen is preserved in the carotid artery.

The technical aspects of clip placement begin to multiply exponentially with aneurysms greater than 1 cm in size. It is mandatory for treatment of giant aneurysms that the carotid artery be temporarily occluded during the placement of the aneurysm clip. With intermediate size aneurysms, temporary carotid occlusion during clipping is often advantageous and should be anticipated prior to the clipping of the aneurysm. In preparation for a carotid occlusion, it is advisable to establish on-line electroencephalography (EEG) monitoring of the effected hemisphere, preferably by direct cortical application of electrodes. Most patients can tolerate 3-5 minutes of ICA occlusion without risk of ischemic compromise, even if EEG changes accompany carotid occlusion.

In treatment of complex and giant aneurysms in this location, periods of occlusion of up to 30 or 40 minutes may be required to complete a difficult clipping. Techniques such as intra-arterial suction/decompression, electroencephalography burst suppression with barbiturate loading, or the use of deep hypothermic circulatory arrest may become necessary.[1,21,24]

Superior hypophyseal aneurysms and aneurysms that project inferior to the carotid artery cannot usually be clipped with standard straight, curved, or angled aneurysm clips. These aneurysms generally have a very broad neck which can include portions of the ICA. Placement of standard clips at right angles to the axis of the artery will produce severe deformities of the carotid artery and usually not lead to satisfactory clipping of the aneurysm. The use of angled fenestrated clips is advantageous, allowing the clip blades to emerge beneath the carotid artery and run parallel to the carotid artery. The ICA is then encompassed in the opening of the clip fenestration.

## Middle Cerebral Aneurysms

### *Anatomy*

The MCA is the continuation of the ICA, distal to the point where the anterior cerebral artery (ACA) originates. The MCA is 70% larger than the ACA and is anatomically the most complex cerebral artery.[9] Its origin is at the medial end of the sylvian fissure, lateral to the optic chiasm, and inferior to the anterior perforated substance. The artery then courses laterally parallel to the sphenoid ridge to enter the sylvian fissure.

The initial segment of the MCA has been termed the M1 segment. This segment continues until the MCA curves sharply to reach the surface of the insula (Figure 14). At the point of the limen insula, the M2 segment begins, usually corresponding to the point of MCA bifurcation into trunks, superior and inferior divisions. Distal to the bifurcation, the trunks turn posterior and superior to reach the surface of the insula, producing a curve known as the genu. The superior or inferior trunks may divide just after the bifurcation, giving the false impression of a trifur-

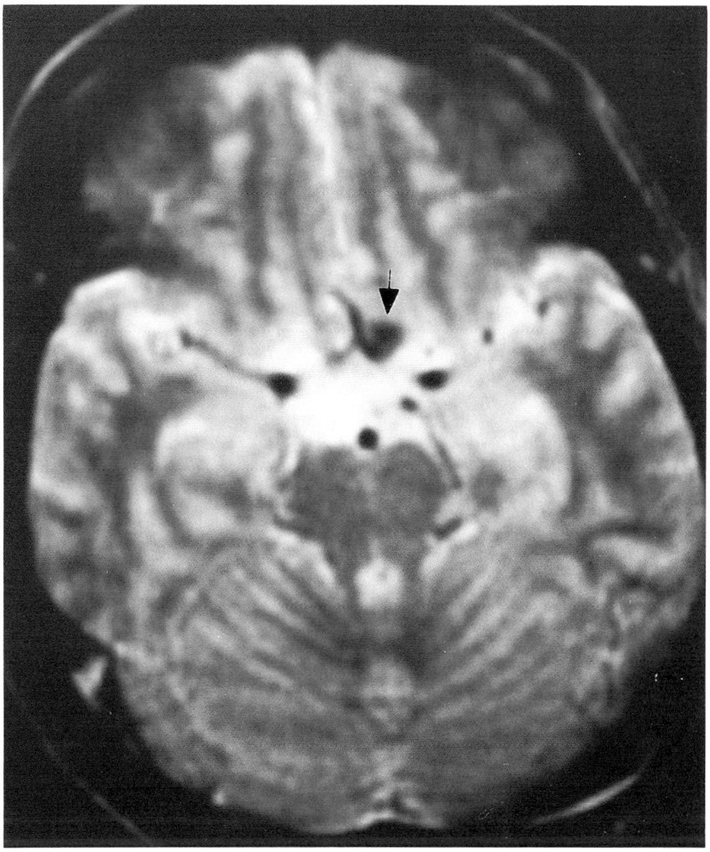

*Figure 13A. Unruptured carotid ophthalmic aneurysm. MRI demonstrates a left carotid ophthalmic aneurysm discovered incidentally. The arrow points to the flow void corresponding to the aneurysm.*

cation; thus, the frequent reference to middle cerebral trifurcation. In Gibo's study, 78% of MCAs divided in a bifurcation, 12% divided in a trifurcation, and 10% divided by giving rise to at least four principle trunks of the MCA.[9] The distal division of the MCA generally occurs in a series of bifurcations to produce the M3 segments of the MCA which extend from the insula to the surface of the sylvian fissure, coursing through the division between the frontal and temporal operculum. The inferior trunk is larger in 32% of cases, the superior is larger in 28% of cases, and the vessels are of equal caliber in 18% of cases. As noted, the other 22% of cases had an aberrant branching pattern.[9] The dominant branch generally carries blood supply to the parietal lobe. The inferior trunk otherwise gives branches that are committed to the temporal lobe, and the superior trunk provides the irrigation to the frontal lobes. The two major trunks, in a highly variable pattern, divide to form between 6 and 11 stem arteries that eventually further divide into the cortical arteries.

## *Operative Technique*

A number of different approaches to MCA aneurysms have been advocated. Most approaches involve splitting the sylvian fissure and either following the MCA distally from the carotid bifurcation to the aneurysm,[16,27,30] or starting at the M3 branches

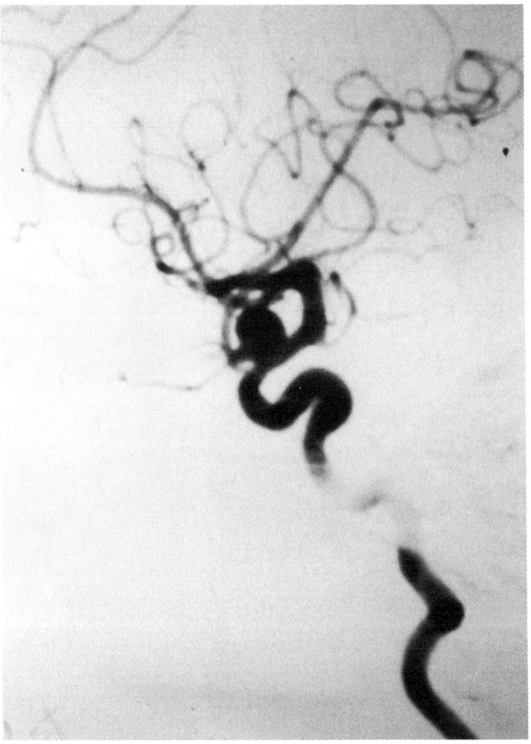

*Figure 13B. Lateral angiogram demonstrates the 1 cm aneurysm just distal to the origin of the left ophthalmic artery.*

of the MCA and following these branches proximally to the middle cerebral bifurcation.[26,32] A transcortical approach through the temporal lobe has also been advocated by some neurosurgeons.[11,12,29]

Transcortical approaches to the middle cerebral aneurysms have the major disadvantage of requiring trauma to otherwise normal temporal lobe structures. The risk of post-traumatic epilepsy in these patients is an issue that has never been resolved. The second disadvantage to transcortical approaches is that often middle cerebral aneurysms project inferiorly and are imbedded into the temporal lobe. This explains why ruptured middle cerebral aneurysms frequently cause an intracerebral hematoma in the temporal lobe. Even when there is an intracerebral hemorrhage, approach through the cortical tissue of the temporal lobe threatens disturbance of the clot that surrounds the dome of the aneurysm and can precipitate rebleeding of the aneurysm.

Although the transcortical approach is a viable one, in the author's experience, this approach is only been used when the frontal and temporal operculam are so densely adherent that no subarachnoid space can be easily developed. In these cases, a subpial resection of the superior temporal gyrus down to the sylvian cistern affords deeper entry into the sylvian fissure and satisfactory exposure of the middle cerebral vessels.

Complete sylvian fissure dissection down to the carotid cistern is seldom necessary for MCA bifurcation aneurysms. Such an approach requires considerable amount of dissection, sylvian fissure opening, and frontal and temporal lobe retraction. The dissection is time consuming, but does have the significant advantage of earlier proximal control of the MCA. This approach is suitable for surgeons not particularly comfortable with sylvian fissure dissection and approach to middle cerebral aneurysms.

In the author's experience, a direct trans-sylvian approach to the middle cerebral bifurcation is the most efficient for MCA aneurysm surgery. With proper brain relaxation, opening the sylvian fissure requires minimal brain retraction to visualize the region of the middle cerebral bifurcation. Of all the intracranial aneurysms, middle cerebral aneurysm surgery requires the least brain retraction (Figure 15). Therefore, a trans-sylvian approach is advantageous, even in poor-grade patients where there may be significant brain swelling.

The trans-sylvian approach keeps the dissection totally in the subarachnoid space and minimizes trauma to any cortical surface. Although some cortical veins that cross the sylvian fissure must be divided, this sacrifice is never of clinical significance. In patients with large temporal hematomas or frontal hematomas from a ruptured MCA aneurysm, the subarachnoid approach eliminates the possibility that the dome of the aneurysm will be disturbed prior to exposure of the neck of the aneurysm which will always reside in the subarachnoid space. The aneurysm is clipped prior to entry into the brain and evacuation of the intracerebral hemorrhage.

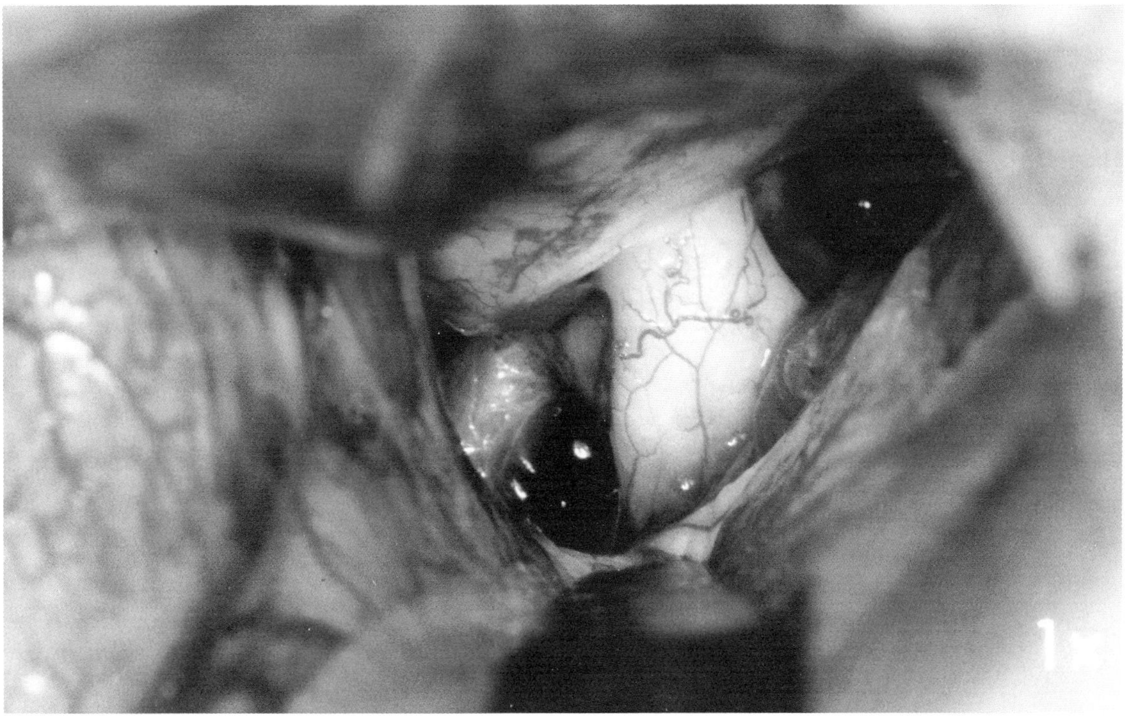

*Figure 13C. Initial operative exposure of the aneurysm before removal of the clinoid. The left optic nerve is expanded by the dome of the aneurysm pushing into the inferior surface of the nerve. Note that the anterior clinoid process hides the proximal portion of the aneurysm neck.*

When there is a large sylvian fissure hematoma, the dissection is greatly simplified by the blood clot expanding the sylvian fissure and separating the frontal and temporal lobes. Care must be exercised to avoid disturbing the clot that is adherent to the dome of the aneurysm. The main negative aspect of a direct trans-sylvian approach is that the neck and dome of the aneurysm are usually encountered before the M1 segment of the MCA has been clearly defined. When the dome of the aneurysm is encountered, the path of least resistance around the dome is taken to advance the dissection down to the base of the aneurysm and the exposure of the M1 artery. Once the distal M1 artery is controlled and prepared for temporary clipping, no deeper dissection is required.

## *Sylvian Fissure Dissection*

The principles of sylvian fissure dissection were presented in a previous section. The amount of sylvian fissure dissection required for middle cerebral aneurysms is often far less than sylvian fissure dissection required to gain exposure of the deeper anterior circulation aneurysms or basilar aneurysms. There is usually no need to disrupt the anterior portion of the sylvian fissure, where the sylvian cistern communicates with the basal cisterns. Middle cerebral aneurysms often lie fairly superficially within the sylvian fissure, adjacent to the lateral part of the sphenoid wing. A relatively shallow dissection within the sylvian fissure is all that is required to expose the neck of the aneurysm.

Yasargil describes a very wide dissection of the entire sylvian fissure for middle cerebral aneurysms and exposure of the basal cisterns, including the lamina terminalis.[32] This amount of dissection appears to be excessive, except in cases of giant aneurysms when maximum exposure will be required. For most small and intermediate size MCA aneurysms, enough dissection of the fissure to visualize

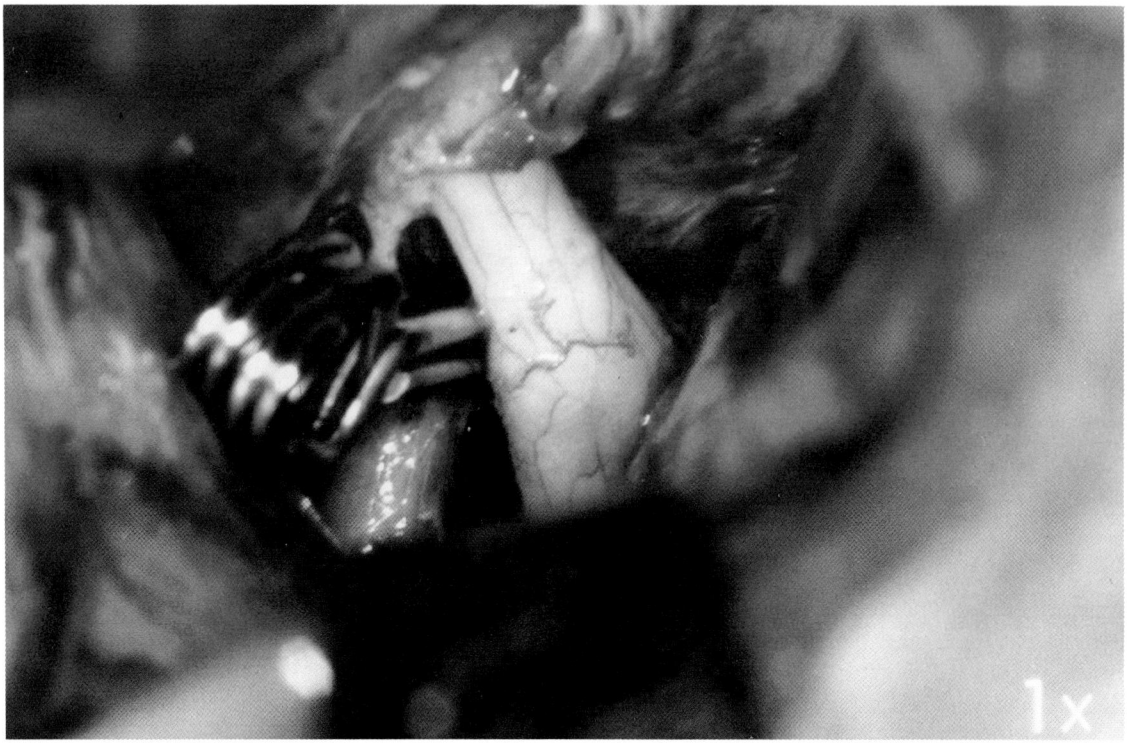


*Figure 13D. Following removal of the anterior clinoid process and the opening of the optic foramen, the aneurysm is easily clipped with two straight clips running parallel to the artery.*

the distal portion of the M1 artery is all that is required to satisfactorily expose and clip aneurysms at the middle cerebral bifurcation.

The difficulty arises in aneurysms that originate on the M1 portion of the MCA in conjunction with an early temporal branch (Figure 14). Aneurysms that arise proximal to the limen insula are more difficult to expose since the aneurysm is proximal to the genu of the MCA. A complete sylvian fissure split is desirable in order to gain access to the region of the carotid bifurcation and allow the surgeon to gain control of the proximal M1 artery. Dissection in this part of the sylvian fissure is more hazardous. Care must be taken to protect the anterior temporal branches and the lenticulostriate arteries which originate along the horizontal portion of the M1 artery.

## *Dissection of the Aneurysm*

Once the M1 section of the MCA proximal to the aneurysm has been exposed, the sylvian fissure dissection can be halted and attention focused on the aneurysm itself. Care must be taken with recently ruptured aneurysms to leave undisturbed pia, arachnoid, and blood clot adherent to the dome of the aneurysm while all of the major branches of the MCA are identified. Most middle cerebral aneurysms arise at a true bifurcation of the M1 segment into the two major M2 branches.

As many as four major M2 branches may be identified from the terminus of the M1 artery. A complete inspection must be made, circumferentially around the neck of the aneurysm to ensure that no unseen branch will be accidentally included in the clipping of the aneurysm neck. With small aneurysms this inspection is generally not challenging. As aneurysms increase in size, and certainly with giant aneurysms, visualization of arterial branches on the opposite side of the dome of the aneurysm may be impossible with the aneurysm fully arterialized.

In a large number of patients, recurrent la-

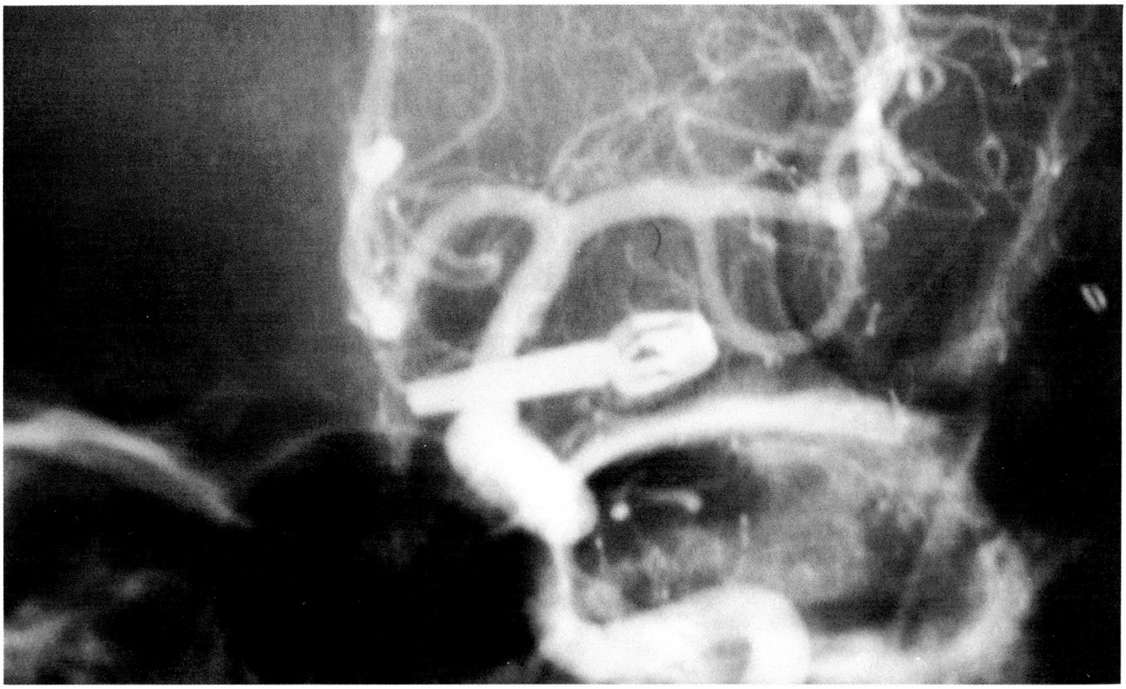

*Figure 13E. Postoperative angiogram demonstrates complete obliteration of the aneurysm with aneurysm clips oriented perpendicular to the artery.*

ticulostriate arteries originate from the major trunks of the M2 segments and return back along the M1 artery to enter the anterior perforated substance. Inadvertent clipping of these arteries is easily possible and must be avoided. Gentle depression on the neck of the aneurysm is usually sufficient to visualize around the posterior aspect of the aneurysm and insure that no striate arteries are adherent to the posterior face of the aneurysm dome. With larger aneurysms and aneurysms with calcification in the neck region, visualization of the contralateral side for major branches and recurrent striate arteries may be impossible without the use of temporary clips (Figure 16).

Temporary clips are very helpful with large complex aneurysms or any aneurysm where there is difficulty visualizing the posterior aspects of the aneurysm neck. Temporary occlusion of the M1 artery will soften the aneurysm and allow gentle retraction. Isolation of the aneurysm by individual clipping of all of the M2 branches as well as M1 is sometimes necessary to completely collapse the

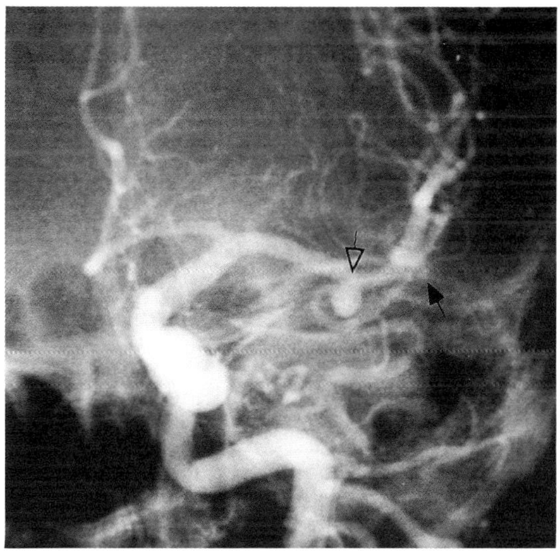

*Figure 14. Anteroposterior angiogram of the left carotid circulation demonstrates a small M1 aneurysm projecting inferiorly at the site of a very proximal origin of an anterior temporal branch. Note that the aneurysm is proximal to the genu of the MCA. The closed arrow points to the genu of the MCA and the termination of the M1 portion. The open arrow points to the position of the aneurysm and the proximal temporal branch.*

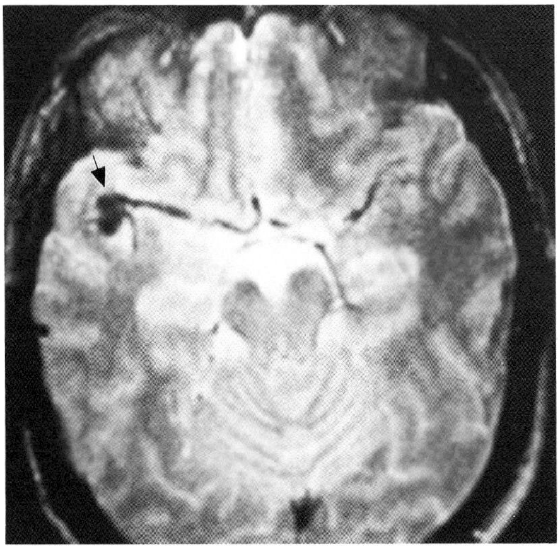

*Figure 15A*. *Axial T2 MRI depicts a middle cerebral bifurcation aneurysm (arrow). Note the proximity of the aneurysm to the cortical surface and the relatively far distance the aneurysm lies outward from the carotid bifurcation.*

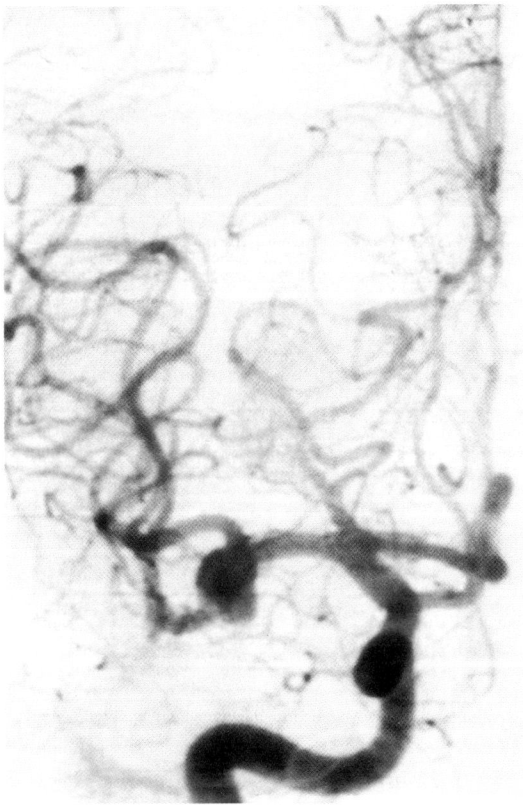

*Figure 15B*. *Anteroposterior angiogram demonstrates a bilobed middle artery bifurcation aneurysm.*

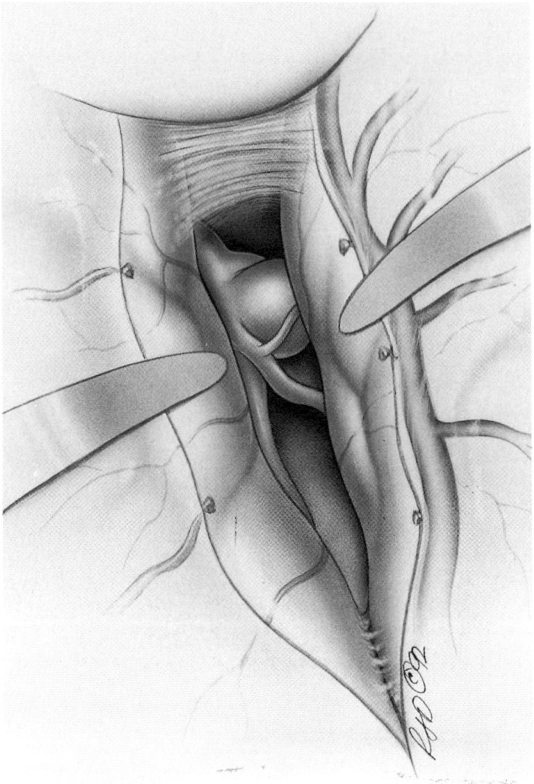

*Figure 16A*. *Drawing of the sylvian fissure partially opened to reveal the region of the middle cerebral bifurcation just distal to the genu of the MCA. Note the three major branches that are visualized, providing a false sense that all of the important middle cerebral branches have been adequately dissected and prepared for clipping.*

aneurysm and make a 360° circumferential dissection. A brief period of temporary occlusion is a safe and effective way to dissect and clip complex MCA aneurysms. In a rare case, deep hypothermic circulatory arrest may be used to permit clipping a giant calcified MCA aneurysm.[24]

Another potential pitfall of middle cerebral aneurysm dissection is failure to recognize the adherence rather than the origin of major vessels to the dome of the aneurysm. Unlike aneurysms in other locations, major M2 or M3 branches can be adherent to the fundus of the aneurysm at a location well distal to the origin of these branches. If sufficient concern has not been paid to these arteries prior to

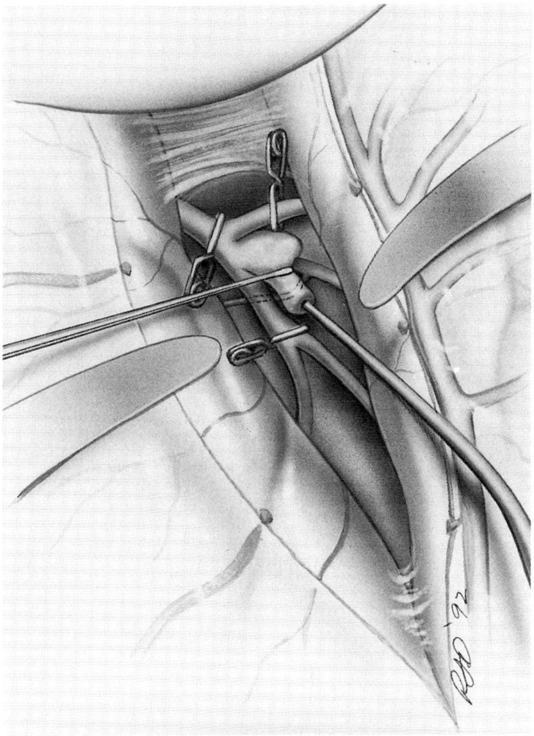

***Figure 16B.*** *Following placement of temporary clips on the major vessels and puncture of the aneurysm dome, the aneurysm is collapsed to reveal a fourth major MCA branch containing a recurrent striate artery. This figure represents the importance of identifying all branches of the middle cerebral bifurcation region and the ease with which a recurrent striate could be inadvertently included in the final clip.*

clipping, and the aneurysm clip is closed, the branch may be stretched, kinked, or even ruptured by the traction of the collapsing aneurysm dome. In some instances, these vessels are so densely adherent to a thin-walled aneurysm that dissection off of the dome of the aneurysm is too hazardous to entertain in the arterialized state. Temporary occlusion is advantageous for the final dissection and clip application.

## *Clip Application*

The principles of clip application for middle cerebral aneurysms are essentially the same as those discussed for carotid aneurysms. Inspection after the clip has been closed insures that the major middle cerebral branches are in not comprised by the clip and also insures that recurrent lenticulostriate arteries have not been inadvertently compromised.

# Anterior Communicating Artery Aneurysms

## *Anatomy*

The ACA is the smaller of the two terminal branches of the carotid artery. Usually the ACA is about one-third smaller than the MCA, but may be as large as the MCA in patients with hypoplasia of the contralateral ACA. The A1 segment courses medially from the carotid artery and somewhat anteriorly to reach the interhemispheric fissure, passing over the optic nerve and chiasm to join with the contralateral ACA through the anterior communicating artery.[8,17]

Normally, a small anterior communicating artery connects two ACAs of equal diameter. However, there is a great deal of variation in the normal structure around the anterior communicating complex, and hypoplastic A1 segments are a frequent occurrence, especially in conjunction with anterior communicating artery aneurysms. In Yasargil's angiographic study of more than 7,000 patients, the A1 segments were equal in 58% of the patients, but 41% of the patients had significant difference in the diameter of the two A2 arteries. In 5% of the patients, one of the A1 arteries was severely hypoplastic or aplastic. In aneurysm series, the incidence of hypoplasia of one of the A1 arteries is extremely common and may be as high as 80%.[31,32] This information underscores the hemodynamic factors that may contribute to aneurysm formation.

At the point where the ACA joins the anterior communicating artery, there is a genu as the subfrontal portion of the artery enters the interhemispheric fissure. The arterial segment distal to the genu and the anterior communicating artery is the A2 segment. The medial portion of the A1 artery and the anterior communicating artery lie within the lamina terminalis cistern. Numerous basal perforating branches arise from the A1, A2, and anterior communicating arteries. These perforating branches course into the anterior perforated substance, the subfrontal area, the dorsal surface of the optic chiasm, the suprachiasmatic area, the hypothalamus, and the sylvian fissure. Commonly, one or two stem vessels originate from the ACA and run a recurrent course before dividing into several fine arteries that penetrate the brain substance.

Two very important perforating branches arise from the A1, A2, or anterior communicating arteries. The first is the recurrent artery of Heubner. This artery arises from the proximal portion of the A2 segment in 78% of patients and from the A1 segment in 14%. It arises directly from the level of the ACOM artery in 8%.[17] The recurrent artery runs back parallel to the A1 segment to the internal carotid artery bifurcation and along the proximal portion of the M1 artery. In this location it enters the anterior perforated substance and has a variable pattern of vascular supply that may include the anterior part of the caudate nucleus, the anterior part of the putamen, a portion of the outer segment of the globus pallidus, and anterior limb of the internal capsule. Occlusion of the recurrent artery has a variable clinical consequence ranging from no neurologic deficits to hemiplegia and mental status changes.

The anterior communicating artery usually has one or more important perforating branches that supply the infundibulum, optic chiasm, and preoptic areas of the hypothalamus. These perforating vessels were not well appreciated until the advent of the operating microscope.[31] The neurosurgical complications of occluding hypothalamic perforating vessels during anterior communicating aneurysm surgery are known to include syndromes involving profound memory disturbance and hypothalamic dysfunction.

The A2 segment of the ACA begins distal to the anterior communicating artery. This segment ascends in the lamina terminalis cistern, in front of lamina terminalis, passing between the two hemispheres to enter the callosal cistern and arc around the genu of the corpus callosum. The callosal marginal artery usually originates just distal to the genu of the corpus callosum to ascend in the interhemispheric fissure and supply the medial side of the frontal lobe.

The callosal marginal artery may arise at variable locations along the A2 segment. In most cases, the distal ACAs are of equal size and supply only the ipsilateral hemisphere. There are, however, numerous anomalies of the distal ACA. Most of the anomalies are not of relevance to anterior communicating aneurysm surgery. However, in 9% of Yasargil's patients, a third A2 branch was discovered, originating from the region of anterior communicating artery.[32] This is a very important anomaly that should be searched for in all cases, since occlusion of this artery can have devastating neurologic consequences. A third A2 segment may represent a very proximal origination of the callosal marginal artery, the orbitofrontal artery, or an aberrant branch, supplying the genu of the corpus callosum and adjacent cortical and hypothalamic structures.

Fenestrated and reduplicated anterior communicating arteries are frequently encountered with anterior communicating aneurysm surgery. These anatomic variants should be suspected when the surgical anatomy appears complicated.

## *Operative Approach*

Some neurosurgeons have advocated an interhemispheric approach for anterior communicating aneurysms.[18,28] This approach through a midline craniotomy has the distinct disadvantage of requiring bilateral frontal lobe retraction. With unilateral interhemispheric approaches, the aneurysm tends to be deep in the base of a very constricted opening. The interhemispheric approach should be reserved for the rare giant aneurysms that project posteriorly and superiorly, well up into the interhemispheric fissure. In all other cases, a unilateral pterional craniotomy is the

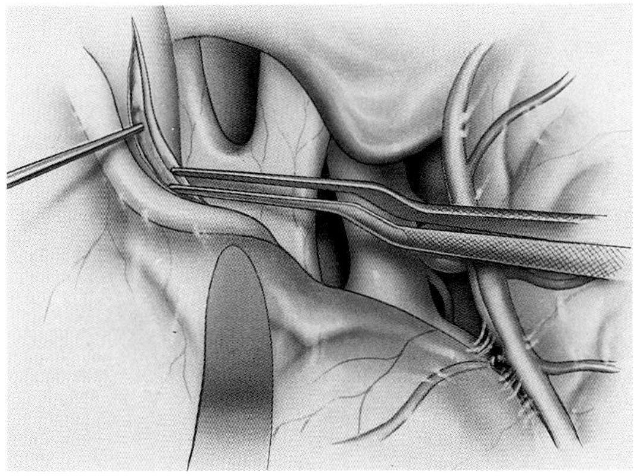

*Figure 17A. Drawing of the operative technique for clipping anterior communicating aneurysms. Gyrus rectus resection is begun using suction and cautery. Note the position of the olfactory nerve just above the gyrus rectus.*

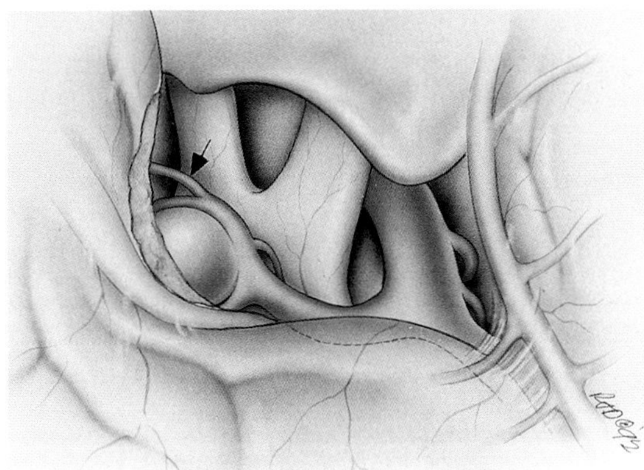

*Figure 17B. Following resection of the gyrus rectus, the region of the aneurysm and the anterior communicating segment is visualized. This patient is depicted as having a hypoplastic left A1 artery (arrow) and a dominant right A1 artery. Also note the small hypothalamic perforating vessel depicted coming off the inferior aspect of the anterior communicating segment, just above the optic chiasm.*

preferred approach to aneurysms of the anterior communicating region.

The initial stages of pterional craniotomy and exposure of the carotid-ophthalmic cisterns is completely analogous to that described for aneurysms of the proximal carotid artery. A sylvian fissure dissection with separation of the anterior parts of the frontal lobe from the temporal lobe improves the retraction down to the communicating complex.

Dissection of the sylvian fissure is not mandatory for the majority of anterior communicating artery aneurysms. With larger aneurysms or those that have a complex orientation, sylvian fissure dissection is beneficial and can be considered a useful adjunct if the sylvian cistern is well established and easily dissected. If difficulty is encountered in performing the sylvian fissure dissection, the procedure can be abandoned and attention directed immediately to the basal cisterns.

The carotid and ophthalmic cisterns on the side ipsilateral to the craniotomy should be widely opened, but it is usually not necessary to carry the carotid artery dissection distally to the carotid bifurcation. After the optic nerve has been totally dissected from the frontal lobe attachments, it is almost always possible to identify the middle section of the A1 artery as it courses over the posterior aspect of the optic nerve, on its way to the interhemispheric fissure. Even if the A1 artery takes a very posterior loop and is not immediately evident following opening of the optic cistern and the cistern of the lamina terminalis, a gyrus rectus resection of the ipsilateral frontal lobe will generally reveal the distal A1 artery on the medial side of the gyrus. The gyrus resection also minimizes the amount of frontal lobe retraction required to visualize the A1 and communicating segments (Figure 17).

Identification of A1 establishes some degree of proximal control as the A1 artery is followed distally into the communicating complex. As soon as the medial portion of the A1 artery is identified, a position should be cleared for placement of a temporary clip prior to exposure of the anterior communicating complex. Care must be taken to insure that the recurrent artery of Heubner and perforating vessels off the A1 artery are not in the field that is prepared for temporary occlusion should this become necessary.

In the rare instance when the ACOM aneurysm projects directly anteriorly and inferiorly into the anterior portion of the optic chiasm, the aneurysm may be identified prior to gyrus rectus resection and enough of the

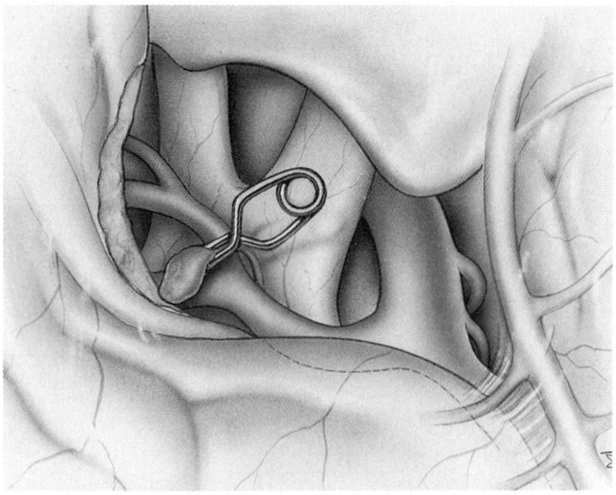

*Figure 17C. Appearance of the aneurysm following application of a short, straight Yasargil clip.*

neck visualized to allow safe clipping of the aneurysm. If the A1-A2 junction on both sides cannot be seen easily without significant frontal lobe retraction, it is always preferable to perform the gyrus rectus resection rather than to place undo traction on the frontal lobe.

The dissection should proceed along the posterior aspect of the A1 artery, searching for the point where the artery makes a sharp turn into the A2 segment. This approach avoids the aneurysm until the ipsilateral A1 and A2 have been identified. The aneurysms generally project in the direction of blood flow of the dominant A1 artery. It is usually wise to approach anterior communicating aneurysms from the side ipsilateral to the dominant A1 artery, and on the side that contains the neck of the aneurysm. Although it is possible to operate on anterior communicating aneurysms from the opposite side, it is always easier to follow the appropriate A1 artery into the point where the aneurysm arises, dissecting the neck prior to visualizing the aneurysm dome. If there appears to be no dominant A1 artery and the aneurysm is truly midline, a right-sided exposure will be preferable for a right-handed surgeon, but left-sided exposures are used when the left A1 artery is the dominant supply to the aneurysm.

Following correct identification and dissection of the ipsilateral A1-A2 junction, the neck of the aneurysm will usually become apparent on the opposite side of the junction of these two arteries. It is then necessary to leave the dome of the aneurysm undisturbed while the dissection continues across the aneurysm neck to the contralateral side. The opposite A1 artery must be identified, and this is usually best seen in the contralateral portion of the chiasmatic cistern over the other optic nerve. The most difficult vessel to identify is usually the contralateral A2 artery, especially with aneurysms that project anteriorly and superiorly since the dome of the aneurysm will overlie the contralateral A2 segment.

Every effort should be made to visualize this vessel prior to clipping. It is usually possible to gently retract the aneurysm to see around to the opposite side and find the contralateral A2 artery. This maneuver is useful to clearly identify the extent of the neck, especially with large and giant aneurysms where it may be extremely difficult to find the A2 artery on the opposite side of the aneurysm.

Whenever possible, an attempt should be made to identify both A1 segments, both A2 segments, the anterior communicating artery, the ipsilateral recurrent artery of Heubner, and the hypothalamic perforating vessel or vessels that originate from the anterior communicating segment. Following identification of all of these vessels, the aneurysm neck should be fully dissected. Even at this point in the operation, other problems can be encountered such as the presence of aberrant vessels, reduplicated anterior communicating arteries, or supernumerary A2 branches. These arteries are often not apparent until an initial aneurysm clip has been placed.

## *Aneurysm Dissection*

With recently ruptured aneurysms of the anterior communicating complex, the overriding principle of aneurysm dissection is to leave the dome of the aneurysm undisturbed. With anterior and inferiorly projecting aneurysms, the dome is often adherent to the optic chiasm, and the contralateral A1 artery may be very difficult to identify. The surgeon must

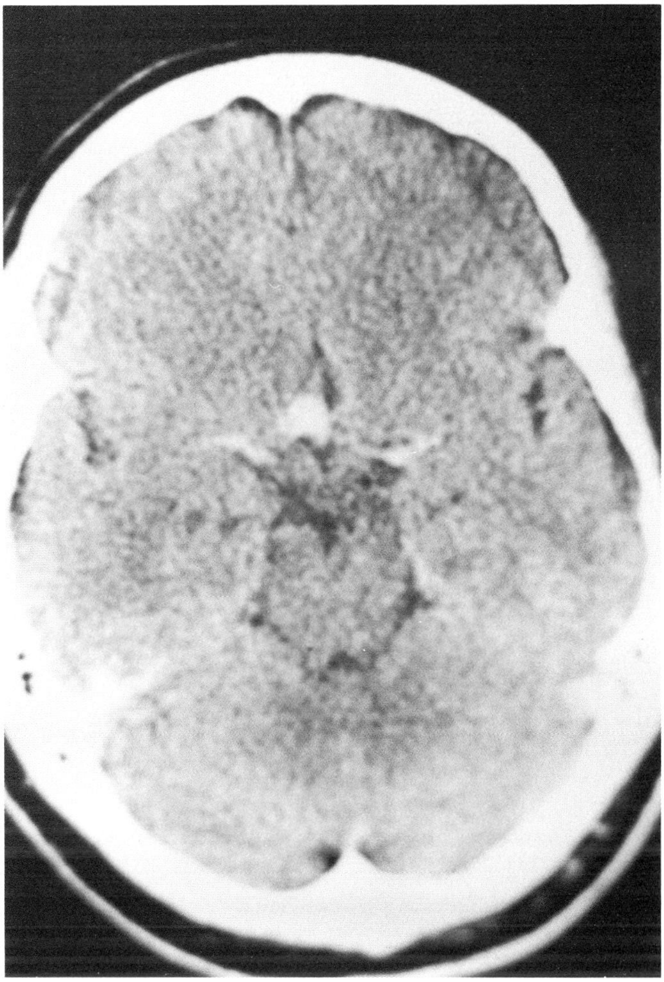

*Figure 18A. Large anterior communicating artery aneurysm. Contrast-enhanced CT scan demonstrates location of anterior communicating artery aneurysm projecting off toward the right hemisphere.*

be careful not to put undo traction on the arteries of the communicating complex and pull the aneurysm off of the chiasm, inciting intraoperative rupture.

With aneurysms that project superiorly and into one of the frontal lobes, retraction of the frontal lobe is hazardous as it may again precipitate rupture of the aneurysm. Gyrus rectus resection should replace brain retraction to gain increased visualization of the neck of the aneurysm and the multiple vessels. The pia, arachnoid, and blood clot on the dome of the aneurysm should be left undisturbed during the dissection around the neck and the communicating complex. Aneurysms in this location often hide the contralateral A2 segment.

Sometimes the A2 arteries are densely adherent to the dome of the aneurysm. This provides particular challenge, since freeing the arteries off the dome can increase the risk of intraoperative rupture. It is often best to clip the aneurysm even before the dissection of the contralateral A2 has been fully completed. Once the aneurysm is clipped, the dissection can proceed without difficulty. If the origin of the A2 vessel has been comprised, the clip can then be adjusted.

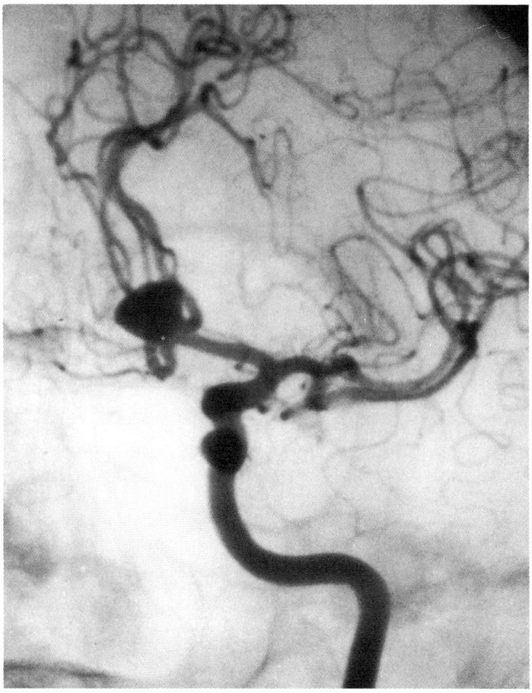

***Figure 18B****. Oblique view of the left carotid angiogram demonstrates a dominant A1 artery filling both A2 arteries as well as the aneurysm. This patient had an aplastic right A1 artery.*

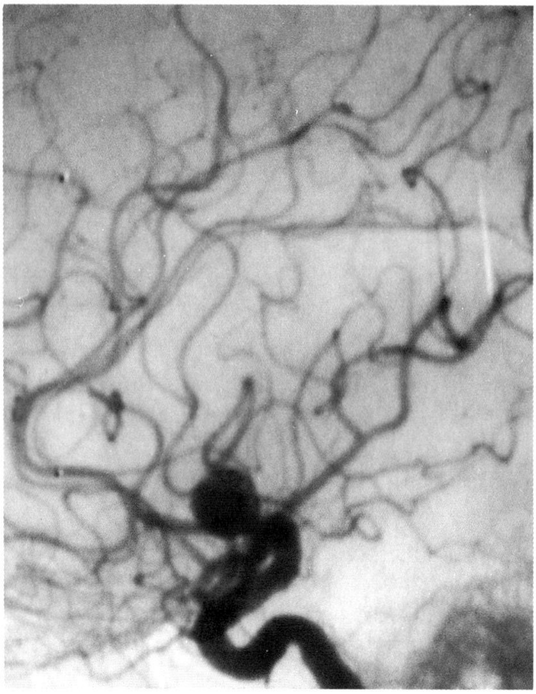

***Figure 18C****. Lateral angiogram demonstrates the upward projection of the aneurysm with the A2 arteries overlying the aneurysm dome.*

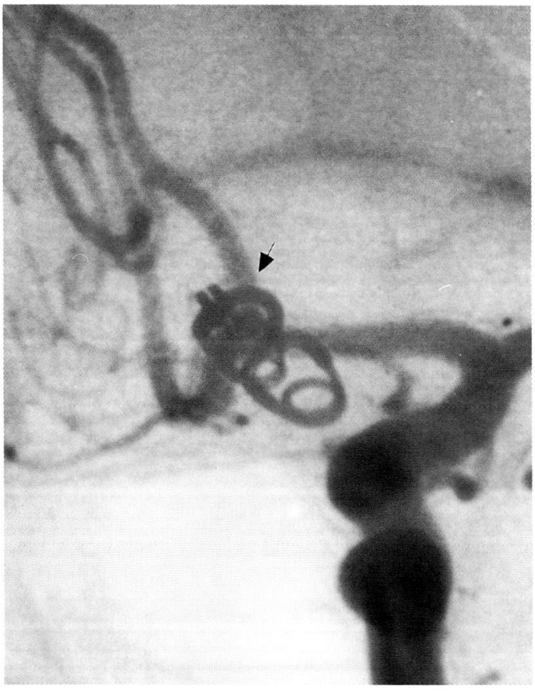

***Figure 18D****. Postoperative angiogram demonstrates the use of a fenestrated clip, obliterating the aneurysm. Note that the left A2 artery is traveling within the clip fenestration (arrow).*

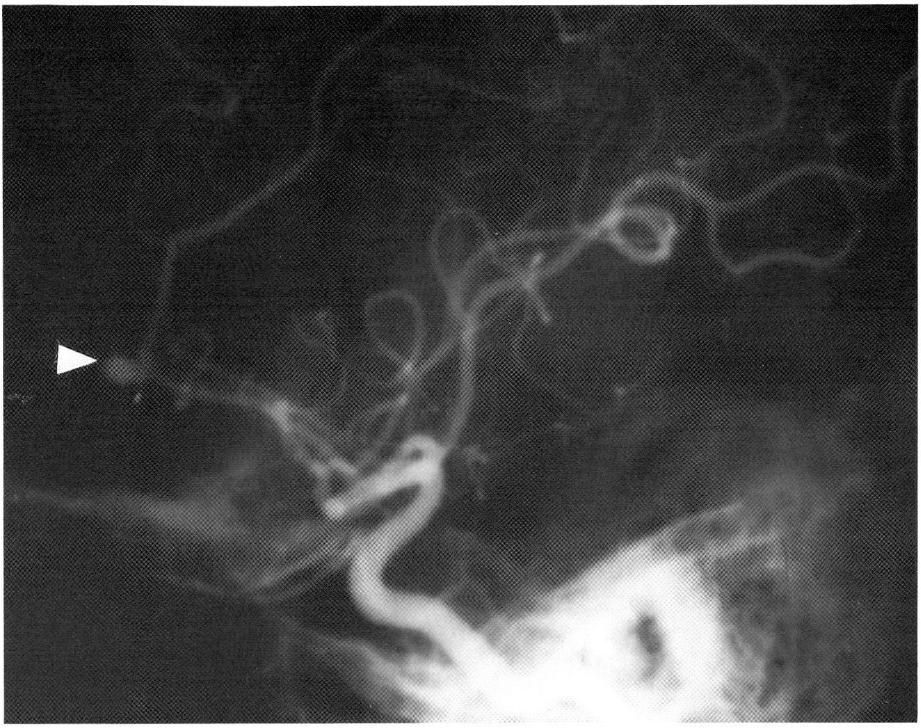

*Figure 19. Lateral carotid angiogram demonstrates a recently ruptured 8 mm pericallosal aneurysm, just anterior to the genu of the corpus callosum (arrow).*

The ipsilateral A2 artery sometimes overlies the mid-portion of the dome of a superior directed aneurysm, and it is very difficult to mobilize the aneurysm enough to get a clip around the A2 artery without significant kinking or risk of rupture of the aneurysm. A straight fenestrated clip may be useful to clip the aneurysm and preserve the A2 in its natural position within the clip fenestration (Figure 18).

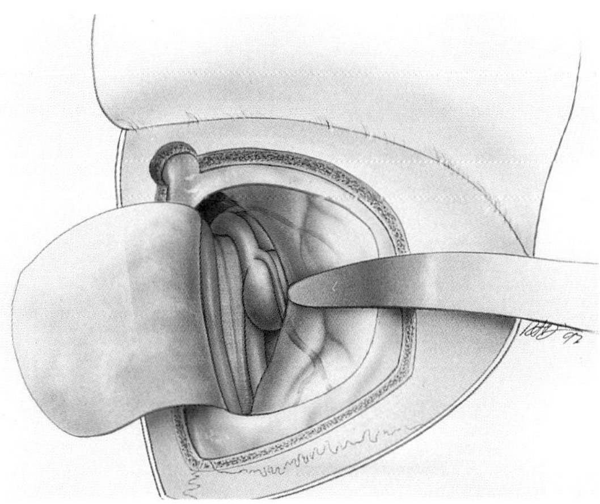

*Figure 20. Drawing of the operative exposure of a distal pericallosal aneurysm on top of the genu of the corpus callosum. The retractor is holding the right hemisphere away from the falx, exposing the pericallosal artery with the aneurysm arising at the origin of the callosal marginal artery.*

With posteriorly projecting aneurysms, the risk to hypothalamic perforators becomes most critical. These arteries are usually stretched around the inferior side of the aneurysm neck and dome, and must be carefully identified and dissected off the aneurysm prior to clip placement. The dissection for posterior projecting aneurysms usually takes place behind the A1 and A2 arteries so that the recurrent artery of Heubner will also be in the field, obstructing somewhat the view of the aneurysm. This artery needs to be carefully identified and kept free from damage during the dissection.

Sometimes the fronto-orbital artery can be mistaken for the recurrent artery of Heubner. This distinction is important to make since

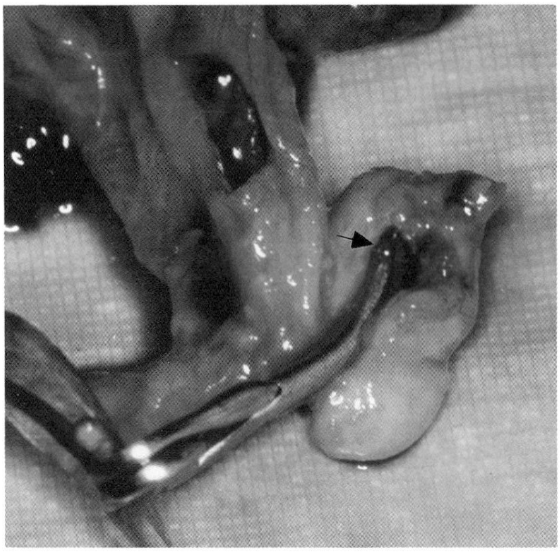

*Figure 21. A postmortem photograph of a patient who died immediately after aneurysm surgery to clip a recently ruptured posterior communicating aneurysm. The clip was incorrectly placed on the dome of the aneurysm, so that the blades ruptured the dome. Attempt to advance the clip blades introduced the blade into the lumen of the aneurysm, preventing eventual proper clipping. The arrow points to the hole in the aneurysm, with the clip blade introduced into the lumen of the aneurysm.*

the frontal orbital artery can be sacrificed with no real risk of neurologic deficit. This artery should not be routinely sacrificed, but if it is densely adherent to the dome of the aneurysm or greatly obstructing the progress of the dissection, it is better to sacrifice the artery or include it in the clip rather than to risk intraoperative aneurysm rupture.

Inferiorly projected aneurysms are usually only seen with fusiform dilatations of the anterior communicating artery and not with the aneurysms projecting off the crotch of one of the major branching points. These aneurysms are particularly difficult to deal with since the hypothalamic perforators often arise directly from abnormal segments of the artery. It is sometimes possible to reconstruct the anterior communicating artery by placing a straight clip behind the A1 and A2 arteries in order to preserve a lumen across the anterior communicating complex to supply the hypothalamic perforators. Such a clipping is impossible is many large aneurysms. The anterior communicating artery should not be trapped bilaterally unless there is already significant hypothalamic damage due to recent rupture. Unilateral clipping of the origin of the anterior communicating artery from the dominant supply to the aneurysm will often be sufficient to induce thrombosis in the aneurysm.

## *Clip Application*

Most of the principles expressed for clip application in other locations in the anterior circulation will apply to the anterior communicating complex. In aneurysms in other locations, it is generally possible to predict from examining the angiogram the type and size of clip that will be necessary. With anterior communicating complex aneurysms, a great deal of flexibility will be required in planning the final clip application. Since there are so many vessels that need to be identified and preserved during the dissection and clip application, the configuration of these arteries in relationship to the aneurysm dome has to be taken into account when planning the final clipping.

A straight clip passed along the axis of the ipsilateral A1 artery is usually sufficient to clip the aneurysm. It may sometimes be necessary to orient a clip almost perpendicular to the direction of the anterior communicating artery in order to clip many superiorly projecting aneurysms. Fenestrated clips may be useful when the ipsilateral A2 artery is obstructing the convenient passage of the clip blades.

Temporary clipping is often not as convenient to accomplish as with carotid aneurysms or MCA aneurysms in view of multiple arterial connections to the region. With clipping of the dominant A1 artery, sufficient softening of the aneurysm dome can usually be achieved to allow the final dissection and clip application. Total isolation of all of the afferent and efferent vessels of the anterior communicating complex by temporary clips is probably not desirable. The great abundance of perforating vessels, including the hypothalamic perforators and the recurrent artery of Heubner, cannot withstand total cessation of blood flow for more than a brief time. If an aneurysm cannot be clipped with the assistance of bilateral A1 temporary occlusion, complete circulatory arrest should probably be considered.

## Pericallosal Aneurysms

Pericallosal aneurysms arise on the distal anterior cerebral artery in relationship to the genu of the corpus callosum (Figure 19). These aneurysms typically arise at the bifurcation of the pericallosal artery and the origin of the callosomarginal artery. Since the aneurysms are well distal within the interhemispheric fissure, the pterional approach to these aneurysms is not a viable option.

The safest and most direct route to pericallosal aneurysms is the interhemispheric approach from a frontal midline craniotomy anterior to the coronal suture (Figure 20). Aneurysms that lie directly anterior and on top of the genu can be easily accessed through this approach. In rare instances, aneurysms arise beneath the genu of the corpus callosum but still too distal in the fissure to be safely visualized from the pterional approach. In these cases, the craniotomy must be very low on the floor of the frontal fossa to make a direct approach underneath the genu of the corpus callosum.

Much like the dissection of the MCA, dissection of pericallosal aneurysm through the interhemispheric fissure requires identification of the distal arteries and dome of the aneurysm prior to visualizing the proximal feeding vessel. Once the pericallosal artery is identified on the surface of the corpus callosum, the artery is followed proximally until the neck of the aneurysm can be seen. Depending on which way the aneurysm is projecting, the dissection will proceed along the path of least resistance towards the proximal side of the aneurysm and establishment of control of the proximal pericallosal artery. As with ruptured aneurysms in other locations, the dome of a ruptured pericallosal aneurysm should not be disturbed until proximal and distal control is established on the ACA.

With aneurysms on the inferior or anterior part of the genu of the corpus callosum, visualization from above will not usually supply satisfactory control of the proximal pericallosal artery. It may be necessary to resect a small portion of the corpus callosum in order to view the pericallosal artery underneath the genu, proximal to the aneurysm. Resection of a small portion of the genu of the corpus callosum will not produce any noticeable neurologic deficit. Once proximal and distal control have been established and the major branches of the ACA have been identified, clipping of pericallosal aneurysms can proceed according to standard principles documented in previous sections of this chapter.

## Intraoperative Aneurysm Rupture

The sequence of steps taken to deal with an intraoperative rupture varies, depending on when in the course of the operation the rupture occurs. If the aneurysm rupture occurs even before the aneurysm is visualized, the most propitious move is to place a temporary clip on the proximal feeding artery. While this maneuver usually will not stop arterial bleeding, it will greatly reduce the blood flow, allowing rapid dissection of the feeding artery to the aneurysm and dissection of either the aneurysm or the artery distal to the aneurysm. Both proximal and distal control can then be achieved.

Fortunately, the most common time for aneurysms to rupture intraoperatively is during aneurysm dissection and clipping. Clipping the aneurysm neck in the event of intraoperative rupture should only be attempted if the aneurysm has been well dissected; poorly placed clips can shear the neck of the aneurysm, making eventual clipping impossible. It is always preferable to use temporary clips on the parent vessels rather than firing clips blindly at a ruptured aneurysm or inducing systemic hypotension.

Sometimes it is not possible to place temporary clips to gain control of a ruptured aneurysm. A large bore suction placed directly on the rupture site can clear enough blood to allow definitive dissection and clipping of the aneurysm. When this maneuver is also impossible, it is best to tamponade the bleeding with small muscle pledgets held with cotton against the rupture site. The muscle will induce thrombosis of the ruptured area and often contain the hemorrhage while the dissection is proceeding. At times, an aneurysm may rupture during placement of the definitive clip. As the clip is being closed, the dome pulls away from the adhering structures and the previous rupture site is reopened. If the dissection has been done properly and the aneurysm clip is moving in the right direction when the rupture occurs, the advance and closure of the clip usually will secure the aneurysm.

A rupture should always be anticipated, since often the bleeding can totally obscure vision during the time that the clip is being manipulated. Rather than backing out of the maneuver, the surgeon who is prepared can continue with the clip even if vision is obstructed by arterial bleeding. In this event, it is advisable to advance the clip further than originally estimated to ensure complete occlusion of the aneurysm. Final adjustments in the clip placement can be made after bleeding has been stopped.

A common error made after aneurysm rupture during clipping is to slightly reopen and advance the clip. This often introduces one of the blades into the lumen of the dome, completely preventing clipping of the aneurysm (Figure 21). The experienced surgeon can often rectify the situation by opening the clip, removing it slightly, and changing its orientation to travel more perpendicular to the neck of the aneurysm. With torrential arterial bleeding, however, it is difficult to evaluate the true nature of the problem. In this event, it is usually better to place temporary clips on the parent artery proximal and distal and to remove the aneurysm clip completely, so that the rupture site can be evaluated and proper clip placement achieved.

There is no magic formula for the approach to intraoperative aneurysm ruptures, but advanced planning is critical to the success of managing this dreaded complication.

## References

1. Batjer HH, Samson DS. Retrograde suction decompression of giant paraclinoidal aneurysms. *J Neurosurg.* 1990;73: 305–306.
2. Dandy WE. *Intracranial Arterial Aneurysms.* Ithaca, NY: Comstock Publishing: 1944.
3. Day AL. Aneurysms of the ophthalmic segment: a clinical and anatomical analysis. *J Neurosurg.* 1990; 72:677–691.
4. Dolenc VV. A combined epi- and subdural direct approach to carotid-ophthalmic artery aneurysms. *J Neurosurg.* 1985;62:667–672.
5. Dott NM. Intracranial aneurysms; cerebral arterioradiography; surgical treatment. *Trans Med Chir Soc Edinburgh.* 1933;112:219–240.
6. Drake CG. On the surgical treatment of ruptured intracranial aneurysms. *Clin Neurosurg.* 1965;13: 122–155.
7. Drake CG. Earlier times in aneurysm surgery. *Clin Neurosurg.* 1985;32:41–50.
8. Dunker RO, Harris AB. Surgical anatomy of the proximal anterior cerebral artery. *J Neurosurg.* 1976; 44:359–367.
9. Gibo H, Carver CC, Rhoton AL Jr, et al. Microsurgical anatomy of the middle cerebral artery. *J Neurosurg.* 1981;54:151–169.
10. Gibo H, Lenkey C, Rhoton AL Jr. Microsurgical anatomy of the supraclinoid portion of the internal carotid artery. *J Neurosurg.* 1981;55:560–574.
11. Heros RC, Ojemann RG, Crowell RM. Superior temporal gyrus approach to middle cerebral artery aneurysms: techniques and results. *Neurosurgery.* 1982; 10:308–313.
12. Höök O, Norlén G. Aneurysms of the middle cerebral artery: a report of 80 cases. *Acta Chir Scand Suppl.* 1958;235:1–39.
13. Keen WW. Intracranial lesions. *Med News (NY).* 1890;57:439–449.
14. McKissock W, Richardson A, Walsh L. Posterior/communicating aneurysms: a controlled trial of the conservative and surgical treatment of ruptured aneurysms of the internal carotid artery at or near the point of origin of the posterior communicating artery. *Lancet.* 1960;1:1203–1206.
15. McKissock W, Richardson A, Walsh L. Middle-cerebral aneurysms: further results in the controlled trial of conservative and surgical treatment of ruptured intracranial aneurysms. *Lancet.* 1962;2:417–421.
16. Peerless SJ. The surgical approach to middle cerebral and posterior communicating aneurysms. *Clin Neurosurg.* 1974;21:151–165.
17. Perlmutter D, Rhoton AL Jr. Microsurgical anatomy of the anterior cerebral-anterior communicating recurrent artery complex. *J Neurosurg.* 1976;45:259–272.
18. Pool JL. Aneurysms of the anterior communicating artery: bifrontal craniotomy and routine use of temporary clips. *J Neurosurg.* 1961;18:98–111.

19. Robinson RG. Ruptured aneurysms of the middle cerebral artery. *J Neurosurg.* 1971;35:25–33.
20. Sahs AL, Perret GE, Locksley HB, et al. *Intracranial Aneurysms and Subarachnoid Hemorrhage. A Cooperative Study.* Philadelphia, Pa: JB Lippincott; 1969.
21. Schucart WA, Kwan ES, Heilman CB. Temporary balloon occlusion of a proximal vessel as an aid to clipping aneurysms of the basilar and paraclinoid internal carotid arteries: technical note. *Neurosurgery.* 1990;27:116–119.
22. Solomon RA, Fukushima T. New aneurysm clip appliers for "key-hole" neurosurgery. *Neurosurgery.* 1991;28:474–476.
23. Solomon RA, Onesti ST, Klebanoff L. Relationship between the timing of aneurysm surgery and the development of delayed cerebral ischemia. *J Neurosurg.* 1991;75:56–61.
24. Solomon RA, Smith CR, Raps EC, et al. Deep hypothermic circulatory arrest for the management of complex anterior and posterior circulation aneurysms. *Neurosurgery.* 1991;29:732–738.
25. Spetzler RF, Lee KS. Reconstruction of the temporalis muscle for the pterional craniotomy. *J Neurosurg.* 1990;73:636–637.
26. Sundt TM Jr. *Surgical Techniques for Saccular and Giant Intracranial Aneurysms.* Baltimore, Md: Williams & Wilkins; 1990.
27. Suzuki J, Kodama N, Fujiwara, et al. Surgical treatment of middle cerebral artery aneurysms: from the experience of 174 cases. In: Suzuki J, ed. *Cerebral Aneurysms.* Tokyo: Neuron Publishing Co; 1979: 278–283.
28. Suzuki J, Mizoi K, Yoshimoto T. Bifrontal interhemispheric approach to aneurysms of the anterior communicating artery. *J Neurosurg.* 1986;64:183–190.
29. Symon L. Surgical management of middle cerebral artery aneurysms. In: Schmidek HH, Sweet WH, eds. *Operative Neurosurgical Techniques: Indications, Methods, and Results.* New York, NY: Grune & Stratton; 1982;2:891–908.
30. Wilson CB, Spetzler RF. Operative approaches to aneurysms. *Clin Neurosurg.* 1979;26:232–247.
31. Yasargil MG. *Microneurosurgery, I: Microsurgical Anatomy of the Basal Cisterns and Vessels of the Brain, Diagnostic Studies, General Operative Techniques and Pathological Considerations of the Intracranial Aneurysms.* New York, NY: Thieme Stratton; 1984.
32. Yasargil MG (ed). *Microneurosurgery, II: Clinical Considerations, Surgery of the Intracranial Aneurysms and Results.* New York, NY: Thieme Stratton; 1984.
33. Yasargil MG, Fox JL. The microsurgical approach to intracranial aneurysms. *Surg Neurol.* 1975;3:7–14.

# CHAPTER 8

# Posterior Circulation Aneurysms: Surgical Management

Fernando G. Diaz, MD, PhD, Jonathan Hodes, MD, and Bernard Vellardo, MD

Aneurysms arising in the posterior circulation present difficult problems of approach due to limited accessibility of the vertebrobasilar system, potential problems of ischemia from damage to the vessels from which the aneurysms arise, or damage to the smaller perforating vessels that originate in the vicinity. Great attention to detail and clear understanding of the operative anatomy of the vertebrobasilar system facilitate the safe and successful approach to these aneurysms. The surgical approaches can be divided into three categories: (1) supratentorial; (2) infratentorial; and (3) transbasal. The various factors determining the preoperative preparation for patients with vertebrobasilar aneurysms, the intraoperative procedures used to facilitate the operations, the three operative categories used to treat these aneurysms, and the potential complications that may develop in the management of aneurysms arising from the posterior circulation will be reviewed. Observations made from the surgical procedures and complications encountered will be analyzed to better understand the occurrence and prevention of these complications.

## Preoperative Considerations

Patients with vertebrobasilar aneurysms may present for evaluation either following an event of subarachnoid hemorrhage (SAH), or following a cerebral angiogram or computed tomography (CT) scan obtained for other reasons.[19,20] These patients should have a thorough medical and neurologic evaluation including complete cerebral angiography, CT scan, and/or magnetic resonance imaging (MRI) of the brain.[22] Patients suffering an SAH require admission to an intensive care unit (ICU) for evaluation and preparation for surgery.

A complete preoperative medical evaluation should be made in elderly patients to minimize and prepare for possible intraoperative cardiac, respiratory, or renal complications resulting from intentionally induced hypertension or hypotension, blood loss, the use of cardiac suppressants such as barbiturates or lidocaine, or the use of diuretics such as mannitol.[22]

Intraoperative hypertension, while not a condition generally required by the surgeon, can occur frequently during the induction of anesthesia. It may not only induce aneurysm rupture prior to the performance of the craniotomy, but may also cause myocardial infarction from the increased tension of the myocardial wall in relation to the pressure in the coronary arteries. Careful monitoring of the arterial blood pressure with an indwelling arterial line will facilitate the pre- and intraoperative management of the blood pressure and prevent any undesirable fluctuations.

Intraoperative hypotension was proposed by Drake[3,4] to facilitate the dissection of cerebral aneurysms and to prevent the onset of intraoperative rupture. Myocardial ischemia may develop in patients with pre-existing chronic hypertension, marginal cardiac function, or severe coronary artery disease. Patients with vertebrobasilar aneurysms are best managed with a Swan-Ganz (S-G) catheter placed to monitor their cardiac function during surgery. An optimum intravascular blood volume may be established preoperatively by the administration of intravenous albumin and the careful monitoring of both the cardiac output and cardiac index.

In patients who chronically have received antihypertensive medication, severe hypotension may occur during induction of anesthesia. This is generally the result of a relative state of hypovolemia, which may be compounded by the sudden vasodilation that follows induction, and may be prevented by the judicious administration of fluids in the preoperative period. Extreme intraoperative bleeding may also be followed by severe hypotension in patients who are normotensive as well as in those who are chronically hypertensive. This problem may be anticipated only by securing blood preoperatively.

Intraoperative administration of barbiturates and lidocaine in preparation for the application of temporary clips has potential problems with myocardial perfusion and respiratory suppression.[2,15] The sudden administration of these agents may be followed by immediate hypotension, which if prolonged, may result in myocardial ischemia. Chronically hypertensive patients and patients with coronary artery disease are more susceptible to hypotension when barbiturates are given. A slow intravenous infusion of barbiturates is less likely to result in significant hypotension. Barbiturates and lidocaine may also result in the onset of hypoventilation and $CO_2$ retention postoperatively. A careful preoperative evaluation of patients with chronic obstructive pulmonary disease or other pulmonary problems may include securing arterial blood gases or pulmonary function tests, in addition to a chest x-ray.

Mannitol has been used to decrease brain volume during surgery, thus requiring less brain retraction. Susuki[21] promoted the use of mannitol in aneurysm surgery because it may protect the brain during brief periods of vessel occlusion. In addition to its diuretic properties, mannitol acts as a membrane stabilizer and free-radical quencher. It must be used carefully in patients with marginal renal function because it can potentiate the development of renal insufficiency from dehydration and crystallization of the mannitol in the renal tubules. Mannitol may precipitate the onset of acute myocardial insufficiency in patients with marginal cardiac function since it produces a transient volume overload prior to the onset of its diuretic effect.

A four-vessel cerebral angiogram must be completed in all patients to determine the aneurysm location, to exclude the presence of multiple aneurysms (which occur in 20% of cases) and to rule out the presence of cerebral vasospasm.[13] A conventional selective arteriogram is the most common form of evaluation, but a selective digital arteriogram is rapidly becoming the preferred form of evaluation. The critical aspect of the arteriogram is the precise acquisition of the arterial anatomy, including small vessels and perforating arteries, and the detailed study of the nature of the aneurysm neck. It is advisable to obtain selective arterial injections of the extracranial vessels in some patients, in anticipation of a possible extracranial-to-intracranial anastomosis.[20,21]

Imaging with CT or MRI is usually necessary to exclude the presence of intra- or extraparenchymal hematomas, and to access the extent of the SAH, the presence of hydrocephalus, and the possibility of intra-aneurysmal clot formation. A partially thrombosed giant aneurysm is potentially a problem because of the possibility of intraoperative embolization and the potential difficulty in securing complete aneurysm clipping. A false sense of security may be gained from an angiogram revealing a small amount of dye filling the aneurysm, when in reality the aneurysm is large and mostly filled with clot.[2,6,13,15,18,19]

The clinical presentation of the patient largely determines the evaluation and preoperative preparation that may be performed. Patients presenting without an SAH may have a more gradual and planned evaluation than patients who present with recent hemorrhage. The decision to proceed with an operation should be based on the clinical condition of the patient, including the neurologic evaluation. Patients with a poor medical condition and good neurologic status should not be operated on any sooner than the patient with a poor neurologic condition and a favorable medical status. A poor condition in either case would likely lead to a poor outcome. The success of the operation depends on careful preoperative planning, as well as the execution of the operation.

## Intraoperative Considerations

The intraoperative preparation of the patient begins in the preinduction area and ends in the recovery room.[22] Patients with posterior circulation aneurysms require careful monitoring of their cardiovascular, pulmonary, and renal functions throughout their stay in the operating room. Several drugs may be administered during surgery as cerebral protective agents, or in anticipation of hypotension or arterial occlusion.

Cardiovascular monitoring is essential in the intraoperative management of patients with vertebrobasilar aneurysms. A radial arterial catheter must be placed preoperatively, and continuous intra-arterial pressure measurements must be maintained intraoperatively. Cardiovascular function should be correlated by the placement of an S-G catheter to record myocardial function. Intraoperative measurements of central venous pressure, pulmonary arterial pressure, pulmonary wedge pressure, cardiac output, and cardiac index facilitate the surgical procedure. Intraoperative intervention with drugs that may affect cardiovascular function can then be monitored, and changes in cardiac performance corrected appropriately.[22]

Preoperative evaluation of the patient with possible pulmonary problems will allow the neuroanesthesiologist to anticipate possible problems with ventilation or gas exchange. Patients with vertebrobasilar aneurysms require, like other neurosurgical patients, a mild state of hyperventilation to keep the $PCO_2$ around 30–35 mm Hg. Dropping the $PCO_2$ below this level will not induce any further cerebral relaxation by vasoconstriction, and may in fact be detrimental by inducing cerebral ischemia. The extent of hyperventilation must also be carefully planned in patients who have any degree of residual vasospasm. Inducing severe hyperventilation in these patients may aggravate cerebral ischemia because of the combined effect of the vasoconstriction induced by the two mechanisms. The possibility of hypoventilation during surgery from intubation in the right main-stem bronchus must be anticipated and prevented. Immediate postoperative hypoventilation from early extubation or too much anesthetic must also be kept in mind in these patients, who would otherwise do very well if their respiratory control was properly coordinated.[22]

Adequate renal function is essential in patients who will undergo a craniotomy. The intraoperative administration of diuretics facilitates cerebral retraction, especially in patients who have an aneurysm in the territory of the basilar artery (BA). Furosemide given 20–40 mg at induction fosters the onset of diuresis, prevents the development of renal tubular casts, and prevents the possible occurrence of myocardial overload from the administration of mannitol. An accurate hourly account of urinary output must be maintained with an indwelling foley catheter. Immediate fluid replacement is necessary once the aneurysm has been clipped and brain retraction is no longer needed.

Anesthesia is induced with intravenous thiopental sodium and maintained with nitrous oxide-oxygen and isoflurane. During induction the patient receives intravenous diphenylhydantoin 15 mg/kg, vancomycin 1000 mg, dexamethasone 10 mg, gentamycin 80 mg, furosemide 20–40 mg, and mannitol 0.5 gm/kg. Spinal fluid drains are not used routinely because drainage of spinal fluid from the cisterns generally has been effective in achieving cerebral relaxation. Arterial blood gases, end expiratory $CO_2$ recordings, and pulse oximetry are monitored throughout the operation. Arterial $PCO_2$ is maintained at about 30–35 mm Hg, $PO_2$ around 95 mm Hg, and oxygen saturation at about 100%. Temperature is maintained at normal with a warming blanket. Arterial pressure is maintained as close to preoperative values as possible. Intraoperative hypotension is seldom used, generally only when proximal control of the BA cannot be accomplished with a temporary clip.

## Operative Approaches

Surgical management of aneurysms in the vertebrobasilar circulation has been difficult and fraught with many potential intraoperative problems. Direct approach has been prevented by the location of the BA immediately adjacent to the clivus and the proximity of the brain stem and cranial nerves. Drake[3,4] was the first to consistently operate on aneurysms arising from the BA, and developed techniques and approaches that have been subsequently followed, as well as modified, by many. Approaches to aneurysms arising in the vertebrobasilar circulation depend on their anatomic location. The operative routes now favored are the supratentorial approach to aneurysms of the tip and distal half of the BA, the suboccipital approach for aneurysms of the vertebral artery (VA) and some vertebrobasilar junction aneurysms, and the transbasal approaches for aneurysms arising from the vertebrobasilar junction and mid-portion of the BA.

### *Supratentorial Approaches*

The surgical management of aneurysms arising from the tip of the BA via the subtemporal approach was made popular by Drake.[3,4,12] Yasargil[23] preferred the trans-sylvian approach, believing that one could obtain better control of the BA and its bifurcation through this route. Sano[13,14] combined both of these approaches and developed a mixed trans-sylvian subtemporal approach, which some call the "one-and-a-half approach."

### *Subtemporal Approach*

The patient's head is placed in a lateral position, and the body in a lateral decubitus, or supine with the right shoulder elevated by a roll. A vertical incision is made generally in the right preauricular area and extended to just above the level of insertion of the temporalis muscle. The skin incision may also be made in a reverse question mark following the hairline. The temporalis muscle is incised vertically along its fibers, which are then transected across the base of the zygoma to facilitate the exposure of the entire squamosal portion of the temporal bone. A round or quadrangular free bone flap is elevated, with the most inferior portion lying flat with the floor of the temporal fossa. The dura is incised in a cruciate manner, and the temporal lobe is elevated to expose the tentorial incisura, taking care to preserve the vein of Labbé. The tentorial incisura is either retracted with sutures to expose the midbrain, or is transected and then retracted. The oculomotor (III) nerve is left adherent to the uncus of the temporal lobe by not releasing it from the arachnoid that binds it to the temporal lobe. This facilitates the upward displacement of the oculomotor nerve and the ipsilateral posterior cerebral artery (PCA) with the temporal lobe retraction. The trochlear (IV) nerve is identified and preserved as it enters the edge of the tentorium and traverses parallel with the superior cerebellar artery (SCA).[3,4,17]

The SCA is followed anteriorly and medially until the BA is identified. The junction of the ipsilateral superior cerebellar, the proximal posterior cerebral (P-1), and the basilar arteries can be seen clearly from this approach.

Aneurysms arising from the basilar bifurcation and from the SCA area can be exposed and clipped. It is generally necessary to place a retractor on the cerebral peduncle to expose the interpeduncular area and see the origin of the perforating arteries arising from the BA.[18,20] Careful dissection of the perforators is necessary to separate them from the dome of the aneurysm, allowing proper clip placement. Aneurysms of the basilar bifurcation may require a fenestrated clip to preserve the ipsilateral P-1.[3,4] Visualization of the contralateral P-1 and SCA is difficult from this approach and has resulted in their occlusion by the clip. Drake[3,4] recommends the use of clips that are tailored to the exact width of the aneurysm neck. To tailor the clip it is necessary to measure the neck and then cut off the unneeded portion of the clip, a technique successful in occluding the aneurysms without clipping the opposite P1. The mechanical cutting of an aneurysm clip, however, changes its ferromagnetic properties, and may lead to its eventual failure.[10]

The subtemporal approach is quick and requires minimal dissection of the surface structures to reach the area of the midbrain. The perforators arising from the BA are easy to identify through this approach and can generally be totally preserved when dissected away from the aneurysm dome. However, there is considerable limitation in the ability to expose the contralateral P-1 and SCAs. It is not always possible to obtain proximal control of the BA because of the limited space available. A distinct advantage to this approach is the ability to perform an intracranial-to-extracranial anastomosis to the superior cerebellar or the posterior cerebral artery, in preparation for the complete occlusion of the BA.[15,20]

The subtemporal approach has been used in a few cases to reach aneurysms arising from the distal half of the BA.[8,17] This exposure is gained through a standard temporal craniotomy, elevating the entire temporal lobe, and transecting the tentorium from the point of entry of the trochlear (IV) nerve to the level of insertion of the tent on the petrous portion of the temporal bone. This permits the exposure of the trigeminal (V) nerve, gasserian ganglion and fossa, and the superior portion of the pons. It is necessary to place a retractor on the pons to expose the BA and then identify the aneurysm, which is generally located against the clivus. In some cases, the superior border of the petrous apex may be removed behind the gasserian fossa and in front of the cochlea.[8] This is a very restrictive approach, with limited proximal control of the BA, and with potential of aneurysm rupture when retracting the belly of the pons. The location of the trochlear and trigeminal nerves generally makes placement of the aneurysm clip very difficult.[17,18]

### *Trans-Sylvian Approach*

The patient is placed supine in a reclining position, with the head rotated 15° to the opposite side and with 15° of head extension supported by skeletal fixation. An incision is made along the frontal hairline from the level of the zygoma to a point approximately level with the ipsilateral mid-pupillary line. The skin and muscle are reflected in one single flap, exposing the entire squamous portion of the temporal bone, the frontalis process of the lateral orbital wall, and the vertical portion of the frontal zygomatic area. Yasargil[23] recommended a complex muscle incision disinserting the temporalis muscle from its anterior attachment and retracting it posteriorly, after separating the fatty tissue containing the frontalis branch of the facial (VII) nerve. This dissection lengthens the operation and does not offer any greater protection to the nerve than does the combined elevation of the skin and muscle in a single flap.

A free bone flap is elevated with a craniotome, centering the craniotomy on the pterion (Figure 1). The pterion is drilled down until the meningo-orbital branch of the middle meningeal artery is exposed. Prior to its opening, the dura is sutured to the skull to prevent epidural bleeding from leaking into the depth of the wound. It is then opened in a semicircular manner with the base on the pterion, and sutured to the temporalis mus-

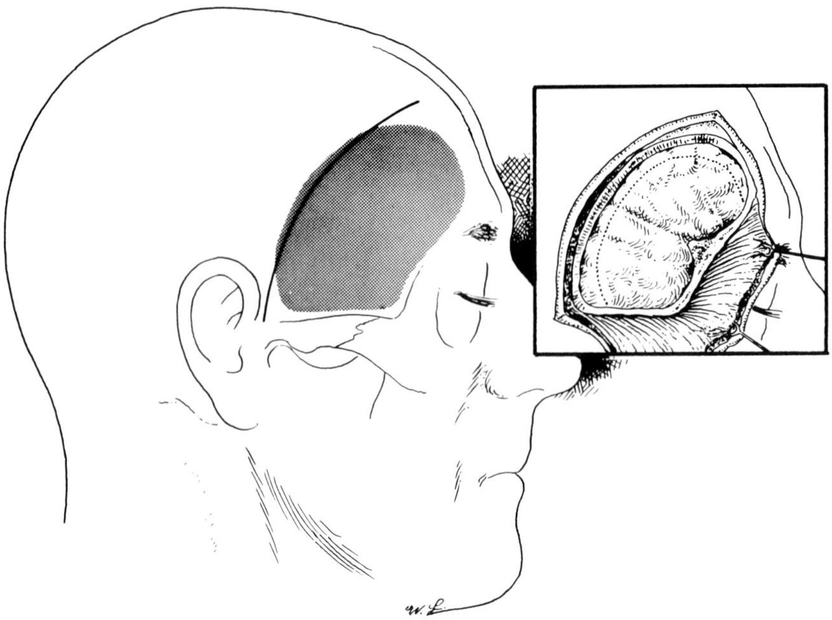

*Figure 1. Pterional craniotomy. The patient's head is positioned in skeletal fixation oriented with 15° of extension and 15° of rotation to the contralateral side. A free bone flap is elevated to include the pterional area, and the entire anterior two thirds of the middle cranial fossa, to facilitate the exposure of the tentorium cerebelli.*

cle. The operating microscope is brought into the field, and the sylvian fissure is opened widely to expose the entire course of the internal carotid and its bifurcation, the optic (II) nerve and optic chiasm, the proximal portion of the anterior cerebral artery (ACA), and the trunk and bifurcation of the middle cerebral artery (MCA) to the level of the limen insulae. All arachnoidal bands are released with sharp dissection to obtain maximum brain relaxation with minimal brain retraction, and to allow spinal fluid drainage from the cisterns. Additional cerebrospinal fluid (CSF) may be obtained by opening the lamina terminalis above the chiasm.

The anterior temporal lobe is retracted laterally while preserving the sylvian veins draining into the sphenopetrosal sinus. The oculomotor nerve is identified as it courses through the interpeduncular cistern to its entry into the cavernous sinus. The arachnoid bands around the oculomotor nerve are released, and the membrane of Lilliquist is opened, exposing the BA and its bifurcation by simply following the oculomotor nerve to the mesencephalon, or following the posterior communicating artery to the PCA. The basilar bifurcation is found immediately medial to either of these two structures as they reach cerebral peduncle. The perforating arteries arising from the posterior communicating artery and from the carotid bifurcation must be carefully dissected and preserved.

Exposure of the BA may be gained through one of several routes of access depending on the anatomy of the carotid artery (Figure 2). When the carotid artery is relatively short or is filled with atheroma, preventing its retraction, access can be gained to the BA through a lateral approach between the oculomotor nerve and the carotid artery (Figure 3). When the carotid artery is normal in length or longer than normal before it bifurcates, it may be retracted laterally and the optic nerve medially, thus gaining access to the BA between the two (Figure 4).[16,23] When this is not possible, the basilar bifurcation may be

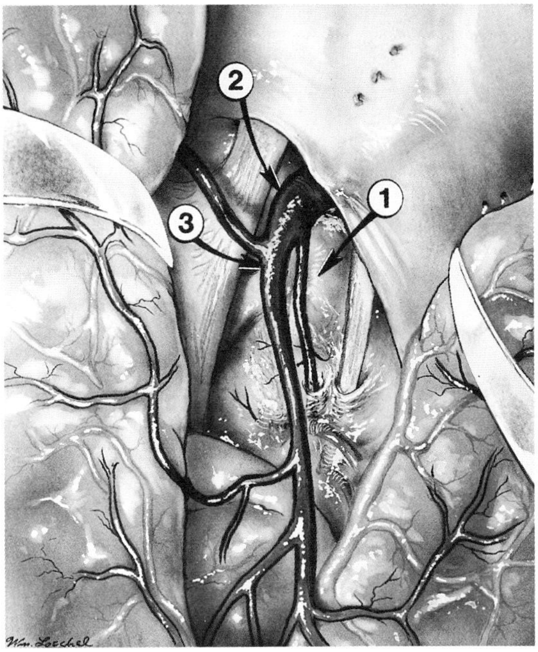


***Figure** 2. Alternatives to reach the basilar tip through a pterional approach. (1) Lateral to the internal carotid artery (ICA) and medial to the oculomotor (III) nerve. (2) Between the ICA and the optic (II) nerve. (3) Above the bifurcation of the ICA, through the perforating arteries. A wide dissection of all basilar cisterns and sylvian fissure is needed to expose the tip of the BA through the pterional approach.*

reached by separating the perforators of the carotid bifurcation, and gaining access to the BA between the trunks of the anterior and middle cerebral arteries (Figure 5).[9] Finally, if this is not possible, and the posterior communicating artery is either hypoplastic or has no prominent branches, the BA may be reached through a lateral approach after the posterior communicating artery has been clipped and transected. This last alternative is the least desirable of all due to the potential development of ischemic changes in the territory of the perforators of the posterior communicating artery.

## *Combined "One-and-a-Half" Approach*

Sano[13] described the combined approach,

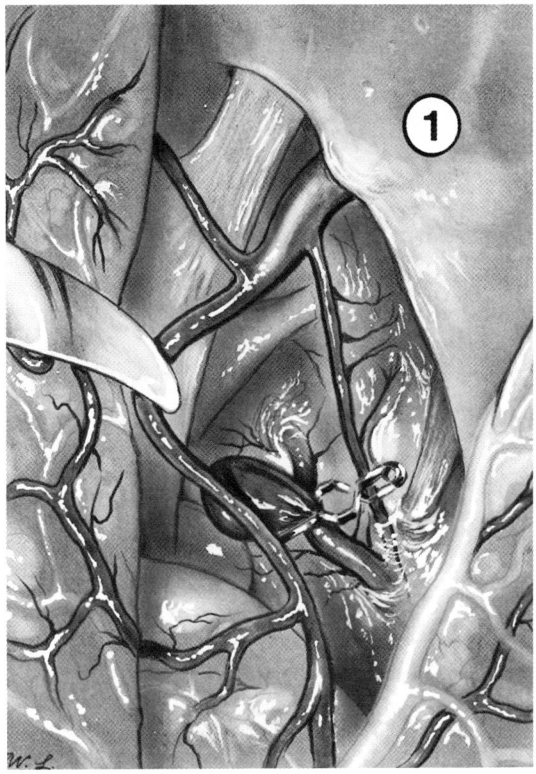


***Figure** 3. Approach to BA tip lateral to the ICA. After the sylvian fissure and basilar cisterns are widely dissected, the ICA is retracted medially, and the posterior communicating artery is followed to the posterior cerebral artery to locate the area of the basilar bifurcation. The membrane of Lilliquist is opened, and the basilar tip is found immediately beneath the membrane. A temporary clip may be applied proximal to the aneurysm in preparation for placement of the permanent clip on the aneurysm neck. The posterior communicating artery may be ligated and transected in some cases with good collaterals.*

which allows access to the basilar bifurcation through either a pure trans-sylvian route, or through a more subtemporal route depending on the circumstances. The skin incision and flap are basically the same as for the trans-sylvian approach described above, although the skin incision is extended to about 1 centimeter below the level of the zygoma. The bone flap is extended to the floor of the middle fossa to develop a flat plane extending from the pterion to the area of the tragus. The pterion is resected in a similar manner to the

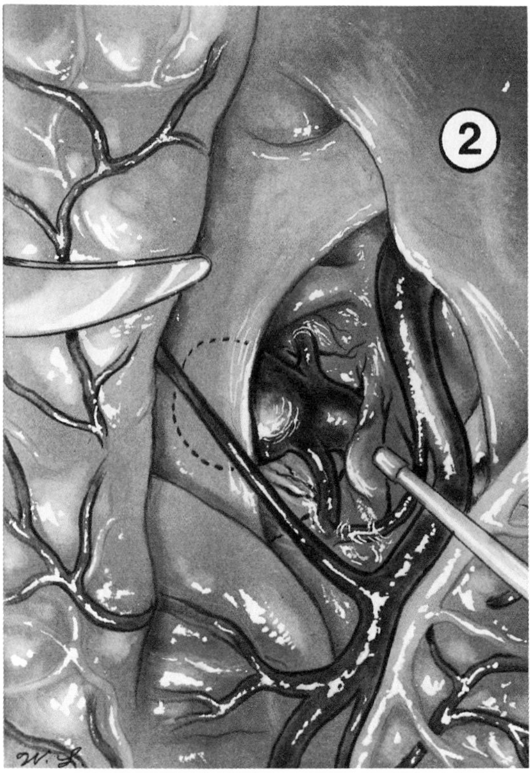


***Figure 4.*** *Approach to the basilar tip between the ICA and the optic (II) nerve. When the ICA is long and redundant before its bifurcation, the space medial to it is enough to dissect the basilar tip and clip the aneurysm. Numerous perforators from the ICA travel through this space and must be carefully identified and preserved. In some cases it is necessary to retract on the optic nerve to visualize the basilar tip well.*

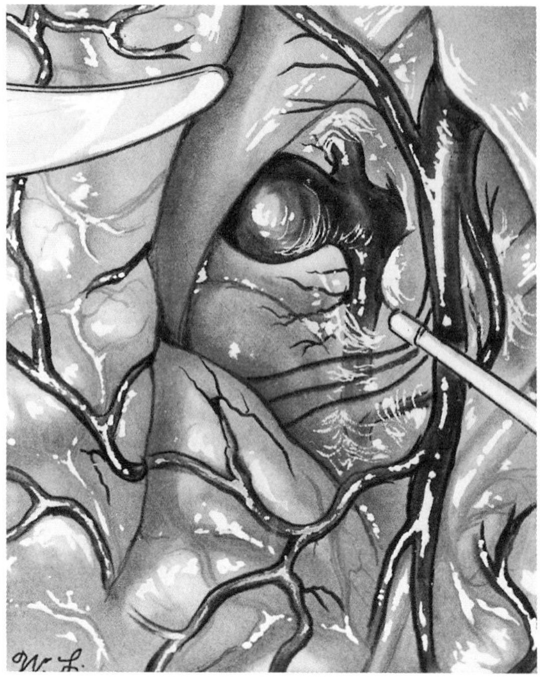

***Figure 5.*** *Approach to the basilar tip above the ICA bifurcation. In some patients the ICA is short and not movable. In these patients it is possible to expose the basilar tip, which separates the small perforators arising from the internal carotid bifurcation, and to open the membrane of Lilliquist through this route. The dissection of the sylvian fissure must be wide and relaxed to permit access to the tip of the BA. The mammillary bodies are usually in the center of the operative field, as well as all perforators arising from the basilar bifurcation. The perforators must be preserved.*

trans-sylvian approach, extending the resection to the floor of the middle fossa. In some cases it will be necessary to transect the orbitomeningeal branch to allow the total removal of the lesser wing of the sphenoid, thus permitting a clear and unobstructed entry to the microscope light. The dura is opened to create a flap, based anteriorly. The sylvian fissure and carotid artery area are dissected as described above. The temporal veins are transected, and the tip of the temporal lobe is retracted superior and posterior, to expose the entire floor of the middle fossa. When the dissection is performed correctly, one can access the area of the basilar bifurcation through a pure trans-sylvian approach, or through a subtemporal approach by merely rotating the patient to the contralateral side about 15°. The exposure of the oculomotor nerve and the lateral aspects of the carotid artery and cavernous sinus is better through this approach. The BA generally can be visualized clearly through this route, permitting the application of temporary clips whenever necessary.

When the basilar bifurcation is located below the level of the dorsum sellae, the bifurcation may be reached by removing the posterior clinoid process, and opening the tentorial incisura farther laterally.[16] When the basilar bifurcation is located much higher than the level of the dorsum sellae, there are two alternatives to reaching the bifurcation through this approach. One is to resect the inferior surface of the temporal lobe, allowing exposure of the proximal portion of the aneurysm neck. This alternative is not desirable because the resection would generally include the most medial portion of the temporal lobe, the uncus, and a portion of the hippocampus. A different alternative is to resect the zygoma and remove the floor of the middle fossa, and if necessary perform a superior and lateral orbitotomy, as described by Maroon[11] for resection of intraorbital tumors. This latter alternative allows the direct exposure of the mammillary body region with minimal brain retraction. Since the resection of bone is more extensive, this permits a shorter distance from the surface of the wound to the area of the basilar bifurcation. For this approach to be effective it is necessary to make a wide dissection of all the basal cisterns, to minimize brain retraction.

## *Suboccipital Approach*

The suboccipital approach was the first used to treat aneurysms of the vertibral artery (VA) and vertebrobasilar junction.[4,6,7] This approach permits wide exposure of the medulla and lateral pons but limits possible access to the more distal and medially located aneurysms. Accessibility of the vertebrobasilar junction is made very difficult by the cranial nerves.

The patient usually is positioned prone on chest rolls, with the head supported on skeletal fixation. The sitting position is seldom used any longer because of the associated risks of significant air embolism and hypotension. The exposure may be obtained either through a pure midline incision or through a unilateral approach. Through a midline incision, the dissection is extended from the level of the inion to about the level of C2–3, separating the paravertebral muscles to expose the entire occipital squama. The dissection is carried farther laterally on the side of the aneurysm to expose the tip of the mastoid process. A craniectomy is completed removing the exposed occipital bone across the midline, but predominantly on the side of the pathology. The bone resection is extended through the foramen magnum to the tip of the mastoid on the side of the aneurysm, and to the edge of the transverse sinus superiorly. It is often advisable to also remove the posterior arch of the atlas. The dura is opened in a Y fashion and sutured to the muscle. The cisterna magna is incised, allowing copious drainage of CSF prior to attempting retraction of the cerebellum or dissection of the VA.

The VA is identified proximally as it enters through its dural ring, and courses ventrally and medially through the fascicles of the spinal accessory (XI) and hypoglossal (XII) nerves. The VA may be followed medially by applying gentle retraction on the cerebellar tonsil. When the aneurysm originates from the posterior inferior cerebellar artery (PICA), the aneurysm will be found immediately in front of the olivary prominence of the medulla. Care must be taken to dissect all small cranial nerve rootlets from the aneurysm, as well as all small perforating branches arising from the PICA to the medulla. Aneurysms in this location generally can be clipped without much difficulty, especially when a temporary clip is placed on the VA prior to the application of the aneurysm clip. Large aneurysms and giant aneurysms of the PICA may require trapping of the VA to achieve satisfactory exclusion from the circulation. The midline approach is not ideal for large or giant aneurysms and is no longer in frequent use.

The lateral or retromastoid approach is the preferred approach for VA aneurysms.[6,7] The patient usually is placed in either the lateral or park bench position, although some prefer the prone position. A "hockey stick" incision is placed halfway between the mastoid process and the midline, from about 5 cm above the level of the mastoid to the level of C2–3. The paravertebral muscles are incised and retracted, exposing the lamina of C2 and C3, the dorsal arch of the atlas, the mastoid process, the suboccipital area, and the posterior edge of the foramen magnum. A craniectomy to the midline and through the foramen magnum is completed to expose the sigmoid and transverse sinuses. It is not always necessary to remove the arch of C1 although this may improve the angle of view below the cerebellar tonsil. The VA is identified extracranially as it courses over the arch of C1 and penetrates the atlanto-occipital membrane. A large vein generally located in that area should be cauterized carefully before the VA can be exposed totally. The dura is opened in a cruciate manner, basing the superior and lateral flaps on the transverse and sigmoid sinuses.

The cisterna magna is incised to allow drainage of CSF, and gentle retraction is applied on the lateral portion of the cerebellar tonsil. In large or giant aneurysms it may be necessary to resect a portion of the cerebellum to prevent postoperative swelling from excessive retraction. The VA is dissected in its intradural portion and followed to the origin of the PICA. The retraction of the cerebellum is generally less through the lateral exposure, and control of the proximal VA is also better. A temporary clip may be applied more easily through this exposure. It is not always possible to reach the distal portion of the VA in the case of a large or giant aneurysm of the PICA. In those cases, Drake[4] recommends the permanent ligation of the VA proximal to the aneurysm. If the VA to be ligated is the dominant vessel, a vessel loop is placed about it and exteriorized so that the VA may be occluded when the patient is awake.[3,4] The same maneuver can currently be performed extraoperatively using endovascular balloons. If there is good contralateral or small VA, it may be occluded directly with a permanent clip. Some aneurysms arising from the vertebrobasilar junction may be reached via this approach. The dissection has to be extended to separate all rootlets of the cranial nerves from nerves VII-XII allowing gentle retraction of the brain stem away from the clivus. Access to the clivus area is difficult through this exposure, and successful obliteration of distal vertebral aneurysms is variable because of the limited space available for aneurysm dissection and clip application.

## *Transbasal Approaches*

The approach of the midbasilar region is the most difficult and most taxing for satisfactory and safe obliteration of aneurysms in this area. Sano[14] described the transoral approach, but Drake[4] discouraged its use because of the potential for infection and the development of CSF leaks. More recently, with increasing interest in access to the posterior fossa via a transmastoid translabyrinthine approach, Giannotta[5] described the transmastoid presigmoid approach to the vertebrobasilar junction. As a result of more aggressive approaches to skull base tumors, it is possible to approach aneurysms of the vertebrobasilar junction through a combined transmastoid supra- and infratentorial approach, which may be more appropriately called the asterional approach.

### *Transclival Approach*

The patient is positioned supine and the head is supported with skeletal fixation. The oropharyngeal area is approached through a Dingman retractor, allowing the mouth to open widely and the tongue to be displaced inferiorly. An oral endotracheal tube is required in these cases, although some prefer to perform a tracheostomy prior to beginning the case. The soft palate may be reflected into the nasopharynx through a suture placed in the uvula and anchored to a red Robinson catheter passed down from one of the nostrils. In cases where the reflection of the soft palate is insufficient to expose the area of the clivus, the soft palate is incised starting lateral to the uvula and extending the incision to the midline until the hard palate is reached. The flaps of soft palate are then reflected laterally and sutured to the tonsillar pillars.

The posterior pharyngeal wall is incised in the midline from the most superior portion of the clivus to and through the anterior rim of the foramen magnum. It is not necessary to extend the incision below the level of the body of C2. The pharyngeal mucosa is reflected from the midline and sutured to the lateral pharyngeal walls. A Crockard retractor may be used to reflect the pharyngeal flaps also. The attachment of the longus coli muscles and the attachments of the cruciate ligament are released from the anterior surface of the clivus, and the clivus is drilled off with a high-speed drill. In most cases it is possible to reach the inferior two thirds of the clivus through this approach. When this is not possible, it is necessary to access the superior portion of the clivus through a combined transnasal and transoral approach, creating a LaForte One disarticulation of the maxilla.[1] A wider and more radical exposure may be obtained by performing a rhinotomy, displacing the nasal pyramid laterally on a vascularized pedicle, performing a maxillotomy, and freeing the entire anterior surface of the clivus from the sphenoid sinus to the arch of C1.

Drilling the clivus down allows a field of exposure that is limited to approximately 3.5 cm in vertical length, and 1 cm in cross-sectional diameter. The dural surface is opened in the midline, and the vertebrobasilar junction and proximal BA are generally midfield. Unfortunately, the aneurysms are also in the middle of the field, and clip application is difficult. The wound is closed in layers. To repair the dural surface, it is necessary to use a fat or fascial graft, fastened with a few sutures and secured to the dural wall with fibrin glue. A spinal CSF drain is necessary for at least 10 days to prevent the development of a CSF leak.

### *Transmastoid Presigmoid Approach*

The transmastoid approach is performed through a mastoidectomy incision placed directly over the mastoid with enough room to expose the entire sigmoid sinus, the most lateral portion of the posterior fossa just below the tentorium. The mastoid is drilled off by an otolaryngologist who can carefully identify and preserve the intrapetrous portion of the facial nerve and the semicircular canals. Once the dura has been exposed, the mastoidectomy resection is extended to include the most lateral portion of the occipital bone. This permits the exposure of the sigmoid sinus in the middle of the wound through a bony exposure of approximately 4 cm in diameter. The dura in front of the sigmoid sinus is incised, and the anterolateral surface of the pons is exposed. When this exposure is not sufficient, the sigmoid sinus is ligated and transected. In order to do this, it is necessary to have planned the operation on the side of the nondominant sigmoid sinus, confirmed by preoperative cerebral angiography with a prolonged venous phase. Once the sinus is transected, the anterior surface of the pons can be exposed with a small retractor placed on the pons. The BA and vertebrobasilar junction can be accessed through this method, although the room available for exposure and dissection of the BA and the aneurysm is limited. Proximal control of the BA is not always possible through this exposure.[5]

### *Asterional Approach*

The retromastoid presigmoid or "asterional approach" is performed through a hockey stick incision placed directly over the mastoid region, extending about 5 cm above the mastoid and to the level of C1. The periosteum is reflected off the mastoid, and the insertion of the sternocleidomastoid muscle is separated in its majority from the mastoid groove. The dissection is extended until the digastric groove is identified. A free bone flap is reflected, centered on the asterion, and straddling the transverse and sigmoid sinuses (Figure 6A). To complete the evaluation of the bone flap it is necessary to place burr holes on either side of the transverse sinus anteriorly and posteriorly, and to connect these holes with a power saw. The resection of the mastoid is then extended to approximately 5 mm posterior to the external or membranous ear canal. The resection is continued to the level of the dura until the entire sigmoid sinus is exposed from the level of the superior petrosal sinus to the jugular bulb. A large mastoid emissary vein is frequently found as the dissection progresses and must be cauterized and transected to permit access to the entire course of the sigmoid sinus.

The dura is sutured to the bone and opened in front of the sigmoid sinus, first above and then below the tentorium. The

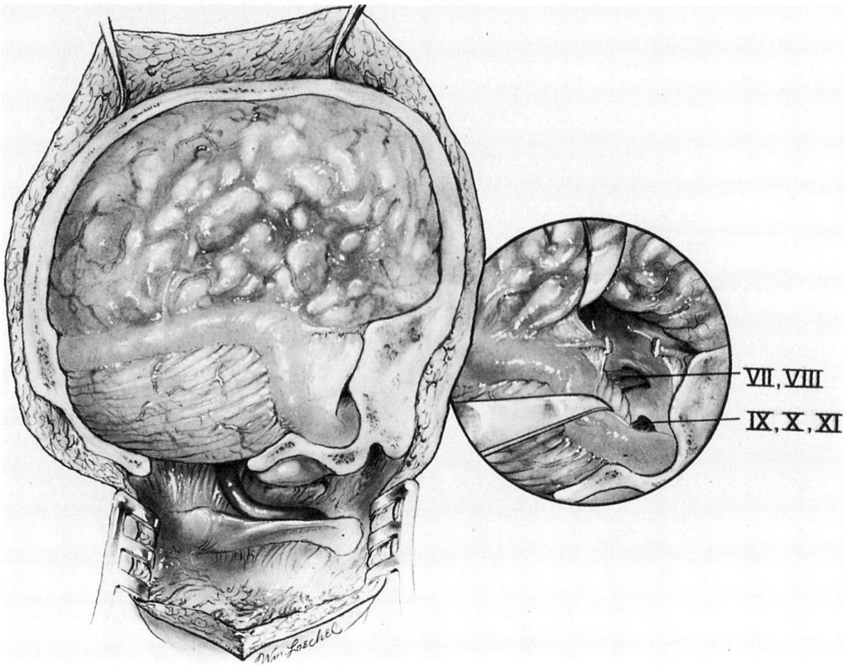


*Figure 6A. Asterional approach to the vertebral and basilar artery. With the patient on the lateral decubitus position, the posterior temporal area, mastoid region, and suboccipital area are approached through a hockey stick incision. The area above and below the transverse sinus, and the dura anterior to the sigmoid sinus are dissected to expose the superior petrosal sinus.*

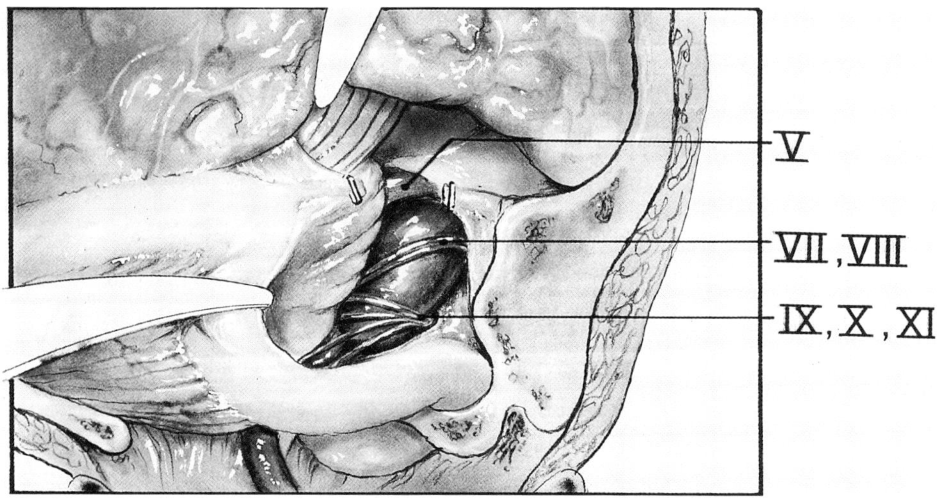


*Figure 6B. The dura above and below the transverse sinus is incised. The superior petrosal sinus and tentorium are transected, exposing the VA from the jugular foramen, the vertebrobasilar junction, and the entire BA from its origin to the SCA. All cranial nerves from trigeminal (V) to hypoglossal (XII) are exposed and easily preserved through this approach.*

incision above the tent is placed anterior to the vein of Labbé. The superior petrosal sinus is dissected, ligated between two sutures, and transected. The infratentorial incision is then extended to the level of the jugular bulb. The tentorium is incised completely until the trochlear nerve can be seen in the ambient cistern. This exposure allows gentle retraction of the temporal lobe superiorly and the belly of the pons posteriorly (Figure 6B). The nerve fascicles of the trigeminal, facial, and vestibulocochlear (VIII) nerves are gently dissected and separated. The most inferior margin of the exposure is the foramen jugulare, superiorly the temporal lobe, anteriorly the dorsum of the petrous apex and clivus, and posteriorly the belly of the pons and medulla.

The distal VA may be followed into the vertebrobasilar junction, and the BA can be seen clearly to just below the origin of the SCAs. Proximal control of both VAs and distal BA may be obtained through this approach. Small and large aneurysms of the midbasilar portion may be accessed this way, without sacrificing a major venous sinus. Gentle retraction may be applied on the pons without problems, and the cranial nerves traversing the area do not interfere with the placement of temporary or permanent clips. Potential problems from this approach consist mostly in the possible damage to the facial nerve in its intrapetrous portion, or damage to the semicircular canals or the cochlea, resulting in permanent hearing loss.

## Clinical Material and Results

Forty-five patients presenting with vertebrobasilar aneurysms have been evaluated by the authors since 1979. There were 33 women and 12 men of ages ranging from 23–67 years. Mode of presentation included SAH (24), incidental angiographic finding (15), and CT finding (6). Hunt-Hess grades following SAH were: I (17), II (5), and III (3). All patients were angiogrammed immediately post-SAH. Location of aneurysms were: basilar tip (27) (Figure 7); basilar trunk (7) (Figure 8); PICA (8); superior cerebellar (2); and posterior cerebral (1). CT scan findings were: SAH (24); possible aneurysm (6); and mass

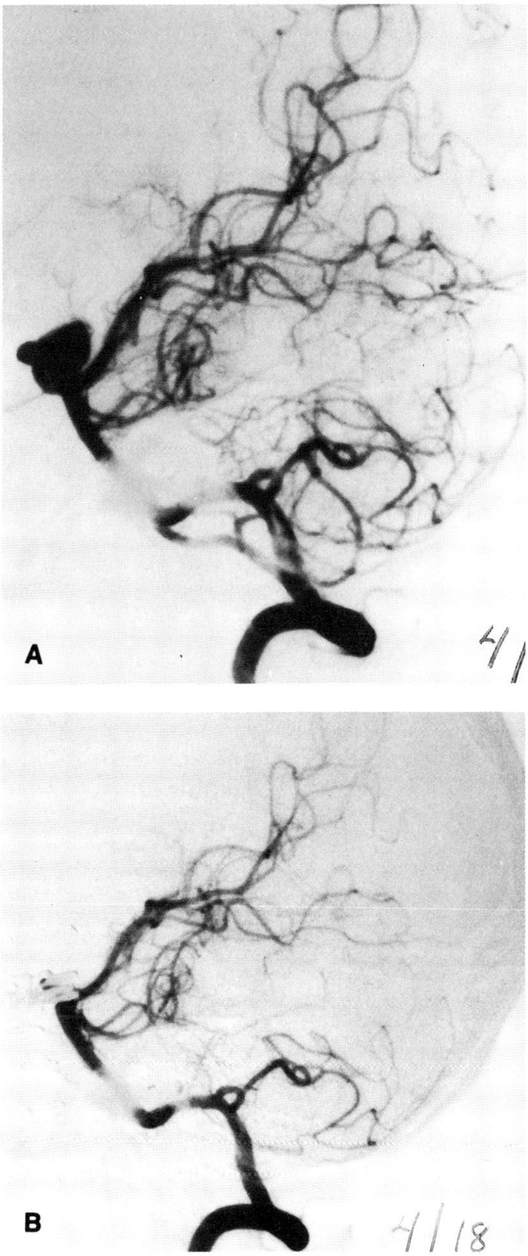


***Figure** 7. 54-year-old Caucasian woman 3 days post hemorrhage. Neurologically intact except for a headache and nuchal rigidity. **(A)** Preoperative angiogram revealed a medium-sized aneurysm arising at the basilar bifurcation, projecting directly superiorly. **(B)** Postoperative angiogram demonstrates the aneurysm to be clipped, but the main perforating artery is missing. The patient developed a severe midbrain infarction immediately postoperatively from which she never recovered. Extreme care must be exercised to identify and separate all perforating arteries.*

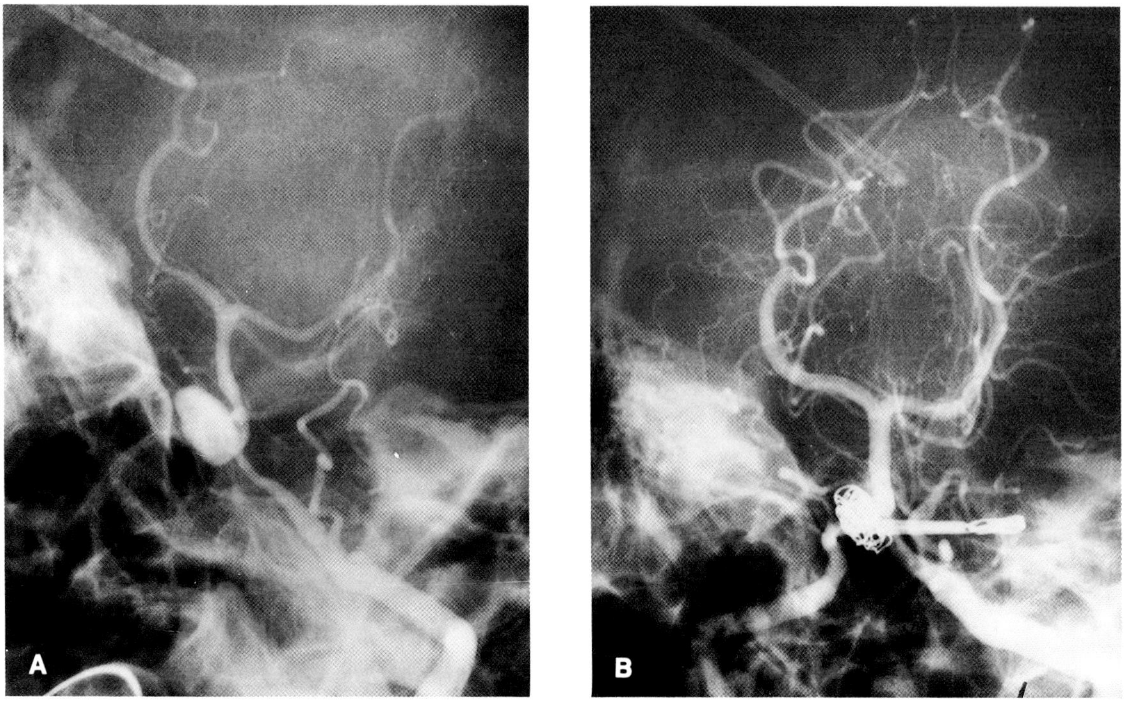


*Figure 8.* *A 52-year-old white woman 5 days posthemorrhage. Moderately obtunded, followed commands and responded to painful stimuli in a purposeful manner. Ventriculostomy placed for moderate hydrocephalus. (A) Preoperative angiogram revealed a vertebrobasilar junction aneurysm of moderate size. (B) Postoperative angiogram showing complete obliteration of the aneurysm obtained by the initial placement of intravascular coils allowing the patient to return to a more normal neurologic state, followed by direct clipping via the asterional approach. The patient regained normal neurologic function.*

effect (4). All patients were maintained in the ICU until their symptoms subsided and operated on generally 2–6 weeks posthemorrhage. One patient rebled and died during the observation period. Complications included: hemiparesis (3) (basilar tip); permanent cranial nerve palsy (3) (trunk, 2; PICA, 1); and mortality (3) (trunk). All other patients have returned to normal or to their preoperative neurologic condition.

## Conclusion

Surgery for aneurysms of the vertebrobasilar system remains the most difficult and challenging aspect of vascular neurosurgery. The high risk of injury to the brain stem and cranial nerves makes any approach fraught with danger. Basilar tip aneurysms are probably best handled through a one-and-a-half approach, a modified pterional trans-sylvian approach to include the anterior and midtemporal areas. Vertebral and PICA aneurysms can be handled satisfactorily through a retromastoid suboccipital approach in cases where the aneurysm is not of giant dimensions. Giant PICA aneurysms, as well as those of the vertebrobasilar junction and trunk of the BA, are best approached through an asterional approach. However, small aneurysms in these areas may also be handled through a transmastoid presigmoid approach. The advent of interventional techniques with intraaneurysmal platinum coils will probably change the surgical approaches now considered to be satisfactory.

## References

1. Archer JD, Young S, Uttley D. Basilar aneurysms: a new transclival approach via maxillotomy. *J Neurosurg.* 1987;67:54–58.

2. Ausman JI, Diaz FG, Mullan S, et al. Posterior inferior to posterior inferior cerebellar artery anastomosis combined with trapping for vertebral artery aneurysm: case report. *J Neurosurg.* 1990;73:462–465.
3. Drake CG. Further experience with surgical treatment of aneurysms of the basilar artery. *J Neurosurg.* 1968;29:372–392.
4. Drake CG. Ligation of the vertebral (unilateral or bilateral) or basilar artery in the treatment of large intracranial aneurysms. *J Neurosurg.* 1975;43:255–274.
5. Giannotta SL, Maceri DR. Retrolabyrinthine transsigmoid approach to basilar trunk and vertebrobasilar artery junction aneurysms: technical note. *J Neurosurg.* 1988;69:461–466.
6. Heros RC. Lateral suboccipital approach for vertebral and vertebrobasilar artery lesions. *J Neurosurg.* 1986;64:559–562.
7. Hudgins RJ, Day AL, Quisling RG, et al. Aneurysms of the posterior inferior cerebellar artery: a clinical and anatomical analysis. *J Neurosurg.* 1983;58:381–387.
8. Kawase T, Toya S, Shiobara R, et al. Transpetrosal approach for aneurysms of the lower basilar artery. *J Neurosurg.* 1985;63:857–861.
9. Kobayashi S, Sugita K, Nakagawa F. An approach to a basilar aneurysm above the bifurcation of the internal carotid artery: case report. *J Neurosurg.* 1983; 59:1082–1084.
10. Kossowsky R, Dujovny M, Kossovsky N, et al. Failure of a Heifetz aneurysm clip. *J Neurosurg.* 1982; 57:233–239.
11. Maroon JC, Kennerdell JS. Surgical approaches to the orbit: indications and techniques. *J Neurosurg.* 1984;60:1226–1235.
12. Peerles SJ. Drake CG. Posterior circulation aneurysms. In: Wilkins RH, Rengachary SS, eds. *Neurosurgery.* New York, NY: McGraw Hill; 1985; 2:1167–1917.
13. Sano K, Asano T, Tamura A. *Acute Aneurysm Surgery.* New York, NY: Springer Verlag; 1987:223–247.
14. Sano K, Jimbo M, Saito I. Vertebro-basilar aneurysms with special reference to the transpharyngeal-transclival approach to the basilar artery aneurysm [in Japanese]. *Noto Shinkei.* 1966;18:1197–1203. English abstract.
15. Spetzler RF, Hadley MN, Rigamonti D, et al. Aneurysms of the basilar artery treated with circulatory arrest, hypothermia, and barbiturate cerebral protection. *J Neurosurg.* 1988;68:868–879.
16. Sugita K, Kobayashi S, Shintani A, et al. Microneurosurgery for aneurysms of the basilar artery. *J Neurosurg.* 1979;51:615–620.
17. Sugita K, Kobayashi S, Takemae T, et al. Aneurysms of the basilar artery trunk. *J Neurosurg.* 1987; 66:500–505.
18. Sugita K, Kobayashi S, Takemae T, et al. Giant aneurysms of the vertebral artery: report of five cases. *J Neurosurg.* 1988;68:960–966.
19. Sundt TM Jr. *Surgical Techniques for Saccular and Giant Intracranial Aneurysms.* Baltimore, Md: Williams & Wilkins, 1990.
20. Sundt TM Jr, Piepgras DG, Houser OW, et al. Interposition saphenous vein grafts for advanced occlusive disease and large aneurysms in the posterior circulation. *J Neurosurg.* 1982;56:205–215.
21. Suzuki J. *Cerebral Aneurysms: Experience with 100 Directly Operated Cases.* Tokyo: Neuron Publishing Co; 1979.
22. Varkey GP, Thompson WR. Anesthetic considerations in the surgical repair of intracranial aneurysms. *Int Anesthesiol Clin.* Summer, 1982;20:159–170.
23. Yasargil MG, Antic J, Laciga R, et al. Microsurgical pterional approach to aneurysms of the basilar bifurcation. *Surg Neurol.* 1976;6:83–91.

# CHAPTER 9

# Giant Cerebral Aneurysms

H. Hunt Batjer, MD, Thomas A. Kopitnik, MD, Phillip D. Pardy, MD, Duke S. Samson, MD, and Dan M. Meyer, MD, PhD

Giant cerebral aneurysms comprise a complex and heterogenous group of cerebrovascular disorders with a myriad of unusual presenting complaints and multiple types of structural lesions. It is likely that giant aneurysms represent the final anatomic result of many inborn and acquired vascular defects. Giant aneurysms may evolve from the simple growth of small aneurysms or from repetitive arterial dissections and intramural hemorrhages. Arbitrarily, this classification of aneurysms includes lesions greater than 25 mm in diameter; as such, it encompasses a number of unusual and morbid ectasias of various arteries.

Since their recognition, giant aneurysms have challenged the ingenuity and talents of neurologists, neurosurgeons, neuroanesthesiologists, and neuroradiologists. Contemporary management of patients with giant aneurysms incorporates each of these disciplines to confront the various potential complications occurring spontaneously and developing following definitive structural therapy. While the problems associated with eliminating small intracranial aneurysms from the circulation have largely been solved by the developments of microsurgery, unique aspects of giant aneurysms defy universal solution.

Pertinent challenges include the incorporation of efferent vessels and perforators into the aneurysmal sac, thrombosis within the lumen, wall calcification, and the achievement of adequate softening to allow successful vascular reconstruction. In many, if not most circumstances, temporary interruption of the involved circulation is required to achieve definitive aneurysm obliteration. This adds iatrogenic cerebral ischemia to the list of potential complications and led to the use of brain protective strategies including rheological agents, pharmacologic metabolic suppression, hypothermia, and profound cooling with systemic circulatory arrest.

In this chapter, we relate our current management strategies to specific anatomic sites involved and advocate a multidisciplinary "team" approach to the formulation and execution of an optimal therapeutic plan for each unique patient.

## Natural History

Clear documentation exists proving that small aneurysms can enlarge to giant size and giant lesions relentlessly progress. Arguments have been proposed suggesting that this growth occurs in a fashion analogous to the enlargement of chronic subdural or chronic parenchymal hematomas.[36] This idea is supported by the presence of highly vascularized membranous walls often found in giant aneurysms. Recurrent hemorrhage into this wall could explain progressive growth. Neuroradiologic evidence of continued growth is dependent on computed tomography (CT) and magnetic resonance (MR) followup because the angiographically patent sac may remain-relatively stable despite dramatic growth of the thrombotic mass.[1]

Massive intraluminal thrombosis may in fact represent the majority or the totality of the lesion volume,[53] a phenomenon initially described by Lyell.[29] Whether this thrombosis results from stasis within the sac or from repeated intramural hemorrhage is not known, but it is quite clear that giant aneurysms represent an unstable and dynamic pathophysiological situation. We observed the progressive enlargement of a completely thrombotic giant distal basilar aneurysm that ultimately occluded a posterior cerebral artery (PCA) and led to death.[5]

Patients harboring giant intracranial aneurysms may present with ischemic neurologic symptoms. In some instances static flow and thrombosis may result in distal embolization, but narrowing and compression of afferent and efferent vessels has also been described.[30] Seizures may be focal or generalized and likely result from cortical compression or hemosiderin deposition from prior hemorrhage.[51] While symptoms of generalized raised intracranial pressure may be seen late in the disease process, acute hydrocephalus due to obstruction of the foramina of Monro, third ventricle, aqueduct, or fourth ventricle may initiate medical consultation.[5,10]

Early observers felt that hemorrhage was rare from giant aneurysms and that symptoms of mass effect or ischemia were the chief risk to the patient. Most large series refute this view, and it is clear that about one-third of all diagnosed giant aneurysms present with acute subarachnoid hemorrhage (SAH).[16,52] Our experience is very consistent with this relative incidence. Many cases without documented prior SAH are found to have diffuse hemosiderin in the subarachnoid space, raising the possibility that the actual aneurysm growth may have related to repetitive subclinical bleeding. It is our distinct impression that the outlook for the patient with a newly diagnosed giant aneurysm is poor, with tendency for relentless progression not rarely halted by acute SAH.

## General Treatment Strategies

### *Medical*

Hypotensive therapy following SAH was commonly employed prior to the microsurgical era. Technical improvements and the threat of delayed ischemia relegated this regimen into historical context. Nevertheless, in 1982 two patients with giant aneurysms were treated with chronically induced hypotension.[43] One patient was 73 years old and presented with visual failure. She was found to have a giant supraclinoid aneurysm; after treatment with hydrochlorothiazide her headache symptoms improved and she suffered no further visual loss. She died less than 1 year later, and no autopsy was performed. A second patient was similarly treated for painful cranial neuropathy from a giant cavernous aneurysm. Her pain dramatically resolved with hypotensive therapy; she had been followed for 4 years at the time of publication and was working as a nurse.[43]

While we do not advocate primary medical therapy for the young patient with an operable aneurysm, this use of hypotension may have some role in symptomatic patients who for some reason are not candidates for invasive therapy or who refuse surgery.

### *Endovascular Therapy*

The 1980s witnessed explosive growth in intravascular technology which forever changed cerebrovascular surgery. Beginning with Serbinenko's report of balloon catheterization and occlusion of major arteries, the stage was set for the development of completely new concepts of care of the giant aneurysm patient.[40] Reports soon followed detailing the use of balloon technology for Hunterian treatment as well as sac occlusion of giant aneurysms.[9,12,13,17,18,22,24,37] More recently, platinum microcoils emerged as an elegant and potentially safer intravascular device for producing clot within aneurysms.[23]

Perhaps the most important contribution of this technology to date is the treatment of giant cavernous aneurysms. Our initial attempts at selective cavernous giant aneurysm occlusion with carotid preservation had less than optimal results, including a few disasters with distal embolization of balloons and one case of fatal SAH due to a ball-valve effect.

More recent experience showed that balloon technology allows trial awake internal carotid occlusion with neurologic and hemodynamic monitoring; if evidence of clinical or regional cerebral blood flow (rCBF) changes develops, the balloon can be immediately deflated. To our surprise 80% to 85% of patients tolerate the abrupt sacrifice of an internal carotid using this protocol. We were also impressed with the clinical response to proximal balloon occlusion in terms of pain relief and cranial nerve recovery. This protocol has also proved valuable in our unit in the treatment of some cases of vertebrobasilar aneurysms, yielding immediate improvement in brain stem compressive symptoms.

The selective occlusion of giant and smaller aneurysms has also been performed with detachable balloons, with some spectacular results and not insignificant complications. In addition to some perioperative morbidity and mortality, incomplete occlusion of the sac led to rerupture and growth of aneurysms over following months. A major question remains regarding whether secure re-endothelialization will occur permitting long-term protection from regrowth.

Reports of selective aneurysm occlusion using microcoils look extremely favorable, although long-term followup is not yet available.[23] It is clear that in certain extremely morbid giant aneurysms, especially those with intraluminal thrombosis, microcoils offer a lower initial therapeutic risk than an open procedure. Whether simply occluding the patent portion of a thrombotic sac will offer long-term benefit from compressive symptoms or protection from enlargement remains to be proven. We saw a patient progressively decline and die from relentless enlargement of a completely thrombosed giant distal basilar artery aneurysm.[5]

With the reservations expressed above, we believe that major contributions to the care of the giant aneurysm patient will emerge from the new intravascular technology. A particular role for selective aneurysm occlusion in the Grade IV or V patient is seen to offer protection in the early post-SAH period from rebleeding and to permit agressive hyperdynamic therapy should ischemic consequences develop. Even if the occlusion is temporary, this early protection could allow neurologic recovery to occur if the initial injury was not too severe.

Additionally, the recurrent difficult giant aneurysm has carried significant morbidity, particularly in the posterior circulation.[6] Microcoils are particularly attractive in this setting, especially in the elderly patient. A very significant role is seen for selective intravascular occlusion in those patients with serious comorbid factors complicating SAH, such as cardiac or pulmonary disease that would preclude general anesthesia.

## *Proximal Ligation*

In 1784, Hunter ligated a popliteal artery for treatment of a peripheral aneurysm,[16] and the principle was established of decreasing the pressure in an aneurysmal sac indirectly by occluding the afferent blood supply. The first intracranial application of this principle was performed by Sir Victor Horsley in 1885 when a middle fossa mass proved to be a giant aneurysm.[27] Internal carotid ligation stopped the hemorrhage and the patient made a good recovery.[15]

Ligation of the common or internal carotid artery became routine in subsequent years, although hemispheric ischemia often developed and commonly caused death or disability. The development of reversible closing clamps was a major breakthrough that allowed immediate access for reperfusion if ischemic symptoms occurred. Embolic complications still developed, however, and led Drake to recommend anticoagulation during this period.[16] This modality finds persistent usage today. For patients with marginal distal tissue perfusion, subtle degrees of clamp closure can be made more exquisitely precise with the use of transcranial Doppler scan.[19]

Application of Hunterian ligation to giant aneurysms was developed by Drake.[16] Lesions with massive distortion of the brain stem could be treated safely and effectively with vertebral ligation. While basilar artery clip ligation was used for distal basilar giant aneurysm, ischemic complications led to the development of the Drake tourniquet.[16] This device could be placed around the basilar artery during an open surgical procedure and the vessel occluded the following day under neurologic surveillance.

Endovascular technology has taken the Hunterian principle to even greater heights with the ability to occlude virtually any extracranial or intracranial vessel reversibly with the patient awake. We use this technique for the management of giant cavernous carotid aneurysms. The vessel is occluded for 30 minutes and neurologic status is carefully monitored. Dual isotope rCBF studies are performed with single photon emission computed tomography (SPECT) before and during carotid occlusion. Patients developing rCBF abnormalities despite preserved neurologic status have proven in our hands to be at risk for the development of cerebral infarction over ensuing days. We now routinely resort to prophylactic revascularization procedures or graded occlusion to minimize risk. Trial occlusion of the vertebral arteries has also proven useful, but trial balloon occlusion of the basilar artery is rarely tolerated due to the occlusion of perforating arteries by the balloon itself in the dead segment.

### *Trapping*

The Hunterian principle of proximal ligation can be expanded to include ligation of the efferent vessel(s). This procedure offers the potential advantage of preventing regrowth or rerupture of a giant aneurysm by reperfusion from collateral sources. While not common, this complication has been well described. In addition, complete isolation of the involved arterial segment allows opening and evacuation of the contents of the aneurysm and decompression of neural and vascular tissues. This principle is used in our unit for those giant carotid cavernous aneurysms with severe visual compromise or for giant vertebral or PICA aneurysms with severe brain stem dysfunction.

### *Definitive Clipping*

Definitive neck clipping represents the gold-standard of aneurysm treatment, eliminating flow into the sac while preserving antegrade flow into all efferent vessels. Due to the pathophysiology of giant aneurysm development, this procedure usually requires temporary interruption of the local circulation. Complicating the picture is the common occurrence of thick, calcific necks which may be complicated by thrombus, as well as the expansion of the origin of efferent vessels out onto the fundus. While newly designed clips with tremendous closing strength have definitely proven advantageous,[49] in many instances it is necessary to either crush the neck with a forcep[16] or temporarily trap the aneurysm and open it widely to evacuate the contents prior to clip reconstruction of the parent vessel.[2,25,39]

In many skull-based lesions, particularly those cavernous in origin, this type of procedure would not be feasible and direct bypass procedures with interposition grafts have been proposed.[45] Direct end-to-end anastomosis has also been possible after excision of certain intracranial giant aneurysms.[44] This variant of direct clipping permits preservation of antegrade flow as well as aneurysm decompression.

## Ischemic Brain Protection

Due to the frequent occurrence of mural calcification and thrombosis and to the frequently dramatic expansion of the base of giant aneurysms, routine permanent aneurysm clips will usually not purchase on the precise neck and have insufficient closing force to obliterate flow into the sac. Following the work of Pool,[34] investigators quickly recognized the advantage of temporarily arresting local circulation to soften the sac and even to open and evacuate the sac. While the availability of extremely strong clips[47,49] improved our ability to deal directly with these sacs, our practice evolved into a routine use of temporary clipping. The now universal availability of safe temporary clips which only rarely produce damage to intracranial vessels has created widespread acceptance of this technique.[26]

The ischemia introduced by temporary occlusion is reversible early on, but can result in cerebral infarction if prolonged. Two major clinical problems are that (1) we do not know precisely the actual safe limits for temporary occlusion, and (2) it is difficult to predict precisely the duration of temporary clipping in planning the individual case. While all intracranial vessels can be safely occluded for very brief periods, a number of strategies have been developed to prolong this safe interval. The barbiturates have been shown to protect the brain in various animal models of ischemia, but with associated cardiotoxicity that can jeopardize blood pressure and collateral circulation at clinical dosage levels.[20,31]

Several years ago, we elected to try etomidate (Abbott Laboratories, North Chicago, Illinois), due to its known cerebral metabolic depressant effects with minimal cardiotoxicity.[3] Like barbiturates, etomidate appears to decrease cerebral metabolic activity by decreasing neuronal activity. This activity, and its absence, may be monitored clinically by electroencephalography (EEG). Laboratory experience has shown that etomidate decreases the cerebral metabolic rate of oxygen ($CMRO_2$) until isoelectricity is reached. Once this level of neuronal depression is achieved, however, the $CMRO_2$ remains stable at 48% of control despite further drug administration.[32,33]

Our protocol evolved into the routine use of this agent at a dosage of 1mg/Kg initially, followed by 10$\mu$g/Kg/min as necessary to maintain burst suppression with EEG monitoring. Systemic conditions of normovolemia, normothermia, normotension, and normoglycemia were maintained throughout the period of elective temporary arterial occlusion. We recently evaluated this protocol to determine the ischemic tolerance as seen in our unit. Over a 2-year period, 121 patients were treated with temporary arterial occlusion. Twenty-one were excluded from analysis due to confounding factors such as emergent temporary occlusion, efferent vessel loss, or the use of a revascularization procedure. The remaining 100 patients were studied as regards age, grade, history of SAH, presence of vasospasm, and size of aneurysm. Technical parameters studied included duration and nature of temporary occlusion, total number of episodes, and specific vascular territory involved.

Several parameters were found to be related to postoperative evidence (clinical and radiographic) of infarction. Patients more than 61 years of age and those in poor neurologic condition had a higher incidence of ischemic complications than did those in better condition. The 95% confidence level for the tolerance of occlusion in patients in Grades I-II was 19 minutes; in Grades III-IV patients, it was 15 minutes. All patients occluded for longer than 31 minutes had both radiographic and neurologic evidence of cerebral infarction. Patients occluded less than 14 minutes routinely tolerated the procedure. In patients occluded for longer that 14 minutes, a trend was demonstrated suggesting a relationship between incomplete trapping and the development of ischemic injury. Trends were also noted suggesting (1) a unique sensitivity to ischemia of the tissue supplied by lenticulostriate and thalamoperforating vessels, and (2) an increasing number of episodes of temporary occlusion may predispose to ischemic injury.

While this study involves a heterogenous group of patients, there is clear demonstration in our setting that the safe limits of temporary occlusion appear to be between 15 and 20 minutes. The frequent need for excessive occlusion times in our referral practice led us to pursue new strategies to prolong tolerance. Experimental data clearly show that hypothermia decreases cerebral metabolism profoundly and does so by a mechanism somewhat different from pharmacologic suppression. Cellular homeostatic mechanisms are impaired by hypothermia, which also has some impact on neuronal activity, whereas the action of commonly used drugs is solely on neuronal activity. This variance in mechanism of action led us to hope that synergism might be possible between etomidate and hypothermia. While mild hypothermia is well tolerated clinically, profound hypothermia requires cardiopulmonary bypass.

The use of deep hypothermia (16° C) and complete circulatory arrest for the treatment of giant cerebral aneurysms has been known for some time.[8,41,42] Early attempts at this technique were often accompanied by exquisite neurovascular reconstruction, only to be complicated by hemorrhagic problems postoperatively. Improvements in cannulation techniques and overall systemic safety precipitated a resurgence of interest in circulatory arrest.[46] Recent work suggests that, in addition to a bloodless field and empty intracranial circulation which often makes the clipping of formidable lesions quite straightforward, the addition of hypothermia to 16° C to the regimen permits circulatory arrest intervals of at least 50 minutes with full neurologic recovery. Even massive and thrombotic giant aneurysms can be evacuated and reconstructed within this time.

It is now our practice that, when the operating surgeon predicts the need for temporary occlusion times between 15 and 20 minutes, mild hypothermia (32° to 33° C) is added to our pharmacologic regimen. This anesthetic addition has not significantly prolonged the operative procedure, although some patients seem to develop a mild coagulopathy that precludes wound closure until normothermia is re-established. When occlusion times of longer than 20 minutes are anticipated, we recommend consideration of global circulatory arrest. While we are still early in our experience with this technique, encouraging results are being seen.

## Specific Anatomic Sites

The preceding discussion addressed some of the conceptual problems associated with giant cerebral aneurysms. The remaining sections of the chapter deal with specific types and locations of aneurysms.

### *Cavernous Carotid Giant Aneurysms*

This group of interesting aneurysms has been the target of renewed interest by innovative skull base surgeons and endovascular therapists. Patients typically present with cranial neuropathy resulting in diplopia, although retro-orbital pain may be a prominent feature. Occasionally patients present with distal ischemic symptoms from thromboembolism or rupture with direct carotid-cavernous fistula. Only extremely rarely does SAH develop through the attenuated roof of the cavernous sinus.

Direct surgical procedures pioneered by Dolenc[14] and others clearly showed that direct exposure and treatment of these lesions is possible, with the chief advantage of maintaining carotid patency in most cases. This achievement is not without cost, however, as Dolenc noted 2 deaths in a series of 7 patients.[14] The surgical procedures were also lengthy, ranging from 3 to 10 hours in duration.[14] We believe that recent literature very much underestimates the frequency of postoperative serious and permanent cranial neuropathy. The catastrophic impact of complete ophthalmoplegia should be kept in mind when recommending a procedure of this type to a patient with subtle symptoms such as a partial sixth nerve palsy.

Detachable balloons appear to offer substantial potential to nonsurgically occlude these aneurysms and preserve carotid patency. Our experience has been less favorable than we had hoped, with distal embolism occurring occasionally and 1 case of fatal SAH 36 hours following the procedure due to an apparent ball-valve effect. New progress with microcoils does appear very promising, with the complete selective exclusion of the sac by filling it with coils. Perhaps in the future, a nonthrombogenic cavernous carotid sleeve placed endovascularly will solve the problem of aneurysms and fistulae in this region.

For the present, however, the safest alternative for patients with adequate collateral potential appears to be internal carotid occlusion. It is surprising that 80% to 85% of patients seem to tolerate abrupt carotid sacrifice. Despite the lack of surgical trapping and deflation, the majority of patients so treated note immediate pain relief and rapid (within weeks) return of function of cranial nerves.

Our regimen involves the performance of an awake trial balloon occlusion. The patient is monitored neurologically as well as hemodynamically (transcranial Doppler) and a dual isotope rCBF study is obtained with SPECT. If the patient remains well neurologically during the 30-minute trial, and the pre- and postocclusion rCBF study remains symmetric, the internal carotid is sacrificed near the skull base to minimize the risk of embolization from the dead segment as described by Heros.[21] Anticoagulation is then tapered within 24 hours. Trapping and decompression is done if visual failure is present from mass effect.

If the patient develops neurologic deficit and rCBF abnormalities during occlusion, a prophylactic revascularization procedure is performed. The patient is then returned to the radiology suite in 2 days for a repeat trial occlusion. If failure again occurs, graded internal carotid artery (ICA) or common carotid artery (CCA) occlusion is performed with the Selverstone clamp. If the patient tolerates occlusion clinically but develops rCBF abnormalities, our recent practice has been to perform a bypass procedure and sacrifice the internal carotid at the same sitting, either surgically or preferably endovascularly. This is a very important subgroup in our experience, as delayed ischemic complications have occurred over the following several days in patients with postocclusion rCBF asymmetry despite clinical tolerance.

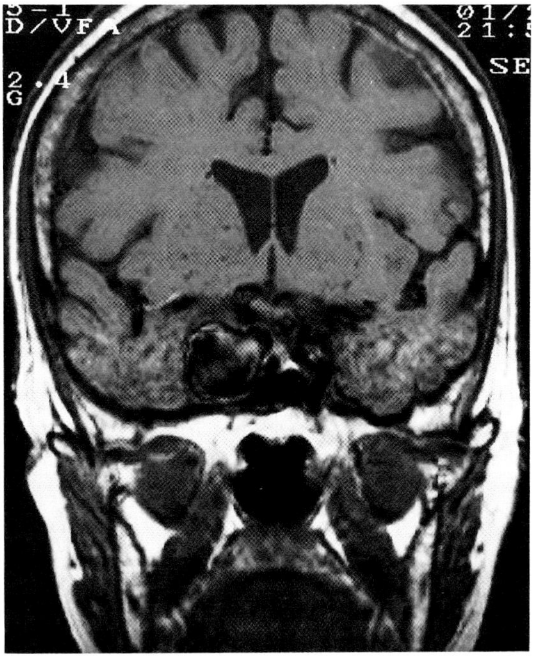

*Figure 1A. This is an elderly woman with a right incomplete abducens and oculomotor nerve palsy. MRI discloses large right cavernous mass.*

We are convinced that rCBF and transcranial Doppler monitoring result in this being an extremely safe protocol. The patient illustrated in Figure 1 demonstrates the utility of the technique. This patient presented with a partial right abducens (VI) and oculomotor (III) nerve palsy. By MRI and cerebral angiography, a right cavernous giant aneurysm was diagnosed (Figures 1A & 1B). She underwent awake trial occlusion which was well tolerated clinically. Her rCBF study, however, clearly showed decreased flow in the right sylvian territory (Figure 1C). She underwent a cortical anastomosis between the superficial temporal artery and a middle cerebral branch. The size of the donor was not large and questions were raised about the adequacy of a graft of this type. She was taken to the neuroradiology suite (still under anesthesia) with EEG monitoring. When the internal carotid was balloon-occluded the EEG remained symmetric, and an impressive flow augmentation was

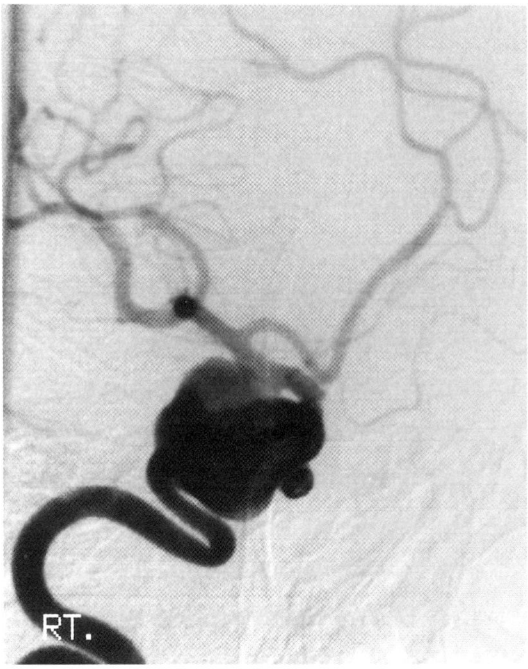


*Figure 1B. Angiography confirms giant aneurysm.*

noted through the bypass graft (Figure 1D), with retrograde perfusion noted to this middle cerebral artery (MCA) bifurcation. Her postoperative rCBF study was perfectly normal and she remained clinically well.

The impact of carotid sacrifice on surrounding vasculature must be carefully anticipated. Since cavernous aneurysms are frequently bilateral, the occlusion of a single carotid in a patient with prominent anterior cerebral collateral flow may result in accelerated enlargement of the contralateral lesion. Consideration should be given to occluding the anterior communicating artery in such a patient if robust collateral is available from the posterior communicating artery.

We lost a young girl who presented with a symptomatic cavernous giant aneurysm from a related hemodynamic error. She had an incidental fusiform basilar aneurysm. She was treated with prophylactic external carotid-internal carotid bypass and trapping of the cavernous segment because visual impairment was present. It was noted postoperatively that the posterior communicating artery was being recruited as a collateral to the impaired middle cerebral territory. She suffered a fatal SAH 1 week later from dramatically enlarged basilar aneurysm.[4]

## *Supraclinoid Giant Carotid Aneurysms*

Giant aneurysms of the intradural carotid artery commonly produce unilateral or

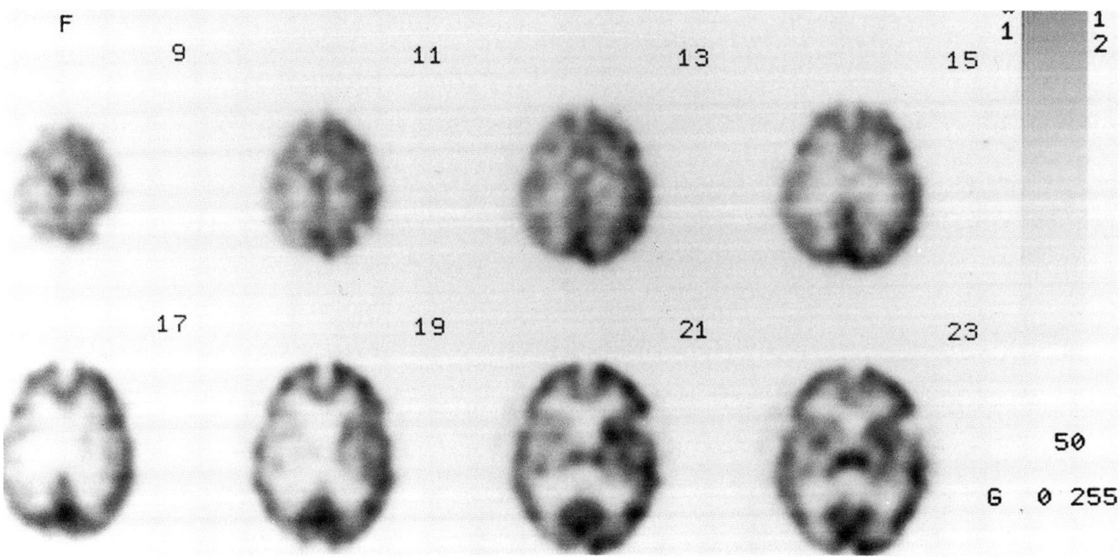


*Figure 1C. SPECT rCBF study done with balloon occlusion of right internal carotid clearly shows decreased flow in right MCA territory.*

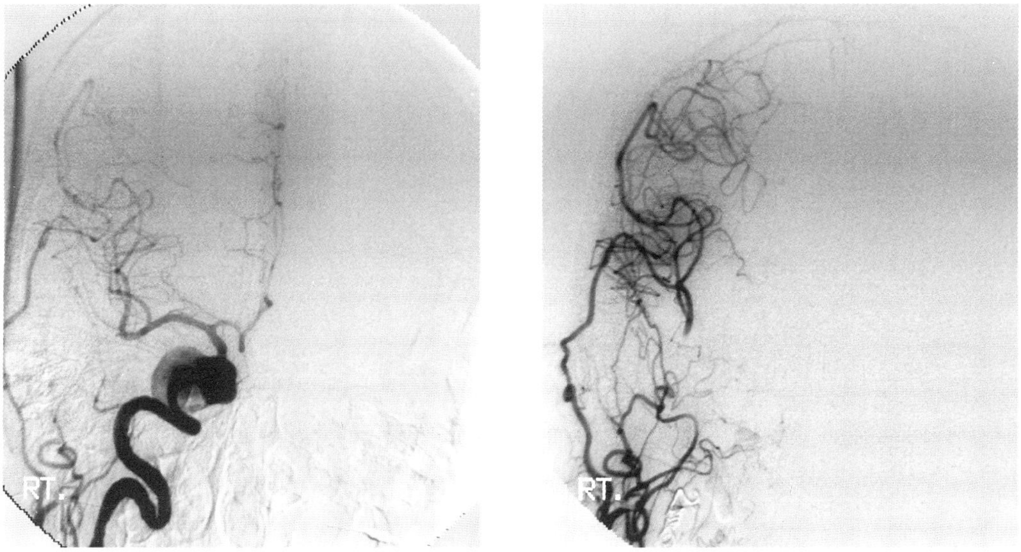


***Figure 1D.*** *Following superficial temporal to middle cerebral bypass, balloon occlusion resulted in dramatic flow augmentation through the bypass and normalization of rCBF.*

bilateral visual impairment and not infrequently present with SAH. Several unique challenges are posed to the surgeon confronted with these lesions: (1) the achievement of proximal arterial control; (2) precise understanding of the site of emergence of the normal carotid from the skull base; (3) adequately deflating the giant sac for definitive clipping; and (4) dissection with minimal manipulation of the already attenuated optic nerve. Despite these problems, almost all such lesions are clippable.

In the majority of giant supraclinoid aneurysms, exposure of an adequate segment of proximal carotid for the placement of a temporary clip intracranially is either not possible or achievable only after extensive bony and dural resection. We believe that the safest alternative is to routinely expose the cervical carotid prior to the performance of craniotomy so that proximal control is obtained prior to brain retraction.

The key to successful carotid clip reconstruction with aneurysm occlusion is the realization that, regardless of aneurysm appearance and projection, the proximal carotid always emerges in intimate association with the lateral aspect of the optic canal. Day carefully delineated the major sites of origin of supraclinoid aneurysms as relating to the ophthalmic artery origin or to the superior hypophyseal artery origin.[11] Giant lesions associated with an ophthalmic origin project largely superiorly, and distort the distal carotid inferiorly and the optic nerve superomedially. Giant aneurysms with a relationship to the superior hypophyseal origin project medially or posteromedially, resulting in the internal carotid being displaced laterally or anterolaterally. The proximal carotid, in both of these situations, emerges and gives origin to the proximal neck immediately adjacent to the lateral aspect of the optic nerve.

The typically broad origin of these aneurysms and the resultant carotid displacement suggests that the proximal neck lies beneath the midportion of the anterior clinoid process. This misperception leads the surgeon to resect more bone than is necessary lateral to the key site. Some giant aneurysms are clippable without bony removal simply by defining and opening the dural component of the optic canal and identification of the ophthalmic artery beneath the optic nerve. This vessel origin almost always implies healthy carotid wall. More commonly, this dural open-

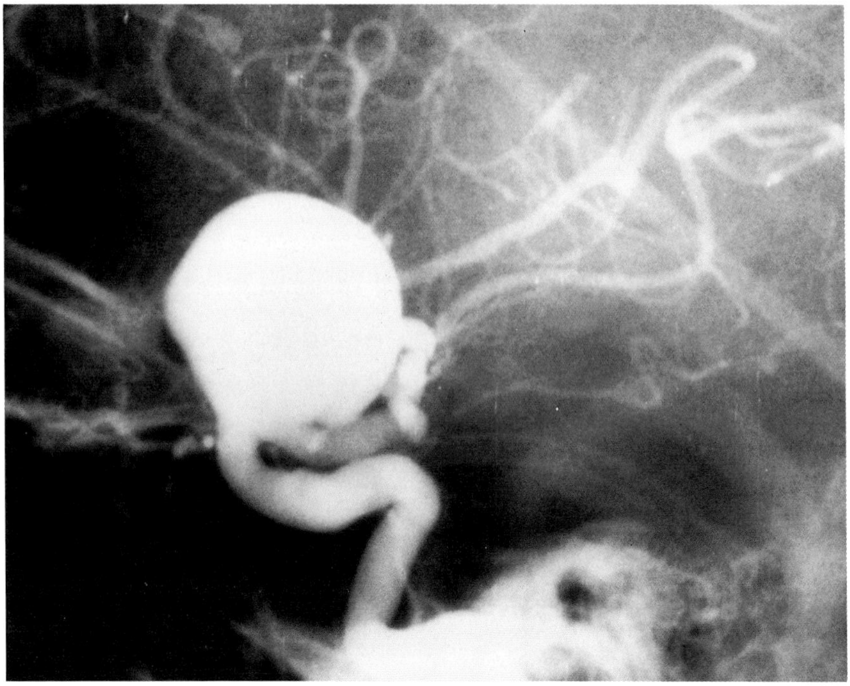

*Figure 2A. The use of retrograde suction decompression via the cervical internal carotid has made most supraclinoid aneurysms manageable with brief episodes of temporary occlusion. Figure shows giant carotid ophthalmic aneurysm with inferior displacement of distal carotid.*

ing should be followed by a focused medial bony resection exposing the dural ring, achieving proximal control and a means to dissect the proximal neck.

Adequate deflation of the giant sac for precise clipping is a problem. All too frequently in our experience, placement of a temporary clamp on the cervical carotid and a distal temporary clip proximal to the posterior communicating artery did not result in adequate softening of the sac and caused attempted clip placements to simply migrate down onto the carotid itself. Opening of the sac in these circumstances was similarly unrewarding, as brisk bleeding occurred due to retrograde flow from the ophthalmic artery and the cavernous branches. The surgeon's nondominant hand was then occupied with keeping the suction over the hole in the aneurysm and unavailable for bimanual dissection.

In response to this problem, we began catheterizing the cervical carotid with an 18-gauge angiocatheter after trapping was performed. Wall suction was then applied to evacuate and deflate the sac in a retrograde fashion.[7] When feasible, the ophthalmic artery can also be temporarily occluded to make the retrograde suction even more effective. This simple technique dramatically improved our handling of proximal carotid aneurysms, and most can be secured with only brief temporary occlusion (Figure 2).

A remarkable case in which this was not possible is illustrated in Figure 3. This patient had been legally blind in his left eye for 2 years and sought medical attention when he began losing vision in his right eye. He was found to have a very unusual thrombotic and partially recanalized proximal carotid aneurysm. A column of contrast passed in a complete loop through the thrombotic sac and emerged into the distal carotid artery. It was apparent that aneurysm deflation would be advisable due to the pre-existent optic compromise. A trial balloon occlusion was tolerated clinically and hemodynamically. Consideration was given to simply trapping the lesion, but it was clear that retrograde flow from the oph-

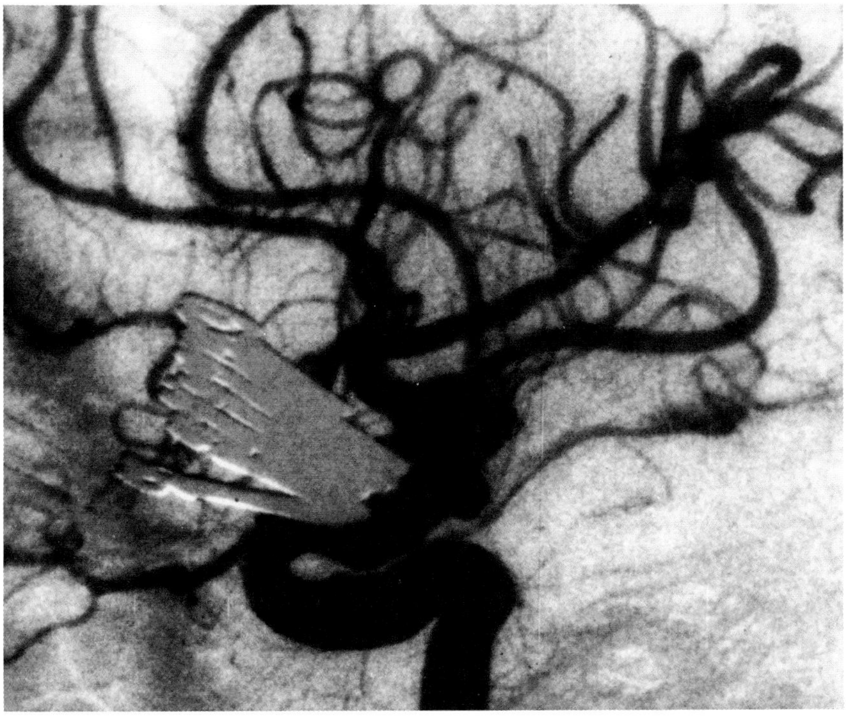

*Figure 2B. Postoperative angiogram confirms aneurysm occlusion with 6 minutes of temporary clipping.*

thalmic artery that was a source of collateral during the trial occlusion would be lost at surgery. We elected to construct a saphenous bypass graft from the origin of the external carotid (so that internal carotid flow would continue during this anastomosis) to the intracranial carotid. The trapped aneurysm was then evacuated with the Cavitron ultrasonic aspirator.

The final problem concerns the manipulation of the optic nerve during dissection. Great care should be exercised to minimize this potentially injurious activity. A key maneuver in our hands has been the wide opening of the optic canal prior to elevating the nerve at all. This maneuver untethers the nerve anteriorly and allows slightly more mobility for the similar degree of retraction.

## *Posterior Carotid Wall Giant Aneurysm*

These lesions are usually relatively straightforward to treat. Proximal control for temporary clipping can usually be safely achieved intracranially in the subarachnoid space. The problems with giant posterior carotid wall

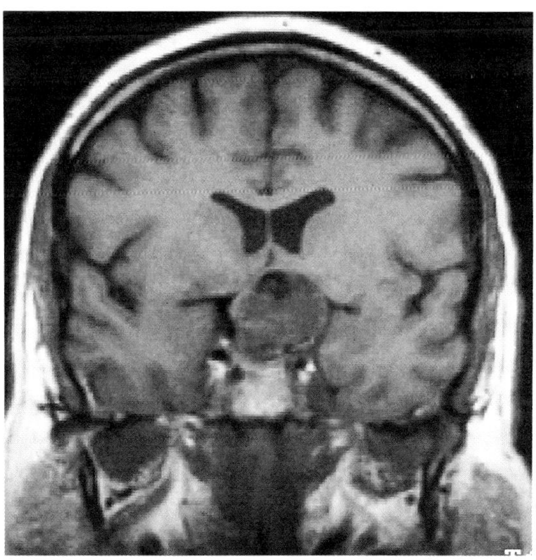

*Figure 3A. This patient was legally blind in the left eye for 2 years and began losing vision in his right eye. Coronal MRI demonstrates partially canalized suprasellar mass. See Figures 3B–E.*

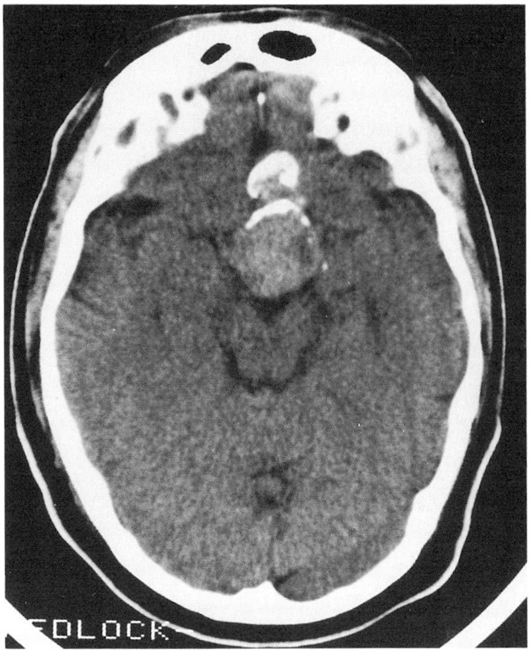

*Figure 3B. Unenhanced CT clearly shows anterior calcification.*

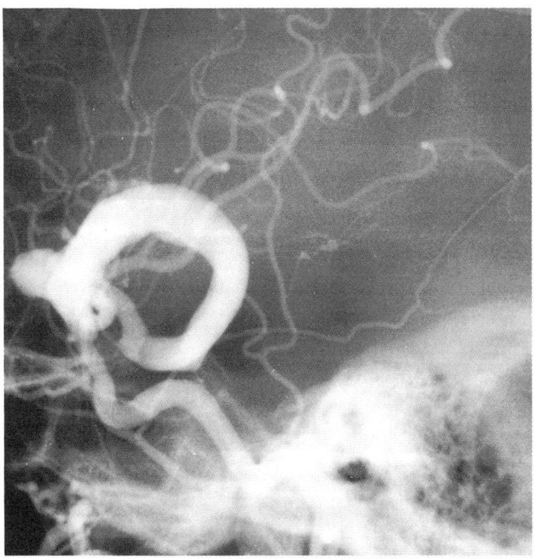

*Figure 3C. Lateral carotid angiogram reveals canalized "loop" through the aneurysm emptying into the distal carotid.*

aneurysms include: (1) difficulty in preserving the anterior choroidal artery, and (2) expansion of much of the circumference of the carotid into the neck precluding traditional clip placement.

The anterior choroidal artery must be gently dissected and absolutely preserved at all cost to avoid devastating neurologic deficit. Temporary trapping of the broad-necked giant aneurysm with deflation has been the surest means in our hands to ensure its preservation.

While occasional giant aneurysms in this site are narrow-necked, they are the minority. Most lesions expand laterally and medially, giving the impression that the carotid simply empties into the sac. The keys to successful reconstruction of an appropriate carotid lumen are temporary trapping, and the use of angled fenestrated clips. Temporary trapping involves clipping the carotid proximally and distally, as well as the posterior communicating artery which is typically medially displaced and seen through the opticocarotid triangle. Angeled fenestrated clips can then be used singly or in series to reconstitute the carotid lumen in the apertures. Persistent aneurysm filling following clipping may occasionally occur from retrograde flow through the posterior communicating artery. If an acceptable P1 is present, the communicating vessel can be permanently clipped to eliminate this problem.

## *Giant Aneurysms of the Middle Cerebral Artery*

Giant aneurysms at this site form a continuum of complexity ranging from the truly saccular, nonthrombotic aneurysm involving the middle cerebral bifurcation, to the thrombotic fusiform lesions involving the entire middle cerebral trunk. Intermediate in difficulty is the thrombotic saccular lesion at the bifurcation.

The most straightforward of these lesions is represented in Figure 4 in which a 2.5 cm aneurysm is seen at the middle cerebral bifurcation with somewhat sluggish flow into the appropriately situated efferent branches. The optimal approach to these lesions in our experience is a lateral trans-sylvian dissection with initial identification of an M2 branch which is judiciously followed to the M1 seg-

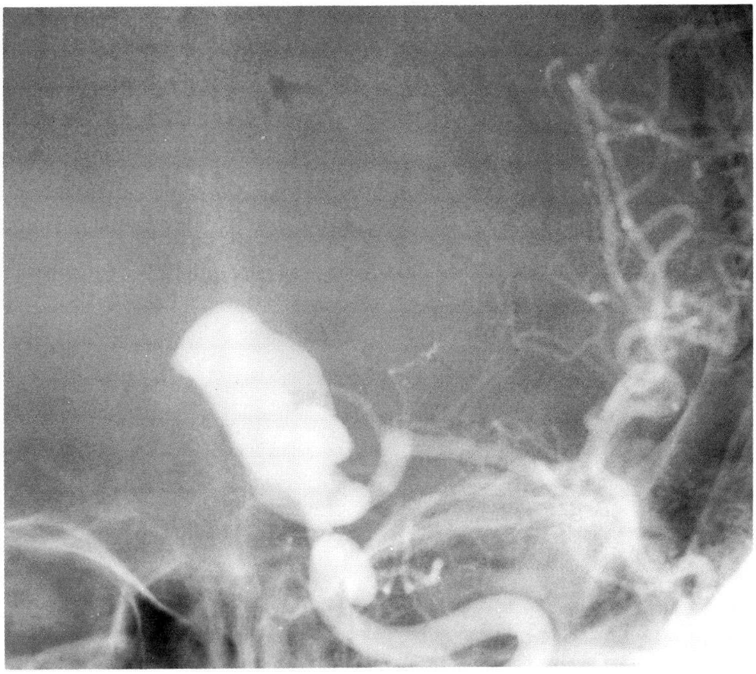

*Figure 3D*. *Anteroposterior angiogram suggests inferolateral displacement of the distal internal carotid artery.*

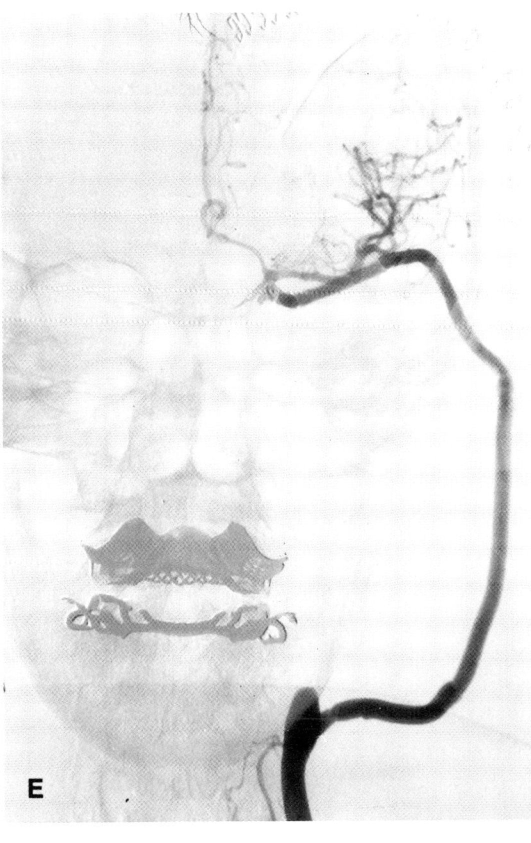


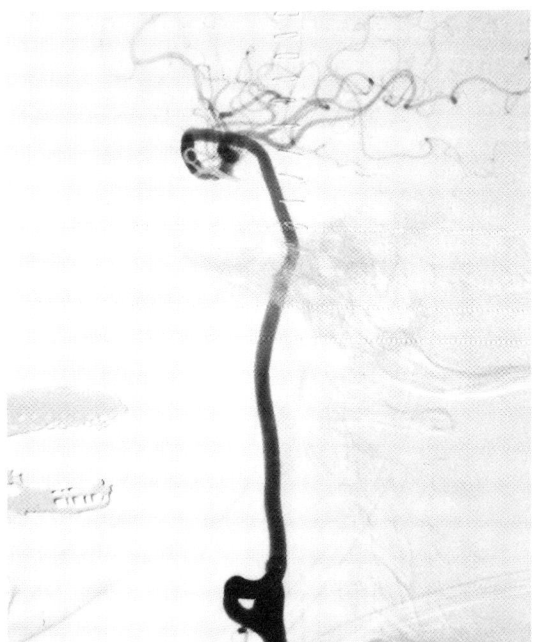


*Figure 3E,F*. *Postoperative anteroposterior (E) and lateral (F) angiogram confirms patency of saphenous bypass graft from external carotid to intracranial internal carotid.*

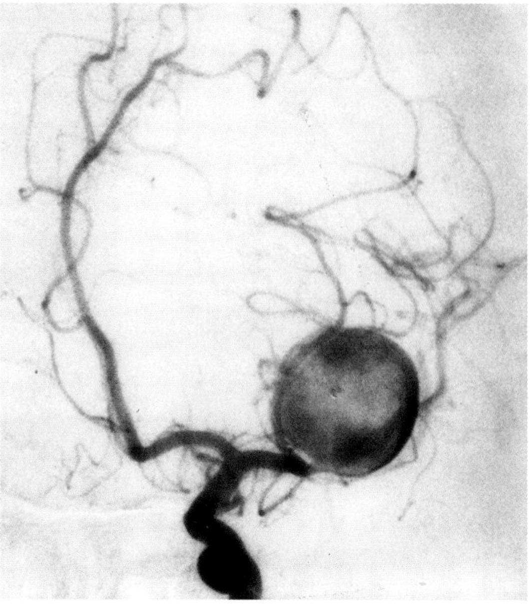

*Figure 4A. This patient is a college student who suffered a minor SAH from this middle cerebral giant aneurysm. Anteroposterior angiogram demonstrates a giant aneurysm at the origin at the middle cerebral bifurcation.*

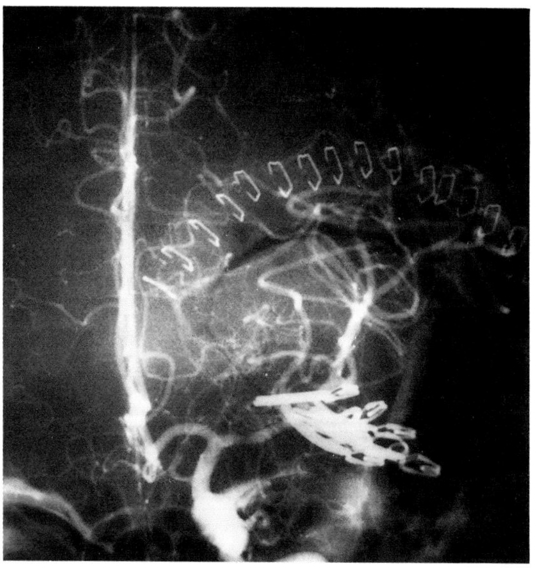

*Figure 4B. Posteroperative angiogram shows complex clip arrangement made possible by temporary trapping and deflation of the sac.*

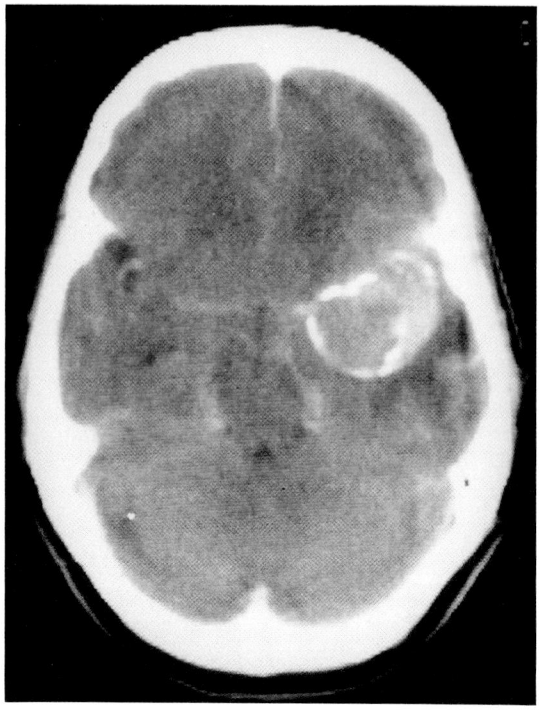

*Figure 5. Calcific middle cerebral giant aneurysm that produced SAH in an elderly woman.*

ment, thus securing proximal control. Occasionally in giant lesions it is helpful to resect a small amount of temporal lobe to safely isolate all M2 branches. Once the afferent and efferent vasculature is dissected, the patient is placed in burst-suppressive coma and temporary clips are applied.

We have had much better results with complete trapping than with simple softening by M1 clipping. The aneurysm is then punctured and deflated. The sac which should now be completely empty can then be clipped preserving outflow. Frequently the empty sac can be secured with a single clip, although the case illustrated in Figure 4 required a more complex arrangement. Time should not be wasted if difficulty is encountered in emptying the sac through a needle puncture wound. An arachnoid knife can be used to create a stab wound through which the sucker can be introduced.

Somewhat more complex is a calcific lesion illustrated in Figure 5. This aneurysm also originates at the middle cerebral bifurcation, but the obvious wall calcification—particularly in the region of the neck—adds difficulty to safe clipping. We used several strategies in this situation with variable success. We crushed the neck with forceps as de-

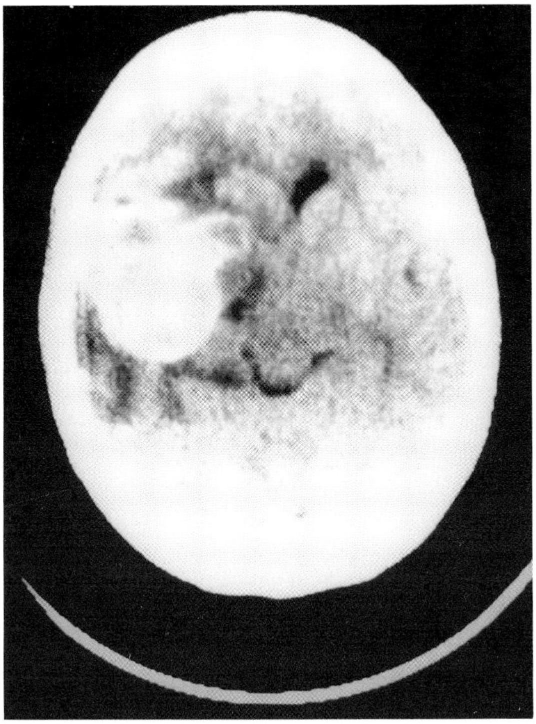

*Figure 6A. A patient presented with increasing headaches and left hemiparesis from this largely thrombotic middle cerebral giant aneurysm. CT shows major mass effect from the thrombotic sac in the middle cranial fossa.*

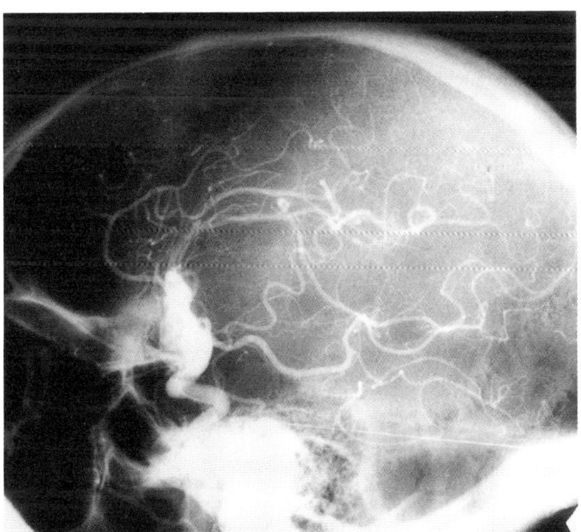

*Figure 6B. Lateral angiogram documents elevation of sylvian vessels with partial filling of aneurysm.*

scribed by Drake[16] and found the Codman hemostat particularly useful. More commonly, it has been helpful to widely incise the sac

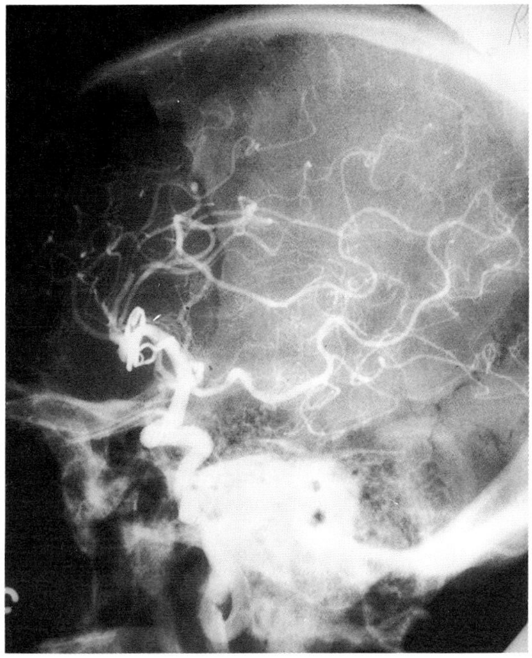

*Figure 6C. Postoperative angiogram shows simple clip arrangement with preservation of the middle cerebral branches.*

and dissect the calcified material out of the wall, leaving more pliable tissue behind. It is extremely important not to be overly aggressive as the dissection enters the mouth of the M1 segment. Injury to intima or plaque in the vessels ultimately to be reconstructed can set the stage for arterial dissection and delayed ischemia. It is better to leave a small amount of abnormal tissue and a bulbous middle cerebral bifurcation than risk a devastating dissection.

Next in levels of increasing complexity is the largely thrombotic middle cerebral giant aneurysm. This lesion typically presents with signs of increasing hemispheric mass effect or distal embolization although seizures, and SAH are not uncommon. Our strategy has been to carefully scrutinize the anatomy to determine the optimal way to achieve proximal and distal control. In cases such as the patient illustrated in Figure 6, profound mass effect from the middle cranial fossa suggests that in concert with a generous trans-sylvian dissection, removal of the residual temporal

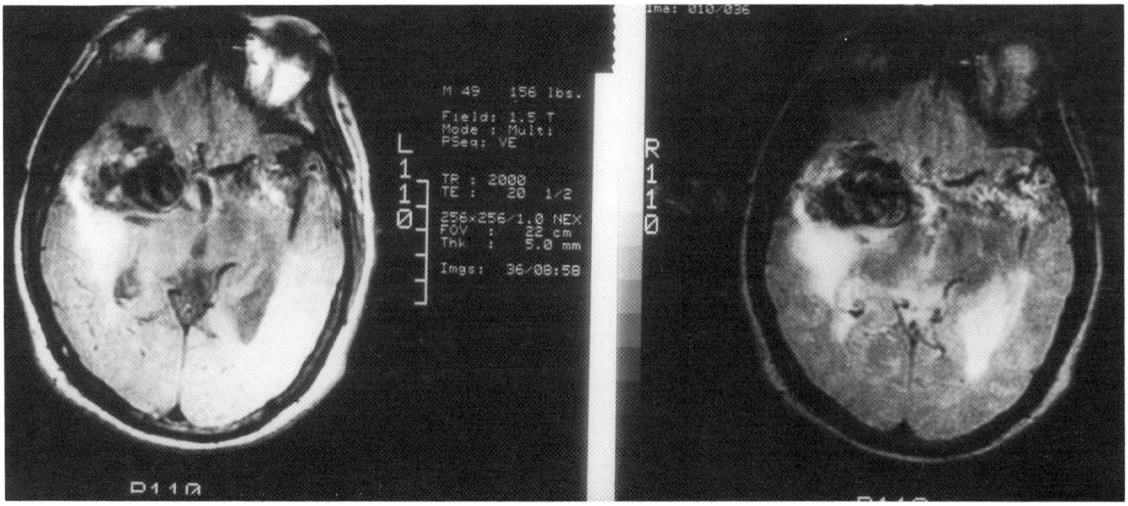


*Figure 7A. This patient presented with ischemic symptoms in the right middle cerebral territory. MRI discloses giant mass with thrombosis along the entire middle cerebral artery.*

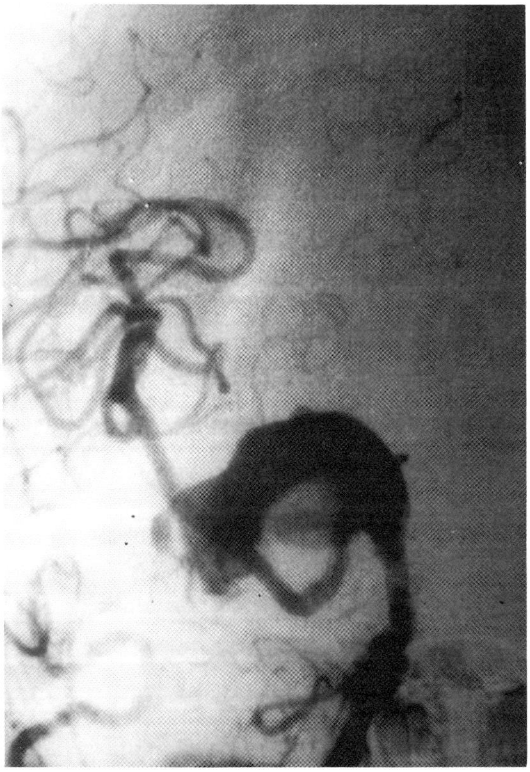

*Figure 7B. Angiography suggests an intact distal M1 segment with aneurysm origin near the carotid bifurcation. At surgery, the entire carotid and middle cerebral arteries were aneurysmal and the angiographic "vessels" were merely channels through the mass.*

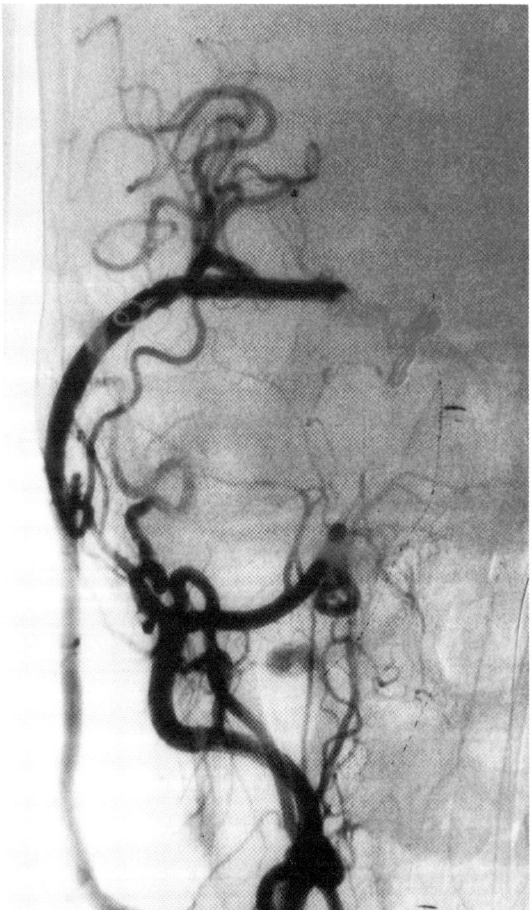

*Figure 7C. Carotid occlusion in the neck and distal saphenous bypass grafting did not prevent devastating infarction.*

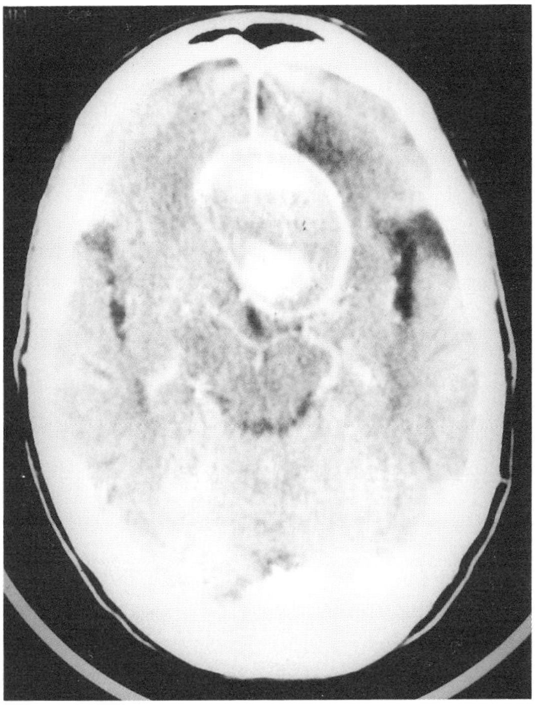

*Figure 8. Giant eccentric, largely thrombotic anterior communicating aneurysm.*

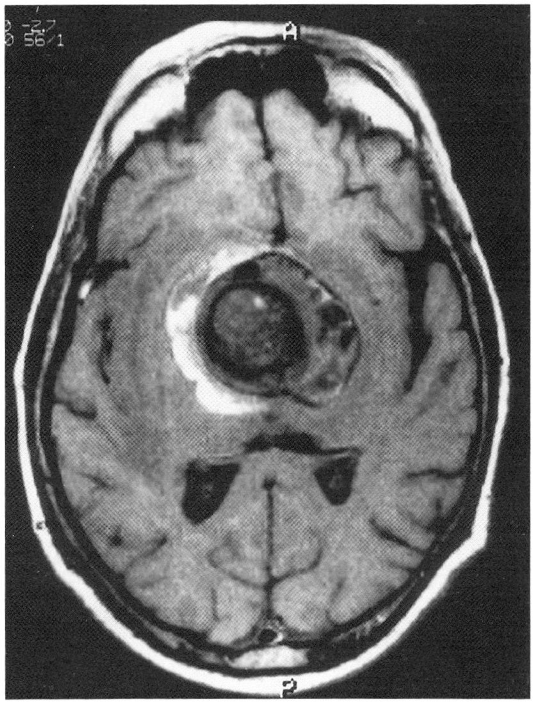


*Figure 9A. This patient in his early 40s became neurologically devastated and was rendered bedridden by the progressive enlargement and final rupture of this largely thrombotic distal basilar artery aneurysm. He had previously been treated with bilateral ventriculoperitoneal shunting. Preoperative MRI demonstrates the magnitude of the thrombotic mass with fresh hemorrhage surrounding the lesion on the right.*

pole would be of benefit. Complete exposure of the aneurysm base is required for what will necessarily be a resection of the aneurysm. After exposure and temporary clipping are established, it is our practice to proceed with immediate amputation of the aneurysm.

Early attempts at limited openings have resulted in poor visualization and undue time wastage out in the fundus. The key to successful clipping and restitution of middle cerebral perfusion is the evacuation of the contents in the neck of the aneurysm. The remaining thrombotic debris can be removed after flow is re-established. To accomplish this goal, we open the sac with a number-11 knife about 1 cm from the surgical neck. Using heavy microscissors, the rest of the aneurysm is circumferentially amputated with great care to leave an adequate cuff to allow clip reconstruction.

After the incision is completed, attention is directed to the neck. Microcurettes can be used to develop a plane between the thrombus and the aneurysm wall. The material may then be removed by progressively peeling it from the wall or by Cavitron aspiration. Again caution should be exercised near the mouth of the M1 to not injure the intima. After final clipping (which can be quite straightforward with a simple cuff of aneurysm remaining) the residual mass can be removed without haste. If under some circumstance the cuff tears or the surgeon fails to leave adequate tissue to reconstruct, suturing the remaining neck can be performed with 8–0 or 9–0 suture.

The middle cerebral giant aneurysm that in our opinion continues to defy solution is the fusiform or thrombotic fusiform aneurysm involving the entire middle cerebral trunk. The most complex types of these lesions, as illustrated in Figure 7, are likely formed as a result of repetitive arterial dissections. The approach to these patients obviously varies with their presenting complaints. Occlusion of the

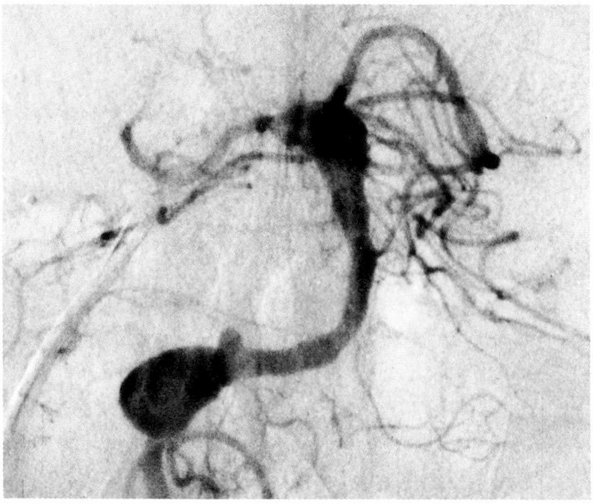

***Figure 9B****. Angiography discloses that the aneurysm was patent only in the region of the neck. Delayed films showed a faint column of contrast passing anteriorly within the sac.*

middle cerebral artery with protective distal bypass has been proposed,[28,50] and has had some success. Rupture of previously unruptured aneurysms has been reported following bypass, however, and Scott et al recommend no delay in the direct approach to the aneurysm.[38] We attempted direct clip reconstruction in certain thrombotic serpentine lesions, with attempts to preserve the origins of lenticulostriates, only to note gangliar and capsular infarction in the postoperative period.

The other frequently performed approach is illustrated by Figure 7. This patient had ischemic symptoms from what we believed was a giant lesion originating at the carotid bifurcation and proximal M1 segment. Exploration revealed, however, that the angiographically apparent carotid and M1 segment were simply channels of patency through the giant mass. At surgery we sacrificed the carotid in the neck and distally revascularized with a long saphenous vein graft. The patient had a devastating infarction postoperatively, which may have resulted from prolonged occlusion time (55 minutes) or the permanent loss of unseen lenticulostriates and anterior choroidal artery, or both.

We remain uncertain how to manage this problem. Endovascular trial occlusion at the origin of the lesion may be helpful, although delayed thrombosis will likely occlude lenticulostriates. Circulatory arrest with the additional time allowed may permit safer reconstruction of the M1 segment, but perforators are still in major jeopardy. Perhaps cervical internal carotid occlusion offers some protection, but this remains controversial.

## *Giant Anterior Communicating Artery Aneurysms*

Giant lesions of the anterior communicating region are briefly addressed, as the principles of repair are identical to those discussed for middle cerebral artery aneurysms. We prefer a pterional exposure, although in cer-

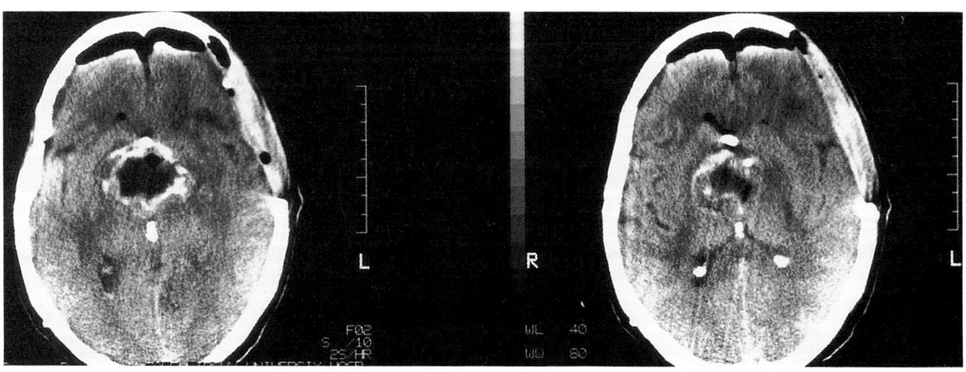


***Figure 9C****. Circulatory arrest under deep hypothermia allowed decompression around the aneurysm neck and successful clipping. A subsequent transcallosal exposure was used to evacuate the sac to maximize the patient's chances of recovery.*

tain situations have used a true subfrontal route. For massive lesions, the subfrontal view may make the A2 segments easier to access. In general, the procedure is planned so that complete control of afferent and efferent vessels is acquired early. For those completely filling aneurysms, simple temporary trapping and needle deflation allows clipping. In more complex lesions (Figure 8), amputation of the fundus is necessary as discussed above, with evacuation of thrombus from the remaining cuff. In general, we approach these lesions with standard burst-suppressive anesthesia as the temporary occlusion times are usually not protracted, although we treated one recent case with circulatory arrest. Due to the size of his lesion and the tenacity of the thrombus circulatory arrest time was 40 minutes and the patient recovered uneventfully.

## *Giant Vertebral Artery Aneurysms*

While the surgical principles do not differ markedly from those previously discussed, the regional anatomy of giant vertebral aneurysms introduces additional sources of morbidity. The common presence of a contralateral vertebral artery, capable of supplying the distal basilar circulation, introduces the excellent surgical alternative of vertebral artery sacrifice. Unfortunately, giant aneurysms in this region also comprise a spectrum from simple enlargement of small aneurysms located just distal to the PICA origin to fusiform and serpiginous variants which may involve much of the lower basilar artery.

Anatomic problems with these lesions involve the necessity to maintain patency of PICA and the intimate relationship of the lower cranial nerves and medulla to the sac. It is critical to perform focused preopertive MRI and contralateral vertebral angiography to clarify the regional anatomy. From a surgical perspective, the patency of a contralateral vertebral allows the comfortable use of even protracted temporary arterial occlusion to permit aneurysm evacuation and vascular reconstruction. We have seen unfortunate morbidity, however, from even straightforward surgical procedures, with lower cranial nerve dysfunction requiring tracheostomy and occasional long tract signs from a shift of the brain stem back into a more anatomic position following aneurysm decompression.

Due to these concerns, surgeons should consider the possibility of using interventional techniques to nonsurgically sacrifice the vertebral artery as a means of circumventing unnecessary morbidity. For the unusual vertebral aneurysms proximal to PICA this is an excellent strategy, as the ipsilateral PICA can be irrigated by the contralateral vertebral artery via the confluens. Tolerance in the awake state can be confirmed before balloon detachment.

For those giant lesions arising immediately distal to PICA in which it is possible to place a clip across the vertebral artery distal to PICA, permanent trapping and evacuation of the sac is an excellent and usually well-tolerated maneuver. Access to the confluens may be difficult and occasionally a contralateral exposure has been necessary to complete the trapping.

The chief problem with giant aneurysms in this region arises with partially thrombotic aneurysms with massive medullary distortion and incorporation of PICA into the mass. In patients with life-threatening deficits due to mass effect, definitive open surgery with temporary (or permanent) trapping with aneurysmnectomy is the treatment of choice.[48] If PICA cannot be preserved, either an occipital artery to PICA bypass or a side-to-side anastomosis with the contralateral PICA will provide adequate supply to the PICA territory. If the patient has only minimal deficits attributable to mass effect, despite the appearance of the MRI, an endovascular occlusion procedure should at least be considered. Some patients are immediately improved by the elimination of pulsations within the mass and actual decompression may occur over years to come. The role of selective microcoil occlusion of the patent portion of the sac remains uncertain.

## *Giant Aneurysms of the Distal Basilar Artery*

We recently reviewed our experience with distal basilar aneurysms,[6] and these data will not be restated. The problems associated with routine aneurysms of the distal basilar artery include (1) the confining space of the interpeduncular cistern, and (2) the vital need to preserve all posterior thalmoperforators emanating from the posterior wall of the basilar artery and the proximal posterior cerebral arteries. Once aneurysms reach giant size, the surgeon's ability to maneuver successfully and preserve vital vascular structures becomes a major challenge.

The successful management of these lesions in our hands has hinged around our ability to achieve definitive proximal and distal arterial control. The use of simple proximal clipping of the basilar artery definitely softens many lesions, permitting more aggressive dissection around the posterior aspect of the sac. If the lesion is partially or largely thrombotic, this maneuver will not permit definitive treatment. We have been repetitively frustrated by the difficulty of temporarily clipping the contralateral P1 from a subtemporal exposure. In some patients the anatomy is favorable, but in most it is not.

The trans-sylvian exposure, with its modification of half-and-half exposure as popularized by Drake, appear in our hands to be the optimal means of exposing and treating distal basilar giant aneurysms. When simple proximal temporary clipping does not permit definitive mobilization of the sac, trapping should be immediately instituted. The aneurysm can then be aspirated and only modest backbleeding from perforators complicates the rest of the dissection. The ultimate exposure of the posterior aspect of the sac to clear perforators can then be performed from a near true lateral exposure when the half-and-half approach is employed.

Two technical points deserve mention. First, many atheromatous basilar arteries are not completely closed by a single temporary clip, resulting in poor aneurysm decompression and impressive bleeding when deflation is attempted. It has become our practice to place two tandem temporary clips on the basilar artery. Second, in complex and thrombotic aneurysms, inclusion of the P1 into the definitive clipping is a very acceptable maneuver if an adequate posterior communicating artery is present. This allows retrograde supply of the perforators arising from the P1. This technique is far superior to the dangerous prolongation of temporary occlusion pushing further attempts to achieve definitive clipping when a P1 clearly arises from a giant sac.

Microsurgery has not completely solved the difficulties with giant distal basilar aneurysms. In complex cases, proximal ligation of the basilar should at least be considered,[35] with bypass protection if trial occlusion fails. Complex, thrombotic aneurysms in this region require more protracted temporary occlusion for definitive treatment than aneurysms in other sites, and as such form an excellent subgroup of the use of hypothermic circulatory arrest (Figure 9). Finally, due to the documented high risk of these lesions treated surgically, careful trials of endovascular therapy should be considered with vigilant follow-up of the patients to determine if such "cures" remain durable. It is our strong opinion that giant distal basilar aneurysms should be treated only in units with a dedicated and experienced neurovascular team composed of neurosurgeons, neuroradiologists, neuroanesthesiologists, and a capable operating room and intensive care facility.

## Summary

We have attempted to highlight some of the complexities and vagaries of giant aneurysm treatment, with some mention of our own prejudices in certain anatomic sites. These biases should be treated as such, but are based on a long and dedicated experience. It is clear that major progress is needed and possible within the field of giant aneurysms; multidisciplinary, co-operative efforts will be required to accomplish that goal.

# References


1. Artmann H, Vonofakos D, Müller H, et al. Neuroradiologic and neuropathologic findings with growing giant intracranial aneurysm. *Surg Neurol.* 1984;21:391–401.
2. Ausman JI, Diaz FG, Sadasivan B, et al. Giant intracranial aneurysm surgery: the role of microvascular reconstruction. *Surg Neurol.* 1990;34:8–15.
3. Batjer HH, Frankfurt AI, Purdy PD, et al. Use of etomidate, temporary arterial occlusion, and intraoperative angiography in surgical treatment of large and giant cerebral aneurysm. *J Neurosurg.* 1988;68: 234–240.
4. Batjer H, Mickey B, Samson D. Enlargement and rupture of distal basilar aneurysm after iatrogenic carotid occlusion. *Neurosurgery.* 1987;20:624–628.
5. Batjer HH, Purdy PD. Enlarging thrombosed aneurysm of the distal basilar artery. *Neurosurgery.* 1990; 26:695–700.
6. Batjer HH, Samson DS. Causes of morbidity and mortality from surgery of aneurysms of the distal basilar artery. *Neurosurgery.* 1989;25:904–916.
7. Batjer HH, Samson DS. Retrograde suction decompression of giant paraclinoidal aneurysms: technical note. *J Neurosurg.* 1990;73:305–306.
8. Baumgartner WA, Silverberg GD, Ream AK, et al. Reappraisal of cardiopulmonary bypass with deep hypothermia and circulatory arrest for complex neurosurgical operations. *Surgery.* 1983;94:242–249.
9. Berenstein A, Ransohoff J, Kupersmith M, et al. Transvascular treatment of giant aneurysms of the cavernous and vertebral arteries. *Surg Neurol.* 1984; 21:3–12.
10. Borrie MJ, Campbell AJ, Caradoc-Davies TH. Obstructive hydrocephalus secondary to giant cerebral aneurysm in the elderly: two case reports of functional improvement after ventricular shunting. *J Am Geriatr Soc.* 1985;33:210–212.
11. Day AL. Aneurysms of the ophthalmic segment: a clinical and anatomical analysis. *J Neurosurg.* 1990; 72:677–691.
12. Debrun G, Fox A, Drake C, et al. Giant unclippable aneurysms: treatment with detachable balloons. *AJNR.* 1981;2:167–173.
13. Debrun G, Lacour P, Caron J-P, et al. Detachable balloon and calibrated-leak balloon techniques in the treatment of cerebral vascular lesions. *J Neurosurg.* 1978;49:635–649.
14. Dolenc V. Direct microsurgical repair of intracavernous vascular lesions. *J Neurosurg.* 1983;58: 824–831.
15. Drake CG. Evolution of intracranial aneurysm surgery. *Can Surg.* 1984;27:549–555.
16. Drake CG. Giant intracranial aneurysms: experience with surgical treatment in 174 patients. *Clin Neurosurg.* 1979;26:12–95.
17. Fox AL, Viñuela F, Pelz DM, et al. Use of detachable balloons for proximal artery occlusion in the treatment of unclippable cerebral aneurysms. *J Neurosurg.* 1987;66:40–46.
18. Gianturco C, Anderson JH, Wallace S. Mechanical devices for arterial occlusion. *AJR.* 1975;124:428–435.
19. Giller GA, Steig P, Batjer HH, et al. Transcranial Doppler ultrasound as a guide to graded therapeutic occlusion of the carotid artery. *Neurosurgery.* 1990; 26:307–311.
20. Goldstein A Jr, Wells BA, Keats AS. Increased tolerance to cerebral anoxia by pentobarbital. *Arch Int Pharmacodyn Ther.* 1966;161:138–143.
21. Heros RC. Thromboembolic complications after combined internal carotid ligation and extra-to-intracranial bypass. *Surg Neurol.* 1984;21:75–79.
22. Higashida RT, Halbach VV, Cahan LD, et al. Detachable balloon embolization therapy of posterior circulation intracranial aneurysms. *J Neurosurg.* 1989;71:512–519.
23. Higashida RT, Halbach VV, Dowd CF, et al. Interventional neurovascular treatment of a giant intracranial aneurysm using platinum microcoils. *Surg Neurol.* 1991;35:64–68.
24. Higashida RT, Halbach VV, Mehringer CM, et al. Giant cavernous aneurysm associated with trigeminal artery: treatment by detachable balloon. *AJNR.* 1987; 8:757–758.
25. Hylton PD, Reichman OH. Endaneurysmal microendarterectomy in the treatment of giant cerebral aneurysms: technical note. *Neurosurgery.* 1988;23: 674–679.
26. Jabre A, Symon L. Temporary vascular occlusion during aneurysm surgery. *Surg Neurol.* 1987;27:47–63.
27. Keen WW. Intracranial lesions. *Med News (NY).* 1890;57:439–449.
28. Lansen TA, Kasoff SS, Arguelles JH. Giant pediatric aneurysm treated with ligation of the middle cerebral artery with the Drake tourniquet and extracranial-intracranial bypass. *Neurosurgery.* 1989;25:81–85.
29. Lyall A. Large aneurysm of the circle of Willis spontaneous cure by thrombosis. *Br Med J.* 1936;2:282.
30. Mehdorn HM, Chater NL, Townsend JJ, et al. Giant aneurysm and cerebral ischemia. *Surg Neurol.* 1980; 13:49–57.
31. Michenfelder JD, Milde JH, Sundt TM Jr. Cerebral protection by barbiturate anesthesia. *Arch Neurol.* 1976;33:345–350.
32. Milde LN, Milde JH. Preservation of cerebral metabolites by etomidate during incomplete cerebral ischemia in dogs. *Anesthesiology.* 1986;65:272–277.
33. Milde LN, Milde JH, Michenfelder JD. Cerebral functional, metabolic, and hemodynamic effects of etomidate in dogs. *Anesthesiology.* 1985;63:371–377.
34. Pool JL. Aneurysms of the anterior communicating artery: bifrontal craniotomy, and routine use of temporary clips. *J Neurosurg.* 1961;18:98–112.
35. Rozario RA, Stein BM. Ligation of the basilar artery as the definitive treatment for a giant aneurysm of the basilar artery apex: case report. *Neurosurgery.* 1980; 6:87–91.
36. Schubiger O, Valavanis A, Wichmann W. Growth-mechanism of giant intracranial aneurysms; demonstrated by CT and MR imaging. *Neuroradiology.* 1987;29:266–271.
37. Scialfa G, Vaghi A, Valsecchi F, et al. Neuroradiological treatment of carotid and vertebral fistulas and intracavernous aneurysms. *Neuroradiology.* 1982;24:13–25.
38. Scott RM, Liu H-C, Yuan R, et al. Rupture of a previously unruptured giant middle cerebral artery aneurysm after extracranial-intracranial bypass surgery. *Neurosurgery.* 1982;10:600–603.
39. Sekhar LN, Nelson PB. A technique of clipping giant intracranial aneurysms with the preservation of the parent artery. *Surg Neurol.* 1983;20:361–368.
40. Serbinenko FA. Balloon catheterization and occlu-

sion of major cerebral vessels. *J Neurosurg.* 1974; 41:125–145.
41. Silverberg GD. Giant aneurysms: surgical treatment. *Neurol Res.* 1984;6:57–63.
42. Silverberg GD, Reitz BA, Ream AK, et al. Operative treatment of a giant cerebral artery aneurysm with hypothermia and circulatory arrest: report of a case. *Neurosurgery.* 1980;6:301–305.
43. Slosberg PS. Symptomatic unruptured giant aneurysms: medical treatment. *Acta Neurochir (Wien).* 1982;62:207–218.
44. Smith RR, Parent AD. End-to-end anastomosis of the anterior cerebral artery after excision of a giant aneurysm: case report;. *J Neurosurg.* 1982;56:577–580.
45. Spetzler RF, Fukushima T, Martin N, et al. Petrous carotid-to-intradural carotid saphenous vein graft for intracavernous giant aneurysm, tumor, and occlusive cerebrovascular disease. *J Neurosurg.* 1990;73:496–501.
46. Spetzler RF, Hadley MN, Rigamonti D, et al. Aneurysms of the basilar artery treated with circulatory arrest, hypothermia, and barbiturate cerebral protection. *J Neurosurg.* 1988;68:868–879.
47. Sugita K, Kobayashi S, Inoue T, et al. Characteristics and use of ultra-long aneurysm clips. *J Neurosurg.* 1984;60:145–150.
48. Sugita KS, Kobayashi S, Takemae T, et al. Giant aneurysms of the vertebral artery: report of five cases. *J Neurosurg.* 1988;68:960–966.
49. Sundt TM Jr, Piepgras DG, Marsh WR. Booster clips for giant and thick-based aneurysms. *J Neurosurg.* 1984;60:751–762.
50. Tognetti F, Andreoli A, Testa C. Giant fusiform aneurysm of the middle cerebral artery treated with extracranial-intracranial arterial bypass and Drake tourniquet. *Surg Neurol.* 1984; 22:33–35.
51. Whittle IR, Allsop JL, Halmagyi GM. Focal seizures: an unusual presentation of giant intracranial aneurysms. *Surg Neurol.* 1985;24:533–540.
52. Whittle IR, Dorsch NW, Besser M. Giant intracranial aneurysms: diagnosis, management, and outcome. *Surg Neurol.* 1984;21:218–230.
53. Whittle IR, Dorsch NW, Besser M. Spontaneous thrombosis in giant intracranial aneurysms. *J Neurol Neurosurg Psychiatry.* 1982;45:1040–1047.

# CHAPTER 10

# Detection, Prevention, and Management of Cerebral Vasospasm

Gregory Hariton, MD, J. Max Findlay, MD, and Bryce Weir, MD

## An Overview

Although ultimately affecting only about 1% of the overall population of North America, aneurysmal subarachnoid hemorrhage (SAH) carries with it a devastating prognosis for the majority of its sufferers. Initial rupture alone is responsible for a mortality or serious morbidity approaching 50%, and a number of complications may affect outcome in remaining survivors. Aneurysmal rebleeding is responsible for the majority of deaths, but other complications include cerebral vasospasm (VSP), hydrocephalus, raised intracranial pressure (ICP), seizures, cardiac or pulmonary dysfunction, and systemic metabolic derangements.

Cerebral VSP or the delayed onset of cerebral arterial narrowing following aneurysmal rupture is both a clinical and radiologic phenomenon. It is defined angiographically as a narrowing of the lumen of major intracranial basal arteries (BAs) due to sustained arterial contraction. Pathologic changes observed in vasospastic cerebral arteries include intense vasoconstriction, and often areas of myonecrosis and endothelial damage. Fibrosis and inflammatory cell infiltration of the arterial wall are minimal. Intimal hyperplasia may occur as a late change. VSP is caused by the deposition of thick subarachnoid blood clot which remains in prolonged contact with basal vessels. It is possible to predict the distribution and severity of VSP by detecting a large SAH in the basal cisterns visualized on computed tomographic (CT) scanning. Symptomatic VSP or delayed ischemic deficit (DID) occurs when arterial narrowing becomes severe enough to cause severe cerebral ischemia and/or infarction.

VSP following aneurysmal SAH is rarely observed within the first 4 days postrupture, and may last for a period of 1–2 weeks. Although most studies report the incidence of angiographic VSP to be in the range of 40% to 50%, the clinical manifestations of VSP are observed in only about one-quarter to a half of these patients. Of this smaller group, some will die or acquire permanent disability due to cerebral ischemia.

On a positive note, it is evident that over the past 10 years many advances in detection, prevention, and management of cerebral VSP have significantly reduced the associated incidence of death and disability.

## Detection

### *Risk Factors and Natural History*

In 1980, it was determined from a large series of patients that VSP rarely occurs within 4 days of SAH and seldom extends past 12 days.[97] Similar findings were reported by Saito and Sano[79] and Kodama et al[53] in smaller series of patients. With the knowledge of a window of opportunity prior to the onset of severe, diffuse VSP, neurosurgeons have sought prophylactic measures to prevent the development of arterial narrowing and/or ischemia.

Suzuki et al[87] reported that patients older than 65 years were not only at a higher risk for angiographic VSP following SAH but had a worse clinical outcome if it developed.

Ljunggren et al[56] in a series of 81 patients suffering aneurysmal SAH found that DID developed in 50% of 18 patients who were hypertensive prior to SAH, compared with only 13% of 65 normotensives. The authors also reported that the hypertensives had a significantly poorer outcome.

Maroon and Nelson[59] were the first to suggest a correlation between hypovolemia and SAH. Following this, other investigators have confirmed a relationship between hypovolemia and symptomatic VSP following SAH. Solomon et al[85] found that 86% of patients with symptomatic VSP had a depression of circulating blood volume as compared to only 13% of asymptomatic patients with angiographic VSP.

Niizuma et al[63] studied the relationship between the aneurysm site and the occurrence of VSP. The authors reported that VSP occurred initially in arteries closest to the aneurysm, followed by extension to other distal sites. Aneurysms near the midline produced a higher incidence of bilateral spasm. In addition, they found that middle cerebral artery (MCA) aneurysms were associated with the highest incidence of VSP.

CT scanning, when performed shortly after aneurysm rupture, is undoubtedly of greatest value in predicting VSP. Fisher et al[27] classified SAHs into 1 of 4 groups, based upon the quantity and distribution of subarachnoid blood visualized on CT scan within 2 days of aneurysm rupture. They then determined, retrospectively, the predictive capability of CT to the subsequent development of VSP. They found that those patients demonstrating thick layers of subarachnoid blood showed severe VSP in all cases. Only 1 in 18 patients with no subarachnoid blood visible on CT developed severe spasm (see Figure 1).

The patient's clinical grade or neurologic condition also correlates with the risk for VSP development.[3] Adams et al, from the Cooperative Aneurysm study, reported that admitting level of consciousness and impaired orientation closely paralleled the predictive power of the admission CT scan.

Other factors of less significance, which closely correlate with the original volume of subarachnoid clot viewed on CT scan, include electrocardiogram (ECG) abnormalities, leukocytosis, elevated blood catecholamines, and a low-grade fever.[11,96] (See Figure 2.)

## Clinical Observation

The clinical diagnosis of VSP is often one of exclusion. Since a wide variety of signs and symptoms are potentially associated with VSP, no entirely specific syndrome exists. Frequently associated with the onset of VSP are worsening headache or meningismus.[26] Objectively, signs such as a low-grade fever[96] and a depression in consciousness are commonly observed.[70] As the severity of the VSP increases, presentation reflects the area of cortex fed by the narrowed vessels. Most commonly affected is the territory of the MCA (75%), followed by that of the anterior cerebral artery (ACA) (25%), and less commonly, the posterior circulation.[70] Predictably, VSP involving a single MCA results in hemiparesis, hemisensory loss, or if the speech dominant hemisphere is affected, aphasia. Alteration in level of consciousness is uncommon with MCA VSP unless narrowing is bilateral or diffuse. In general, spasm involving the M1 segment of the MCA results in more severe symptoms than that of the more distal segments. In contrast, patients presenting with VSP of the ACA frequently develop early changes in sensorium, followed by incontinence, abulia, and motor weakness of the lower extremities.[70] The less common occurrence of unilateral ACA spasm with A2 involvement results in milder symptoms,

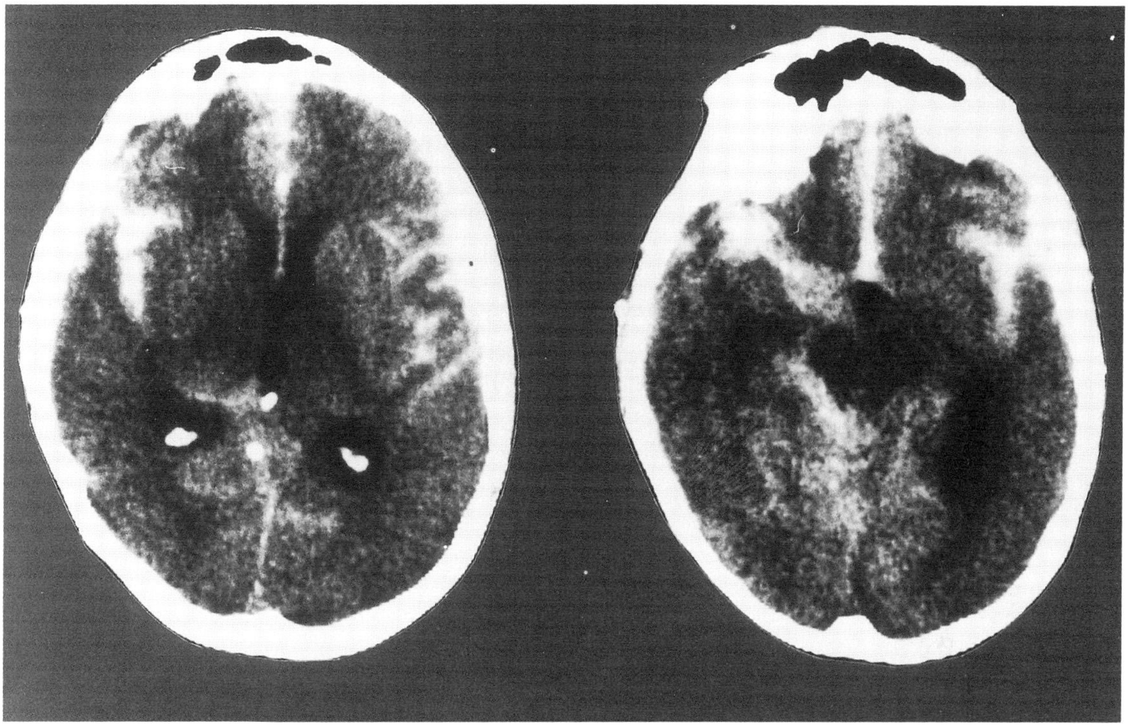

*Figure 1. Noncontrast-enhanced CT scan of a patient with a severe SAH due to a ruptured intracranial aneurysm. A thick subarachnoid clot can be seen filling the basal, sylvian, and insular cisterns as well as the frontal interhemispheric fissure.*

usually causing only motor weakness of the contralateral leg.

Peerless,[70] when examining a series of 420 patients with delayed deterioration following aneurysmal SAH, found the causes to be: 30% VSP, 14% hydrocephalus, 18% hyponatremia and volume depletion, and 6% recurrent subarachnoid or other intracranial bleeding. Other less common causes included aseptic meningitis, vascular occlusion and brain swelling, hypoxia, seizures, cardiac arrest, and pulmonary embolus.

## Angiography

In 1951, Ecker and Riemenschneider[14] described angiographic VSP following SAH for the first time. Discrepancies in cerebral arterial caliber on repeat angiograms were demonstrated in six patients suffering aneurysmal SAH. They noted that maximal spasm generally occurred at the aneurysm site, and that involvement of the major vessels may be associated with neurologic deterioration.

The overall incidence of angiographically demonstrable VSP in patients following aneurysmal SAH remains controversial, with reports varying from 21% to 62%.[63] This wide variation may be due to differences in criteria for defining VSP, experience of the radiologist, and technical quality of the films. (See Figure 3.)

Several large studies of patients suffering SAH, analyzed with similar angiographic criteria for the diagnosis of VSP, indicated that the incidence ranged from 31% to 51%.[81] This probably reflects the truest estimation as to the angiographic incidence of VSP following SAH.

Attempts have been made at a classification scheme of angiographic VSP, defining both type and severity.[68,81,98] This may be useful in predicting overall prognosis or in determining those patients at risk for developing focal

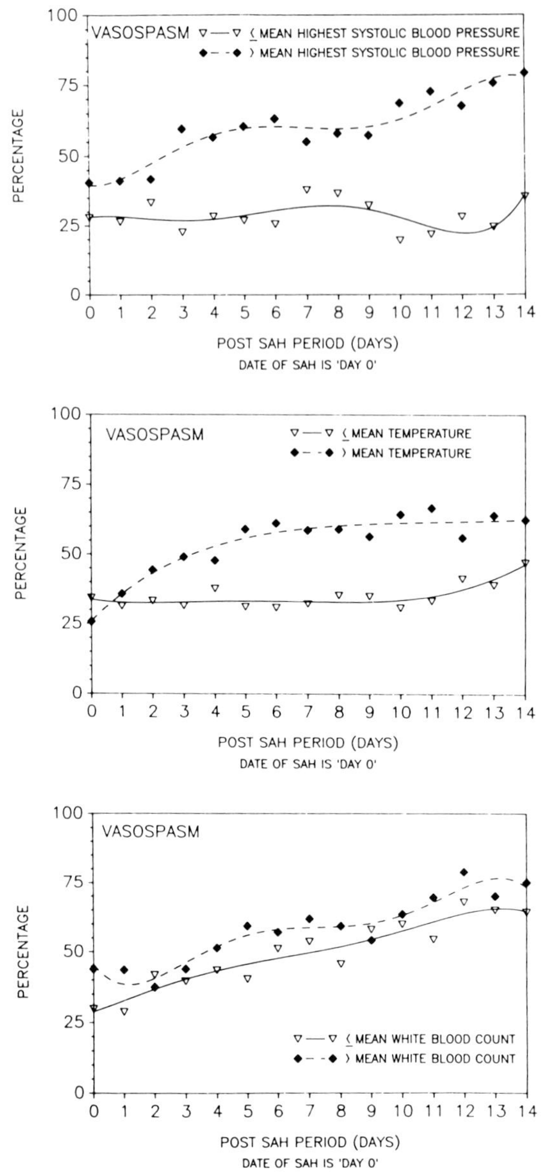


***Figure 2.*** *The percentage of patients who were either above or below the means for highest daily systolic blood pressure, temperature, and white blood cell count and who developed vasospasm is shown. For instance on day 3 post-SAH those with blood pressure above the mean had about a 50% chance of developing clinical vasospasm while those with blood pressure below the mean had about a 25%.*

neurologic deficits. Sano and Saito[81] described 3 types of angiographic VSP: type 1, extensive diffuse (worst prognosis); type 2, multisegmental (intermediate prognosis); and type 3, localized (favorable prognosis). In a smaller series of patients, Ohta et al[68] classified angiographic VSP into five types: diffuse, segmental, nodular, tapering, and centrally sparing. The authors found that the diffuse type was associated with the worst prognosis.

Fisher et al[27] developed a grading system in an effort to correlate severity of VSP with development of DIDs. They classified VSP into five types: Grade 0, no narrowing; Grade 1, lumen greater than 1 mm, Grade 2, lumen approximately 1 mm and distinct; Grade 3, lumen narrowed to approximately 0.5 mm with distinct borders; and Grade 4, lumen less than 0.5 mm and minimal forward flow. It was concluded that a strong propensity to develop VSP existed in the patient with grade 3 or 4 and not in those with the better grades 0, 1, and 2.

In summary, although angiography remains our most sensitive test in the diagnosis of VSP, newer adjunctive methods including transcranial Doppler (TCD) and cerebral blood flow (CBF) monitoring may help in reducing its use. Cerebral angiography is essential in preoperative localization of the aneurysm site in patients suffering SAH, and for now remains the gold standard to which other methods in the diagnosis of VSP are compared. Hopefully noninvasive magnetic resonance (MR) angiography or CT angiography will continue to improve with new technologic advances.

## *CT Scan*

In the Cooperative Aneurysm Study, Adams et al[2] examined CT scans of 1,378 patients following SAH and found that 96% showed evidence of bleeding on the day of the rupture. By day 3 post-SAH, CT scans with detectable intracranial blood had decreased to 74%. Similar results were shown by Findlay,[18] who reported a diagnostic success of 83% in early detection of SAH.

In addition to the diagnosis of SAH, the initial CT scan also demonstrates the location and quantity of subarachnoid blood, essential information in predicting those patients at risk of developing VSP.[27,51] (See Figure 4.)

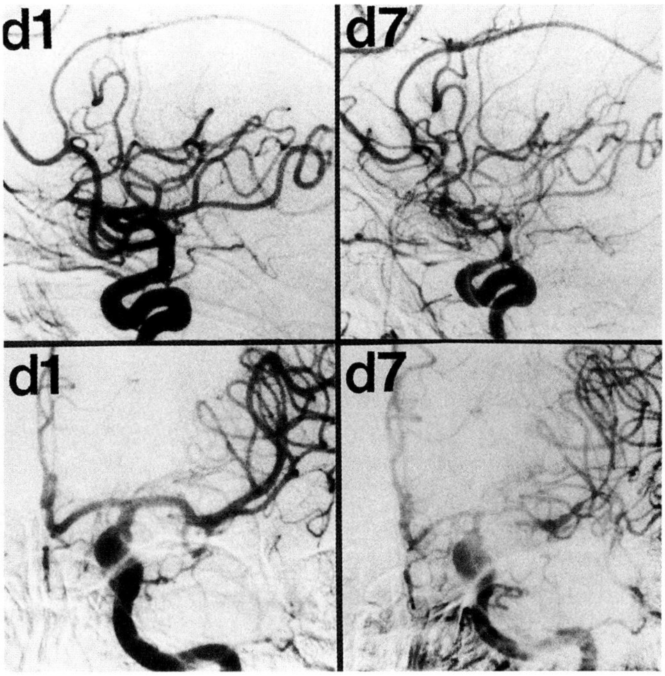


*Figure 3. Cerebral angiography (left carotid injection, anteroposterior and lateral views) demonstrating the development of severe vasospasm in the distribution of the left MCA, ACA, and distal internal carotid, 7 days from the initial hemorrhage.*

Japanese neurosurgeons were the first to demonstrate a relationship between the quantity of subarachnoid blood visualized on CT scan and the development of VSP.[50] Takemae et al[88] reported in 1978 on their series of 39 patients undergoing CT within 4 days following the onset of SAH. Vasospasm developed in 83% of the patients with high density areas in the basal cisterns and in none of the patients lacking high density areas on CT scan.

Fisher et al[27] in 1980 performed a retrospective analysis of 47 patients with SAH. The authors found a positive correlation between the amount and distribution of subarachnoid blood detected on CT scan and the delayed development of VSP. The CT scans were classified into four groups: Group 1, no blood detected; Group 2, diffuse blood greater than 1 mm thick; Group 3, localized clots greater than 1 mm thick; and Group 4, diffuse or no subarachnoid blood but with intracerebral or intraventricular clots. The authors found that 96% of those patients in Group 3, or with thick subarachnoid clot, developed VSP; and of those with no detectable subarachnoid blood on CT, only 1 of 18 patients developed severe VSP.

In a prospective study involving 41 patients, Kistler et al,[51] utilizing the same group classification, reported similar results. In 20 of 22 patients with thick subarachnoid clot (Group 3), severe VSP was correctly predicted, whereas in 14 of 19 patients with no blood, diffuse blood, or blood outside of the subarachnoid space, the absence of VSP was correctly predicted. Early recognition of patients in jeopardy of developing severe VSP allows for early implementation of prophylactic therapeutic measures.

The CT scan also plays a major role in the evaluation of patients for symptomatic VSP. Other etiologies of neurologic deterioration aside from VSP (hydrocephalus, rebleeding, intracranial hematoma, edema) should be ruled out with the aid of the CT scan. Finally, the CT scan can also be of use in identifying the extent and location of cerebral infarctions secondary to VSP. (See Figure 5.)

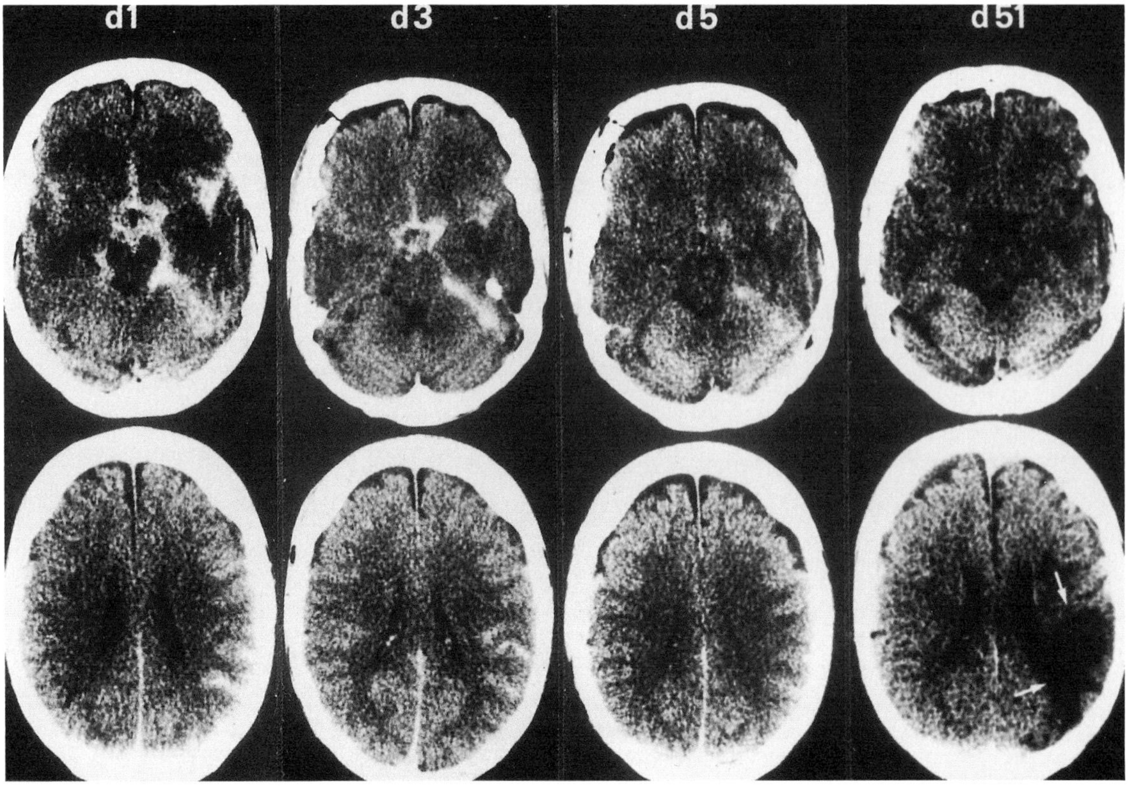


*Figure 4. The preoperative day 1 post-SAH CT scan showed that the most blood was contralateral to the posteriorly directed proximal internal carotid posterior-communicating aneurysm on the right. The amount of clot remained the same in the immediate postoperative CT scan done by day 3 post-SAH. Most of the subarachnoid blood was gone by day 5 post-SAH which was the day that delayed onset dysphasia and hemiparesis developed. On day 51 an infarct due to vasospasm was visible (see arrows).*

## *Transcranial Doppler*

Early detection of cerebral VSP was made possible in 1982 with the introduction to neurosurgery of TCD sonography by Aaslid et al.[1] The advent of a noninvasive technique of detecting, as well as assessing the severity and location of cerebral VSP was welcomed enthusiastically. There are several advantages of the TCD method over cerebral angiography including lower cost, no risk, and the possibility for repetitive examinations.[42]

The TCD is not a direct measurement of vessel diameter, but rather a measure of blood flow velocity. It is based on the principle that measurements of the mean blood flow velocity will be inversely proportional to changes in the vessel diameter. With the TCD method both peak and mean velocities are recorded and may be used to describe the arterial blood flow velocity. Considered to carry more physiologic significance, the mean flow velocity is less dependent on cerebral cardiovascular parameters and correlates more closely with perfusion. Although satisfactory intracranial recordings are possible in all basal vessels, the most useful information has been gained from examination of the MCA.[58] Studies have demonstrated a clear correlation between MCA diameter, as measured by angiography, and MCA mean flow velocity, as evidenced by TCD.[1,35] In a series of 50 healthy patients, Aaslid et al,[1] using the TCD method, reported a mean velocity of 62 cm/sec with a range of 33–90 cm/sec for the MCA. Seiler et al,[84] in an analysis of 39 patients following SAH, conducted serial TCD examinations to evaluate its diagnostic capability of VSP. The authors reported that maximal mean flow velocities

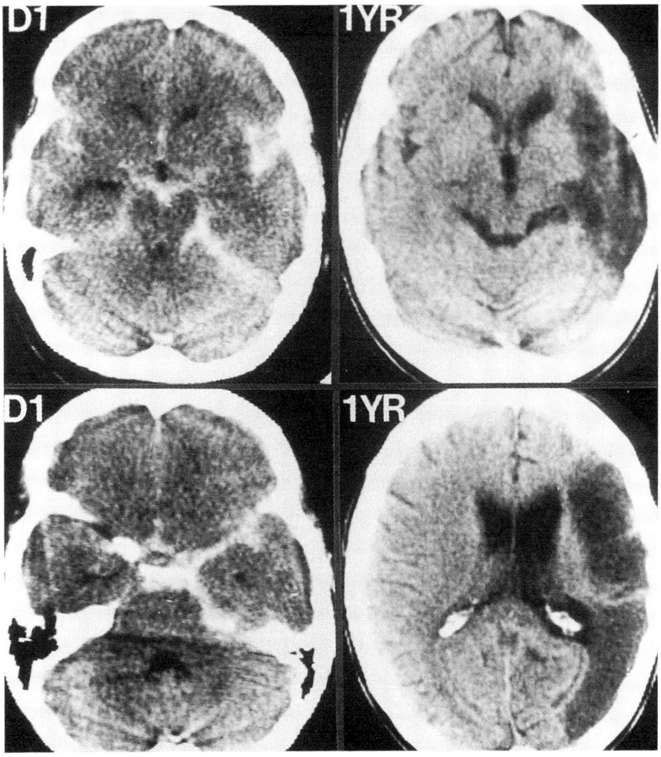


*Figure 5. Patient with severe SAH as seen on CT scan at day 1. The effects of severe vasospasm have resulted in a massive left-sided cerebral infarction apparent on CT scan at 1 year.*

greater than 200 cm/sec were usually associated with symptomatic ischemia and infarction, whereas all patients with velocities measuring less than 140 cm/sec remained asymptomatic. (See Figures 6 and 7.)

TCD studies which have followed the time course of cerebral VSP following SAH have closely paralleled studies utilizing angiography.[35] Klingelhofer et al[52] evaluated cerebral VSP by TCD and simultaneous ICP measurement in a series of 76 patients suffering aneurysmal SAH. The authors reported that a pronounced elevation in ICP was accompanied by reduction of mean velocities, and that the evaluation of time course and severity of VSP, based entirely upon the TCD measurement of mean flow velocity in the presence of raised ICP, can result in false-negative results.

Current recommendations for TCD include an early baseline evaluation prior to the onset of VSP.[78] This should be followed by daily recordings throughout the first 2 weeks post-SAH. Particular attention should be paid to a daily elevation in mean velocity.

## *Cerebral Blood Flow*

Numerous studies have demonstrated the relationship between diminished CBF and the development of delayed neurologic deficits secondary to cerebral VSP.[104,107] Many of these deficits due to ischemia are potentially reversible if sufficient blood flow is restored prior to cerebral infarction. Various methods have been sought to assess and quantify the regional CBF, thereby differentiating reversible from irreversible neurologic deficits.[91]

Several technologies exist for the clinical measurement of CBF in patients suffering aneurysmal SAH.[105] The earliest studies using radiolabeled xenon ($^{133}Xe$) were only possible through intra-arterial injections, thereby limiting use of this technique. With the advent of intravenously and inhalationally

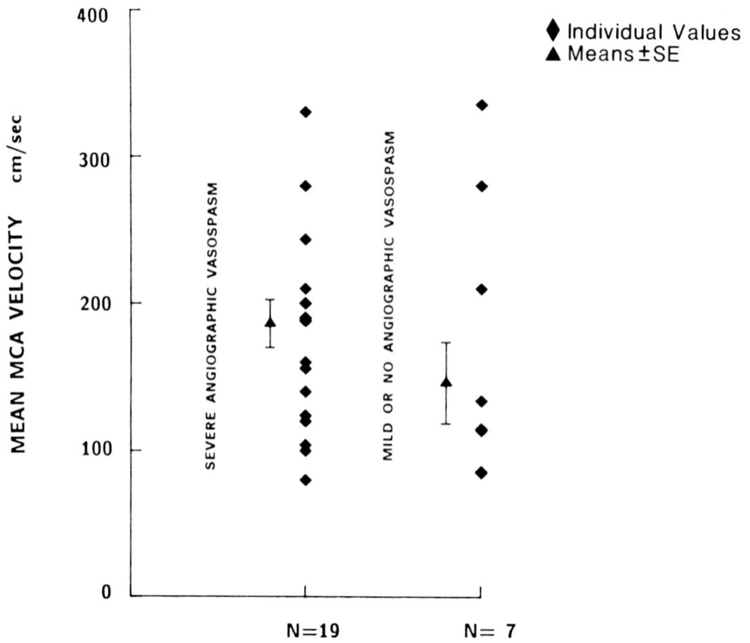


*Figure 6. The highest daily mean MCA velocity (as measured by TCD) for each case with severe angiographic vasospasm and with no or mild angiographic vasospasm. The means of the two groups are not significantly different.*

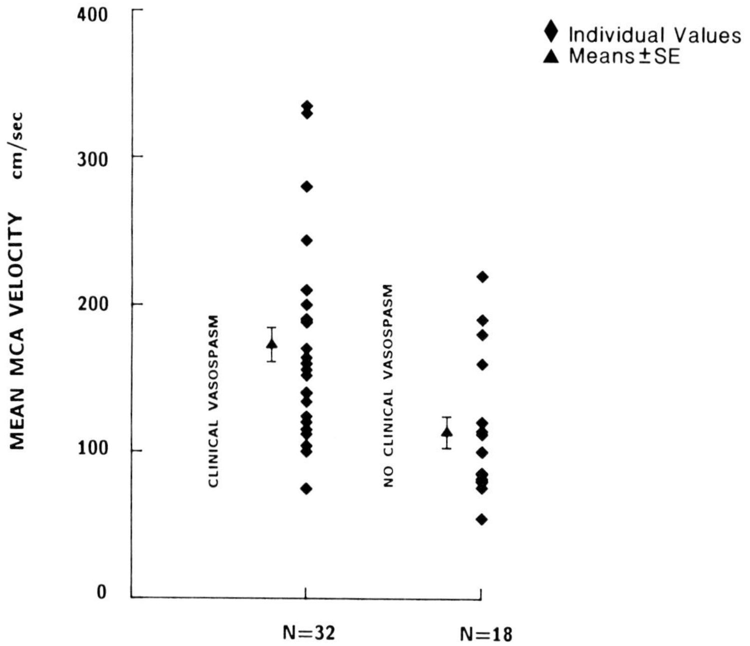


*Figure 7. The highest daily mean MCA velocity (as measured by TCD) for each case with a diagnosis of clinical vasospasm or no clinical vasospasm. The difference was highly significant. Many of these symptomatic episodes were transient.*

administered $^{133}$Xe, which provides stable xenon-enhanced CT, CBF studies gained popularity[95] due to their good resolution and accurate quantitative information.[91]

The more recent development of positron emission tomography (PET), in addition to the quantitative measure of CBF, provides information on the regional cerebral metabolic rate of oxygen and oxygen extraction fraction.[77]

As VSP becomes increasingly severe, regional blood flow falls, resulting in compensatory peripheral vasodilation of intracerebral vessels, thus increasing cerebral blood volume.[30] As oxygen delivery to the ischemic tissue fails, relatively more oxygen is extracted and the oxygen extraction fraction increases.

Yamakami et al[104] in a series of 35 patients suffering aneurysmal SAH, examined the relationship between regional CBF and angiographically demonstrable VSP. The authors observed a significant flow reduction in those patients demonstrating severe VSP, whereas patients with mild VSP showed no decrease in blood flow. There was also a strong correlation between the development of DIDs and severe VSP.

Despite the usefulness of CBF measurements in demonstrating the causal relationship between reduced CBF and both angiographic and symptomatic VSP, the time, expense, and complexity of the technique still limit its use in routine clinical practice.[95]

## Prevention

### *Calcium Channel Antagonists*

While many therapies aimed at the prevention of VSP remain experimental, the use of calcium channel blockers has been an effective means in improving clinical outcome as well as decreasing the incidence of infarction in clinical trials. Except for nicardipine there has been no evidence that calcium channel blockers significantly prevent large vessel narrowing following SAH, which suggests that they might have an effect in vasodilating smaller vessels in the parenchyma, or have a neuronal protective action.[74]

Although a variety of calcium channel blockers are commercially available, nimodipine, and more recently nicardipine have been used in the area of neurovascular studies due to their relative neurovascular selectivity. Nimodipine, a dihydropyridine, is structurally related to nifedipine. Nimodipine is lipophilic and therefore crosses the blood-brain barrier easily, demonstrating relative selectivity for blocking the influx of extracellular calcium into cerebrovascular smooth muscle (*Nimodipine,* American Hospital Formulary Service, Drug Information Supplement B. 1989:12B–18B).

In 1983, Allen et al[6] reported the first prospective trial of nimodipine following SAH. The study was prospective, double blind, randomized, placebo-controlled, and involved the initiation of nimodipine versus placebo therapy within 96 hours of SAH. In addition to daily assessments, the final neurologic outcome was determined through a detailed neurologic exam performed within 7 days following completion of treatment. Severe deficits associated with cerebral VSP occurred in 8 of 60 (13%) patients receiving the placebo and in only 1 of 56 (2%) patients receiving nimodipine. Other investigators have reported similar results demonstrating that nimodipine clearly reduces morbidity in patients following SAH.[74,75]

Petruk et al[74] demonstrated that the use of oral nimodipine in poor grade aneurysm patients resulted in a decreased incidence and severity of DIDs. In a series of 157 patients the authors reported the incidence of permanent neurologic deficits to be 29% of 72 patients in the nimodipine group versus 47% of 82 patients in the control.

The largest study to date, published by Pickard et al,[76] was a multicenter British trial involving 554 patients. The authors reported that although mortality did not differ between the 2 groups, those receiving nimodipine had a significant reduction in both poor outcome and cerebral infarction. In assessing incidence and severity of angiographic VSP, they found no intergroup differences.

Despite the proven clinical benefit of nimodipine following SAH, its mechanism of action remains uncertain. Hypotheses include (1) increased microcirculatory collateral flow, not angiographically detectable,[29] and (2) a direct neuronal cytoprotective effect.[74]

The newest cerebrovascular selective calcium channel blocker to be studied clinically is nicardipine.[31] Haley et al[31] in a randomized, double blind, multicenter study administered either nicardipine or placebo to patients following acute aneurysmal SAH. The authors reported that in addition to demonstrating a 30% reduction in symptomatic VSP in the nicardipine group, there was also a 20% reduction in angiographic VSP.

## Clot Removal

One of the first clinical studies suggesting that subarachnoid clot in the proximity of the basal vessels plays a major role in the causation of VSP was carried out by Suzuki et al.[87] In a series of 413 patients admitted with aneurysmal SAH, patients with surgical repair and clot removal within 24 hours had an improved outcome and a decrease in the incidence of postoperative VSP. The authors hypothesized that early operation and clot removal allowed for control of ICP and prevention of VSP.

In another study, a variety of spasmogenic factors resulting from blood clot breakdown were identified and demonstrated experimentally to induce VSP.[92] It was therefore predicted that early operation and removal of the subarachnoid blood clot in the acute stage following SAH could decrease the incidence of VSP and improve outcome.

Mizukami and associates[61] performed surgery within 4 days and attempted radical clot removal in 64 patients suffering SAH. Follow-up analysis was carried out by CT scan to determine the effectiveness of clot removal, and angiography was used to determine the incidence and severity of VSP. In areas where blood clot was effectively removed, only mild or no VSP occurred and all patients remained neurologically intact. In approximately 10% of the patients, when it was surgically impossible to remove portions of the clot (i.e. frontal interhemispheric fissure and posterior aspect of the insular cisterns), permanent delayed neurologic deficits secondary to VSP sometimes occurred.

Taneda,[89] in a series of 239 patients, studied the effect of both the timing of surgery and the extent of clot removal on the incidence of VSP and clinical outcome. Of 101 patients operated on within 48 hours with extensive clot removal, only 11% developing DIDs suffered morbidity or mortality. Among the 94 patients operated on within the same time period but with limited clot removal, 28% had poor outcome. In the final group, operation was delayed for 10 days or more and among these patients a poor outcome was seen in 25% of 44 patients.

At the University of Alberta, studies have been conducted examining both the effect and timing of clot removal in a primate model of SAH.[34,65] Nosko et al randomized 24 monkeys into 3 groups undergoing either sham operation, clot placement only, or clot placement and removal within 24 hours. All of the animals in which the clot was left in place demonstrated significant VSP, whereas none of the animals in the sham operated or clot removal groups demonstrated significant VSP. Furthermore, 25% of the animals in the clot group developed severe ischemic deficits versus none in the other groups.

As a followup to this study, Handa et al,[34] using the same model, evaluated the timing of clot removal in preventing VSP. Thirty monkeys were randomized into 1 of 5 groups: (1) sham operated; (2) clot removal at 48 hours after SAH; (3) clot removal at 72 hours; (4) clot removal at 96 hours; and (5) clot placement only. The authors found no significant VSP in any of the cerebral arteries in the 48 hours or sham groups. In contrast, significant VSP was seen in all cerebral vessels of the 96-hour group and in the internal carotid artery (ICA) and ACA of the 72-hour group.

Despite these encouraging studies, several difficulties exist. It is widely believed that total clot removal from the basal cisterns is both technically difficult and potentially dangerous to the patient.[43] For these reasons, mechanical clot removal is not widely practiced in North America.

## *Fibrinolytic Agents*

The problems with mechanical clot removal have encouraged the utilization of pharmacologic agents introduced intrathecally in the hope of lysing clot and preventing VSP.

Using a feline model of cerebral VSP, Peterson et al[71] injected a combination of streptokinase and streptodornase into the intrathecal space of cats 1 hour following experimental SAH. After 3 hours each animal was sacrificed and examined for the quantity of remaining clot. Although the authors found a complete dissolution of clot in all animals, the animals suffered severe meningoencephalitis. Alksne et al[4] in a pig model of SAH, reported a decrease in post-SAH vasculopathy following the single intrathecal injection of plasmin.

Kodama et al[54] in a clinical trial of 179 patients suffering SAH, grades II–IV, used a continuous intrathecal infusion of urokinase and ascorbic acid. Following early operation and mechanical clot removal, irrigating catheters were placed into one or both sylvian fissures and into the preclinoid or internal carotid cistern. Twelve hours following the operation a continuous intrathecal infusion of urokinase and ascorbic acid in a Ringer's solution was begun. The duration of therapy ranged from 4–14 days with a mean of 9.6 days. The authors reported that only 3 of 83 patients (3.1%) in the drug-treated group developed symptomatic VSP versus 37 of 96 control patients (38.5%).

Utilizing the primate model of experimental SAH, Findlay et al demonstrated the safety and efficacy of intrathecally administered recombinant tissue plasminogen activator (rt-PA) in clot dissolution and prevention of VSP.[20,22,23,25] Their first study was a randomized, controlled, blinded design, involving 3 intrathecal injections of 0.5 mg of rt-PA over a 24-hour period, in monkeys who had undergone experimental SAH.[25] The injections began 1 day following the induction of SAH; 7 days later angiography was repeated and the animals sacrificed. The authors found that in the rt-PA–treated group virtually all of the clot was dissolved and VSP was prevented, whereas all of the placebo group demonstrated large remaining subarachnoid clots and severe VSP. In followup studies using the same model and design, they have also shown that rt-PA injected intrathecally from a unilateral site was effective in diffusing through the basal cisterns and lysing a bilateral clot.[20] Finally, in 2 studies involving the timing and dosage of rt-PA administration, it was determined that 0.75 mg injected intrathecally was sufficient to completely lyse a 5-ml clot if administered within 72 hours of the hemorrhage.[23]

Stemming from the clear evidence that rt-PA is both safe and efficacious in lysing subarachnoid clot and preventing VSP, several clinical trials are under way and preliminary results have been favorable.[24,60,66,106]

## *21-Aminosteroids*

Recent experimental trials of the nonglucocorticoid 21-aminosteroid U74006F or tirilazad mesylate were based upon the suggestive evidence of the involvement of free radical generation and lipid peroxidation in the pathogenesis of VSP.[82]

During conversion of oxyhemoglobin to methemoglobin in the perivascular clot, a number of oxygen-free radicals are liberated[80] including superoxide anion, hydrogen peroxide, and singlet oxygen. These free radicals can cause damage to the cerebrovascular endothelium, alteration in vascular tone, and initiation of lipid peroxidation. This latter pathway leads to the production of lipid peroxides which have been shown experimentally to be potent cerebral vasoconstrictors.[80,82]

Hall and Travis[32] showed that the 21-aminosteroid U74006F, a potent inhibitor of iron-catalyzed lipid peroxidation, retarded development of post-SAH cerebral hypoperfusion in a feline model. The authors speculated that the mechanism was threefold: (1) improved mean arterial blood pressure and cerebral perfusion pressure (CPP); (2) inhibition of lipid peroxidative damage to the cerebral vasculature; and (3) control of post-SAH rise in ICP.

Steinke et al[86] evaluated the efficacy of U74006F in the prevention of angiographic VSP in a primate model of SAH. Twenty hours following experimental SAH, therapy was begun with U74006F and continued just prior to sacrifice on day 7. They reported a significant reduction in angiographic VSP in the treatment group versus placebo. Zuccarello et al,[109] in a similar experimental design, demonstrated that pretreatment with U74006F completely prevented SAH-induced VSP in rabbits.

Kanamaru et al[46] of the University of Alberta evaluated various dosages of U74006F in preventing VSP in the primate model following SAH. They reported that each of the 3 dosages (0.3 mg/kg, 1.0 mg/kg, or 3.0 mg/kg) was equally effective in preventing chronic VSP. More recently the authors have also demonstrated a significant reduction in malondialdehyde (a by-product of lipid peroxidation) in the clot of U74006F-treated monkeys versus placebos, 7 days following experimental SAH.[47]

Currently, the safety and efficacy of this agent is being investigated in clinical trials.[19]

### *Other Strategies*

Some evidence has suggested a link between chronic cerebral VSP following SAH and the inflammatory response.[9] The data are based largely upon the detection of increased concentration and activity of various inflammatory mediators such as eicosanoids, prostaglandins, cytokines, as well as circulating immune complexes, and the inherent ability of these agents to cause vasoconstriction and/or vascular damage.[9] These observations have led to a number of investigations in the use of NSAIDs and steroids in the prevention of VSP.

Chyatte et al[10] in a series of 21 patients suffering aneurysmal SAH, evaluated the use of high-dose methylprednisolone in preventing cerebral VSP. All patients in the study were judged to be of high risk to develop VSP based on admission CT scan or clinical grade. The authors reported that methylprednisolone-treated patients demonstrated a lower morbidity and mortality than those not receiving steroids. More recently, in a canine model of SAH these authors have shown that both ibuprofen and methylprednisolone could prevent or significantly reduce angiographic VSP.[8]

The prophylactic value of the immunosuppressive agent cyclosporin in preventing SAH-induced cerebral VSP has recently been evaluated in animals. Peterson et al[72] reported that cyclosporin A led to a reduction in both incidence and severity of angiographic VSP in a canine model. Differing results were reported by Handa et al[33] in a primate model of SAH.

Although early experimental evidence has demonstrated favorable results with anti-inflammatory agents in preventing VSP and improving outcome in animals, further randomized clinical trials are required.

## Management

Without question, the ideal means of managing VSP is prevention. Unfortunately this is not always possible. For those patients developing symptomatic VSP there are a number of effective and widely used treatment modalities which limit further neurologic deterioration, such as hypertensive, hypervolemic, hemodilutional therapy, and nimodipine.

### *Management of ICP and Ventilation*

Measurements of ICP following aneurysmal SAH have been documented extensively in the literature.[37,38,64,93,94] During most cases of acute aneurysmal rupture there is a sudden rise in ICP, followed by a gradual decline to baseline levels.[93]

Continuous ICP measurement in patients suffering aneurysmal SAH was pioneered by

Nornes and Magnaes.[64] In a series of 9 patients they described 2 types of pressure patterns recorded during aneurysm rupture. Type 1 involved a sudden pressure peak followed by the immediate decline in pressure to the baseline. Type 2, associated with a more severe bleed, was described as a sudden increase in pressure, dramatic clinical deterioration, and sustained pressure elevation.

Hayashi et al[38] monitored the ICP in 12 patients with diffuse VSP following aneurysmal SAH. They reported an early decline of ICP at the onset of VSP, followed by a gradual secondary rise in ICP, believed to be due to ischemic brain swelling or infarction.

Voldby and Enevoldsen[94] while monitoring the ICP in 52 patients suffering aneurysmal SAH, found a close relationship between increased ICP and decline in neurologic status. They also reported reversal of neurologic deficits through the control of ICP in patients with angiographically mild VSP.

Fearnside and Adams[17] advocated the use of ventricular drainage and mannitol infusion in an effort to maintain the ICP below 25 mm Hg as a first line of management. Other treatment methods include elevation of head of bed to 30 degrees with minimal angulation of neck, muscle paralysis, hypothermia, and barbiturate coma.[96] Ventilatory goals should include maintenance of $pCO_2$ at the lower limit of normal and provision of $pO_2$ sufficient to achieve maximal oxygen delivery.

Mechanical ventilation of the patient suffering aneurysmal SAH is generally reserved for those patients in poor clinical grades. Intubation and mechanical ventilation provide airway protection and manipulation of ventilatory parameters. Positive end-expiratory pressure may prevent atelectasis and other pulmonary complications.[95] Of specific concern to those patients with VSP is the reduction in reactivity of the cerebral vessels to $CO_2$.[13,36]

Petruk et al[73] in a primate model of VSP performed correlative studies of CBF and vessel diameter during graded $pCO_2$ changes. They found a significant augmentation in CBF in response to profound hypercapnia which was independent of changes in vessel diameter.

## *Induction of Hypertension, Hypervolemia, and Hemodilution*

The first published observation of further neurologic deterioration following hypotension in patients suffering cerebrovascular accidents was made by Denny-Brown in 1951.[12] He noted that in patients with severe structural narrowing of cerebral vessels, the concomitant presence of hypotension produced clinical worsening. He theorized that by initiating steps to raise systemic blood pressure, it was possible to prevent or treat recurrent cerebrovascular symptoms.

The above observations were substantiated in patients suffering cerebrovascular insufficiency.[16,101] Through efforts to increase systolic blood pressure with volume expanders and/or vasopressors, it was possible to reverse neurologic symptoms secondary to cerebral ischemia.[16,101]

Consequent to each of these treatment modalities is improvement in CBF. This may result from an increase in the CPP or an improvement in flow states achieved through a decrease in blood viscosity or hemodilution.[39] CPP may in turn be increased through a decrease in ICP, a rise in systemic blood pressure, or both.[39]

Studies have suggested that improvement in CBF in vasospastic arteries may have a greater dependence upon blood pressure and viscosity.[19,104] Therefore investigators have focused their attention upon the improvement in cardiac output by augmentation of preload and increasing cardiac contractility, in addition to decreasing blood viscosity through hemodilution.[19]

In a series of 7 patients suffering symptomatic VSP following SAH, Kosnik and Hunt[55] were successful in reversing ischemic deficits in 6, using a combination of vasopressor-induced hypertension and volume expansion.

Giannotta et al[28] examined a series of 17 patients presenting with severe neurologic compromise from postoperative VSP. In all patients, the central venous pressures (CVPs) were monitored and an initial attempt was made to reverse symptoms through volume expansion. Phenylephrine and/or dopamine were employed only in cases failing hypervolemic therapy. The authors reported complete reversal of symptoms in 12 patients and partial reversal in 3 patients.

Kassell et al[49] in a large series of patients were able to permanently reverse the neurologic deterioration in 43 of 58 patients with angiographically confirmed VSP following SAH. The treatment, which was generally continued for a period of 7 days, consisted of induced arterial hypertension, volume expansion, and vagal blockade. Systolic blood pressure was raised as high as 240 mm Hg in those patients with surgically secured aneurysms and to 160 mm Hg in patients prior to surgery. Despite rigorous monitoring, they reported a number of therapy-induced complications, including aneurysmal rebleeding (19%), pulmonary edema (17%), dilutional hyponatremia (3%), coagulopathy (3%), pneumothorax (2%), and myocardial infarction (2%).

More recently, Awad et al[7] treated a series of 113 SAH patients of whom 36% demonstrated subsequent symptomatic VSP with a similar regimen of hypertension and hypervolemia. CVP was maintained between 10–12 mm Hg, and systolic blood pressure kept between 110–200 mm Hg. Eighty-four percent of cases with clinical VSP who were treated showed either improvement in neurologic symptoms or no further deterioration, whereas only 16% demonstrated clinical worsening despite therapy. Overall, serious morbidity and mortality from VSP was less than 7%.

Solomon et al[85] reported a series of 56 patients considered to be high risk for development of VSP. Utilizing a protocol of hypervolemic and hypertensive therapy they were able to prevent the development of delayed neurologic deterioration in 46 patients (82%).

Wood et al[102,103] have suggested the additional rheologic advantage of dilutional hypervolemia with the use of low molecular weight dextran and/or albumin in preventing symptomatic VSP. This theory suggests that through a decrease in blood viscosity there is a decrease in cerebrovascular resistance and a resultant augmentation of CBF. While reviewing rheologic therapy in acute cerebral ischemia, Wood suggested[102] that a hematocrit of approximately 30% would be ideal for both oxygen transport and improved flow states.

The rapidity with which dopamine increases blood pressure makes it our preferred initial pressor therapy following hypervolemia. Swan-Ganz catheters are generally inserted in patients whose deterioration is known to be due to VSP not immediately responding to moderate blood pressure elevation and fluid manipulation, and in any patient with compromised cardiac or pulmonary function.

## *Balloon Angioplasty*

Transluminal angioplasty is gaining increasing usage as a treatment of symptomatic VSP. This technique was first reported by Zubkov et al[108] who performed a total of 105 dilatations in a series of 33 patients utilizing transluminal angioplasty. They reported successful regression of neurologic deficits in all patients. Eskridge reported 12 patients with symptomatic VSP who underwent balloon angioplasty.[15] The results demonstrated sustained improvement in symptoms in 75% of the patients within 48 hours of the procedure. Higashida et al[41] achieved success in 71% of 14 patients using balloon angioplasty to reverse the acute effects of cerebral ischemia.

Despite the success of this procedure to treat acute neurologic deficits secondary to VSP, it is generally accepted that it should be reserved for a highly selected patient population.[40] Specific guidelines suggested by

Eskridge et al[15] include: (1) the new onset of neurologic deficit post-SAH not attributable to other causes; (2) no evidence of infarction on a recent CT scan; (3) neurologic deficit not reversed by hypervolemic and hypertensive therapy; (4) angiographically apparent VSP in a location that could be responsible for the deficit.

To achieve maximal success with balloon angioplasty with an acceptable complication rate, the procedure should be performed as quickly as possible following the onset of symptoms in patients with secured aneurysms by experienced interventional angiographers.

The complications include conversion of pale infarcts into hemorrhagic ones, rupture of blood vessels and incompletely clipped aneurysms, and the displacement of clips from aneurysms. A disadvantage of the method is the difficulty and increased risk in catheterizing A1 and M1 and more distal, smaller vessels which may be spastic.

## *Vasodilators*

Since it has been assumed that VSP results from persistent contraction, a number of investigators have sought agents capable of producing direct vasodilation.[70] Unfortunately, potential problems exist with the use of these agents. In the presence of acute VSP with marginal ischemia, the systemic administration of vasodilators may induce systemic hypotension and aggravate ischemia.[39] Therefore there has been an increasing interest in the intrathecal, topical, or local intra-arterial administration of these agents.[95,100]

Wilkins reviewed a wide variety of vasodilatory drugs that have been studied experimentally and clinically. Aside from the cerebrovascular selective calcium channel blockers, results for the most part have been generally disappointing. Isoproteronol, salbutemal, phentolamine, propranolol, reserpine, aminophylline, prostacyclin, nipride, and papaverine are agents demonstrated to be partially effective in reducing VSP either through the direct dilatation of cerebral arteries or the antagonism of their constriction.[100]

Recently, clinical studies involving the agents calcitonin-gene-related peptide administered intravenously[45] and intracisternal papaverine[83] have reported encouraging results in reversing VSP. The ability to deliver higher concentrations of drugs by super-selective catheterization and intra-arterial infusion to arteries most involved will lead to advances in therapy. (See Figure 8.)

## *Summary*

Over the past decade, significant progress has been made in the areas of detection, prevention, and management of cerebral VSP following aneurysmal SAH. Recent advances have significantly reduced the resultant mortality and serious morbidity to less than 25%. As the understanding of the pathophysiology of cerebral VSP improves, so too will our ability to prevent and treat its occurrence.

Patients with large volume SAH are more likely to have a poor initial grade and to develop after several days progressive contraction of the larger basal conducting arteries. This can last from days to several weeks and may so reduce flow that ischemic infarction develops. Early surgery and secural of the ruptured aneurysm not only prevents rebleeding but permits removal by mechanical means of as much clot as possible, probably reducing the risk of VSP. It also permits the safer use of hypertension, hypervolemia, intra-arterial vasodilators, and balloon angioplasty if severe clinical manifestations of VSP develop. The early use of calcium antagonists and the maintenance of optimal fluid balance are helpful. New compounds such as the 21-aminosteroids may act to ameliorate the effects of SAH. The intrathecal instillation of fibrinolytic agents such as rt-PA may prevent VSP by promoting the rapid dissolution and absorption of the clot. Super-selective catheterization and intra-arterial delivery of high concentration of vasodilators may be helpful in reversing established VSP.

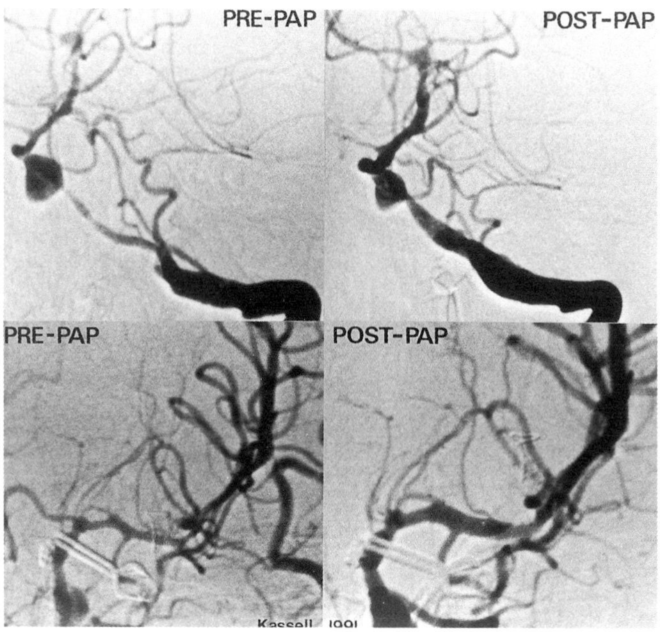


***Figure 8.*** *Top: Cerebral angiography demonstrating severe vasospasm of the distal left vertebral and proximal basilar arteries* ***(left)****. Following intra-arterial papaverine infusion normal patency of the vertebral basilar system is apparent* ***(right)****.* ***Bottom:*** *Anteroposterior view of the left ICA demonstrating severe vasospasm involving the distal carotid and middle cerebral arteries* ***(left)****. Following intra-arterial papaverine normal patency of these vessels can be observed (right).*

# References


1. Aaslid R, Markwalder T-M, Nornes H. Noninvasive transcranial Doppler ultrasound recording of flow velocity in basal cerebral arteries. *J Neurosurg.* 1982;57:769–774.
2. Adams HP Jr, Kassell NF, Torner JC, et al. CT and clinical correlations in recent aneurysmal subarachnoid hemorrhage: a preliminary report of the Cooperative Aneurysm Study. *Neurology.* 1983; 33:981–988.
3. Adams HP Jr, Kassell NF, Torner JC, et al. Predicting cerebral ischemia after aneurysmal subarachnoid hemorrhage: influences of clinical condition, CT results, and antifibrinolytic therapy: a report of the Cooperative Aneurysm Study. *Neurology.* 1987;37:1586–1591.
4. Alksne JF, Branson PJ, Bailey M. Modification of experimental post-subarachnoid hemorrhage vasculopathy with intracisternal plasmin. *Neurosurgery.* 1986;19:20–25.
5. Alksne JF, Branson PJ, Bailey M. Modification of experimental post-subarachnoid hemorrhage vasculopathy with intracisternal plasmin. *Neurosurgery.* 1988;23:335–337.
6. Allen GS, Ahn HS, Preziosi TJ, et al. Cerebral artery spasm: a controlled trial of nimodipine in patients with subarachnoid hemorrhage. *N Engl J Med.* 1983;308:619–624.
7. Awad IA, Carter LP, Spetzler RF, et al. Clinical vasospasm after subarachnoid hemorrhage: response to hypervolemic hemodilution and arterial hypertension. *Stroke.* 1987;18:365–372.
8. Chyatte D. Prevention of chronic cerebral vasospasm in dogs with ibuprofen and high-dose methylprednisolone. *Stroke.* 1989;20:1021–1026.
9. Chyatte D. Anti-inflammatory agents and cerebral vasospasm. *Neurosurg Clin North Am.* 1990;1:433–450.
10. Chyatte D, Fode NC, Nichols DA, et al. Preliminary report: effects of high dose methylprednisolone on delayed cerebral ischemia in patients at high risk for vasospasm after aneurysmal subarachnoid hemorrhage. *Neurosurgery.* 1989;21:157–160.
11. Cruickshank JM, Neil-Dwyer G, Brice J. Electrocardiographic changes and their prognostic significance in subarachnoid hemorrhage. *J Neurol Neurosurg Psychiatry.* 1974;37:755–759.
12. Denny-Brown D. The treatment of recurrent cerebrovascular symptoms and the question of "vasospasm." *Med Clin North Am.* 1951;35:1457–1474.
13. Diringer MN, Heffez DS, Monsein L, et al. Cerebrovascular $CO_2$ reactivity during delayed vasospasm in a canine model of subarachnoid hemorrhage. *Stroke.* 1991;22:367–372.
14. Ecker A, Riemenschneider PA. Arteriographic demonstration of spasm of the intracranial arteries. *J Neurosurg.* 1951;8:660–667.

15. Eskridge JM, Newell DW, Pendleton GA, et al. Transluminal angioplasty for treatment of vasospasm. *Neurosurg Clin North Am.* 1990;1:387–398.
16. Farhat SM, Schneider RC. Observations on the effect of systemic blood pressure on intracranial circulation in patients with cerebrovascular insufficiency. *J Neurosurg.* 1967;27:441–445.
17. Fearnside MR, Adams CBT. The treatment of raised intracranial pressure following aneurysm surgery. *J Neurol Neurosurg Psychiatry.* 1980; 43:957–961.
18. Findlay GFG. Computer-assisted (axial) tomography in the management of subarachnoid hemorrhage. *Surg Neurol.* 1980;13:125–128.
19. Findlay JM, Macdonald RL, Weir BKA. Current concepts of pathophysiology and management of cerebral vasospasm following aneurysmal subarachnoid hemorrhage. *Cerebrovasc Brain Metab Rev.* Winter,1991;3:336–361.
20. Findlay JM, Weir BKA, Gordon P, et al. Safety and efficacy of intrathecal thrombolytic therapy in a primate model of cerebral vasospasm. *Neurosurgery.* 1989;24:491–498.
21. Findlay JM, Weir BKA, Kanamaru K, et al. Arterial wall changes in cerebral vasospasm. *Neurosurgery.* 1989;25:736–746.
22. Findlay JM, Weir BKA, Kanamaru K, et al. Intrathecal fibrinolytic therapy after subarachnoid hemorrhage: dosage study in a primate model and review of the literature. *Can J Neurol Sci.* 1989;16:28–40.
23. Findlay JM, Weir BKA, Kanamaru K, et al. The effect of timing of intrathecal fibrinolytic therapy on cerebral vasospasm in a primate model of subarachnoid hemorrhage. *Neurosurgery.* 1990;26:201–206.
24. Findlay JM, Weir BKA, Kassell NF, et al. Intracisternal recombinant tissue plasminogen activator after aneurysmal subarachnoid hemorrhage. *J Neurosurg.* 1991;75:181–188.
25. Findlay JM, Weir BKA, Steinke D, et al. Effect of intrathecal thrombolytic therapy on subarachnoid clot and chronic vasospasm in a primate model of SAH. *J Neurosurg.* 1988;69:723–735.
26. Fisher CM. Clinical syndromes in cerebral thrombosis, hypertensive hemorrhage, and ruptured saccular aneurysm. *Clin Neurosurg.* 1975;22:117–147.
27. Fisher CM, Kistler JP, Davis JM. Relation of cerebral vasospasm to subarachnoid hemorrhage visualized by computerized tomographic scanning. *Neurosurgery.* 1980;6:1–9.
28. Giannotta SL, McGillicuddy JE, Kindt GW. Diagnosis and treatment of postoperative cerebral vasospasm. *Surg Neurol.* 1977;8:286–290.
29. Godfraind T, Miller R, Wibo M. Calcium antagonism and calcium entry blockade. *Pharmacol Rev.* 1987;38:321–416.
30. Grubb RL Jr, Raichle ME, Eichling JO, et al. Effect of subarachnoid hemorrhage on cerebral blood volume, blood flow, and oxygen utilization in humans. *J Neurosurg.* 1977;46:446–453.
31. Haley EC, Turner JC, Kassell NF, et al. Cooperative randomized study of nicardipine in subarachnoid hemorrhage: preliminary report. In: Sano K, Takakura K, Kassell NF, et al, eds. *Cerebral Vasospasm.* Tokyo: University of Tokyo Press; 1990: 519–525.
32. Hall ED, Travis MA. Effects of the nonglucocorticoid 21-aminosteroid U74006F on acute cerebral hypoperfusion following experimental subarachnoid hemorrhage. *Exp Neurol.* 1988; 102:244–248.
33. Handa Y, Hayashi M, Takeuchi H, et al. Effect of cyclosporine on the development of cerebral vasospasm in a primate model. *Neurosurgery.* 1991; 28:380–386.
34. Handa Y, Weir BKA, Nosko M, et al. The effect of timing of clot removal on chronic vasospasm in a primate model. *J Neurosurg.* 1987;67:558–564.
35. Harders AG, Gilsbach JM. Time course of blood velocity changes related to vasospasm in the circle of Willis measured by transcranial Doppler ultrasound. *J Neurosurg.* 1987;66:718–728.
36. Hassler W, Chioffi F. $CO_2$ reactivity of cerebral vasospasm after aneurysmal subarachnoid hemorrhage. *Acta Neurochir (Wien).* 1989;98:167–175.
37. Hayashi M, Kitano T, Handa Y, et al. Changes of intracranial pressure, cerebral blood flow and clinical status in patients with diffuse cerebral vasospasm after rupture of intracranial aneurysm [in Japanese]. *Neurol Med Chir (Tokyo).* 1979; 19:1139–1148. English abstract.
38. Hayashi M, Marukawa S, Fujii H, et al. Intracranial pressure in patients with diffuse cerebral arterial spasm following ruptured intracranial aneurysms. *Acta Neurochir (Wien).* 1978;44:81–95.
39. Heros RC, Zervas NT, Negoro M. Cerebral vasospasm. *Surg Neurol.* 1976;5:354–362.
40. Higashida RT, Halbach VV, Cahan LD, et al. Transluminal angioplasty for treatment of intracranial arterial vasospasm. *J Neurosurg.* 1989;71:648–653.
41. Higashida RT, Halbach VV, Dormandy B, et al. New microballoon device for transluminal angioplasty of intracranial arterial vasospasm. *AJNR.* 1990;11:233–238.
42. Hutchison K, Weir B. Transcranial Doppler studies on aneurysm patients. *Can J Neurol Sci.* 1989; 16:411–416.
43. Inagawa T, Yamamoto M, Kamiya K. Effects of clot removal on cerebral vasospasm. *J Neurosurg.* 1990;72:224–230.
44. Johnson RJ, Potter JM, Reid RG. Arterial spasm and subarachnoid hemorrhage: mechanical considerations. *J Neurol Neurosurg Psychiatry.* 1958; 21:68. Abstract.
45. Johnston FG, Bell BA, Miller JD. Calcitonin gene related peptide in delayed cerebral ischaemia. In: Sano K, Takakura K, Kassell NF, et al, eds. *Cerebral Vasospasm.* Tokyo: University of Tokyo Press; 1990:396–399.
46. Kanamaru K, Weir BKA, Findlay JM, et al. A dosage study of the effect of the 21-aminosteroid U74006F on chronic cerebral vasospasm in a primate model. *Neurosurgery.* 1990;27:29–38.
47. Kanamaru K, Weir BKA, Simpson J, et al. Effect of 21-aminosteroid U-74006F on lipid peroxidation in subarachnoid clot. *J Neurosurg.* 1991; 74:454–459.
48. Kassell NF, Haley EC, Torner JC, et al. Nicardipine and angiographic vasospasm. *J Neurosurg.* 1991; 74:341A. Abstract.
49. Kassell NF, Peerless SJ, Durward QJ, et al. Treatment of ischemic deficits from vasospasm with intravascular volume expansion and induced arterial hypertension. *Neurosurgery.* 1982;11:337–343.

50. Katada K, Kanno T, Sano H, et al. Computed tomography of ruptured intracranial aneurysm in acute stage [in Japanese]. *No Shinkei Geka.* 1977;5:955–963. English abstract.
51. Kistler JP, Crowell RM, Davis KR, et al. The relation of cerebral vasospasm to the extent and location of subarachnoid blood visualized by CT scan: a prospective study. *Neurology.* 1983; 33:424–436.
52. Klingelhöfer J, Sander D, Holzgraefe M, et al. Cerebral vasospasm evaluated by transcranial Doppler ultrasonography at different intracranial pressures. *J Neurosurg.* 1991;75:752–758.
53. Kodama N, Mizoi K, Sakurai Y. Incidence and onset of vasospasm. In: Wilkins RH, ed. *Cerebral Arterial Spasm.* Baltimore, Md: Williams & Wilkins; 1980:361–365.
54. Kodama N, Sato M, Yamanobe K, et al. Prevention of vasospasm cisternal irrigation therapy with urokinase and ascorbic acid. In: Sugita K, Shibuya M, eds. *Intracranial Aneurysms and Anteriovenous Malformations — State of Art.* Nagoya: Nagoya University COOP Press; 1990:151–155.
55. Kosnik EJ, Hunt WE. Postoperative hypertension in the management of patients with intracranial arterial aneurysms. *J Neurosurg.* 1976;45:148–154.
56. Ljunggren B, Brandt L, Kågström E, et al. Results of early operations for ruptured aneurysms. *J Neurosurg.* 1981;54:473–479.
57. MacDonald RL, Weir BKA, Runzer TD, et al. Etiology of cerebral vasospasm in primates. *J Neurosurg.* 1991;75:415–424.
58. Mani RL, Eisenberg RL. Complications of catheter cerebral arteriography: analysis of 5,000 procedures, II: relation of complication rates to clinical and arteriographic diagnosis. *AJR.* 1978;131:867–869.
59. Maroon JC, Nelson PB. Hypovolemia in patients with subarachnoid hemorrhage: therapeutic implications. *Neurosurgery.* 1979;4:223–226.
60. Mizoi K, Yoshimoto T, Fujiwara S, et al. Prevention of vasospasm by clot removal and intrathecal bolus injection of tissue-type plasminogen activator: preliminary report. *Neurosurgery.* 1991;28:807–813.
61. Mizukami M, Takemae T, Tazawa T, et al. Value of computed tomography in the prediction of cerebral vasospasm after aneurysm rupture. *Neurosurgery.* 1980;7:583–586.
62. Newell DW, Winn HR. Transcranial Doppler in cerebral vasospasm. *Neurosurg Clin North Am.* 1990;1:319–328.
63. Niizuma H, Kwak R, Otabe K, et al. Angiographic study of cerebral vasospasm following the rupture of intracranial aneurysms, II: relation between the site of aneurysm and the occurrence of vasospasm. *Surg Neurol.* 1979;11:263–267.
64. Nornes H, Magnaes B. Intracranial pressure in patients with ruptured saccular aneurysm. *J Neurosurg.* 1972;36:537–547.
65. Nosko M, Weir KA, Lunt A, et al. Effect of clot removal at 24 hours on chronic vasospasm after SAH in the primate model. *J Neurosurg.* 1987; 66:416–422.
66. Öhman J, Servo A, Heiskanen O. Effect of intrathecal fibrinolytic therapy on clot lysis and vasospasm in patients with aneurysmal subarachnoid hemorrhage. *J Neurosurg.* 1991;75:197–201.
67. Ohta H, Ito S, Yasui N, et al. Extensive evacuation of subarachnoid clot for prevention of vasospasm: effective or not? *Acta Neurochir (Wien).* 1982; 63:111–116.
68. Ohta T, Kawamura J, Osaka K, et al. Angiographic classification of so-called cerebral vasospasm: correlation between existence of vasospasm and postoperative prognosis in subarachnoid hemorrhage [in Japanese]. *No To Shinkei.* 1969;21:1019–1027. English abstract.
69. Osaka K. Prolonged vasospasm produced by the breakdown products of erythrcytes. *J Neurosurg.* 1977;47:403–411.
70. Peerless SJ. Pre- and postoperative management of cerebral aneurysms. *Clin Neurosurg.* 1979;26:209–231.
71. Peterson EW, Choo SH, Lewis AJ, et al. Lysis of blood clot and experimental treatment of subarachnoid hemorrhage. In: Wilkins RH, ed. *Cerebral Arterial Spasm.* Baltimore, Md: Williams & Wilkins; 1980:625–627.
72. Peterson JW, Nishizawa S, Hackett JD, et al. Cyclosporin A reduces cerebral vasospasm after subarachnoid hemorrhage in dogs. *Stroke.* 1990;21: 133–137.
73. Petruk KC, Weir BK, Overton TR, et al. The effect of graded hypocapnia and hypercapnia on regional cerebral blood flow and cerebral vessel caliber in the rhesus monkey: study of cerebral hemodynamics following subarachnoid hemorrhage and traumatic internal carotid spasm. *Stroke.* 1973;5:230–246.
74. Petruk KC, West M, Mohr G, et al. Nimodipine treatment in poor-grade aneurysm patients: results of a multicenter double-blind placebo-controlled trial. *J Neurosurg.* 1988;68:505–517.
75. Philippon J, Grob R, Dagreou F, et al. Prevention of vasospasm in subarachnoid hemorrhage: a controlled study with nimodipine. *Acta Neurochir (Wien).* 1986;82:110–114.
76. Pickard JD, Murray GD, Illingworth R, et al. Effect of oral nimodipine on cerebral infarction and outcome after subarachnoid hemorrhage: British aneurysm nimodipine trial. *Br Med J.* 1989;298: 636–642.
77. Powers WJ, Grubb RL Jr, Baker RP, et al. Regional cerebral blood flow and metabolism in reversible ischemia due to vasospasm. *J Neurosurg.* 1985; 62:539–546.
78. Romner B, Ljunggren B, Brandt L, et al. Transcranial Doppler sonography within 12 hours after subarachnoid hemorrhage. *J Neurosurg.* 1989;70:732–736.
79. Saito I, Sano K. Vasospasm after aneurysm rupture: incidence, onset, and course. In: Wilkins RH, ed. *Cerebral Arterial Spasm.* Baltimore, Md: Williams & Wilkins; 1980:294–301.
80. Sano K. Cerebral vasospasm and aneurysm surgery. *Clin Neurosurg.* 1983;30:13–58.
81. Sano K, Saito I. Timing and indication of surgery for ruptured intracranial aneurysms with regard to cerebral vasospasm. *Acta Neurochir (Wien).* 1978; 41:49–60.
82. Sasaki T, Tanishima T, Asano T, et al. Significance of lipid peroxidation in the genesis of chronic vasospasm following rupture of an intracranial aneurysm. *Acta Neurochir Suppl (Wien).* 1979;28:536–540.

83. Segawa H, Saito I, Okada T, et al. Efficacy of intracisternal papaverine on symptomatic vasospasm. In: Wilkins RH, ed. *Cerebral Vasospasm.* New York, NY: Raven Press; 1988:433–441.
84. Seiler RW, Grolimund P, Aaslid R, et al. Cerebral vasospasm evaluated by transcranial ultrasound correlated with clinical grade and CT-visualized subarachnoid hemorrhage. *J Neurosurg.* 1986; 64:594-600.
85. Solomon RA, Fink ME, Lennihan L. Early aneurysm surgery and prophylactic hypervolemic hypertensive therapy for the treatment of aneurysmal subarachnoid hemorrhage. *Neurosurgery.* 1988; 23:699–704.
86. Steinke DE, Weir BKA, Findlay JM, et al. A trial of the 21-aminosteroid U74006F in a primate model of chronic cerebral vasospasm. *Neurosurgery.* 1989;24:179–186.
87. Suzuki A, Yasui N, Hadeishi H, et al. Causes of poor results of early surgery for ruptured intracranial aneurysms in elderly patients [in Japanese]. *Neurol Med Chir (Tokyo).* 1988;28:1157–1162. English abstract.
88. Takemae T, Mizukami M, Kin H, et al. Computed tomography of ruptured intracranial aneurysms in acute stage: relationship between vasospasm and high density on CT scan [in Japanese]. *No To Shinkei.* 1978;30:861–866. English abstract.
89. Taneda M. Effect of early operation for ruptured aneurysms on prevention of delayed ischemic symptoms. *J Neurosurg.* 1982;57:622–628.
90. Toda N, Shimizu K, Ohta T. Mechanism of cerebral arterial contraction induced by blood constituents. *J Neurosurg.* 1980;53:312–322.
91. Touho H, Karasawa J, Shishido H. Vasospasm and local cerebral blood flow in patients with ruptured intracranial aneurysm. In: Sano K, Takakura K, Kassell NF, et al, eds. *Cerebral Vasospasm.* Tokyo: University of Tokyo Press; 1990:35–37.
92. Towart R. The pathophysiology of cerebral vasospasm, and pharmacological approaches to its management. *Acta Neurochir (Wien).* 1982;63:253–258.
93. Voldby B, Enevoldsen EM. Intracranial pressure changes following aneurysm rupture, I: clinical and angiographic correlations. *J Neurosurg.* 1982; 56:186–196.
94. Voldby B, Enevoldsen EM. Intracranial pressure changes following aneurysm rupture, II: associated cerebrospinal fluid lactacidosis. *J Neurosurg.* 1982; 56:197–204.
95. Weir B. *Aneurysms Affecting the Nervous System.* Baltimore, Md: Williams & Wilkins; 1986:505–569.
96. Weir B, Disney L, Grace M, et al. Daily trends in white blood cell count and temperature after subarachnoid hemorrhage from aneurysm. *Neurosurgery.* 1989;25:161–165.
97. Weir B, Grace M, Hansen J, et al. Time course of vasospasm in man. *J Neurosurg.* 1978;48:173–178.
98. Weir B, Rothberg C, Grace M, et al. Relative prognostic significance of vasospasm following subarachnoid hemorrhage. *Can J Neurol Sci.* 1975; 2:109–114.
99. White RP, Hagen AA, Robertson JT. Effect of nonsteroid anti-inflammatory drugs on subarachnoid hemorrhage in dogs. *J Neurosurg.* 1979;51:164–171.
100. Wilkins RH. Attempts at prevention or treatment of intracranial arterial spasm: an update. *Neurosurgery.* 1986;18:808–825.
101. Wise G, Sutter R, Burkholder J. The treatment of brain ischemia with vasopressor drugs. *Stroke.* 1972;3:135–140.
102. Wood JH. Hypervolemic hemodilution: rheologic therapy for acute cerebral ischemia. *Contemp Neurosurg.* 1982;4:1–6.
103. Wood JH, Simeone FA, Kron RE, et al. Rheological aspects of experimental hypervolemic hemodilution with low molecules weight dextran: relationships of cortical blood flow, cardiac output, and intracranial pressure to fresh blood viscosity and plasma volume. *Neurosurgery.* 1982;11:739–753.
104. Yamakami I, Isobe K, Yamaura A, et al. Vasospasm and regional cerebral blood flow (rCBF) in patients with ruptured intracranial aneurysm: serial rCBF studies with xenon-133 inhalation method. *Neurosurgery.* 1983;13:394-401.
105. Yonas H. Cerebral blood measurements in vasospasm. *Neurosurg Clin North Am.* 1990;1:307–318.
106. Zabramski JM, Spetzler RF, Lee S, et al. Phase I trial of tissue plasminogen activator for the prevention of vasospasm in patients with aneurysmal subarachnoid hemorrhage. *J Neurosurg.* 1991; 75:189–196.
107. Zingesser LH, Schechter MM, Dexter J, et al. On the significance of spasm associated with rupture of a cerebral aneurysm: the relationship between spasm as noted angiographically and regional cerebral blood flow determinations. *Arch Neurol.* 1968;18:520–528.
108. Zubkov YN, Nikiforov BM, Shustin VA. Balloon catheter technique for dilation of constricted cerebral arteries after aneurysmal SAH. *Acta Neurochir (Wien).* 1984;70:65–79.
109. Zuccarello M, March JT, Schmitt G, et al. Effect of the 21-aminosteroid U-74006F on cerebral vasospasm following subarachnoid hemorrhage. *J Neurosurg.* 1989;71:98–104.

# CHAPTER 11

# Endovascular Treatment of Aneurysms and Cerebral Vasospasm

Leo N. Hopkins, MD, Lee R. Guterman, PhD, MD, Kimberly Livingston, MD, Kevin J. Gibbons, MD, and Arvind Ahuja, MD

Endovascular neurosurgery represents a hybridization of neurosurgery, interventional neuroradiology, and neuroscience critical care. The successful development of an endovascular neurosurgical service requires active participation of multiple disciplines in the hospital environment. Both neurosurgeons and radiologists skilled in cerebral vessel catheterization have contributed to the evolution and growth of this field over the past 20 years. Technologic feats accomplished in the catheter industry have propelled this specialty into the limelight of the neurosurgical world. Development of microcatheters and guide wires capable of providing access to cerebral vessels 1 mm in diameter has allowed neuro-interventionists to treat lesions of the intracranial circulation without craniotomy. Application of digital storage and image enhancement technology to cerebral angiography has revolutionized endovascular neurosurgery. Ability to perform a cerebral angiogram and store the digital image has produced a template over which realtime fluoroscopic images can be superimposed. As a result, a roadmap of cerebrovascular anatomy can be used to guide the microcatheter into regions of the brain previously accessible only through surgical exposure.

Two American corporations were responsible for the rapid growth of this field since the mid-1980s. Interventional Therapeutics Corporation of South San Francisco, California, pioneered the development of silicone balloon technology for aneurysm thrombosis and angioplasty. Target Therapeutics of San Jose, California, created microcatheter and guide wire systems that enabled canalization of cerebral vessels of 1 mm in diameter. Target also developed platinum microcoils that promote thrombosis in cerebral vessels.

This chapter presents a chronologic history of the development of endovascular techniques for the treatment of aneurysms and cerebral vasospasm. The authors' philosophy concerning patient selection is described. The techniques presently available for the endovascular treatment of cerebral aneurysms are reviewed. The postoperative management of intensive care unit patients and the importance of long-term followup for patients receiving experimental therapeutic intervention are discussed.

## Historical Background

The first description of a catheter-based treatment of a cerebral aneurysm was published in 1964 by Luessenhop and Velasquez.[35] They reported an unsuccessful attempt to induce aneurysm thrombosis by placing a silicone balloon into an aneurysm of the supraclinoid carotid artery.

## *Balloons*

In 1973, Serbinenko performed the first successful treatment of a saccular aneurysm with a detachable latex balloon. The aneurysm cavity thrombosed while patency of the lumen of the parent artery was maintained. One year later, Serbinenko[43] reported 300 cases of balloon catheter occlusion of major cerebral vessels. Catheter placement was achieved by direct puncture of the internal carotid artery (ICA). Only 3 of the 300 reported cases involved successful treatment of cerebral aneurysms with detachable balloons. Treatment of 1 basilar artery (BA) and 2 supraclinoid carotid artery aneurysms was described. No followup was reported. Before these 3 successful cases, 2 deaths during treatment of BA aneurysms were reported. Serbinenko described the use of a temporary balloon occlusion catheter to provide proximal occlusion in a vessel harboring an aneurysm. The balloon could be deflated while a polymer or coagulant was injected. Reinflation of the balloon would facilitate flow direction of the coagulant substance into the aneurysm cavity. No details were described concerning the system used for detachable balloon occlusion of aneurysms.

In 1981, Debrun et al[7] reported 9 patients with unclippable giant aneurysms treated with detachable balloons. Four patients had a superficial temporal artery to middle cerebral artery (MCA) bypass before sacrificing the parent vessel by detachable balloon occlusion. One patient had an arterial ligation without bypass. Debrun concluded that sacrifice of the parent artery appeared safer than direct aneurysm obliteration.

Also, in 1981, Hieshima et al[16] published a technical note describing a detachable balloon for therapeutic transcatheter occlusions. An inflatable silastic balloon was secured to a coaxial catheter system via miter valve.

In 1982, Romodanov and Shcheglov[41] reported 137 intravascular occlusions of saccular aneurysms of the cerebral arteries using a detachable balloon catheter. Between 1974 and 1980, 119 patients were treated. Followup varied between 1 month and 6 years. Fifteen patients had the parent vessel obliterated. Only 2 patients were treated following subarachnoid hemorrhage (SAH). One hundred and four patients presented in "satisfactory neurologic condition" before embolization. Complete obliteration of the aneurysm cavity without compromise of the parent vessel was achieved in 93 patients. Only 3 of 119 patients experienced recanalization of the aneurysm lumen. Four deaths were reported, 3 from thrombosis of the ICA and 1 from pneumonia. Details of patient followup were not provided.

In 1984, Berenstein et al[4] reported 14 patients with giant aneurysms of the cavernous-carotid and vertebral arteries. The lumen of the parent vessel was sacrificed in all cases. In one instance, an attempt was made to treat the aneurysm cavity; this resulted in recanalization, and the parent artery was subsequently sacrificed.

In 1986, Hieshima et al[18] placed two detachable silicone balloons into a left carotid-ophthalmic artery aneurysm. After 8 months, complete angiographic obliteration of the aneurysm was maintained. In that same year, Hieshima et al[19] reported balloon occlusion of a distal BA aneurysm with proximal BA stenosis. Balloon angioplasty was employed to widen the proximal BA and facilitate placement of the silicone balloons. The patient developed slight dysmetria, and the proximal posterior cerebral arteries were noted to be narrowed bilaterally. In 1987, Higashida et al[26] reported a patient who was asymptomatic 1 year after balloon embolization of a giant cavernous-carotid artery aneurysm. No followup angiogram was obtained.

In 1987, Fox et al[11] published a series of 68 patients with unclippable aneurysms. Thirty-five had an extracranial-intracranial arterial bypass (EIAB) prior to balloon occlusion of the artery that harbored the aneurysm. Balloon placement was either proximal and/or distal to the aneurysm orifice. No attempts were made to treat the aneurysm cavity directly.

Later that year, Hieshima[20] reported balloon occlusion of an anterior cerebellar artery aneurysm that had bled repeatedly. After placement of two balloons, the patient developed a subtle right hemiparesis and was placed on sodium warfarin. Followup angiography 3 months later demonstrated obliteration of the aneurysm cavity with preservation of the lumen of the parent vessel. In 1988 Higashida et al[25] reported 80% occlusion following balloon embolization of a carotid ophthalmic artery aneurysm in which attempted EIAB, clipping, and wrapping had failed.

In 1988, Goto et al[13] reported development of a polymer (2-hydroxy-ethyl-methacrylate, HEMA) that, when injected into a silicone balloon within an aneurysm cavity, resulted in permanent solidification of the inflated balloon shape. Initiating the polymerization reaction was simple, reproducible, and facilitated at physiologic temperatures. Later that year, Higashida et al[24] reported complete obliteration of a cavernous-carotid artery aneurysm with a silicone balloon filled with HEMA. After 1 year, the aneurysm remained occluded.

In 1989, Higashida et al[22] published a series of 25 patients with 26 aneurysms of the posterior circulation. Fifteen patients had previous SAH, and 10 had mass effect. In 17 cases, the lumen of the parent artery was preserved. Nine cases required total occlusion of the parent artery. There were 5 deaths, 3 strokes, and 3 transient ischemic attacks. Patients were heparinized during the procedure. Protamine was used to normalize the coagulation process afterwards. Sixty percent of the patients were neurologically intact and stable from 2–43 months following the procedure.

In a 1990 review article, Hieshima et al[17] cited a 4% morbidity and 6% stroke rate in over 200 patients treated with balloon embolization of intracranial vascular abnormalities. There was radiologic evidence of a decreased mass effect following balloon placement. Preliminary data indicated that if an aneurysm was occluded after 6 months, there was a decreased risk of rebleeding. Only 1 patient was reported to have had SAH 6 months after balloon occlusion of an aneurysm.

In 1990, Higashida et al[21] reported a series of 84 patients with intracranial aneurysms treated with detachable silicone balloons, 59 in the anterior circulation and 25 in the posterior circulation. Thirty-one patients presented with acute SAH. The time interval between initial bleed and balloon embolization was not reported. This treatment was restricted to patients who either failed surgical clipping, could not tolerate general anesthesia, or those with anatomically inaccessible aneurysms (cavernous-carotid, midbasilar region). Balloon embolization was felt to be the sole option for intervention in this group. Fifteen deaths were reported, 10 of which resulted from growth and rupture of the aneurysm cavity following balloon placement. There were 9 strokes following balloon placement, the majority caused by liberation of fresh thrombus within the aneurysm cavity during placement of the detachable balloon. In one case, the HEMA liberated from a ruptured balloon migrated distally into the cerebral circulation, resulting in thrombotic stroke. Nineteen of the 84 aneurysms treated were greater than 3 cm in diameter. Sixty-five were totally occluded by placement of 1 or more balloons. Nineteen were subtotally treated, occluding at least 85% of the aneurysm cavity.

In 1990, Shcheglov[44] presented the results of the Kiev experience at the Stonwin lectures in Scarsdale, New York. During a 14-year period, 725 endovascular procedures were performed on intracerebral aneurysms using latex balloon embolization. In each case, the shape of the balloon was tailored to the angiographic appearance of the aneurysm. In 91% of cases, the aneurysm was treated without compromising the lumen of the parent vessel. Seventeen of the 725 cases were performed less than 3 weeks post-SAH. Aneurysms greater than 5 cm in diameter were treated with multiple balloons followed by surgical clipping. Of the 617 patients, the outcome was reported as "good" in 80% and "fair" in 20%. Thirty-three patients died, a mortality rate of 5.4%. The definitions of "good" and "fair" are not provided in the report. At the same conference, Serbinenko presented the Moscow experience of 267 patients treated over a 19-year period.[30] Most procedures involved inoperable aneurysms. In 67% of cases, the aneurysm was occluded from the parent vessel with "good" results. Thirty-seven patients had EIAB prior to endovascular therapy. Thromboembolism of cerebral vessels occurred in 7.9% of cases. Postoperative mortality was 7.5%.

### *Coils*

In 1988, Target Therapeutics marketed a series of platinum coils designed to induce thrombosis after delivery into an aneurysm cavity via the Tracker® catheter system. The authors' experience demonstrated that these coils were easily placed within the body of the aneurysm. Unfortunately, the thrombogenic potential of the platinum was variable, and coil migration out of the aneurysm cavity into the distal cerebral circulation was reported.[40] In 1989, Target improved the thrombogenicity of the coils by incorporating Dacron® threads into the tertiary coil structure. Although the thrombogenicity improved and the amount of postplacement migration decreased, control during coil placement was limited. Once the coil was ejected from the catheter tip, its final position was flow directed with no mechanism available for retrieval.

Since the introduction of microcoils there has been insufficient time for large patient series with followup to be reported. The majority of case reports and small series have been presented at national meetings. During the 1991 meeting of the American Society of Neuroradiology, more than 50 patients with intracranial aneurysms treated by thrombogenic microcoils were reported. Pruvo et al[40] reported 15 patients treated with Target coils. Eleven aneurysms were angiographically obliterated, 4 were subtotally treated. In 3 patients, coils migrated out of the aneurysm after placement, resulting in regressive complete motor paralysis. Lemme-Plaghos et al[32] reported 11 aneurysms treated with Target Flower™ coils. Six were intracavernous. Of these, 3 were subtotally occluded and 2 were angiographically obliterated. One patient had a fatal bleed shortly after treatment. Fox et al[10] reported treatment of 5 patients with Target Flower coils. Four procedures were performed in the acute phase post-SAH. After treatment, all aneurysms were left with residual necks. Casasco et al[6] reported 16 patients treated with microcoils. Five were asymptomatic and 11 had experienced previous SAH. In 12 patients, greater than 90% of the aneurysm was angiographically occluded, with no recurrent hemorrhage after 1 year.

In 1991, Guglielmi et al[14,15] introduced an electrothrombotic detachable coil system that enabled readjustment of coil position before final detachment. They reported treatment in 15 patients, 21–69 years of age. Eight patients had experienced recent SAH. Electrothrombotic coils were placed to occlude between 70% to 100% of the aneurysm cavity. One parent artery harboring an aneurysm was thrombosed. No patients experienced permanent neurologic deficit. Aneurysms of the posterior circulation were subtotally occluded, while aneurysms of the anterior circulation were radiographically obliterated.

## Patient Selection

All endovascular techniques presently used for the treatment of intracranial aneurysms are experimental. Although they have been used for years, few have the approval of the Food and Drug Administration (FDA). As a result, the availability of catheters and embolic material is controlled, and distribution presently is restricted to approved centers involved in FDA protocols. The experimental nature of these procedures requires prior approval by each institution's Internal Review Board. A detailed consent outlining the experimental nature of the procedure and all possible complications must be drafted and distributed to participants. To date, the total number of cases performed with any one device is too low to assign statistical significance to complications. Aneurysms in different locations of the cerebral circulation carry different risks. Patients and their families must understand these facts before the procedure is performed.

Patients with unruptured intracranial aneurysms undergo embolization procedures in an awake, yet sedated state so that repeated neurologic examination can be performed during the procedure. An acute deterioration in neurologic status helps determine the course of endovascular therapy and patient management. Although the endpoint for endovascular treatment of aneurysms is angiographic obliteration, acute compromise of vital vascular anatomy can quickly change the focus of therapy. It is crucial that patients remain still while fluoroscopy is being performed. The majority of patients with freshly ruptured aneurysms are agitated, and sedation levels required to control movement and pain often produce unacceptable respiratory depression. Intubation assures adequate control of the patient's airway and provides a mechanism for hyperventilation. Unfortunately, the ability to perform an adequate neurologic exam during the procedure is lost. The UCLA group has utilized EEG monitoring during embolization procedures, but this can be awkward and limit angiographic visualization of vital vascular structures (personal communication: Viñuela F, Madison, Wisconsin, March 1991). Intubation and sedation also facilitate tight blood pressure control and permit induced hypotension.

In acute SAH and cases where general anesthesia is required or where repeated neurologic examinations are not possible, the authors feel that endovascular treatment of patients requires incorporation of principles used during open surgery. Monitoring by ventriculostomy can provide warning of an acute rise in intracranial pressure (ICP) and can maximize cerebral blood flow by drainage. Endovascular treatment of aneurysms following acute SAH should be performed under induced hypotension, i.e. the mean arterial pressure should be reduced by at least 20% to 30% prior to placement of the delivery catheter. Induced hypotension serves to prevent rapid changes in transmural pressure and can decrease the tension in the aneurysm wall.

### *Preoperative Preparation*

Preoperative preparation for elective endovascular intervention includes a complete blood count, partial thromboplastin and activated partial tissue thromboplastin, bleeding time, blood chemistry, urinalysis with microscopic exam, electrocardiogram (ECG), and chest x-ray. Patients are admitted 24 hours before the procedure and are hydrated with dextrose normal saline. Intravenous lines are established, and a Foley catheter is inserted before the procedure. Sixty milligrams of nimodipine is administered orally every 4 hours, and 4 mg of dexamethasone is given intravenously every 6 hours. Both sides of the groin are shaved and prepped before the procedure. A thorough neurologic exam is documented.

On arrival to the angiography suite, the patient is placed on an automated recycled blood pressure cuff for continuous blood pressure monitoring. A radial arterial line is placed when needed. ECG is monitored, and a pulse oximeter is used throughout the procedure. A nitroprusside drip, intravenous labetalol, and nitroglycerine are available for blood pressure control. Hydromorphone hydrochloride, morphine, midazolam hydrochloride, and premixed inotropic solutions are also at hand. After the guide catheter has been positioned, the patient is given 3,000–5,000 units of intravenous heparin, followed by 1,000 units every hour. All arterial flush packs are prepared with 1 unit of heparin/ml of normal saline. Activated clotting time is monitored throughout the procedure to ensure adequate anticoagulation.

## Treatment Techniques and Devices

Presently, three endovascular techniques dominate the treatment of intracranial aneurysms: balloons, coils, and electrothrombotic coils. All require placement of a large caliber guide catheter after percutaneous cannulation of the femoral artery. Typically, an 18-gauge needle is introduced into the femoral artery using the Seldinger technique.[42] A short, polymer-coated guide wire is then inserted through the needle and the needle is removed. A 7-9 French introducer sheath is placed over the wire into the femoral artery and flushed with heparinized saline via pressurized container. A large caliber angiography catheter with a polymer-coated guide wire is inserted through the sheath into the aorta, and guided into the ascending aorta under fluoroscopic visualization. The choice of guide catheter is dictated by the endovascular system in use, the tortuosity of the patient's vasculature, and the condition of the patient's vessels. This catheter is advanced distally into the cervical carotid or distal vertebral vessel harboring the aneurysm. A rotating hemostatic adapter is attached to the proximal end of the guide catheter and continuously flushed with heparinized saline (Figure 1). The rotating hemostatic adapter provides a three-way connection, as well as an adjustable gasket seal, for introduction of smaller caliber catheters into the guide catheter.

Placement of the delivery catheter into the distal cerebral circulation is facilitated by superimposition of a realtime fluoroscopic image onto a digitized and stored cerebral angiogram. The latter provides a road map for the fluoroscopic image of the advancing catheter. The delivery system then can be directed into small intracranial vessels, reducing the risk of perforation. Realtime visualization of the advancing delivery system into the body of the aneurysm cavity minimizes the probability of aneurysm rupture.

## *Balloons*

Placement of the guide catheter for the silicone balloon system (Interventional Therapeutics Corporation) uses an 8 French coaxial catheter system. The inner catheter is longer and more flexible than the outer catheter (Figure 2). The system is positioned using a polymer-coated guide wire over which the inner catheter is placed into the distal circulation. The coaxial balloon catheter system is then assembled (Figure 3). Silicone balloons contain a miter valve that permits introduction of a catheter for inflation (Figure 4). Upon withdrawal, the valve closes, maintaining the inflation pressure and desired size and shape. Once the catheter system is assembled, isosmotic metrizamide is used to inflate the balloon and purge the system of air. Inflation of the balloon with contrast enables visualization during fluoroscopy. Silicone balloons are made of a semipermeable membrane, there-

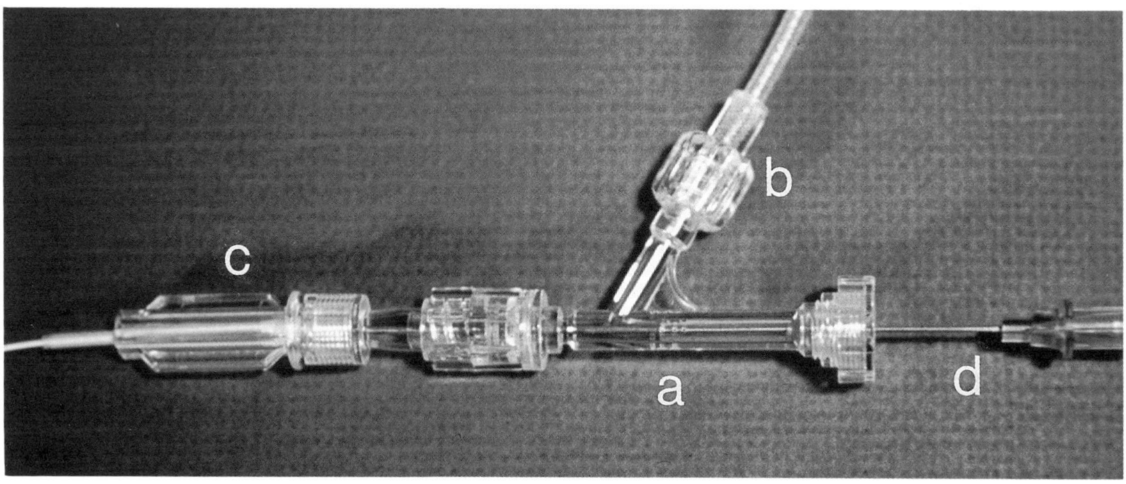


***Figure 1.*** *Rotating hemostatic adapter **(a)**, heparinized saline flush pack **(b)**, guide catheter **(c)**, Tracker® catheter **(d)**.*

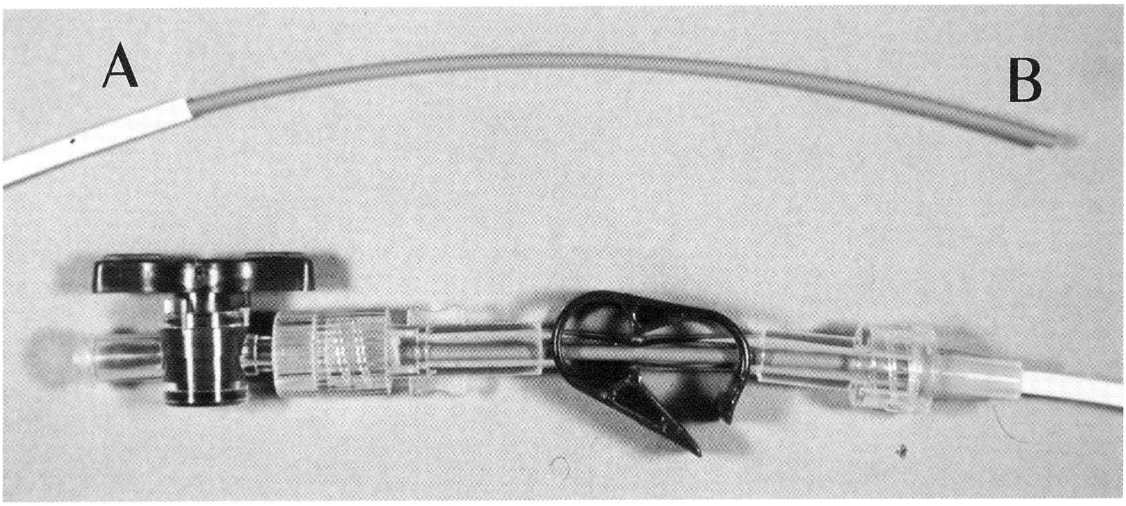


*Figure 2. Interventional Therapeutics Corporation balloon guide catheter. Note the coaxial system. A guide wire is used to advance the system. The inner catheter (B) is then removed, and the outer catheter (A) acts as a guide for the balloon catheter.*

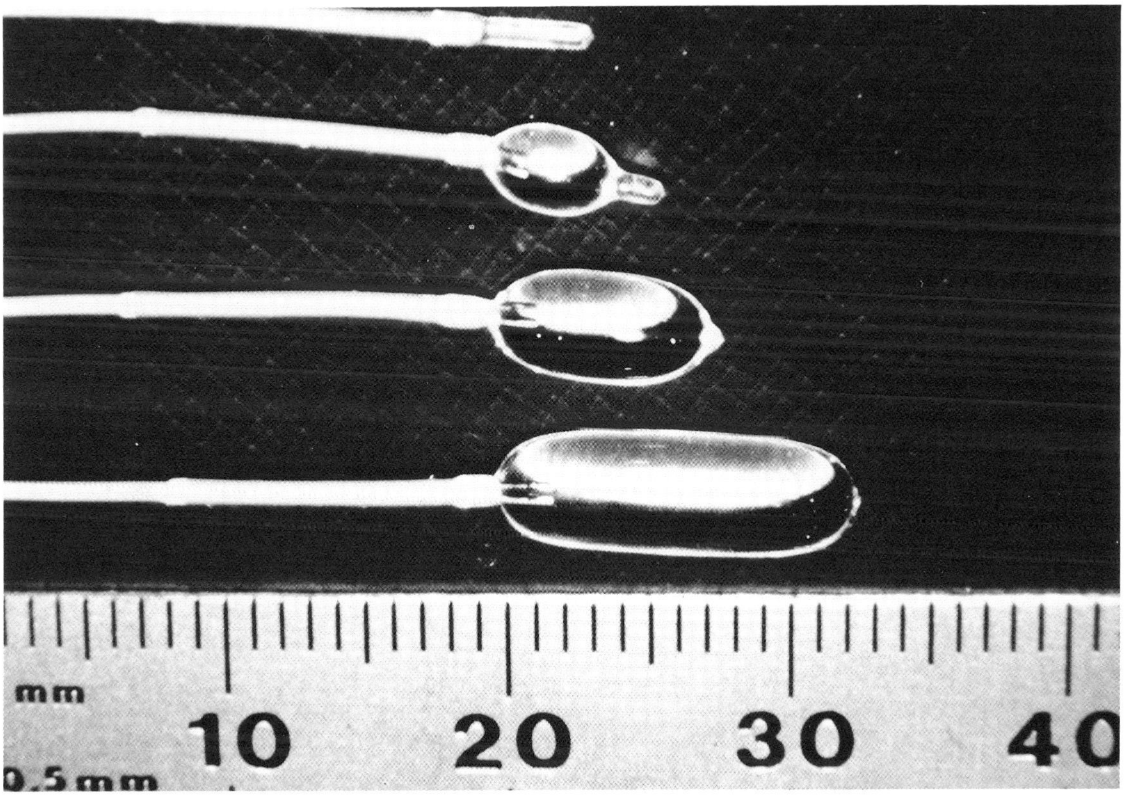


*Figure 3. Interventional Therapeutics Corporation balloon system, uninflated top, and fully inflated bottom.*

fore, mixture of the metrizamide solution must produce an isosmotic solution to prevent swelling of the balloon after intravascular inflation.

Placement of the balloon into the aneurysm cavity can be challenging. Tortuous vessels with areas of stenosis proximal to the aneurysm orifice can block access to the body of

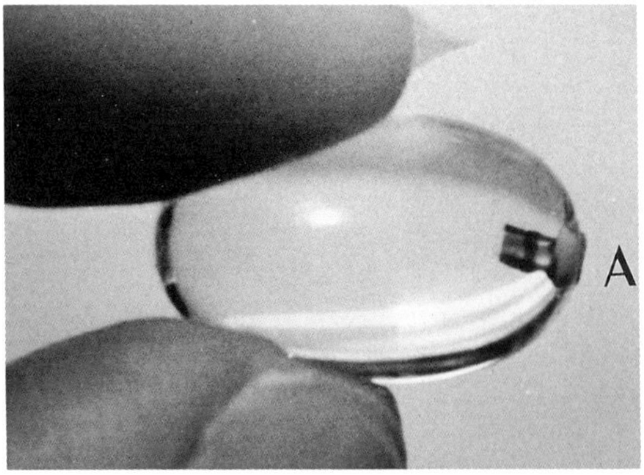


*Figure 4. Interventional Therapeutics Corporation silicone balloon after detachment from catheter. Note the miter valve (A) through which the catheter is inserted.*

the aneurysm. It has not been possible to utilize a guide wire for direction of the balloon into the aneurysm. Placement relies on flow direction. As a result, the utility of this system is limited in some circumstances. Recently Nelson,[38] reporting the use of a Tracker® 18 catheter with a Goldvalve Latex Balloon, outlined a method for incorporating a guide wire into the detachable balloon system. He commented that the silicone balloons produced by Interventional Therapeutics Corporation could be placed onto the Tracker® 18 catheter and positioned with a guide wire.

Once the balloon has been placed into the aneurysm cavity, it is inflated according to its volumetric specifications. After detachment, balloons filled with metrizamide have been reported to deflate. If this occurs before aneurysm thrombosis, the potential for distal embolization of balloon debris could result in infarction. To prevent deflation and rupture, Goto et al[13] developed a permanent inflation system using a hydrophilic polymerizing system. When the balloon had been inflated within the aneurysm cavity, metrizamide was exchanged with a mixture of HEMA, initiator, and catalyst. A polymerization reaction turning methacrylate monomers into polymethyl-methacrylate occurred within the balloon, forming a solid cast of the balloon. Thus, premature deflation was avoided.

Giant aneurysms require multiple balloons to induce thrombosis (Figure 5). Motion of balloon within the aneurysm cavity can result in aneurysm rupture. A ball-valve effect can result if a balloon allows entry of blood into the aneurysm cavity during systole but blocks egress of blood during diastole. The resulting expansion of the aneurysm cavity ends in rupture. In some cases, migration of the HEMA-filled balloon has been documented within an organized thrombus.

## *Coils*

A significant technologic advancement in catheter design that facilitated access to distal branches of the cerebral circulation was realized with the Tracker® catheter system. Target Therapeutic's tapered catheter design and flexible, high torque-ability guide wire system facilitates direct placement of a 1- or 2-mm catheter tip into the body of the aneurysm. Target developed a platinum coil system that could be delivered into the aneurysm cavity through their Tracker® catheters (Figures 6, 7). Coils of various tertiary structures are available and are believed to be thrombogenic. Animal experiments and initial patient experiences indicated that after ejection from the Tracker® catheter, the coils would migrate within the aneurysm cavity. Dislodged coils have embolized into the cerebral circulation (personal communication: Strother C, March 1991, Madison, Wisconsin). Changes in the size and shape of the coils did not affect their thrombogenicity. To increase the thrombogenic capacity of the coils, small Dacron® threads were added to the coil matrix (Figures 8, 9). In animal models, these coils migrated less and seemed to be more thrombogenic. There also was less incidence of recanalization of the aneurysm cavity when coils with Dacron® threads were used.

When the Tracker® catheter has been positioned, the coils are loaded into the proximal end of the catheter and a gold-tipped guide wire is used to push the coils through the catheter into the aneurysm cavity. Once the coil leaves the distal end of the catheter, its final position cannot be controlled. Of greater im-

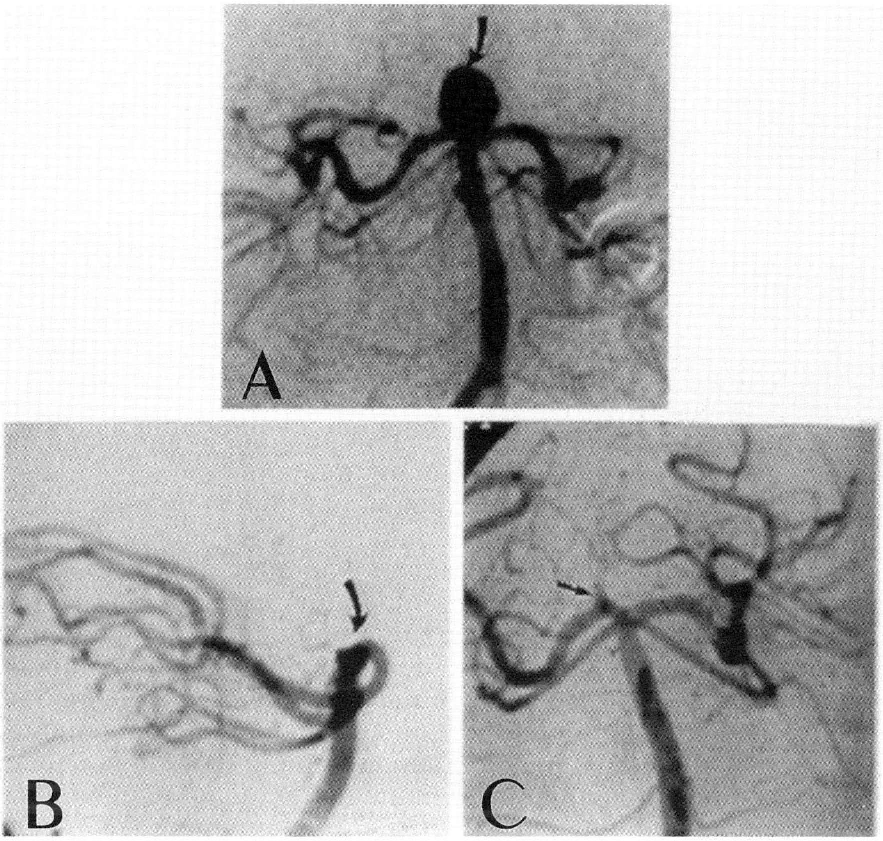


*Figure 5. Balloon embolization of giant basilar tip aneurysm. Aneurysm before embolization, 8 x 10 x 13 mm (A). Lateral (B) and anteroposterior (AP) (C) angiogram of aneurysm after placement of 2 detachable silicone balloons. Reprinted with permission from Higashida et al. Treatment of intracranial aneurysms with preservation of the parent vessel: results of percutaneous balloon embolization in 84 patients. AJNR 1990;11:638.*[21]

portance, the coil cannot be repositioned when released. Ejected coils tend to circulate within the body of a giant aneurysm. This continues until an adequate number of coils have been released to create an anchoring mass. This lack of control of coil placement has potentially devastating consequences for the patient, i.e. a circulating mass of coils can liberate calcified emboli from within the aneurysm cavity and cause intimal tears and vessel wall dissections. Numerous small series have been reported in abstracts and case reports over the past 2 years, but no large patient series have been reported.[29,40] Four cases have been reported of distal embolization of coils following release within the aneurysm cavity. The small size of these coils and lack of control severely limits their utility.

## *Electrothrombotic Coils*

Electric current produces thrombosis in blood when electrons migrate from anode to cathode. The movement of electrons through a viscous medium results in local heating caused by frictional forces. These microscopic temperature gradients promote clotting. In addition, the positive surface potential generated on the coil during current flow attracts high molecular weight, negatively charged proteins that are themselves thrombogenic. External application of an electric

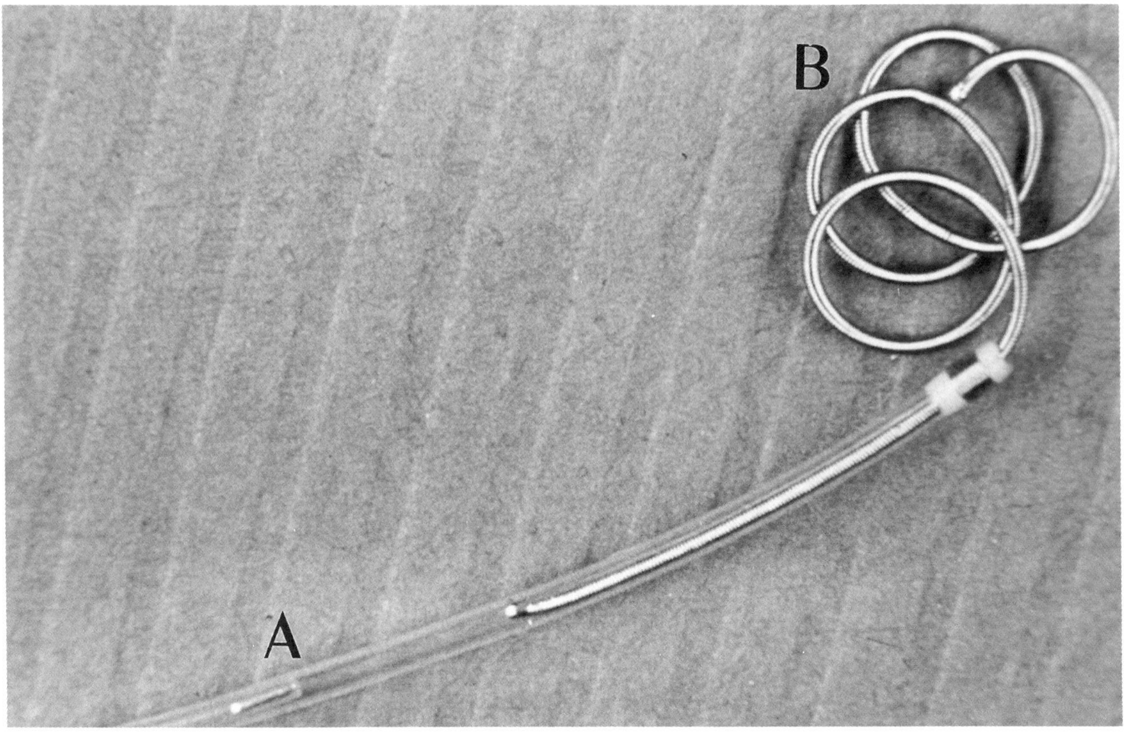


*Figure 6. Target Therapeutics Tracker® with platinum coil, (B). Notice the gold-tipped coil pusher (A) in the catheter. The coil assumes a predetermined tertiary structure after ejection from the catheter tip.*

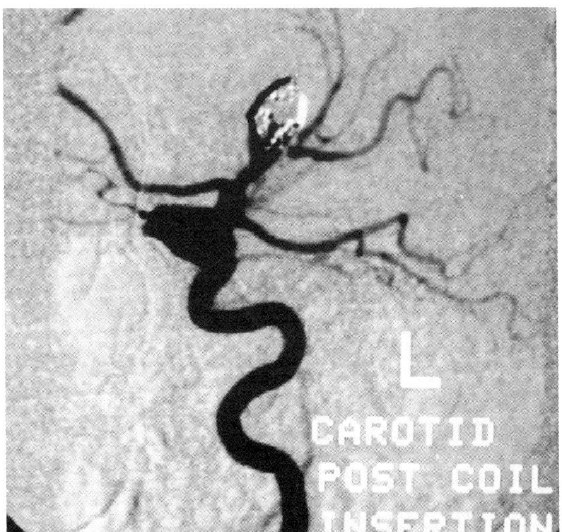


*Figure 7. Flower™ coil embolization of a giant MCA aneurysm. The neck is only partially occluded. Over 30 coils were required to obtain this degree of thrombosis.*

field leads to subtotal thrombosis of the aneurysm cavity. In a canine model, application of an electric field to vessels in the extremity resulted in total thrombosis. Studies on the material properties of metals have demonstrated that platinum provides excellent conductance with minimal degradation during current flow.

Guglielmi et al,[14] in conjunction with engineers at Target Therapeutics, began development of an electrothrombotic coil system in 1990 (Guglielmi Detachable Coil [GDC]). At that time, the inherent flaws in the use of platinum coils for aneurysm thrombosis were the inability to control delivery and final positioning of the coil, and the migration of coils after placement. To overcome these obstacles, coils were attached to a guide wire by a solder junction with a stainless steel core. As current is run from cathode to anode in a conducting solution, the stainless steel degrades, resulting in detachment of the coil from the guide wire. The stainless steel junction must be outside the delivery catheter to ensure exposure of the surface to conducting solution for electrolysis. In addition, coils were increased in length from 2–40 cm (Figure 10), thus permitting

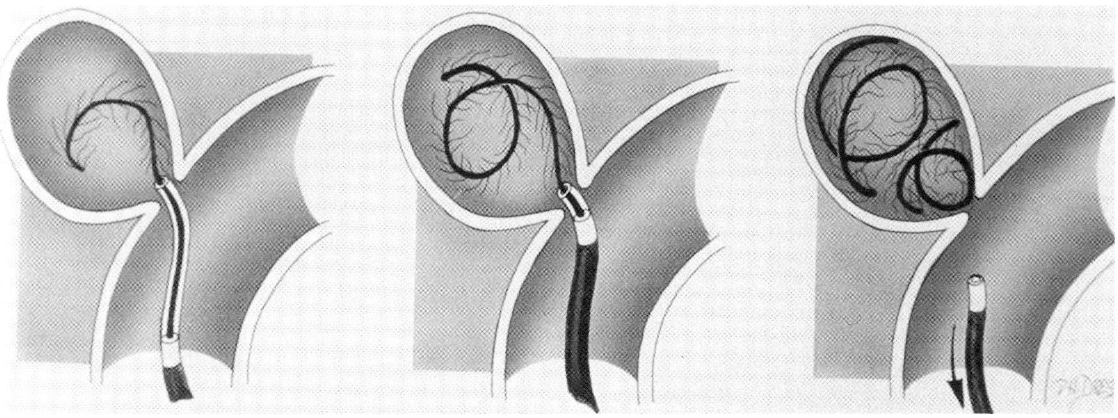

*Figure 8.* *Schematic representation of Tracker® catheter and Flower™ coils. Note the position of the catheter at the neck of the aneurysm. Coils are laid into the body of the aneurysm until the aneurysm has been angiographically obliterated.*

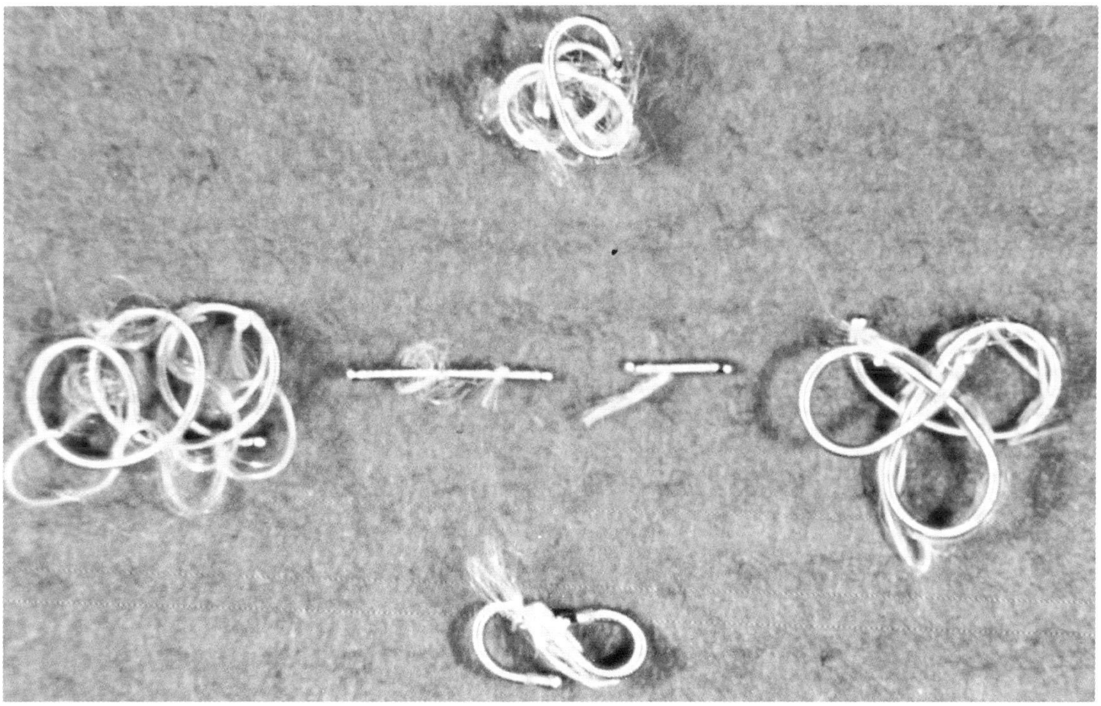

*Figure 9.* *Target Therapeutic Flower™ coils. Platinum coils with Dacron® threads wrapped into the secondary structure of the coil. Note different shapes and sizes available.*

delivery of a large mass of coils into the body of the aneurysm and decreasing the chance of migration out of the aneurysm after release. The coil's tertiary structure is compliant, assuming the shape of the aneurysm into which it is delivered. Multiple coils of various sizes can be delivered into an aneurysm in an attempt to completely thrombose the aneurysm cavity. If during delivery, loops of coil bulge into the lumen of the parent vessel, or delivery threatens rupture of the aneurysm cavity, coils can be retrieved before detachment.

Determination of the aneurysm size is crucial in selection of the appropriate coils for delivery. The authors routinely place 1-cm washers on the anterior and lateral aspect of

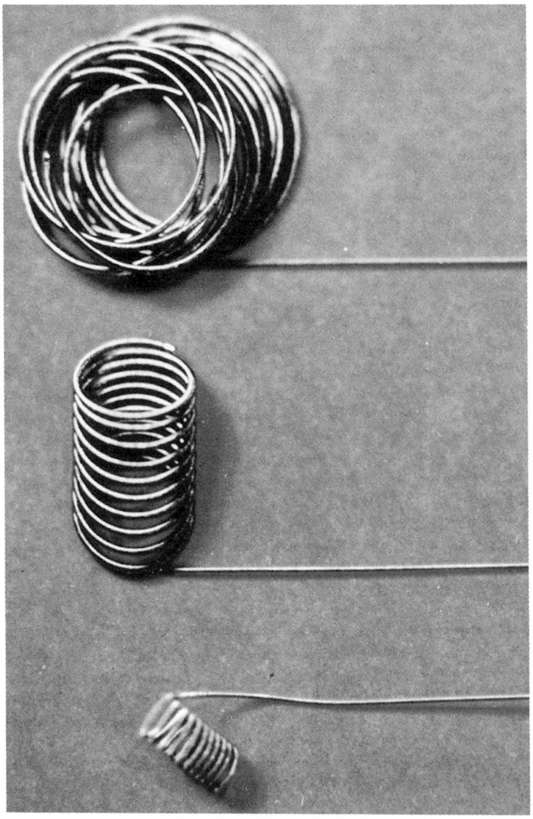

*Figure 10. Electrothrombotic coils (Guglielmi Detachable Coil [GDC] System).*

the forehead during digital angiography (personal communication: Hieshima G, Keystone, Colorado, August 1990). These act as a standard of measure for approximating aneurysm size. As with other systems, the guide catheter is positioned and connected to a rotating hemostatic adapter and heparinized saline flush pack. The GDC Tracker® catheter is positioned so that the distal tip projects into the aneurysm cavity just proximal to the dome of the aneurysm. Delivery of the coil into the aneurysm is performed during direct visualization. The coil should flow out of the catheter without resistance and assume a tertiary structure that conforms to the shape of the aneurysm body. Once the coil has been delivered and the solder junction between coil and guide wire is outside the catheter tip, the current can be applied. The current generator operates in a current clamp mode maintaining 0.5 milliamperes (mA) of current delivery by varying the voltage applied between anode and cathode. As the stainless steel junction begins to degrade, a higher voltage is automatically applied between anode and cathode to maintain the 0.5 mA level. The progress of detachment can be monitored in this way. Once the coil is detached, the guide wire can be removed and an angiogram is performed.

The choice of appropriate coil length is determined by estimates of the aneurysm dimensions. The number and length of successive coils placed into an aneurysm must be individualized on a patient-by-patient basis. The initial coils should be as long as possible to create an anchored matrix in the aneurysm cavity. Successive shorter coils are introduced above the initial coil, pushing it down toward the aneurysm neck. In this way, the largest single bulk of coil is subjected to the most turbulent region of blood flow, which minimizes coil migration out of the aneurysm body. Turbulent blood flow can remodel coil morphology during the first 24–48 hours postplacement. As a result, repeated angiography may demonstrate incomplete treatment of the aneurysm neck. Additional coils can be added at that time.

To date, only cerebral aneurysms that are considered unclippable, secondary to their size or the medical condition of the patient, have been treated (Figure 11). In the initial 100 patients, most aneurysms were in the posterior circulation (personal communication: Guglielmi Detachable Coils/Target Therapeutics Meeting, San Diego, California, November 1991). Although initial results demonstrated a low morbidity and mortality, many of these aneurysms were not completely obliterated angiographically. The decision to leave an aneurysm rest or untreated neck resulted from fear of thrombosing the parent vessel or obliterating perforating branches to the brain stem. Once coils have been placed into an aneurysm cavity, the pattern of flow through the aneurysm is changed, in some cases, becoming more turbulent. The forces generated by turbulent flow have been implicated as the driving forces in formation and growth of aneurysms.

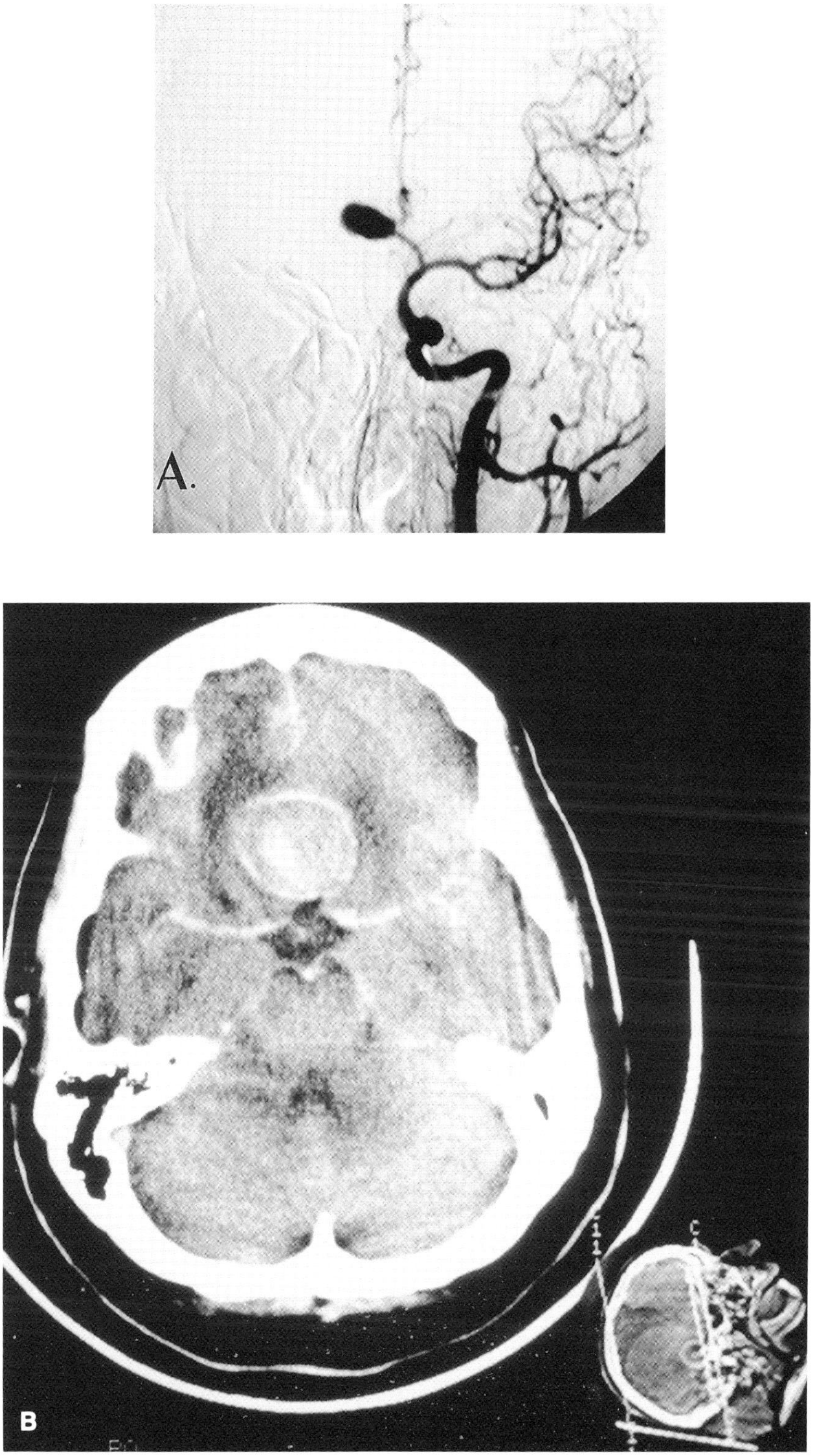


*Figure 11A,B.* *Large anterior communicating aneurysm. AP cerebral artery angiogram before embolization (A) and preoperative computed tomography (CT) scan with contrast (B).*

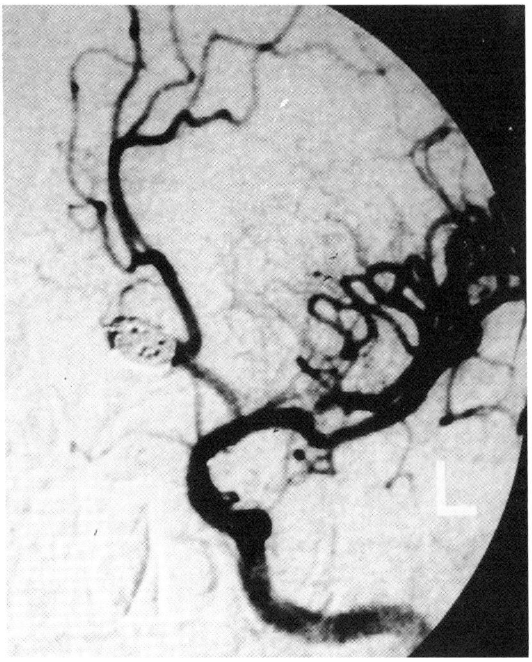


*Figure 11C. The same aneurysm shown in Figure 11A,B after embolization with Guglielmi Detachable Coils (GDC).*

The untreated portion of the aneurysm cavity has potential to thrombose, remain unchanged, or grow. The thrombus formed during the coil procedure is a dynamic entity, its size and histologic components varying over time. The fine equilibrium governing the formation and lysis of thrombus remains incompletely understood. Therefore, it is difficult to predict the fate of an incompletely treated aneurysm. Coil procedures are performed in anticoagulated patients. Disinhibition of the heparin effect on antithrombin III over time or by administration of protamine should affect the growth of existing thrombus within the aneurysm cavity. Aneurysms that appear subtotally obliterated after initial treatment with coils may go on to thrombose over time. A case can be made to err on the side of subtotal treatment, with followup inspection and retreatment if necessary. Alternatively, it is possible that partially treated aneurysms are protected from rebleed. This fact becomes of tantamount importance if coils are used to treat patients acutely post-SAH. Placement of coils from the aneurysm dome downward toward the neck induces formation of a mass of thrombus limiting blood flow into the most fragile portion of the aneurysm, namely the dome. The high wall tension within the aneurysm dome qualifies it as the most likely site for rupture. Therefore subtotal treatment may protect the aneurysm from initial hemorrhage or rebleed.

In his Stonwin lecture, Shcheglov[44] reported 17 patients treated with latex balloons in the acute phase following SAH. There was no mortality. He stated:

> acute phase occlusions require special preparations, including soaking the latex in thrombin and oil, occluding the aneurysm cavity without dangerously increasing intraluminal pressure, and leaving the catheter in for 24 hours. After occlusion of the aneurysm has been verified, we do not hesitate to use induced hypertension to overcome the effects of vasospasm or anticoagulation to mitigate against symptoms thought to result from embolic or thrombogenic events.

His comments imply that introduction of a thrombin-soaked latex balloon protects against rebleed if the aneurysm has been angiographically obliterated. However, 17 patients do not provide adequate numbers from which to draw statistically significant conclusions. The potential for patient deterioration and death following rebleeding further complicates this issue. Only repeated angiography at regular intervals will determine the fate of endovascularly induced aneurysm rests.

In a 1990 editorial, Luessenhop[34] commented that "only complete angiographic obliteration of an aneurysm is a success, and 'good' or 'near complete' occlusion also are procedural failures." This implies that subtotal treatment of aneurysms does not ensure protection from rebleeding. He stressed that it was inappropriate to have a patient endure two management risks, i.e. endovascular and surgical. He stated that "a small group of lesions, mostly large or giant aneurysms on the vertebrobasilar and proximal internal carotid circulation, is suitable for selective ballooning, with or without simultaneous occlusion of the parent artery." It is possible that the effectiveness of this in terms of mortality and morbidity is equal to or better than direct sur-

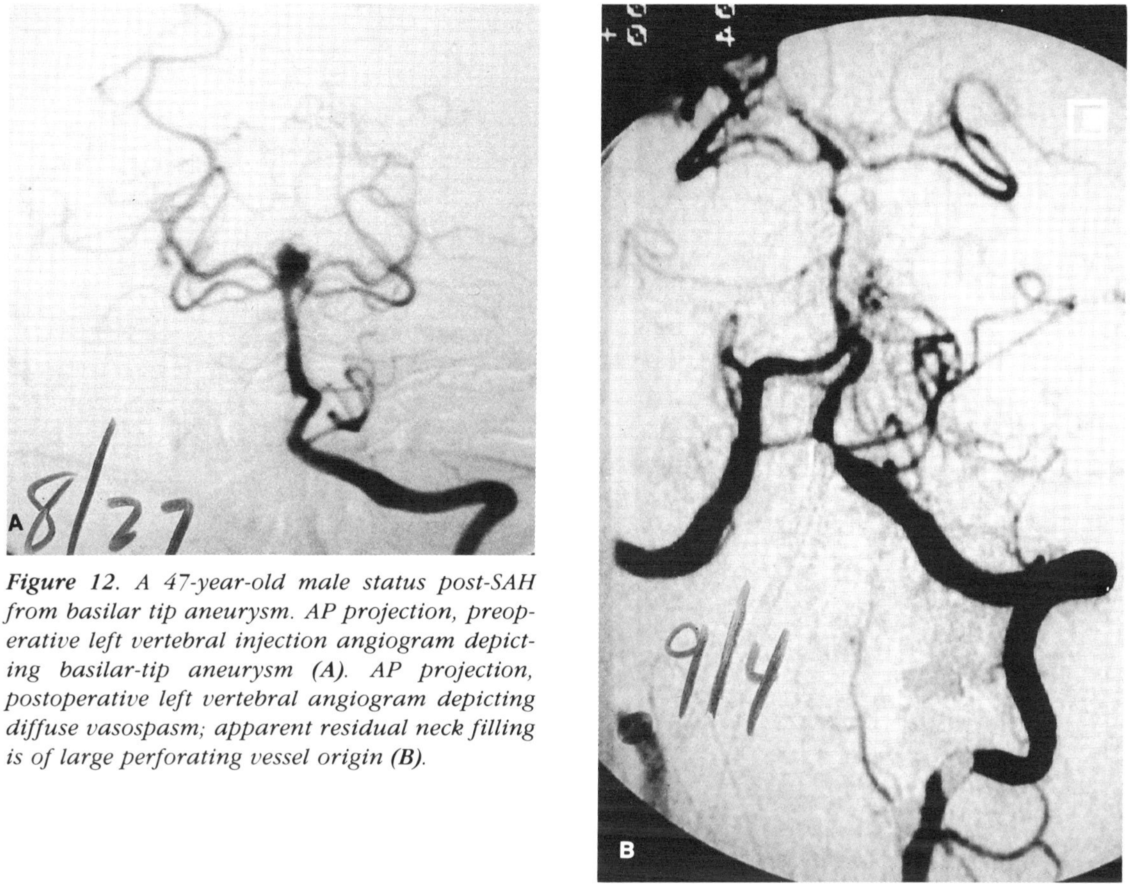


*Figure 12. A 47-year-old male status post-SAH from basilar tip aneurysm. AP projection, preoperative left vertebral injection angiogram depicting basilar-tip aneurysm (A). AP projection, postoperative left vertebral angiogram depicting diffuse vasospasm; apparent residual neck filling is of large perforating vessel origin (B).*

gery in the most experienced hands. If Higashida's results[21,22] are interpreted with consideration to the outcome of patients with untreated inoperable aneurysms, the 18% mortality and 11% stroke rates become more acceptable. Extension of endovascular techniques for treatment of "clippable" aneurysms must await reduction of morbidity and mortality to near zero level.

# Postoperative Treatment

## *Anticoagulation*

After placement of the final coil, activated clotting time is measured and an appropriate bolus of protamine is administered intravenously. Activated clotting time is monitored until it reaches normal levels. A repeat angiogram is obtained to evaluate the relationship between degree of aneurysm thrombosis and caliber of the parent vessel lumen. If the patient has tolerated the procedure and demonstrates no new neurologic deficits, the femoral sheath is removed, and the patient is returned to the intensive care unit.

Growth of the thrombus after completion of the procedure can result in loss of neurologic function secondary to parent vessel occlusion. When this occurs, immediate repeat angiography is essential. If a growing thrombus can be identified angiographically as the cause of neurologic deterioration, thrombolysis must be employed to reduce its mass. This can be accomplished by placement of a Tracker® catheter adjacent to the aneurysm, and infusion of a pharmacologic fibrinolytic. The degree of organization within the thrombus determines the efficacy of this procedure. Fresh, unorganized thrombi can be lysed by direct infusion of 500,000 to 1,000,000 units of urokinase via the Tracker® catheter. This

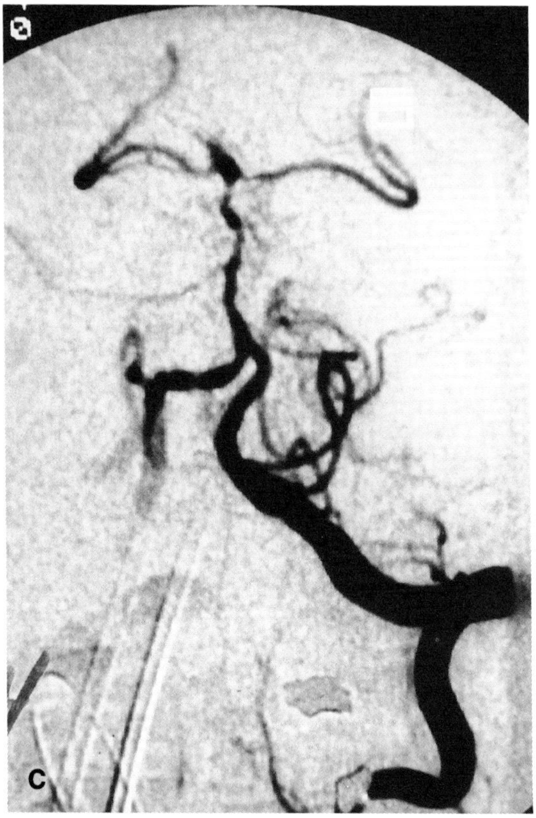


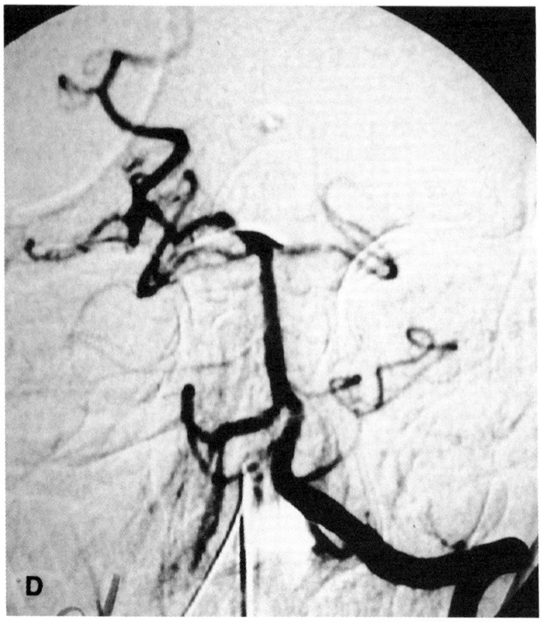


*Figure 12C,D. (C) AP projection, left vertebral angiogram following intra-arterial injection of papaverine 120 mg showing improvement in vessel caliber. AP projection, left vertebral angiogram 4 days postangioplasty depicting persistence of normal vessel caliber and flow (D).*

technique has been used to successfully restore neurologic function lost postoperatively. Patients remain anticoagulated for days or weeks and slowly undergo normalization of their activated partial tissue thromboplastin time.

### *Angiography and Imaging*

Patients undergo repeat angiography at 24 and 72 hours after endovascular treatment of aneurysms. Further studies are obtained at 6 months and 1 year following the initial procedure. The decision to place additional coils into newly formed or old aneurysm rests must be individualized to the angiographic appearance of the rest. In the future, magnetic resonance angiography (MRA) may augment cerebral angiography as a method for followup of aneurysms treated with coils or balloons. Presently the resolution of MRA is inadequate to perform this task. Many coils introduce magnetic artifacts distorting the magnetic resonance appearance of aneurysms.

## Discussion

Any aneurysm is potentially clippable. The neurosurgeon must weigh the risk of radical dissection and potential associated neurologic deficit against the benefits of protection from hemorrhage. The decision to treat an aneurysm by catheter-based intervention, rather than by conventional surgical techniques, requires multidisciplinary input. In most institutions, catheter technologies are performed by neuroradiologists. In the authors' institution, neurosurgeons perform all endovascular procedures. Ideally a team effort is preferred.

Patients with intracranial aneurysms have been referred to the authors' endovascular service for numerous reasons. Endovascular treatment of aneurysms is reserved for patients that are not surgical candidates. Poor surgical risks, i.e. cardiac or pulmonary abnormalities that prevent induction of general anesthesia, would be better served by an endovascular approach, assuming embolization can be performed in the awake patient. Intracavernous aneurysms that require extensive skull base dissection resulting in cranial nerve dysfunction are well treated endovascularly by microcatheter techniques. Surgically inaccessible giant aneurysms of the anterior or posterior circulation whose anatomy precludes reconstruction of a neck are best treated endovascularly, as are aneurysms that have been explored and either unsuccessfully clipped, wrapped, or surgically aborted. BA aneurysms that are felt to be inoperable have routinely been treated by endovascular techniques. The patient series previously cited in this chapter, using balloons or coils to treat aneurysms, have relied on these guidelines for patient selection. In any team approach to the treatment of patients with intracranial aneurysms, the technical ability, experience, and judgment of the participants will govern the choice of intervention.

Endovascular treatment of patients in the acute phase following SAH is a controversial topic. The Kiev experience reported 17 patients that were treated with balloon embolization following acute SAH.[41,44] Soaking the latex in thrombin prior to embolization facilitates clotting in the aneurysm cavity. If the aneurysm is angiographically obliterated, are patients considered protected from rebleeding? In Higashida's series[22] of posterior circulation aneurysms treated with silicone balloons, over 50% of procedures were performed on patients following SAH. The time interval posthemorrhage was not reported. Clearly, patients with fresh blood in the subarachnoid space are less stable and present numerous treatment dilemmas, independent of surgical or endovascular intervention. It is well documented that the highest risk of rebleeding from ruptured intracranial aneurysms occurs within the first 24 hours following the initial bleed. Most delayed rebleeds occur within the first 2 weeks. Surgical placement of an aneurysm clip across the neck of an intracranial aneurysm virtually guarantees protection from rebleeding. Preliminary data suggest that endovascular treatment of acutely ruptured aneurysms may likewise protect the patient from rebleeding. Unfortunately, the number of patients treated following acute SAH is too low to be conclusive.

Kwan et al[31] reported 2 patients with BA aneurysms treated by intra-aneurysmal balloon occlusion. In one case, followup angiography demonstrated aneurysmal enlargement of a subtotally treated aneurysm neck. In the second case, a HEMA-filled balloon migrated distally into the sac of a midbasilar artery aneurysm. This patient rebled and later died. In Higashida's series,[22] 10 of the 15 deaths were from rebleeding following balloon embolization. At the State University of New York at Buffalo, 1 patient treated with electrothrombotic coils rebled and died 4 weeks after coil embolization (personal communication: Hopkins LN, Buffalo, New York, February 1992).

The uncertainty surrounding the maturation of thrombus after embolization complicates the postoperative management of patients with acutely ruptured aneurysms that have been treated with balloons or coils. In the authors' intensive care unit, patients with inoperable freshly ruptured intracranial aneurysms who have been treated by endovascular therapy are sedated and placed under rigid blood pressure control to avoid fluctuations in systolic blood pressure. Sedation and mechanical ventilation are used if needed. The question arises whether endovascular therapies should be considered protective against rebleeding. The definitive answer will require statistical analysis of a large series of patients.

The management of patients who develop vasospasm following endovascular therapy is problematic. In surgical patients who develop delayed ischemic deficit, the authors institute an aggressive course of hypervolemia and hypertension via fluid resuscitation and inotropic support. If an acutely ruptured aneurysm treated with balloons or coils is not considered protected from rebleeding, can volume expansion and hypertension be safely induced? This question is presently unanswered. A more liberal application of angioplasty could provide an adequate alternative for patients with vasospasm and embolized aneurysms.

## Endovascular Therapy of Vasospasm

Symptomatic vasospasm occurs in at least 30% of patients following SAH. Onset begins around day 4 and patients continue to be at risk until at least 12 days following the initial event. The clinical sequelae of vasospasm include altered sensorium, focal neurologic deficit, or coma, leading to stroke or even death.

Although aggressive medical management, including hypertensive/hypervolemic therapy and calcium channel blockers, can ameliorate its incidence and sequelae, vasospasm remains a major cause of the high mortality and morbidity associated with SAH. Transluminal angioplasty has been shown to reverse both clinical and angiographic manifestations of vasospasm. This section will review the present literature and patient series. In addition, the clinical signs and symptoms used as an impetus for angioplasty procedures will be outlined.

### *History*

Percutaneous transluminal angioplasty for peripheral atherosclerotic disease was first described by Dotter and Judkins in 1964.[8] Zubkov et al[47] in 1984 described transluminal angioplasty for vasospasm associated with aneurysmal SAH in 33 patients. Using a latex balloon, 105 vascular territories were successfully treated. After 3 months, patients had no further deterioration in neurologic status.

In 1989, Barnwell et al[2] reported 2 angioplasty procedures in 1 patient. The patient developed a focal deficit and underwent angioplasty in the MCA and ICA. Twenty-four hours later, the patient deteriorated neurologically and was found to have basilar and posterior cerebral artery vasospasm. Although the second procedure was performed 24 hours after the onset of neurologic deficit, the patient did not develop a hemorrhagic infarct. The patient eventually returned to work and resumed an independent life-style.

In 1990, Higashida et al[23] described percutaneous transluminal angioplasty for vasospasm in 40 vascular territories in 14 patients using Interventional Therapeutics Corporation's silicone microballoon device. In 11 patients, vasospasm was due to aneurysmal SAH. In 3 patients, spasm occurred following detachable balloon embolization of an intracranial aneurysm. In 10 of the 14 cases, balloon dilatation resulted in improvement of neurologic function within minutes to hours following the dilatation. One patient died from hemorrhage into a basal ganglia infarct 24 hours following MCA angioplasty.

In 1991, Eskridge[9] reported 30 patients treated with transluminal angioplasty, two-thirds of whom have shown sustained improvement. An upgrade on the Hunt and Hess scale or a 2-point increase on the Glasgow Coma score was the criterion used to define improvement. There was 1 death and 1 small MCA infarct directly attributable to the procedure. Morbidity and mortality rate was under 10%. After 3 years, no delayed complications have been noted.

Also in 1991, Alexander et al[1] reported latex balloon angioplasty of 89 consecutive patients with delayed ischemic deficit and radiographic confirmation of vasospasm. Fifty-eight percent underwent dilatation with unclipped aneurysms; 18% were treated postoperatively. Eight percent of patients underwent simultaneous angioplasty and detachable balloon occlusion of ruptured aneurysm. Fifty-three percent underwent dilatation in a single vascular tree, whereas 47% had bilateral carotid or carotid-basilar angioplasty. Improvement of focal neurologic deficits, level of consciousness, or both, was achieved in 78% of patients.

Fujii et al[12] reported angioplasty of 26 cases of vasospasm, 70% of which were clinically improved. The delay between the evolution of neurologic deficits and angioplasty demonstrated a strong correlation to outcome. Patients treated within 8 hours of the onset of neurologic deficit had better outcome after angioplasty.

## *Indications*

The use of cerebral angioplasty for the treatment of vasospasm is a controversial topic. The optimal time interval between the onset of neurologic deficit and catheter-based intervention has not been established. The authors' service has adopted the criteria of Newell et al.[39] Patients must have a delayed ischemic deficit without hydrocephalus, mass effect, or evidence of new infarction, and have failed medical management of vasospasm (hypertensive and hypervolemic therapy, ventriculostomy, etc). Most important, angiographic demonstration of spasm in a vascular distribution that corresponds to the deficit must be established.

Unfortunately, delay in performing angioplasty has been shown to negatively impact on outcome. Maximizing medical management can take more than 24 hours and severely compromise the window of opportunity for successful angioplasty. Delay can result in ischemic infarct; subsequent angioplasty can produce hemorrhagic infarct.

It must be stressed that before consideration of angioplasty patients must have failed to improve after maximal medical intervention. Once medical therapy has been maximized, the patient should display a rapid response. If improvement in neurologic function is not realized, the patient should be considered for immediate angioplasty. In this way, angioplasty will provide the maximum improvement in neurologic function, while minimizing the risk of reperfusing irreversibly ischemic central nervous system tissue.

## *Technique*

Patients are prepared as outlined earlier. A femoral introducer sheath is placed. With systemic heparinization, a 7.3 French polyethylene guide catheter is positioned into the internal carotid or vertebral artery through which the angioplasty catheter system is to be introduced. All catheters are continuously flushed with heparinized saline via rotating hemostatic adapter. Angioplasty of intracerebral vessels is performed with a nonvalved, nondetachable silicone microballoon (0.85 mm in diameter before inflation) attached to a No. 2 French polyethylene catheter, or to a Tracker® or Stealth® microcatheter (Target Therapeutics). To facilitate selective catheterization, the polyethylene catheter may be steamed so the tip retains a desired shape, while the Tracker® may be used with a steerable guide wire. The authors have found that the Tracker® catheter/guide wire, with nondetachable balloon (Interventional Therapeutics Corporation), provides the most easily positioned system, usually allowing access to all major branches of the cerebral circulation. The catheter is advanced using a digitally subtracted "road map." Dilatations are performed by briefly (less than 5 seconds) and repeatedly inflating and deflating the balloon with 0.05–0.10 ml of iodinated contrast material. Following this maneuver, the balloon catheter is slowly advanced. The inflated volume of angioplasty balloons varies. Careful approximation of the vessel diameter and the angioplasty balloon inflated diameter is crucial. Overinflation of the angioplasty balloon can cause vessel rupture. Angiographic assessment of the progress of the angioplasty can be accomplished by injecting contrast material into the No. 7.3 French guide catheter, which is proximal to the working end of the angioplasty catheter.

## *Pathology*

Muscular contraction within vessel walls does not solely account for luminal changes associated with the clinical vasospasm. Alterations reported in human necropsy and intraoperative arterial specimens following SAH include subendothelial fibrosis, intimal thickening or swelling, myonecrosis, increased myofibroblasts, and increased collagen content in the media.[27,45]

Fujii et al[12] have used a canine hemorrhage model to study the influences of balloon angioplasty on the BA. Angiographically, angioplasty was most effective during the peak phase of vasospasm, and the increased vessel diameter was maintained several weeks after the procedure. Histologic changes seen immediately following angioplasty included denudation of endothelial cells and stretching of internal elastic lamina without disruption of muscle layer. All changes cleared within 4 weeks. No sclerotic changes, such as intimal hyperplasia, remained.

Yamamoto[46] described electron microscopic findings following polyethylene (Stealth catheter) balloon dilation of MCAs from human autopsy specimens. The normal structure of collagen fibers in the vessel walls was disrupted following angioplasty, but it should be noted that the system used (developed for atherosclerotic angioplasty) generated pressures far and above those used in the clinical setting of vasospasm: 22–44 psi versus 5–8 psi employed with in vivo silicone balloon angioplasty.[3]

## *Arterial Rupture*

Brothers et al[5] described a case of fatal rupture of an MCA cortical branch complicating vasospasm angioplasty. They subsequently analyzed the technical factors contributing to this, particularly the pressure/volume characteristics of the balloon and the inherent difficulties in control over balloon diameter in distal cerebral angioplasty. Fifteen balloons were tested, both during unrestricted inflation and during inflation within rigid 8 and 9 French catheters, in an attempt to mimic conditions during in vivo angioplasty. Diameter, pressure, and volume measurements were collected. Minimal (20%) inflation of the unrestricted balloon led to an abrupt pressure peak of about 350 mm Hg, which on further inflation diminished and leveled off to about 280 mm Hg near full inflation. Restricting the inflation diameter within a 2 mm 9 French catheter lumen resulted in steady increase in pressure after the initial peak, reaching 600 mm Hg at 60% and 1400 mm Hg at 100% inflation. With dangerously high pressures generated early in a diameter-restricted setting, they concluded that the elongation behavior of the balloon does not provide protection against arterial rupture. Distal angioplasty may require inflation volumes far less than the maximum 0.1 ml.

Linskey et al[33] reported fatal rupture of the intracranial carotid artery during transluminal angioplasty for vasospasm induced by SAH in a patient with a clipped aneurysm. The rupture, they proposed, most likely resulted from a small portion of aneurysm neck which remained unclipped, thereby leaving an area of structural weakness in the arterial wall at the clipping site and adjacent to the angioplasty. They suggested that angiographically occult aneurysm rests represent contraindications to angioplasty. Rests proximal or distal to stenotic segments have the potential to rupture during angioplasty.

## *Papaverine*

There are some instances in which balloon angioplasty may be technically more dangerous, namely in the distal circulation, or in areas immediately adjacent to treated or untreated aneurysms. In these situations, papaverine can be employed to combat vasospasm as the sole agent or as an adjunct to angioplasty.

Papaverine has been shown to decrease tone in all smooth muscle and has been used to treat cerebral and peripheral ischemia, myocardial ischemia, and ureteral, biliary, and gastrointestinal colics.[36] Helm et al reported a preliminary study of 7 patients with severe cerebral vasospasm secondary to SAH, who underwent superselective injection of 60–150 mg of papaverine over 30–60 minutes (personal communication: Helm G, Meekin G, Phillips D, et al. Intra-arterial papaverine for treatment of cerebral vasospasm. Congress of Neurological Surgeons, October 1991, Orlando, Florida). Three patients had marked increase in vessel diameter angiographically and improved function neurologically. One patient had mild angiographic but marked clinical improvement. None of the patients had adverse cardiovascular or neurologic side effects. The response to papaverine resulted in normalization of flow velocity for a 5-day period, as verified by transcranial Doppler.

Although vasodilator properties of papaverine have been observed both centrally and peripherally, these effects on cerebral arterial spasm are short-lived. However this transient vasodilatory effect is well suited to selective intra-arterial injection as an adjunct to angioplasty in cases where severe vasospasm otherwise precludes adequate positioning of the balloon catheter. Additionally, papaverine-induced vasodilation may lessen subsequent trauma to the blood vessel wall induced by the inflation of the angioplasty balloon.

Kaku et al[28] reported percutaneous transluminal angioplasty in 20 distal vascular territories, using silicone balloon proximally and followed by selective intra-arterial injection of 6.0 mg of 0.2% papaverine hydrochloride, 0.5 mg nicardipine. Five of 7 patients showed improvement of neurologic function afterward.

The authors use intra-arterial papaverine as an adjunct to transluminal angioplasty. Superselective injection of papaverine can temporarily alleviate spasm, permitting distal progression of the balloon angioplasty in some cases, especially in situations where severe spasm initially precludes passage of the angioplasty catheter (Figure 12).

## Conclusion

Catheter-based systems presently available for the treatment of intracranial aneurysms will not replace surgical clipping. The complication rate of patients treated with balloons and platinum coil devices is higher than the complication rate of patients treated with surgical clipping of aneurysms by a vascular neurosurgeon. However, the potential for refinement of existing embolic materials and improvement in catheter design is unlimited. New catheter-based technologies for the treatment of intracranial aneurysms are continuously being developed. Developments in interventional cardiology are providing a framework for the creation of new technologies with direct application in the cerebral circulation. Stents, cylindrical structures placed into arteries harboring cerebral aneurysms, can provide a pathway for distal blood flow, while excluding flow into the aneurysm cavity. Manipulation of the clotting cascade within the body of the aneurysm cavity may provide a means of thrombosis without coils or balloons. Polymers, capable of inducing thrombosis, may one day be delivered directly into the body of the aneurysm cavity without fear of distal embolization. Recently, Macfarlane et al[37] described a catheter-based optical fiber capable of transmitting pulsed-dye laser light into a cerebral vessel and reversing vasospasm. The same treatment, used prophylactically, prevented the onset of vasospasm.

Future innovations for the treatment of cerebral aneurysms and vasospasm will evolve from a collaboration among engineering, physical science, and neuroscience. The exponential growth of computer science and imaging capabilities will stimulate the creation of definitive and permanent catheter-based systems to prevent SAH and cerebral vasospasm.

## References


1. Alexander LF, Zubkov YN, Benashvili GB. Cerebral angioplasty following aneurysmal subarachnoid hemorrhage. *Neuroradiology.* 1991;33(suppl):S154. Abstract.
2. Barnwell SL, Higashida RT, Halbach VV, et al. Transluminal angioplasty of intracerebral vessels for cerebral arterial spasm: reversal of neurological deficits after delayed treatment. *Neurosurgery.* 1989; 25:424–429.
3. Bell J. Comment on: Yamamoto Y, Smith RR, Bernanke DH. Mechanism of action of balloon angioplasty in cerebral vasospasm. *Neurosurgery.* 1992;30:1–6.
4. Berenstein A, Ransohoff J, Kupersmith M, et al. Transvascular treatment of giant aneurysms of the cavernous carotid and vertebral arteries: functional investigation and embolization. *Surg Neurol.* 1984; 21:3–12.
5. Brothers MF, Hedlund LW, Friedman AH. Arterial

rupture during "distal" vasospasm angioplasty. *Neuroradiology.* 1991;33(suppl):S155. Abstract.
6. Casasco A, Rogopoulos A, Aymard A, et al. Endovascular treatment of surgical and nonsurgical intracerebral aneurysms with metallic coils. *Neuroradiology.* 1991;33(suppl):S145. Abstract.
7. Debrun G, Fox A, Drake C, et al. Giant unclippable aneurysms: treatment with balloons. *AJNR.* 1981;2:167–173.
8. Dotter CT, Judkins MP. Transluminal treatment of arteriosclerotic obstruction: description of a new technique and a preliminary report of its application. *Circulation.* 1964;30:654–670.
9. Eskridge J. Angioplasty for cerebral vasospasm. *Neuroradiology.* 1991;33(suppl):S137.
10. Fox AJ, Lownie SP, Drake CG. Endovascular therapy of aneurysms with platinum coils following subarachnoid hemorrhage. *Neuroradiology.* 1991;33(suppl):S145.
11. Fox AJ, Viñuela F, Pelz DM, et al. Use of detachable balloons for proximal artery occlusion in the treatment of unclippable cerebral aneurysms. *J Neurosurg.* 1987;66:40–46.
12. Fujii Y, Takahashi A, Yoshimoto T, et al. Balloon angioplasty for vasospasm after SAH - experimental study and clinical experiences. *Neuroradiology.* 1991;33(suppl):S155. Abstract.
13. Goto K, Halbach VV, Hardin CW, et al. Permanent inflation of detachable balloons with a low-viscosity, hydrophilic polymerizing system. *Radiology.* 1988;169:787–790.
14. Guglielmi G, Viñuela F, Sepetka I, et al. Electrothrombosis of saccular aneurysms via endovascular approach, I: electrochemical basis, technique, and experimental results. *J Neurosurg.* 1991;75:1–7.
15. Guglielmi G, Viñuela F, Dion J, et al. Electrothrombosis of saccular aneurysms via endovascular approach, II: preliminary clinical experience. *J Neurosurg.* 1991;75:8–14.
16. Hieshima GB, Grinnell VS, Mehringer CM. A detachable balloon for therapeutic transcatheter occlusions. *Radiology.* 1981;138:227–228.
17. Hieshima GB, Higashida R, Halbach VV. Intravascular treatment of aneurysms. *Clin Neurosurg.* 1990;36:338–343.
18. Hieshima GB, Higashida RT, Halbach VV, et al. Intravascular balloon embolization of a carotid-ophthalmic artery aneurysm with preservation of the parent vessel. *AJNR.* 1986;7:916–918.
19. Hieshima GB, Higashida RT, Wapenski J, et al. Balloon embolization of a large distal basilar artery aneurysm: case report. *J Neurosurg.* 1986;65:413–416.
20. Hieshima GB, Higashida RT, Wapenski J, et al. Intravascular balloon embolization of a large mid-basilar artery aneurysm: case report. *J Neurosurg.* 1987;66:124–127.
21. Higashida RT, Halbach VV, Barnwell SL, et al. Treatment of intracranial aneurysms with preservation of the parent vessel: results of percutaneous balloon embolization in 84 patients. *AJNR.* 1990;11:633–640.
22. Higashida RT, Halbach VV, Cahan LD, et al. Detachable balloon embolization therapy of posterior circulation intracranial aneurysms. *J Neurosurg.* 1989;71:512–519.
23. Higashida RT, Halbach VV, Dormandy B, et al. New microballoon device for transluminal angioplasty of intracranial arterial vasospasm. *AJNR.* 1990;11:233–238.
24. Higashida RT, Halbach VV, Hieshima GB, et al. Cavernous carotid artery aneurysm associated with Marfan's syndrome: treatment by balloon embolization therapy. *Neurosurgery.* 1988;22:297–300.
25. Higashida RT, Halbach VV, Hieshima GB, et al. Treatment of a giant carotid ophthalmic artery aneurysm by intravascular balloon embolization therapy. *Surg Neurol.* 1988;30:382–386.
26. Higashida RT, Halbach VV, Mehringer CM, et al. Giant cavernous aneurysm associated with trigeminal artery: treatment by detachable balloon. *AJNR.* 1987;8:757–758.
27. Hughes JT, Schianchi PM. Cerebral artery spasm: a histological study at necropsy of the blood vessels in cases of subarachnoid hemorrhage. *J Neurosurg.* 1978;48:515–525.
28. Kaku Y, Yonekawa Y, Tsukahara T, et al. Percutaneous transluminal angioplasty for vasospasm—superselective intra-arterial infusion of papaverine. *Neuroradiology.* 1991;33(suppl):S155. Abstract.
29. Kohne D, Nahser HC. Staged endovascular treatment of cerebral aneurysms with coils. *Neuroradiology.* 1991;33(suppl):S145. Abstract.
30. Konovalov AN, Serbinenko FA, Filatov JM, et al. Endovascular treatment of arterial aneurysms. *AJNR.* 1990;11:225. Abstract.
31. Kwan ESK, Heilman CB, Shucart WA, et al. Enlargement of basilar artery aneurysms following balloon occlusion: "water-hammer" effect. *J Neurosurg.* 1991;75:963–968.
32. Lemme-Plaghos LA, Schonholz CJ, Ceciliano AL. Transarterial platinum coil embolization of aneurysms. *Neuroradiology.* 1991;33(suppl):S144. Abstract.
33. Linskey ME, Horton JA, Rao GR, et al. Fatal rupture of the intracranial carotid artery during transluminal angioplasty for vasospasm induced by subarachnoid hemorrhage: case report. *J Neurosurg.* 1991;74:985–990.
34. Luessenhop AJ. Interventional neuroradiology: a neurosurgeon's perspective. *AJNR.* 1990;11:625–629.
35. Luessenhop AJ, Velasquez AC. Observations on the tolerance of intracranial arteries to catheterization. *J Neurosurg.* 1964;21:85–91.
36. McEvoy GK, ed. *AHFS Drug Information.* Bethesda, Md: American Society of Hospital Pharmacists; 1991:1046–1047.
37. Macfarlane R, Teramura A, Owen CJ, et al. Treatment of vasospasm with a 480-nm pulsed-dye laser. *J Neurosurg.* 1991;75:613–622.
38. Nelson M. A versatile, steerable, flow-guided catheter for delivery of detachable balloons. *AJNR.* 1990;11:657–658.
39. Newell DW, Eskridge JM, Mayberg MR, et al. Angioplasty for the treatment of symptomatic vasospasm following subarachnoid hemorrhage. *J Neurosurg.* 1989;71:654–660.
40. Pruvo JP, LeClerc X, Soto Ares G, et al. Endovascular treatment of 16 intracranial aneurysms with microcoils. *Neuroradiology.* 1991;33(suppl):S144. Abstract.
41. Romodanov AP, Shcheglov VI. Intravascular occlu-

sion of saccular aneurysms of the cerebral arteries by means of a detachable balloon catheter. *Ad Tech Stand Neurosurg.* 2. New York, NY: Springer-Verlag; 1975;2:25–49.
42. Seldinger SI. Catheter replacement of the needle in percutaneous arteriography. *Acta Radiol.* 1952;39: 368–376.
43. Serbinenko FA. Balloon catheterization and occlusion of major cerebral vessels. *J Neurosurg.* 1974; 41:125–145.
44. Shcheglov VI. Endosaccular detachable balloon catheter treatment of cerebral saccular aneurysms. *AJNR.* 1990;11:224–225. Abstract.
45. Smith RR, Clower BR, Grotendorst GM, et al. Arterial wall changes in early human vasospasm. *Neurosurgery.* 1985;16:171–176.
46. Yamamoto Y, Smith RR, Bernanke DH. Mechanism of action of balloon angioplasty in cerebral vasospasm. *Neurosurgery.* 1992;30:1–6.
47. Zubkov YN, Nikiforov BM, Shustin VA. Balloon catheter technique for dilatation of constricted cerebral arteries after aneurysmal SAH. *Acta Neurochir (Wien).* 1984;70:65–79.

## Editorial Comments

The authors have presented a comprehensive review of the many advances in endovascular surgery in the past decade, applying to the treatment of aneurysms and cerebral vasospasm. Cases treated to date with these modalities have mostly included inoperable patients or aneurysms not amenable to direct clipping, and cases with cerebral vasospasm who have failed maximal medical therapy. The outcomes reported, together with associated morbidity and mortality, must be interpreted in light of this unfavorable bias. Yet, it may not necessarily follow that these techniques will have better performance in cases amenable to conventional therapy. There are to date no controlled data on the results of endovascular surgery in patients amenable to open surgery. Uncontrolled data suggest that endovascular surgery—even when associated with parent artery occlusion, is highly effective and safer than open surgical options for intracavernous and possibly for posterior circulation giant aneurysms. The use of endovascular surgery for other aneurysms remains experimental, and limited by protocols to cases where surgery is not feasible or is contraindicated.

The above raises the important question as to what aneurysm is truly inoperable, and who should decide on criteria of operability. There are situations where a neurologist, a radiologist or a less experienced neurosurgeon may be intimidated by the size or appearance of an aneurysm which is clearly clippable in experienced hands. In conjunction with this question, there may be a host of open surgical approaches, and a spectrum of endovascular options for a single lesion. Who should decide regarding the advantages of each and the "justifiable risk" in a given situation? Should a case which was "explored and the aneurysm found unclippable" be automatically considered for endovascular therapy regardless of the level of experience and expertise of the operating surgeon? These are critical questions which will frequently arise in practical situations. We agree with the authors that a truly multidisciplinary approach is indicated, involving a cohesive team with *strong and credible* neuroradiologic and neurosurgical viewpoints. Such a multidisciplinary approach is the best practical guarantee that the patient will be provided all reasonable options with mature and well-balanced guidance. Well-controlled prospective studies, careful analysis of ongoing personal and published experience, and responsible application of rapidly evolving technical advances should strongly influence the operation of such teams.

Once a given interventional modality is chosen by the patient and the treating team, there remain many questions about preoperative management; periocclusion events including propensity to thrombosis, embolism, or hemorrhage; and short- and long-term management after the procedure. There are many questions about the durability and long-term effectiveness of many endovascular procedures, especially those aiming at preserving the parent vessel. Furthermore, there is a relevant question as to whether the parent vessel should be preserved at any cost, especially in view of such uncertainties and in cases where collaterals allow tolerance to parent vessel occlusion.

In cases of symptomatic vasospasm intractable to medical therapy, it is not known when endovascular therapy should be initiated and what modalities to use and in what order. Clearly, early intervention would be desirable before irreversible brain parenchymal ischemic changes which may predispose to reperfusion complications. Yet endovascular treatment, notably the angioplasty of branches of the circle of Willis, may be associated with dreadful complications, frequently including lethal vessel rupture. Papaverine infusions appear to be much less risky than angioplasty, and may be justified quite early in the course of symptomatic vasospasm, and may be in asymptomatic preocclusive stenoses. Future refinements of endovascular techniques will likely lower the morbidity of intervention substantially so as to justify early and widespread use in the course of vasospasm.

Despite the above questions and concerns, it is evident that endovascular techniques have introduced a new dimension to the management of cerebral aneurysms. Endovascular techniques can enhance conventional surgical procedures by providing endovascular proximal control (and suction decompression), preoperative information about tolerance to occlusion of a parent vessel, or intraoperative superselective angiography and verification of the results of vascular reconstructions. The symbiotic interaction of endovascular and open surgical options offers the patient with a difficult aneurysm problem the best chances for effective therapy with the least risk. A firm commitment to such an interaction should underlie the philosophy of collaboration of interventional neuroradiologists and neurovascular surgeons within multidisciplinary teams entrusted with the management and scientific investigation of difficult aneurysms.

*Issam A. Awad, MD, MS, FACS*

# CHAPTER 12

# Infectious, Traumatic, and Other Unusual Aneurysms

Nelson Oyesiku, MD, and Daniel L. Barrow, MD

Most intracranial aneurysms, commonly referred to as "saccular aneurysms," arise in the vicinity of the circle of Willis and are congenital or arteriosclerotic in origin. Less commonly, aneurysms may arise secondary to infection, tumor, trauma, or other disorders. These peculiar lesions present an unusual diagnostic and sometimes therapeutic challenge to the neurosurgeon who is more accustomed to managing saccular aneurysms. However, several distinctive features of these lesions and a growing repertoire of therapeutic options allow us to be better prepared in meeting their challenge.

## Infectious Intracranial Aneurysms

Infectious intracranial aneurysms are uncommon, comprising only 2.6% to 6.0% of all intracranial aneurysms.[146,172] These aneurysms occur as a result of an ***intravascular*** source of infection. The majority of infectious intracranial aneurysms occur in patients with bacterial endocarditis. More rarely, infectious aneurysms may develop from an *extravascular* infection, such as meningitis, cavernous sinus thrombophlebitis, osteomyelitis, or pharyngitis.

Although infectious aneurysms are uncommon, rupture of these lesions is a common presentation and carries a grave prognosis with a mortality ranging from 60% to 90%.[24,81,110,146,173] Infectious aneurysms are treatable, but their early recognition requires a high index of suspicion.

Although the relative incidence of infectious aneurysms may be decreasing, the increasing use of corticosteroids, antibiotics, and antimetabolites may account for the growing number of reports of fungal aneurysms and infectious aneurysms of extravascular origin.[11,35,58,85,184]

### *Pathophysiology*

Karsner[81] classified infectious aneurysms into three types depending on the method of spread to the affected artery. The first and most common is due to emboli of vegetations from an infected cardiac valve, and thus is of ***intravascular*** origin. The most frequent organism cultured from patients with bacterial aneurysms due to endocarditis is *Streptococcus*. The second and far less common mode of spread is by extension from a neighboring infection. This ***extravascular*** source may result from meningitis, cavernous sinus thrombophlebitis, osteomyelitis of the skull, facial sinus infection or a postoperative infection.[12,62,69,73,130,151,172] The third form of infectious aneurysm is the ***primary or cryptogenic mycotic aneurysm,*** occurring in the absence of an obvious inflammatory process elsewhere in the body. The diagnosis of these rare lesions is presumptive and is based on the clinical situation and angiographic appear

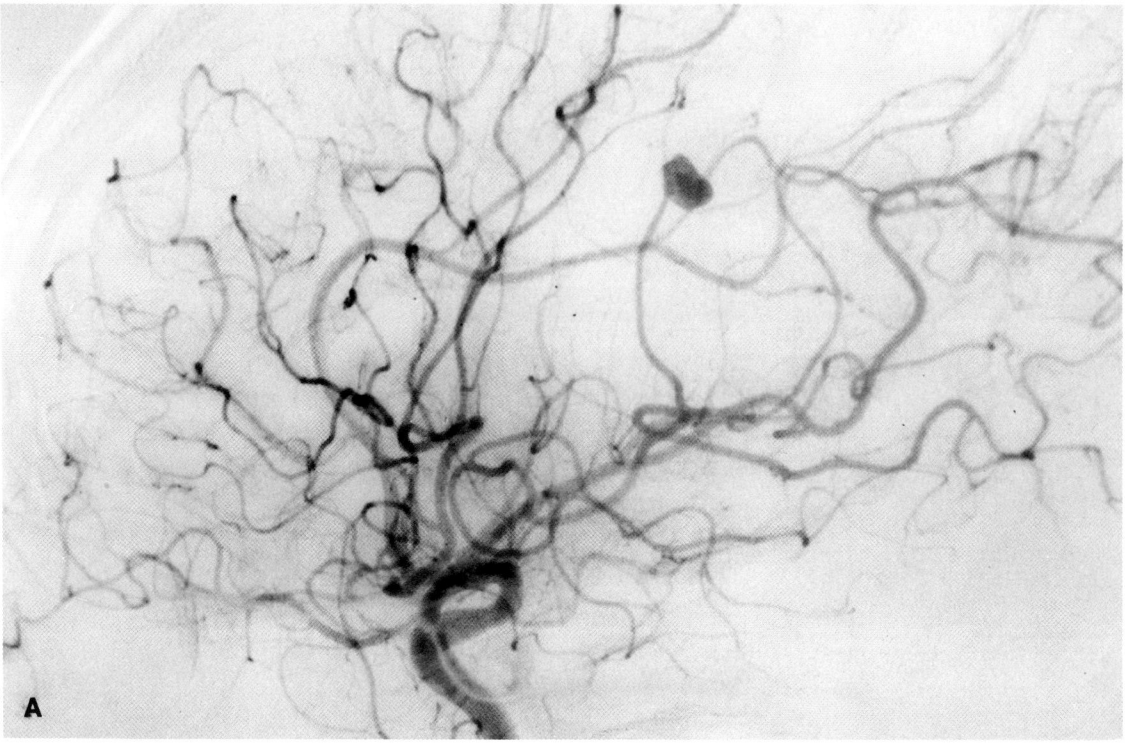


*Figure 1. Lateral (A) and AP (B) left carotid angiograms demonstrate an infectious aneurysm on a distal branch of the middle cerebral artery in a patient with infective endocarditis.*

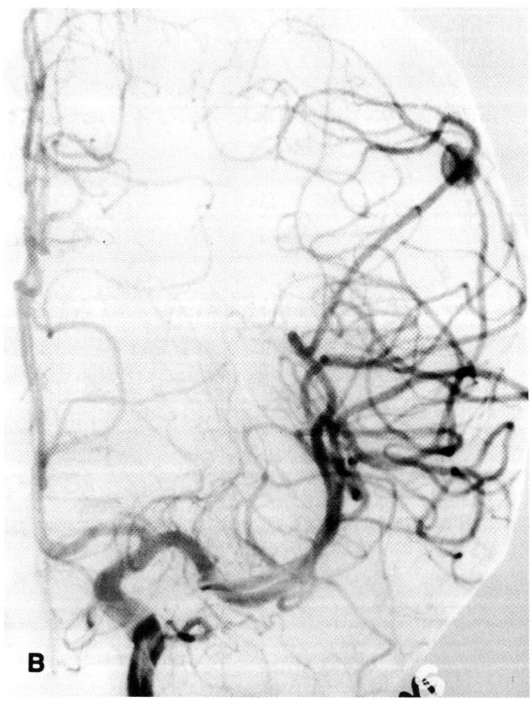


ance. Blood cultures are frequently negative, making these aneurysms difficult to treat with antibiotics.

Early controversy regarding the genesis of these aneurysms may have been dispelled by the findings of Molinari et al, who studied an animal model of septic cerebral embolization and demonstrated, as have others, that the inflammatory response proceeded from the adventitial surface toward the media, with the internal elastic membrane and intima being affected last.[46,109,120]

Infectious intracranial aneurysms of ***intravascular*** origin usually occur more peripherally in the vascular tree than do saccular aneurysms; they are commonly multiple. The high incidence of these aneurysms in the distal branches of the middle cerebral artery (MCA) reflects relative flow through this vessel and the likely sites for septic emboli to lodge and to produce an arteritis (Figure 1).[16,47]

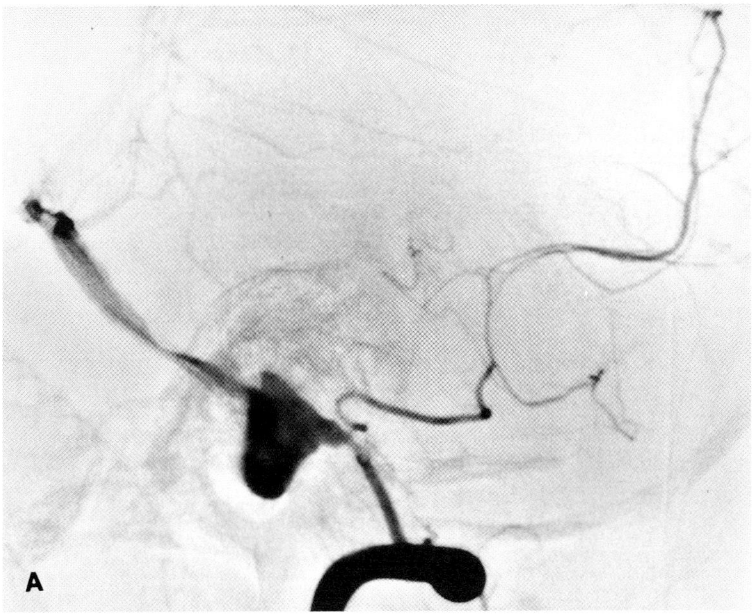


*Figure 2. Lateral (A) and AP (B) vertebral angiogram reveals a large distal vertebral artery aneurysm in a 4-year-old patient who developed a postoperative* Aspergillus *infection following craniectomy for a pilocytic cerebellar astrocytoma. The patient expired and at autopsy this aneurysm was found to contain* Aspergillus *fungal elements in the wall. (Reprinted with permission from Barrow DL, Prats AR. Infectious intracranial aneurysms. Comparison of groups with and without endocarditis.* Neurosurgery. *1990;27:562-573.)*

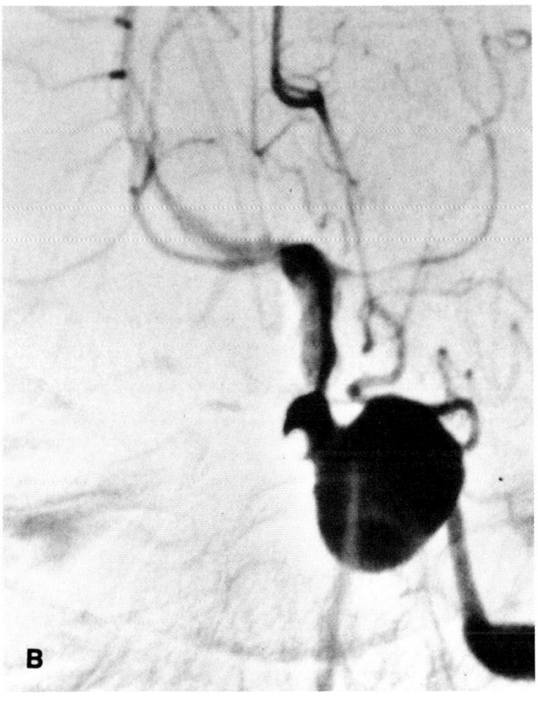


If the aneurysm originates *extravascularly,* it tends to be located more proximally, probably due to the presence of large vessels at the base of the brain where the infection is most intense (Figure 2).[69,80,172]

Fungal or "true" mycotic aneurysms are rare, nearly always occur in immunosuppressed patients, and are almost uniformly fatal.[11,35,47,106,127,128] Fungal aneurysms, unlike bacterial aneurysms, are frequently located proximally with neighboring thrombosed arteries (Figure 3)[73,184] and usually develop over a more protracted course. This period frequently lasts months prior to rupture, during which time the patient is often afebrile. This indolent course makes fungal aneurysms extremely difficult to diagnose.

## *Microbiology*

The majority of bacterial aneurysms asso-

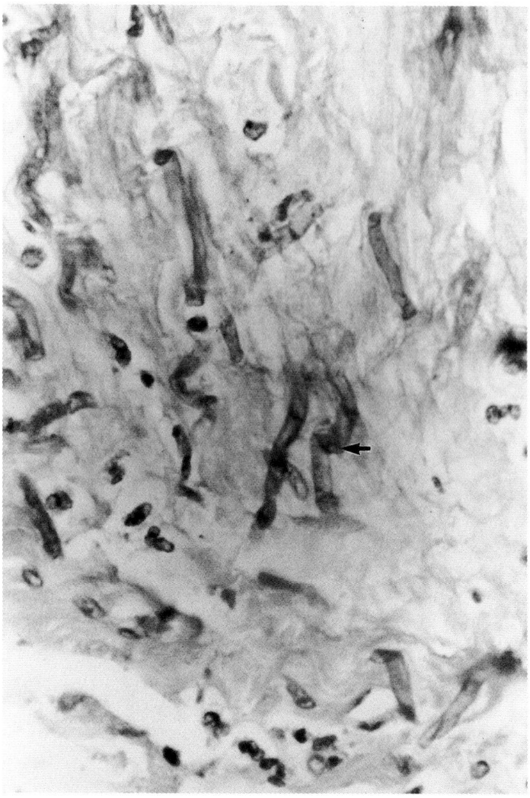

*Figure 3. Photomicrograph of aneurysm from case illustrated in Figure 2 demonstrates fungal elements in wall of aneurysm (arrow).*

ciated with infectious endocarditis are caused by *Streptococcus* or *Staphylococcus*. Ojemann et al reviewed 81 cases of infectious aneurysms from endocarditis and found the following incidence of causative organisms: *Streptococcus* (44%), *Staphylococcus* (18%), multiple organisms (4.8%), and negative cultures (10%). The incidence of staphylococcal endocarditis is increasing, whereas the incidence of alpha hemolytic streptococcal and pneumococcal endocarditis is diminishing.[127,128] Anaerobic bacterial and fungal infections are also increasing in prevalence, possibly due to the more widespread use of antibiotics, corticosteroids, and other immunosuppressants.[3,58,85,142]

Fungal intracranial aneurysms nearly always occur in the setting of immunosuppression. The most common organisms involved in mycotic aneurysms are *Aspergillus,* which usually spread from the facial sinuses or appear following cranial surgery,[11,106] *Candida albicans,* usually in the setting of *Candida* endocarditis, and Phycomycetes, most often found in diabetic patients. *Candida* and *Aspergillus* are highly angioinvasive, which may account for their predominance as causal agents of fungal aneurysms.

## *Clinical Manifestations*

Most infectious aneurysms occur in patients with bacterial endocarditis. The mean age of these patients is about 40 years; men and women are equally affected, and many have congenital or rheumatic heart disease. The incidence of infectious aneurysms in patients with bacterial endocarditis is from 2% to 10%.[16,143,190] The actual incidence may be much higher, as some lesions are asymptomatic; others spontaneously resolve, but some patients die before diagnosis.[16,127,128,190]

A significant number of patients with bacterial endocarditis without neurologic symptoms or signs present with a life-threatening hemorrhage from an infectious aneurysm. In Ojemann's review of 81 patients with bacterial intracranial aneurysms and definite or probable endocarditis reported between 1959 and 1980, 52% presented with hemorrhage.[128] In the series reported by Roach and Drake, all 5 patients (100%) presented with hemorrhage.[146] Ten of the 12 patients (83%) reported by Barrow and Prats bled as the initial manifestation.[11]

Despite this high incidence of hemorrhage and few premonitory neurologic signs or symptoms, neurologic symptoms are common in patients with bacterial endocarditis and often are the presenting symptoms of an infectious aneurysm. Neurologic symptoms are from septic emboli causing ischemia, suppuration, hemorrhage, meningoencephalitis, or abscess. Such symptoms occur in 29% to 39% of patients with endocarditis.[27,54,143] Cates and Christie found that 35% of patients with bacterial endocarditis had major visceral emboli, and 43% of these were to the brain.[27]

In 4% of their reported 442 cases of bacterial endocarditis hemorrhage from an infectious intracranial aneurysm contributed to death, and 21% of these patients had a clinically recognizable embolic event prior to hemorrhage. Frazee et al found warning signs or symptoms in all 13 patients in their series, the most common being headache followed by various focal neurologic complaints.[47] Often, in retrospect, a prior sign or symptom is elucidated from the history which, if interpreted correctly, would have led to earlier diagnosis.

The presentation of patients with infectious aneurysms of extravascular origin depends on the exact etiology. Many times the underlying disease or disorder overshadows the clinical manifestations of the aneurysm. In patients with intracavernous infectious aneurysms from cavernous sinus thrombophlebitis, the predominant symptoms and signs are exophthalmos, ophthalmoplegia, and ocular pain (Figure 4).

## *Diagnostic Studies*

The diagnosis of infectious endocarditis is made by history and physical examination, blood cultures, and lumbar punctures when not contraindicated by the presence of an intracranial space-occupying lesion. The diagnosis should be suspected in a febrile patient with precipitous neurologic signs.[54] The recognition of premonitory signs or symptoms prior to hemorrhage is important in early identification of infectious aneurysms and in reducing morbidity and mortality.

Computed tomography (CT) or magnetic resonance imaging (MRI) should be performed to exclude an intracranial mass. The CT scan or MRI should be obtained without and with contrast to demonstrate an associated abscess or cerebritis. This is followed by lumbar puncture with bacteriologic evaluation. Angiography is performed if there is a hemorrhage or if an aneurysm is suspected

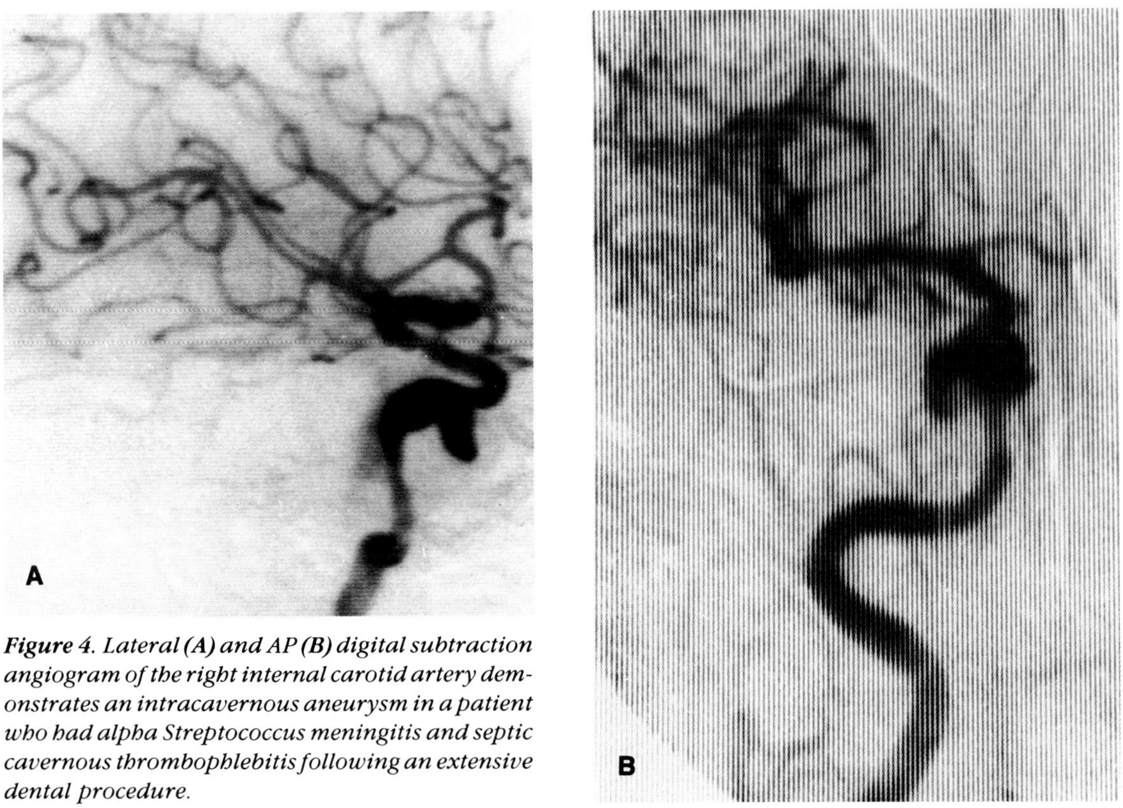


*Figure 4. Lateral (A) and AP (B) digital subtraction angiogram of the right internal carotid artery demonstrates an intracavernous aneurysm in a patient who had alpha Streptococcus meningitis and septic cavernous thrombophlebitis following an extensive dental procedure.*

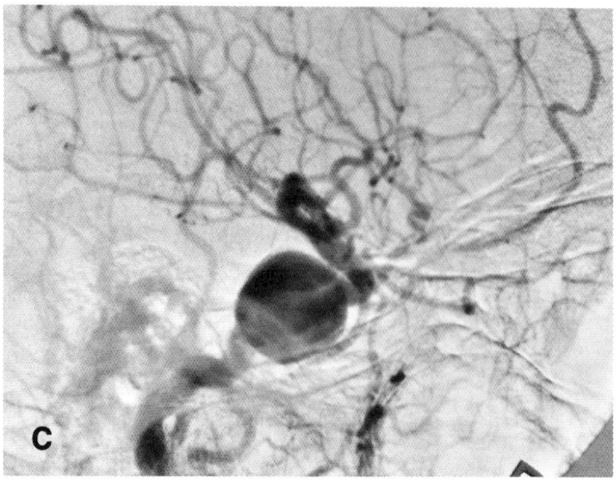

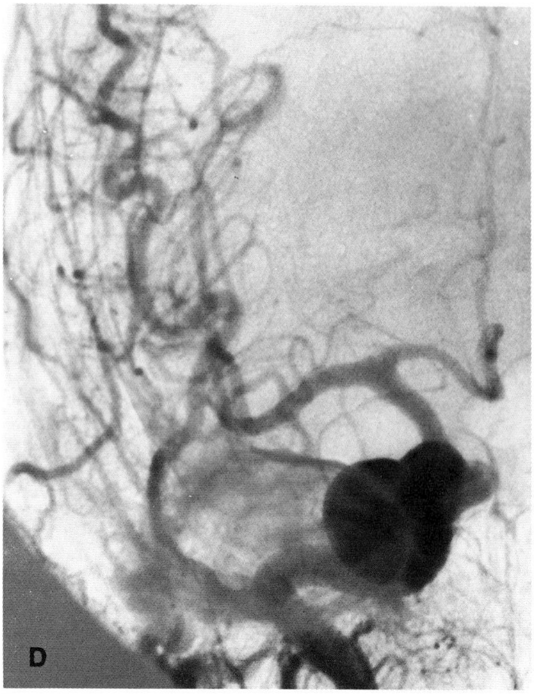

***Figure 4.*** *After antibiotic treatment, followup angiography (C* ***and*** *D) shows a significant enlargement of the aneurysm, which was then treated by endovascular occlusion of the internal carotid artery and aneurysm. (Reprinted with permission from Barrow DL, Prats AR. Infectious intracranial aneurysms. Comparison of groups with and without endocarditis.* **Neurosurgery**. *1990;27:562-573.)*

clinically or radiographically (Figure 5). The presence of small peripheral lesions, multiple aneurysms, or aneurysms with poorly defined necks should suggest an infectious cause.

Given the variable and unpredictable course of this disorder, the angiogram must be repeated at regular intervals to monitor the response to medical or surgical treatment.

## *Natural History*

The clinical course of infectious intracranial aneurysms may result in spontaneous cure, enlargement or reduction in size of the aneurysm, or development of new aneurysms.[16,24,40,47,82,114,183,199] The prognosis is extremely poor once the aneurysm ruptures. In this situation, the mortality ranges from 60% to 90%.[16,63,146]

## *Treatment*

The presence of an infectious aneurysm is not an absolute indication for surgery, as the aneurysm may resolve with antibiotics, often with preservation of the parent artery.[113] If the aneurysm does not resolve after a full course of antibiotics and certainly if it enlarges during or after treatment, surgery should be strongly considered. Although earlier surgery is an option for a readily approachable infectious aneurysm, delaying surgery during antibiotic therapy may allow for reparative fibrosis that will facilitate surgical repair.[11,24]

In their demonstrated propensity to bleed, ruptured infectious aneurysms often require a more aggressive surgical approach. The presence of a life-threatening intracranial hematoma is an indication for surgery, and preferably the aneurysm should be treated simultaneously (Figure 6).

Single, distal, ruptured infectious intracranial aneurysms in medically stable patients should be treated by excision. Proximally located bacterial aneurysms, unruptured aneurysms involving arteries where excision is likely to cause a serious neurologic deficit, or multiple aneurysms, should be treated by antibiotics and monitored with serial angiography repeated every 10 to 14 days and

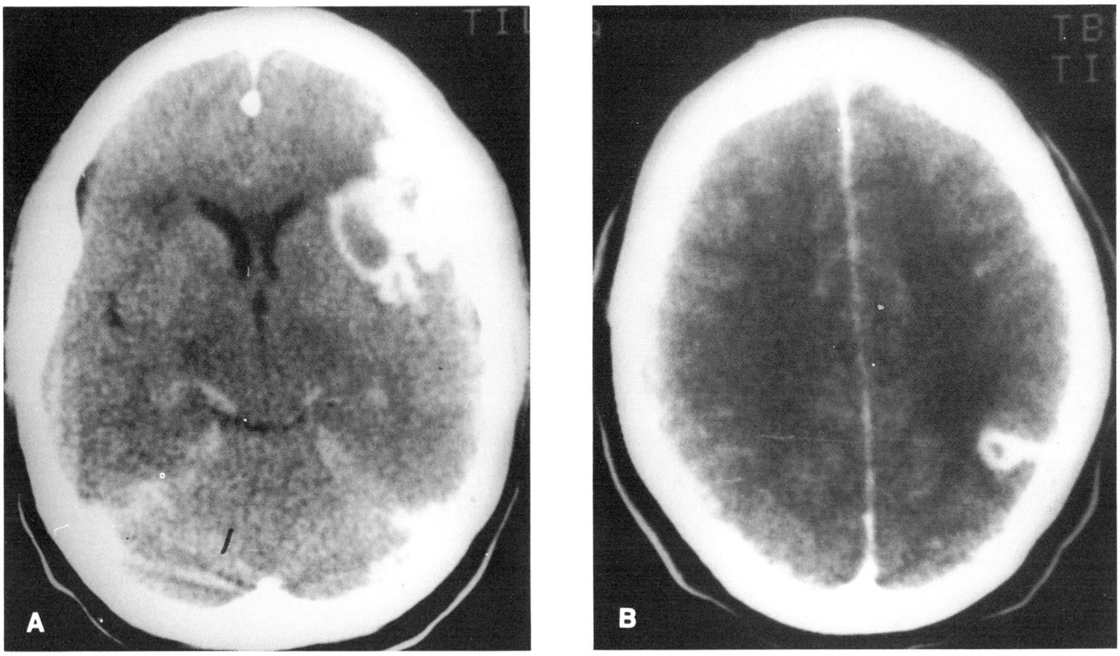


*Figure 5. (A) Axial CT demonstrates an area of hemorrhage near the left sylvian fissure and higher cut (B) shows a smaller hematoma in the posterior parietal area. This patient with subacute bacterial endocarditis was suspected to have infectious aneurysm as documented by left carotid angiography. (C) One aneurysm shows up on the early arterial phase of the lateral angiogram (arrow).*

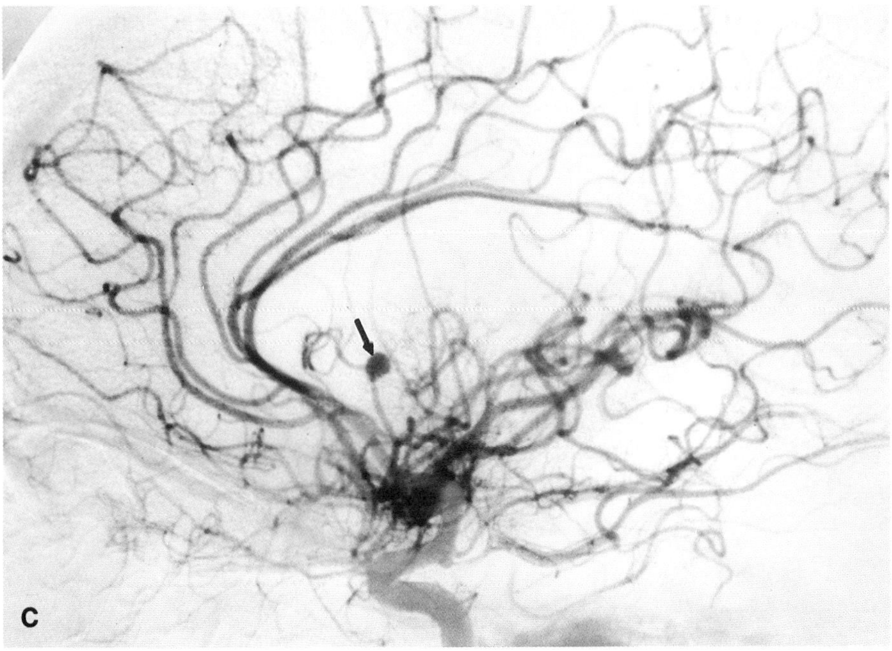


again at the end of the antibiotic course. If the aneurysm does not resolve after antibiotic treatment, surgery is usually recommended (Figure 7).[127,128]

In operating on infectious aneurysms, the surgeon may have to be innovative once the sac is exposed, as the surgical repair of these lesions can be extremely difficult. Preserva-

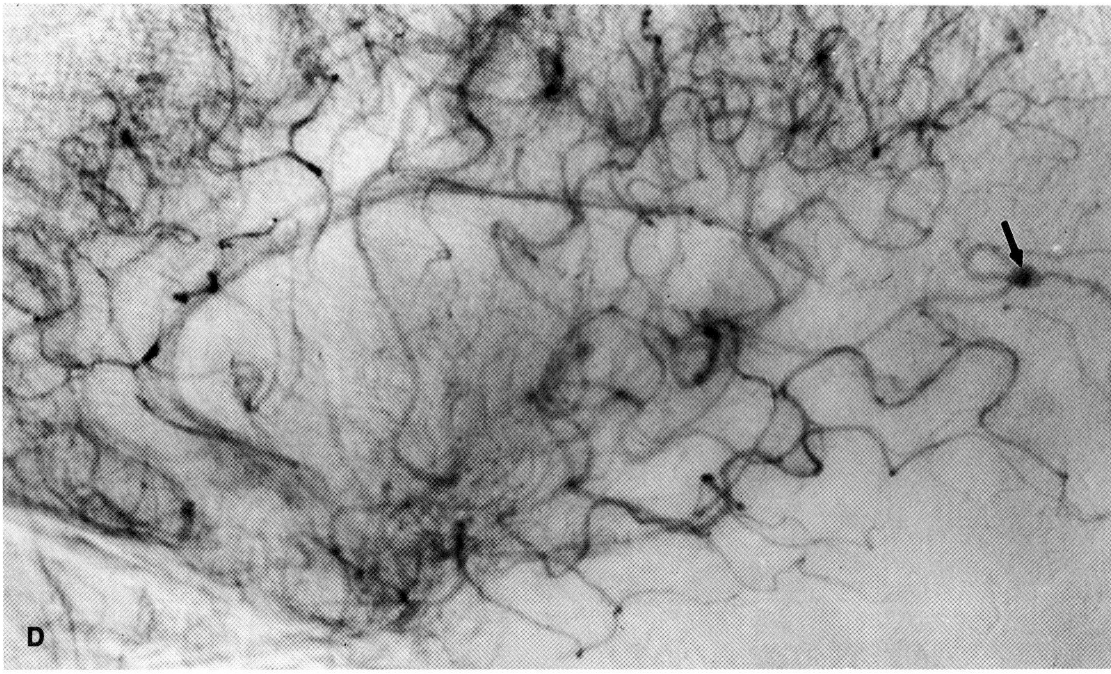


*Figure 5D. Same patient as in Figure 5A–C with another aneurysm appearing in a later phase of the lateral angiogram.*

tion of the normal vessel lumen while excluding the aneurysm from the circulation may be impossible for several reasons: the entire circumference of the vessel may be involved without the presence of a clippable neck, or the vessel may be extremely friable and unclippable. Furthermore, the wall of the aneurysm is frequently composed solely of gliotic, compressed brain tissue, making dissection hazardous. If the lesion is on a small distal branch, the vessel may be sacrificed with little or no neurologic deficit. If an important parent vessel or proximal artery must be sacrificed, an extracranial-to-intracranial bypass may be necessary to prevent infarction.[35,40,58]

## Traumatic Aneurysms

Traumatic intracranial aneurysms are infrequent lesions.[13,39,57,77,78,134,145,154,161,195] In a review of 912 operated intracranial aneurysms only 3 (0.3%) were classified as traumatic.[122] Fewer cases of traumatic aneurysms have been reported since 1976 since CT has replaced cerebral angiography as the primary evaluation of head injury.[122] Despite their rarity, the probability of rupture, combined with a readily available surgical cure, makes early diagnosis imperative.[60,84,100,178,195] Most traumatic aneurysms are located in the supratentorial compartment at sites other than branching points. Rarely are they infratentorial or multiple.

Traumatic aneurysms may be situated on the extradural internal carotid or vertebral artery,[7,13,15,61] the middle meningeal artery,[90] or on intracerebral arteries.[23,152] Traumatic aneurysms of intracerebral arteries are usually peripherally located—the most common location is a cortical branch of the middle cerebral artery (MCA).[23,28,33,61,152,195] Traumatic aneurysms have also been reported on the anterior cerebral, pericallosal,[20] and anterior choroidal artery.[34] Together, the middle cerebral and anterior cerebral artery locations account for 88% of cases.[195] Less than 10% of traumatic intracranial aneurysms involve the posterior circulation.[23,43,104,145,178,195] These aneurysms have been reported on the posterior inferior cerebellar artery (PICA),[104,178] the basilar

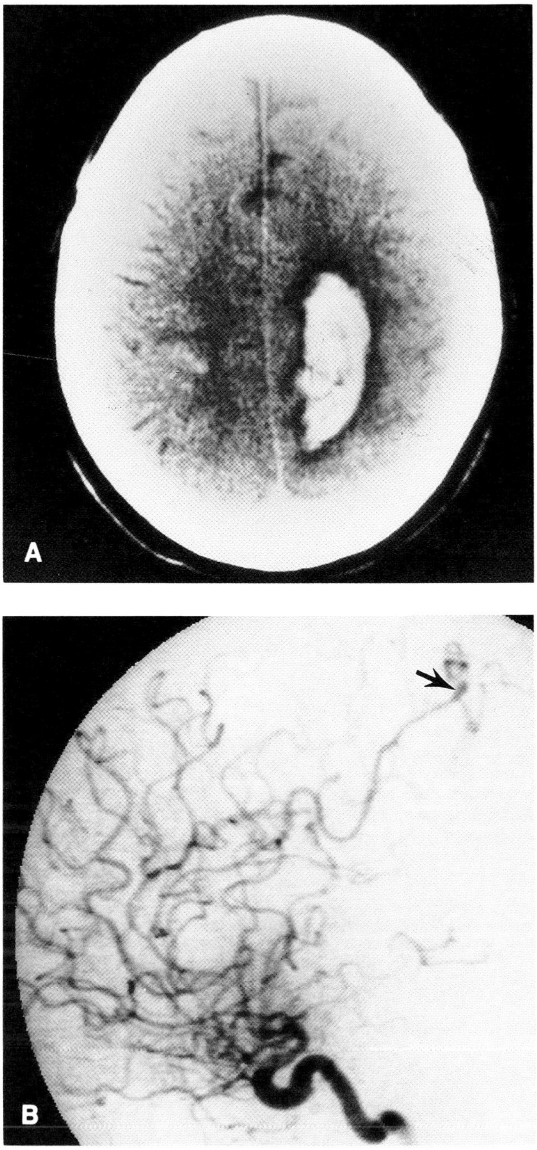


*Figure 6. (A) Axial CT demonstrates a large hematoma in this patient with known bacterial endocarditis. Because of his poor neurologic condition, he was taken directly to surgery without an angiogram. After evacuation of the hematoma, an intraoperative angiogram (B) demonstrated the aneurysm (arrow), which was then clipped.*

artery,[43] the superior cerebellar artery (SCA),[145] and the posterior cerebral artery (PCA).[153]

## Pathogenesis

The majority of traumatic aneurysms are caused by blunt injuries to the head (62%); other causes include penetrating wounds (27%) and iatrogenic trauma during intracranial surgery (11%).[13,97]

Intracranial traumatic aneurysms from direct injury usually result from penetrating bone fragments or from other missiles and weapons (Figure 8).[1,13,19,25,28,57,84] Direct iatrogenic traumatic intracranial aneurysms may be secondary to transnasal surgery, craniotomy, trephination, or repeated fontanelle taps (Figure 9).[32,41,67,75,131,137,160,186] Indirect arterial trauma can occur with severe closed head injuries; in these injuries vessels are damaged by striking the falx, tentorium, or bony prominences[61] during major brain shifts, or the vessel may be involved in an area of focal brain necrosis.[17] For instance, post-traumatic pericallosal aneurysms are probably caused by injury at the edge of the falx, and post-traumatic aneurysms of the MCA probably occur from the vessel striking the sphenoid ridge. Traumatic aneurysms, therefore, are invariably associated with skull fractures or other evidence of severe brain injury such as acute subdural hematoma,[57,98] cerebral contusions and hematomas,[57,77] and lacerations.[88,104,134]

Superficial cerebral arteries may be torn at the point where they adhere to or supply the dura. Surface arterioles that accompany bridging veins or densely adhere to the dura may be injured during acceleration or deceleration of the brain.[37] Superficial vessels may also be trapped within a fracture line, resulting in vessel wall injury. Although skull base traumatic aneurysms most commonly involve the petrous and cavernous carotid artery (CCA),[21] basilar skull fractures involving the clivus may lead to a traumatic aneurysm of the PICA, and a fracture of the sella turcica has been reported to result in a traumatic aneurysm.[88,104] Finally, giant traumatic aneurysms of the internal carotid artery (ICA) have resulted from skull base injuries at the site of aneurysm formation.[170]

Extracranial cervical carotid aneurysms may result from violent puncture wounds, angiography, endarterectomy, or as a delayed result of dissection (Figure 10).

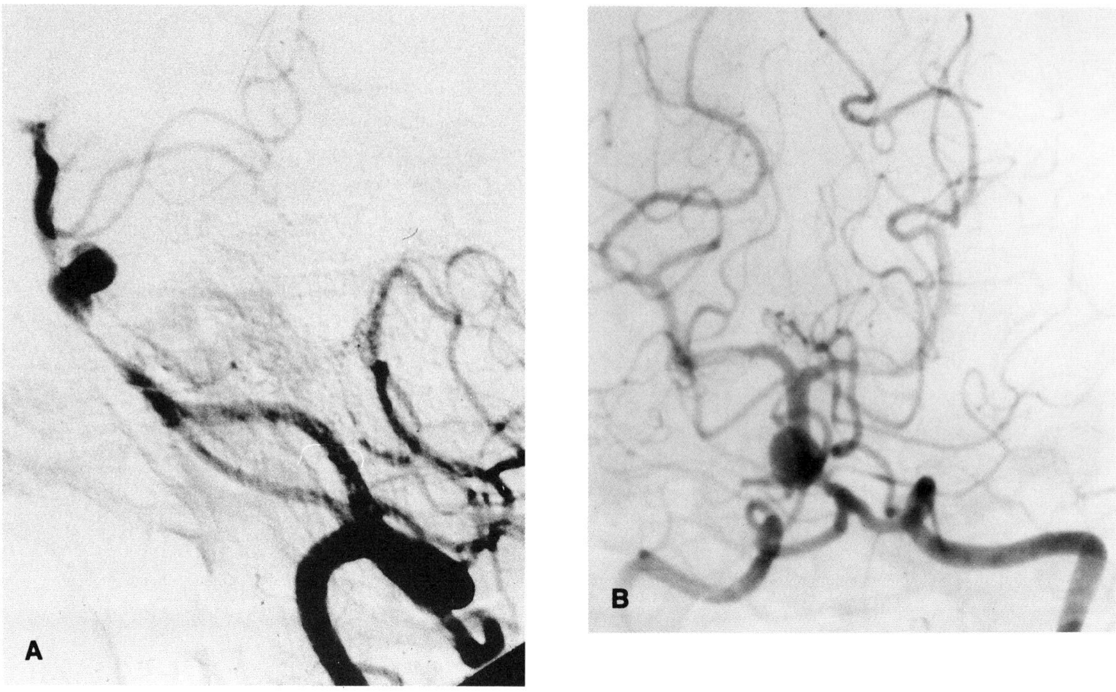


*Figure 7.* *Lateral (A) and AP (B) vertebral angiogram of infectious midbasilar artery aneurysm that developed after treatment of Pseudomonas meningitis. When the aneurysm did not resolve with antibiotic treatment, the sac was surgically treated as documented on postoperative angiography* ***(C and D)****. (Reprinted with permission from Barrow DL, Prats AR. Infectious intracranial aneurysms. Comparison of group with and without endocarditis.* Neurosurgery*. 1990;27:562-573.)*

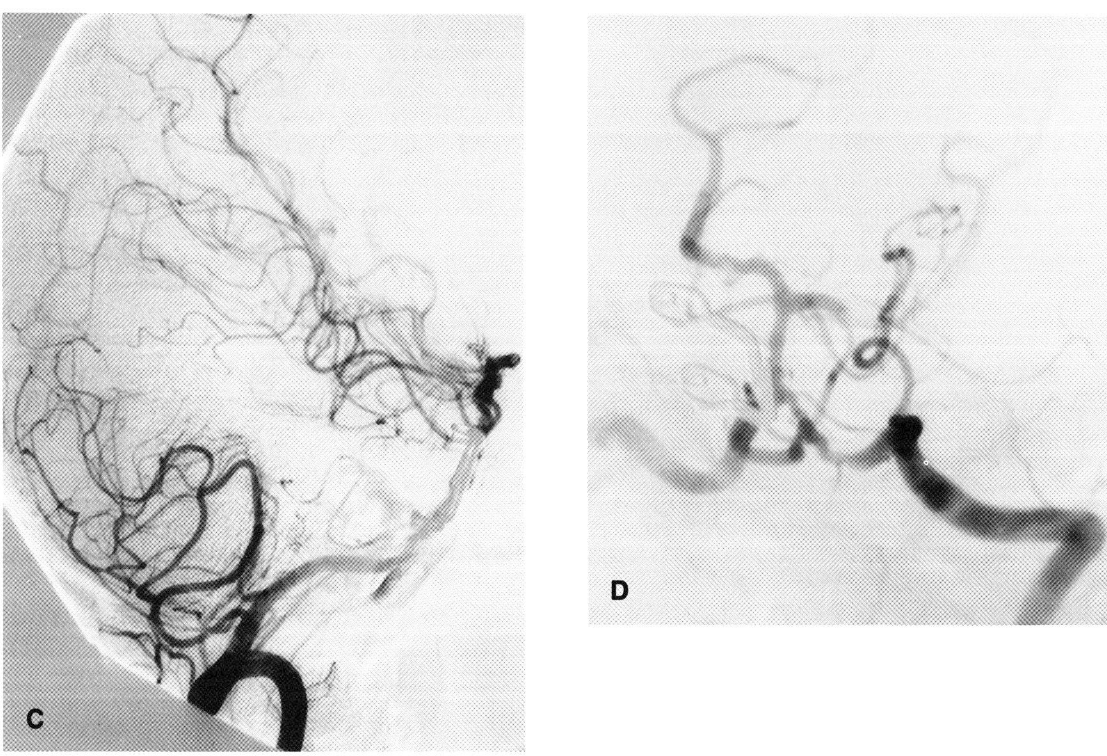

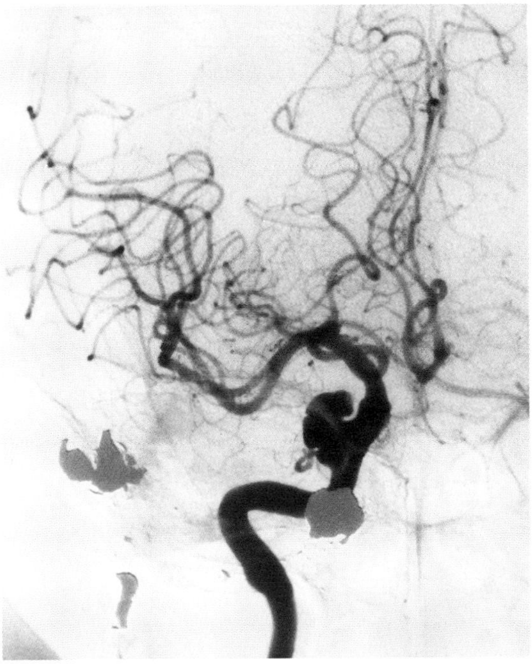

*Figure 8.* *AP right carotid angiogram reveals a traumatic intracavernous aneurysm (arrow) following a gunshot wound. Note metallic bullet fragments (arrowheads). The patient was treated with trapping and a petrous-to-supraclinoid carotid saphenous vein bypass.*

Traumatic meningeal aneurysms may arise by at least two different mechanisms. When the middle meningeal artery enters the cranial cavity, its histologic appearance changes to that of a cerebral artery and medial defects are very common.[65] A temporal skull fracture may bruise the wall of the middle meningeal artery and cause extravasation of blood, which is initially contained in the outer dural laminae. Fibrosis of this overlying tissue results in a false aneurysm.

Other meningeal artery aneurysms may be found on the inner dural membrane and are attached to both the inner dural membrane and the cerebral cortex. Markwalder and Huber[96] considered these aneurysms to be the consequence of traction on small bridging vessels between the meningeal and cerebral vessels produced by displacement of the brain at the moment of impact. Aneurysms of these thin-walled, poorly supported vessels may expand silently and rupture. These authors also implicate the fibrinolytic action of cerebro-

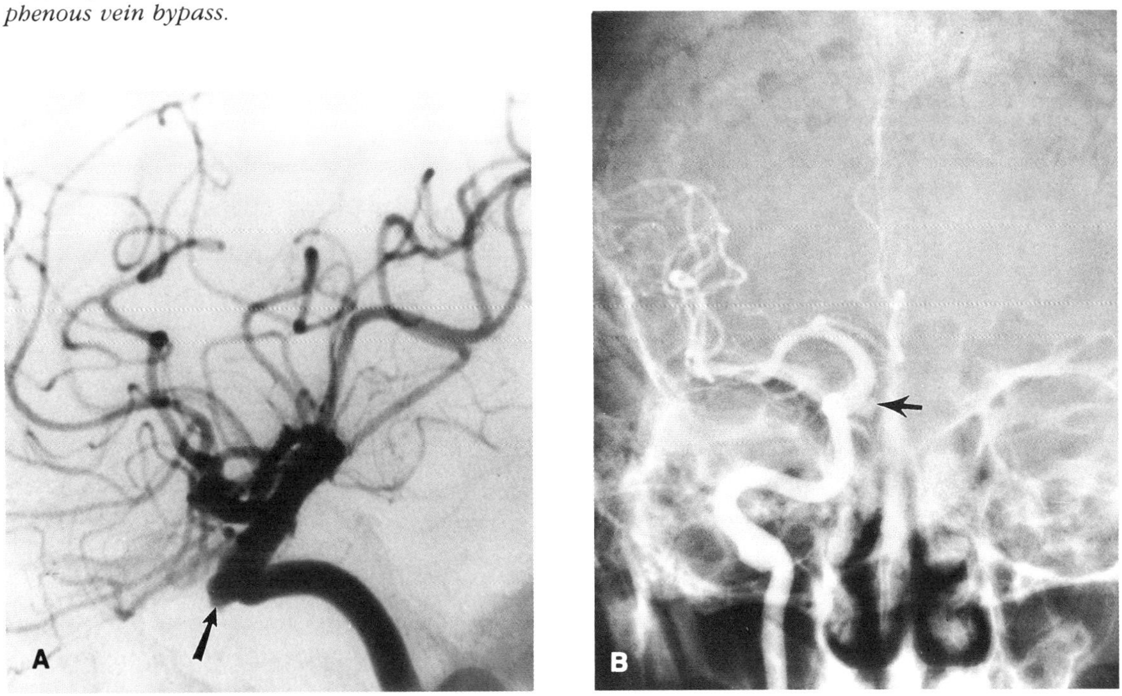


*Figure 9.* *Lateral (A) and AP (B) right carotid angiograms demonstrate a small intracavernous aneurysm (arrow) in a patient who presented with massive epistaxis following trans-sphenoidal removal of a pituitary adenoma. He was treated by STA–MCA bypass followed by endovascular carotid occlusion.*

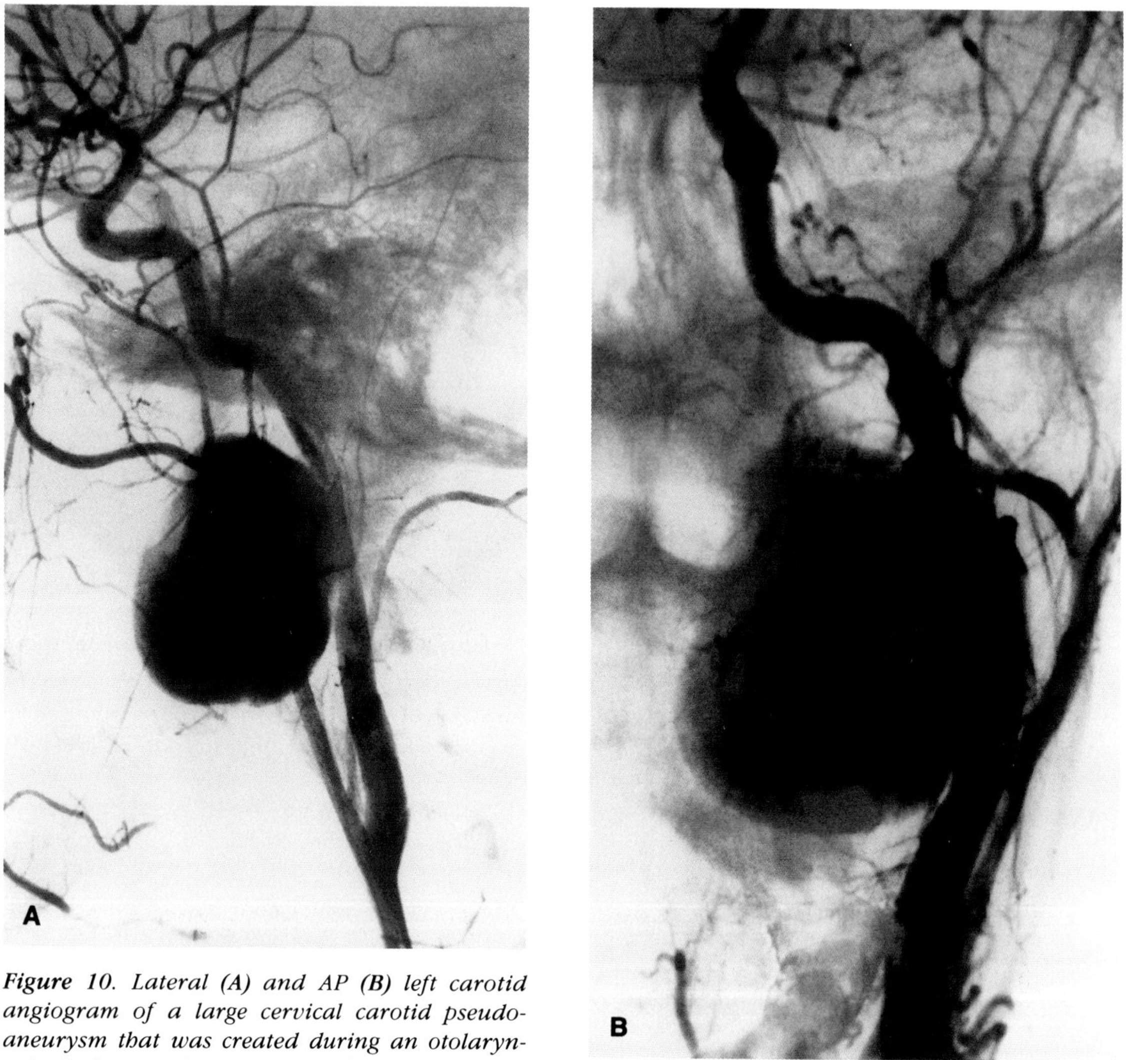


*Figure 10. Lateral (A) and AP (B) left carotid angiogram of a large cervical carotid pseudoaneurysm that was created during an otolaryngological operative procedure. The patient was treated with endovascular coil occlusion of the carotid artery after a balloon-test occlusion and SPECT demonstrated adequate collateral circulation (see Figure 14).*

spinal fluid (CSF) in the early rupture of these meningeal aneurysms.[96]

Traumatic aneurysms may also be classified pathophysiologically as true to false aneurysms. "True" aneurysms develop when the chief arterial injury is to the internal elastic lamina, resulting in slow aneurysmal dilatation. The more common lesion is the "false" aneurysm in which there is hemorrhage from a small, full-thickness arterial rent into local brain tissue, followed by formation of a fibrous sac. Mixed varieties, with rupture of a "true" aneurysm giving rise to a secondary "false" aneurysm[23] and dissecting traumatic aneurysms of cerebral arteries[38,141] have also been reported.

Traumatic intracranial aneurysms in childhood are rare. They may arise from various mechanisms. Penetrating trauma occurs most commonly in teenage boys from gunshot wounds. Nonpenetrating injuries result from motor vehicle injuries and falls, and these aneurysms may be located at the skull base or the periphery. Proximal aneurysms show a predominance in teenage boys, whereas peripheral aneurysms tend to occur in younger children and show less of a male preponderance.[21]

## Natural History

The natural history of traumatic aneurysms is unpredictable. They may enlarge[57,170] or resolve spontaneously as in 8 of 94 (8.5%) cases reported by Yokota et al.[195] The most common presentation is hemorrhage.[9,45,153] This usually occurs after the initial injury in an otherwise stable patient. The interval between the antecedent head trauma and the rupture of a traumatic aneurysm is highly variable and may range from hours to years.[28] One review of more than 40 cases showed a mean interval from injury-to-rupture of three weeks.[45] Burton et al[23] found a mortality of 54% in the literature on peripheral traumatic aneurysms to 1968; from 1968 to 1975, however, mortality dropped to an estimated 18% of published cases.[45]

There are relatively few reports of uneventful recovery from rupture of a traumatic intracranial aneurysm, suggesting that early diagnosis and treatment are important in preventing significant morbidity and mortality. Rupture of traumatic aneurysms tends to be more catastrophic than the hemorrhage from saccular aneurysms, with a mortality ranging from 27% to 50%.[2,9,43,45,153]

## Diagnosis

The diagnosis of a traumatic aneurysm requires a high index of suspicion as the sequelae of the initial trauma frequently mask any evidence of the aneurysm. Most traumatic intracranial aneurysms come to the clinical attention only after they rupture. The diagnosis should be suspected in any patient who deteriorates after initial recovery from a head injury. A computed tomography (CT) scan will frequently reveal fresh blood from the aneurysmal hemorrhage (Figure 11). Enlarging aneurysms may present as a result of mass effect. Intracavernous traumatic aneurysms may produce massive epistaxis because the intracavernous carotid is in close anatomic relationship to the sphenoid and nasal fossae. These aneurysms may result in fatal (52) or several epistaxis,[60,187] but more commonly present with ophthalmoplegia due to compression of intracavernous cranial nerves or visual loss (Figure 12). In a recent report of 6 patients presenting with delayed visual loss after head trauma, the etiology was an aneurysm or pseudoaneurysm or carotid cavernous fistula. Visual loss occurred from 1 day to 13 years after the initial injury and the pathogenesis of visual loss with the aneurysms and pseudoaneurysms was either direct optic nerve or chiasmal compression and intracranial hematoma (Figure 12).[189] Rupture of a middle meningeal artery aneurysm may present with an epidural or subdural hemorrhage.[89] Extracranial carotid aneurysms may present with embolic symptoms or symptoms due to mass effect such as hoarseness, dysphagia, dyspnea, ocular pain, or Horner's syndrome.

Cerebral angiography provides a definitive diagnosis. The traumatic intracranial aneurysm is differentiated angiographically from saccular aneurysms by its peripheral location away from branching points, its delayed filling and emptying, the absence of a well-formed neck, and an irregular contour. Traumatic aneurysms are frequently less opaque than saccular aneurysms and are occasionally missed on initial angiography, only to become apparent on a later study. The traumatic aneurysm of the middle meningeal artery, in addition to the above generic characteristics, also presents distinctively as an aneurysmal shadow on the floor of the middle cranial fossa displacing the ipsilateral MCA.[89] The diagnosis of traumatic aneurysms may be overlooked in the presence of associated life-threatening hematomas,[134] since angiography has been replaced by CT in the initial evaluation of head injury.[122]

With further experience, magnetic resonance (MR) imaging may play an important role in identifying traumatic aneurysms. The authors have used MR angiography as a

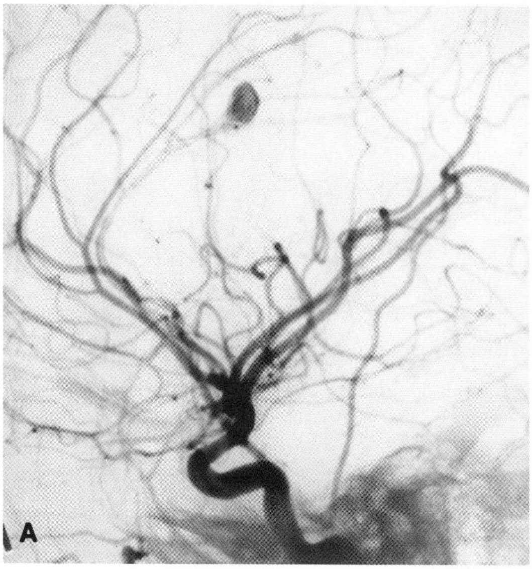


*Figure 11. Lateral (A) and AP (B) carotid angiogram of a traumatic distal anterior cerebral artery pseudoaneurysm that was discovered in a patient who deteriorated after initial improvement following a closed head injury. CT revealed fresh blood in the region of the aneurysm. The aneurysm was treated by trapping.*

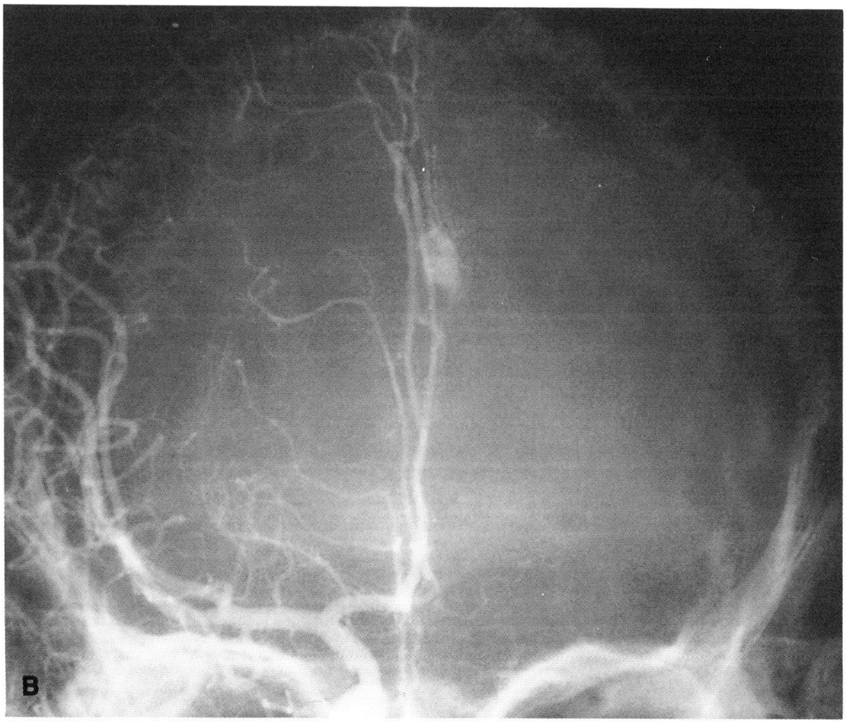


means of following extradural traumatic aneurysms noninvasively.

## *Treatment*

There is a significantly lower mortality for surgically treated patients with traumatic intracranial aneurysms than for patients treated nonsurgically.[2,9,45,134,195] Surgical mortality ranges from 18% to 30%, depending on whether the lesion has bled, whereas mortality for nonoperative management ranges from 40% to 75%.[9,45,195] This difference may reflect a selection bias with patients in poor condition more often being treated nonoperatively.

Craniotomy should provide adequate exposure with proximal and distal control of the injured vessel. The goal of surgery is to eliminate the aneurysm from the circulation and preserve the parent artery. Direct clipping of these aneurysms may be difficult, as the wall is fragile and the neck, if present, is often broad-based or ill-defined.[100,135] When direct

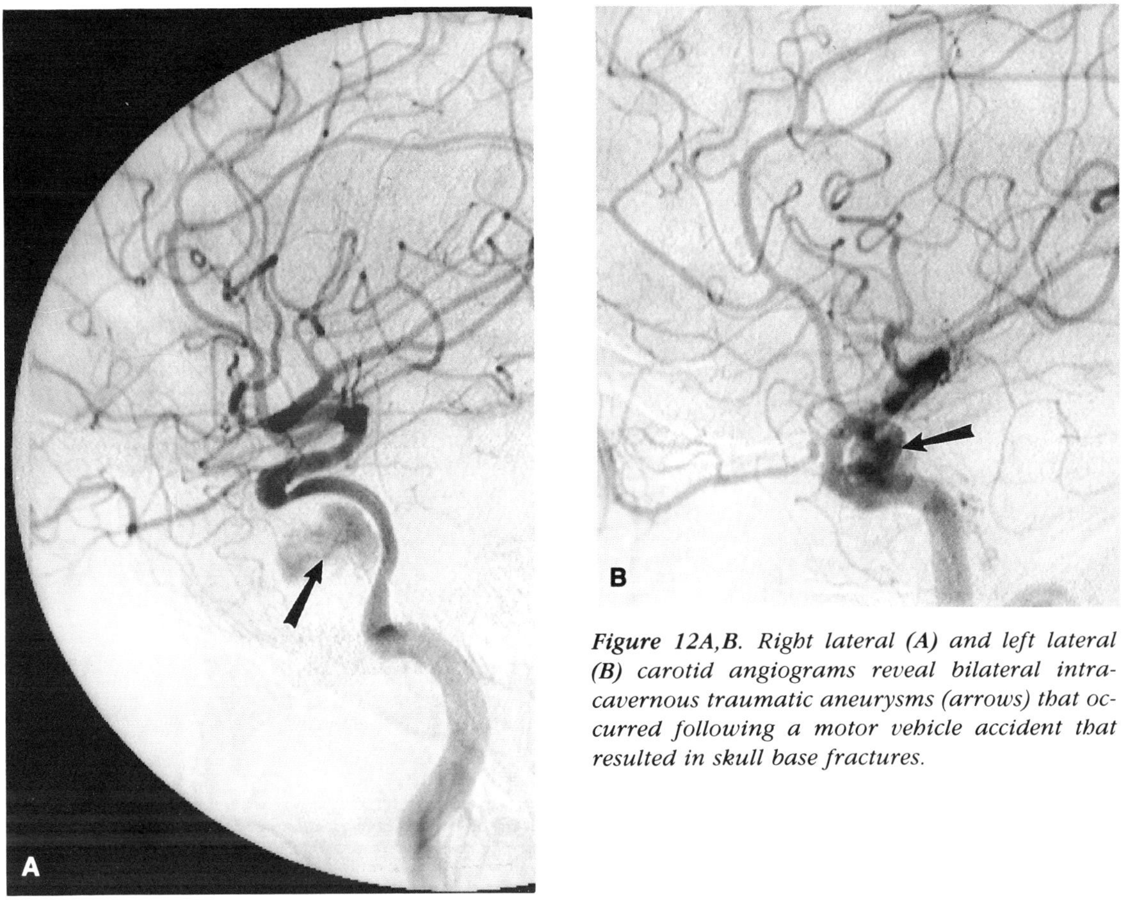


*Figure 12A,B. Right lateral (A) and left lateral (B) carotid angiograms reveal bilateral intracavernous traumatic aneurysms (arrows) that occurred following a motor vehicle accident that resulted in skull base fractures.*

clipping cannot be accomplished, a circumferential sleeve clip, such as the Sundt clip graft, may eliminate the lesion. The peripheral location of these aneurysms will sometimes allow for resection of the lesion and sacrifice of the parent artery without neurologic deficit. Often, the cerebral tissue distal to the site of arterial injury and the aneurysm is already infarcted. Other surgical strategies include cauterization, trapping,[57,75] wrapping with muslin, and excision with microvascular bypass grafting.[60]

Traumatic pseudoaneurysms of the extracranial carotid or vertebral arteries may be treated with antiplatelet therapy to reduce the change of embolization.[141] Definitive surgical therapy may involve direct repair of the aneurysm or endovascular occlusion of the sac, often along with the parent artery (Figure 13). Particularly for pseudoaneurysms of the carotid artery located in the high neck or near the base of the skull,[53] an endovascular approach with occlusion of the sac (and often the parent artery) with detachable coils is less traumatic for the patient (Figure 14). Prior to endovascular treatment, a balloon-test occlusion, combined with measurement of cerebral blood flow by either single photon emission computed tomography (SPECT) or Xenon computed tomography, is performed to assess the patient's ability to tolerate sacrifice of the parent artery. If the patient does not tolerate the test occlusion clinically or if the CBF drops significantly during temporary occlusion, the vessel must be spared, reconstructed, or a bypass procedure performed such as a superficial temporal artery (STA)-to-middle cerebral artery (MCA) bypass or external carotid-to-MCA vein graft bypass.

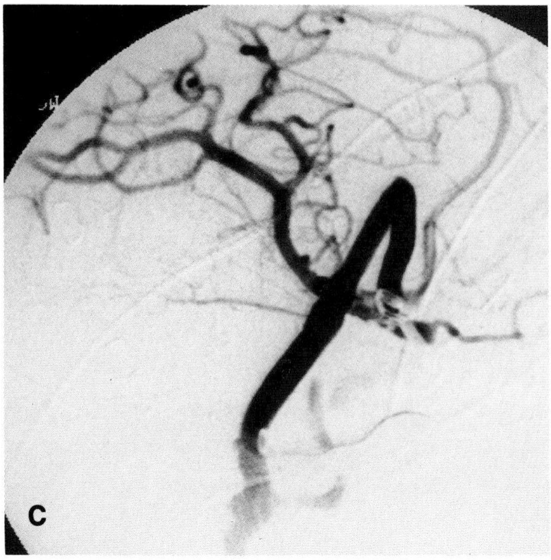


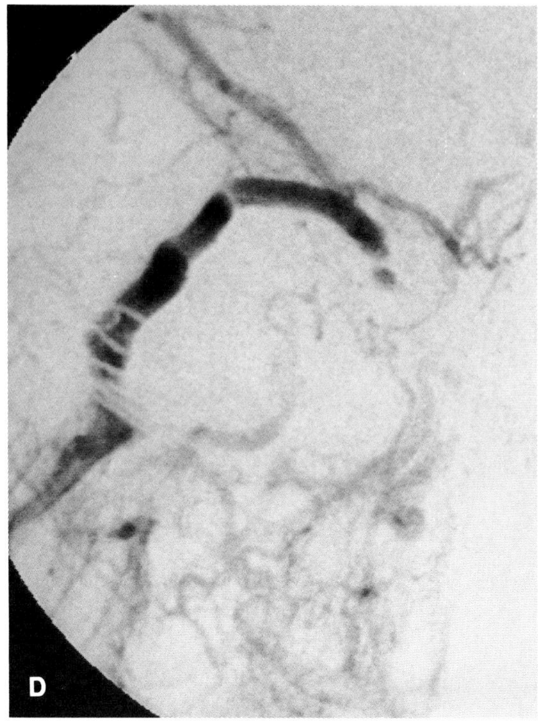


*Figure 12C,D. This large, right-sided lesion was treated by trapping and petrous carotid-to-supraclinoid carotid vein graft bypass, as shown on the lateral (C) and AP (D) intraoperative angiograms.*

## Dissecting Aneurysms

Dissecting aneurysms may affect any part of the extracranial or intracranial arterial tree. Dissecting aneurysms are more common in the extracranial arteries, especially the cervical carotid. Intracranial dissecting aneurysms usually involve the supratentorial anterior circulation (65.7%) and less commonly the posterior circulation (34.3%). Most intracranial dissecting aneurysms are located on the MCA (36.8%) and less commonly on the anterior cerebral artery (7.8%), or vertebrobasilar arteries (22.3%), and 31.6% are multiple, involving two or three main branches.[121]

### *Pathogenesis*

Dissections may be spontaneous or traumatic[167] and usually occur in otherwise healthy people. Males are more commonly affected than females. Lesions in the cervical arteries and the posterior circulation tend to occur in young to middle-aged patients. Children are more prone to anterior circulation dissections. Marfan's syndrome, syphilis, moyamoya disease, polycystic kidney disease, and fibromuscular dysplasia predispose to dissections and, as discussed earlier, closed head injury with neck torsion is a common cause of cervical carotid artery and anterior circulation dissections. Other etiologic factors include spontaneous arteritis, wall defects, polymyositis, pregnancy, or arterial wall necrosis.[52,66,86,99,126,139,169,181,196] Arterial dissections begin as a breach in the endothelium and subjacent layers, resulting in extrusion of the advancing blood column into the arterial wall, separating the layers and collapsing the true intima upon itself. In type 1 dissections, the arterial dissection is between the internal elastic lamina and the media. In type 2 lesions the dissection plane is through the media into and through the adventitia, resulting in subarachnoid hemorrhage (SAH).

Intracranial dissecting aneurysms are located predominantly on the middle cerebral artery, and they usually originate subintimally.[168] On the contrary, extracranial carotid artery dissections usually originate in the media.

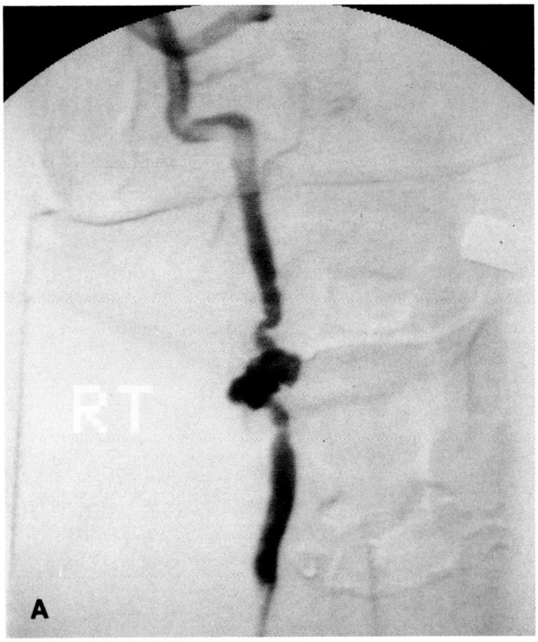


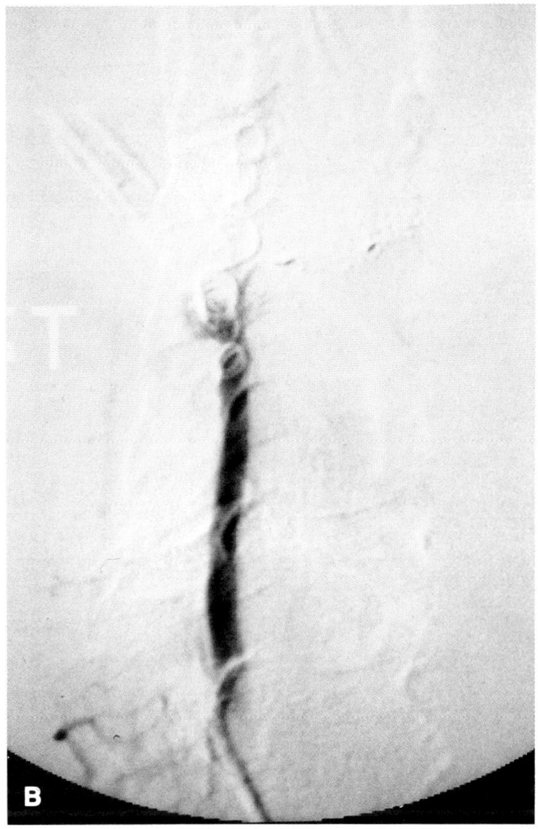


*Figure 13. Right AP vertebral angiogram demonstrates a vertebral artery pseudoaneurysm created by a wound (arrow). This lesion was treated by endovascular coil occlusion (arrow) of the vertebral artery and aneurysm after patency of the contralateral vertebral artery was documented.*

Extracranial vertebral dissections are less common than intracranial vertebral or cervical carotid artery dissections. Posterior circulation dissecting aneurysms occur mostly in males (2.6:1), with a mean age of 36 years. Etiologic factors include trauma, syphilis, and hypertension, or they may arise spontaneously.[94] Dissecting aneurysms of the vertebral artery usually develop between C2 and the foramen magnum.

Yokota et al reviewed 94 vertebral artery aneurysms in 86 patients. Twenty-six (28%) were dissecting aneurysms, 81% of these bled, and 24% of these rebled,[195] confirming an earlier impression that most dissecting aneurysms with SAH are likely vertebral or basilar in location.[48,105,162,198]

## *Clinical Presentation*

The clinical presentation of dissecting aneurysms may be the result of embolization and induced cerebral ischemia. Other patients may present with hemorrhage or local compressive symptoms from enlargement of the aneurysm. Headache is a common initial symptom of intracranial dissecting aneurysm and usually antedates the more serious ischemic or hemorrhagic strokes.[193]

Intracranial dissecting aneurysms result in intraparenchymal or SAH[48] and death more frequently than extracranial dissecting aneurysms.[125] Traumatic dissections of the extracranial carotid artery most commonly present with delayed focal cerebral ischemic symptoms; less common is a focal unilateral headache associated with oculosympathetic paresis or bruit. In fact, following a head injury, the abrupt onset of focal cerebral symptoms after an initial recovery should suggest an arterial injury. The delayed ischemic symptoms from a dissecting aneurysm are usually due to embolization.[108,180]

Vertebral artery dissecting aneurysms

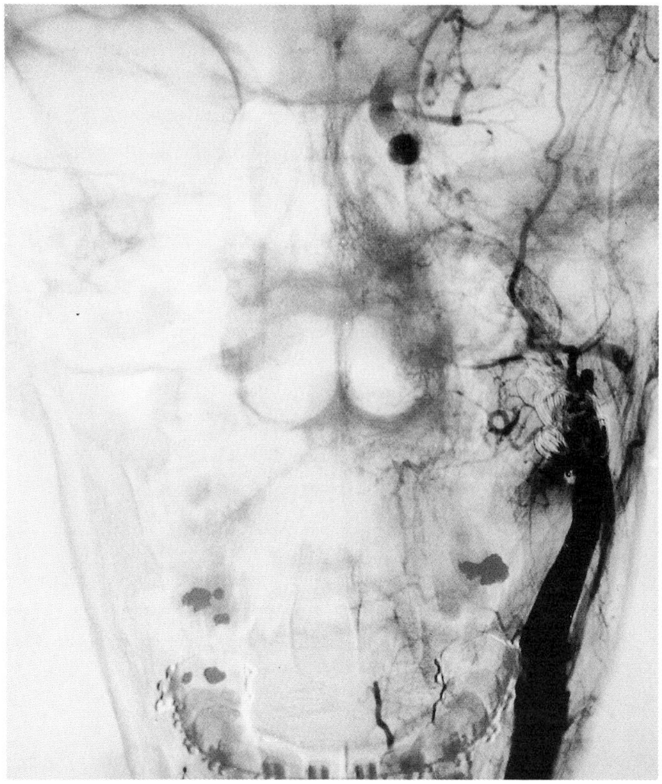

*Figure 14. Left AP angiogram illustrates endovascular coil occlusion of a large cervical carotid pseudoaneurysm (see Figure 10).*

may cause symptoms ranging from suboccipital pain to profound neurologic deficits from extension of the dissection or distal emboli.[14,116,177,194] Intracranial vertebral dissections were found by Caplan et al to have four overlapping presentations: (1) brain stem infarcts due to subintimal dissection extending into the basilar artery that affected younger patients and were often single fatal events; (2) SAH due to subadventitial or transmural dissection; (3) aneurysms causing mass effect on the brain stem and lower cranial nerves; and (4) chronic dissections due to connective tissue defects causing extensive bilateral aneurysms, repeated transient ischemic attacks, small strokes, and SAH.[26] Dissecting aneurysms of the basilar artery are rare and usually present with brain stem ischemia rather than SAH.[74]

## *Diagnostic Imaging*

Angiographic findings typical of dissecting intracranial aneurysms include (1) fusiform dilatation of the vessel with narrowing proximally and distally to the dilatation (pearl-in-a-string sign); (2) retention of contrast within the aneurysm into the late capillary or venous phase; (3) double lumen.[48,92,163] Other angiographic findings in extracranial dissections include aneurysm, stenosis of the lumen, occlusion, intimal flap, and distal branch occlusion (embolization), and slow internal carotid-to-MCA flow.[108] An initial angiogram may be normal, only for the dissecting aneurysm to become apparent on a repeat study.[119] MR angiography is also useful in delineating dissecting aneurysms,[164] and may demonstrate intimal flaps, intramural hematoma, and hematoma adjacent to the parent artery.[4]

### *Natural History*

The natural history of intracranial dissecting aneurysms is nebulous, partly because of the small number of cases and partly because the aneurysms have been mainly diagnosed by postmortem histologic examination. Dissecting aneurysms of the vertebral artery seem to carry a high rate of bleeding and brain stem infarction leading to a high morbidity and mortality.[95,177] The risk of bleeding as estimated from a review of 26 dissecting aneurysms of the vertebral artery was about 81%, and the risk of rebleeding in those patients was 24%.[194] This rate of rebleeding was confirmed by Aoki et al to be approximately 30% in another review of 60 vertebral artery dissecting aneurysms. Most of these rebleeding episodes occurred acutely.[6]

Some dissecting aneurysms have resolved spontaneously with complete remission.[95]

The natural history of dissecting aneurysms is determined in part by the plane of dissection. Evidence for this is derived from an autopsy series of 110 patients with SAH in which the incidence of dissecting aneurysms was 4.5% (5 cases) and all 5 cases had progressed rapidly to death from massive SAH. Subintimal dissections resulted in terminal occlusion from intramural hematoma and usually extended into the basilar artery with brain stem infarction. Subadventitial dissections usually resulted in massive SAH with the dissection confined to the vertebral artery.[157]

### *Treatment*

The management of dissecting aneurysms is controversial. Surgically accessible lesions may be treated by aneurysmorrhaphy, or resection and end-to-end anastomosis or resection and interposition of a vein graft. Operative repair is usually followed by antiplatelet or anticoagulant therapy.

Inaccessible carotid lesions may be treated by carotid ligation with or without external-to-internal carotid bypass grafting.[86] Ligation of the artery or endovascular balloon occlusion proximal to the dissection decreases intravascular pressure and promotes thrombosis and vessel occlusion. This option is available for the nondominant vertebral artery[116,174,177,194] but carries a significant or even prohibitive risk for the basilar, middle cerebral, or anterior cerebral arteries, unless good collateral circulation can be unequivocally demonstrated. Alternatively, inaccessible lesions with embolic symptoms may require only antiplatelet and anticoagulant therapy.[94] Although basilar artery dissections often do poorly even with treatment,[191] there are more encouraging reports of dissecting aneurysms of the basilar artery, including one case treated conservatively and another operative treatment by wrapping of the aneurysm.[74] Vande Kelft et al also report a case of dissecting aneurysm of the basilar artery treated conservatively with complete resolution.[181] Patients who present with a sudden complete stroke are probably beyond treatment, whereas patients presenting with transient ischemic attacks or strokes-in-evolution may benefit from treatment.

## Sickle-Cell Anemia and Aneurysms

Neurovascular complications of sickle-cell anemia are not uncommon and include intracerebral hemorrhage, infarction, and SAH with or without aneurysm formation.[140] Patients with sickle-cell anemia and SAH from ruptured aneurysms range in age from 18 to 42 years, with an average of 29 years, which is much younger than the average age of onset of SAH in patients with aneurysms encountered in most clinical series.[191]

### *Pathogenesis*

Sickled erythrocytes adhere abnormally to the endothelial cells of the vessel wall, result-

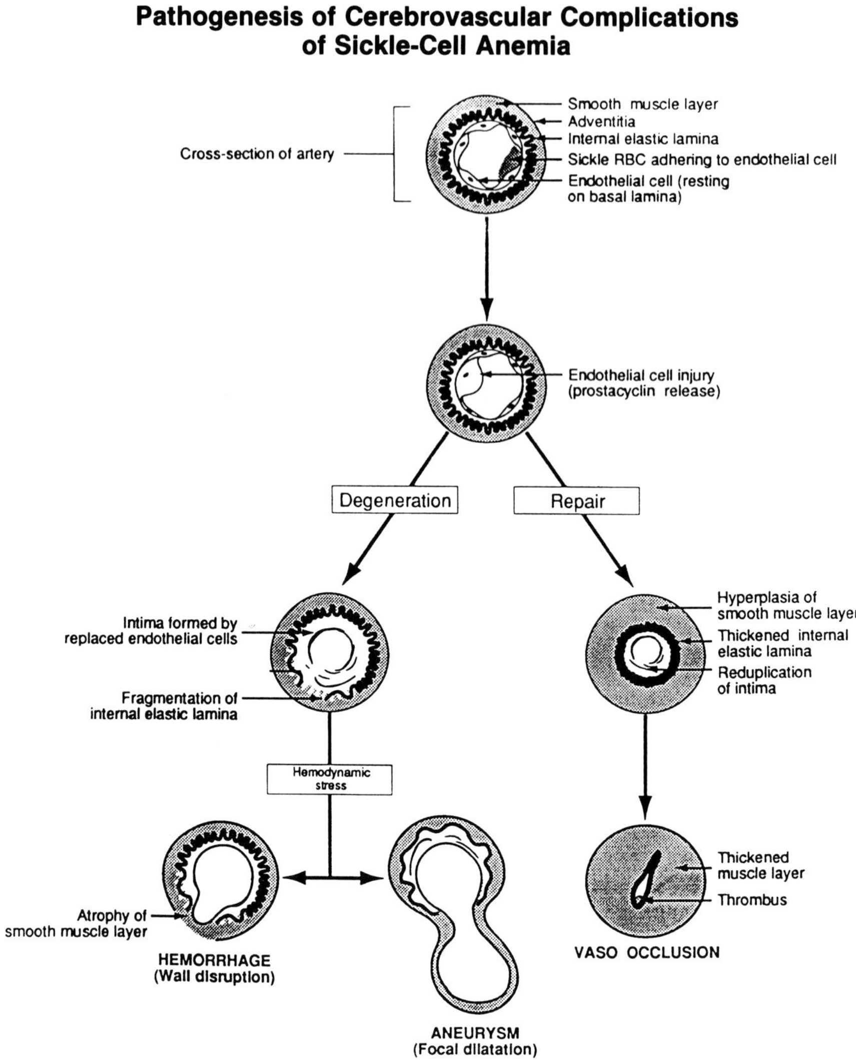


*Figure 15. Proposed pathogenesis of cerebrovascular complications of sickle-cell anemia, including aneurysm formation. (Reprinted with permission from Oyesiku NM, Barrow DL, Eckman JR, et al. Intracranial aneurysms in sickle-cell anemia: clinical features and pathogenesis.* J Neurosurg. *1991;75:356-363.)*

ing in endothelial cell injury.[68] Biochemical evidence of endothelial injury includes the observation that prostacyclin, which is produced by endothelial cells and hence is a biochemical marker of endothelial injury, is released in a fashion that correlates positively with abnormal erythrocyte adhesion.[188] The arterial degeneration in sickle-cell anemia is therefore initiated by endothelial injury from adhesion of the sickled erythrocyte to the endothelial cell. Furthermore, this adherence of abnormal sickled erythrocytes may disrupt the diffusion of oxygen and nutrients across the endothelial cell membrane,[198] exacerbating endothelial or medial cell damage. Finally, hemodynamic stress at the sites of arterial wall injury probably results in aneurysm formation (Figure 15).[132,168]

## *Multiplicity of Aneurysms*

There is some evidence for an increased

incidence of multiple aneurysms in sickle-cell anemia. In one series, a total of 30 aneurysms were found in 15 patients.[132] Although these are small numbers, the incidence of multiple aneurysms was high: in a report of 9 patients with 15 multiple aneurysms (60%), 6 patients had single aneurysms, 5 had 2 aneurysms, 3 had 3 aneurysms, and 1 patient had 5 aneurysms.[132] Review of published experience to 1992 shows that 18 of 41 (43.9%) patients with sickle-cell disease and intracranial aneurysms had multiple aneurysms.[5,29,132]

Many of the aneurysms associated with sickle-cell anemia are found in unusual locations. For example, there are reports of these lesions on the P1 segment of the PCA, the basilar artery at the union of the vertebral arteries, and bilateral mirror aneurysms of the posterior communicating artery (Figure 16).[29,132]

## *Perioperative Management*

The principles of perioperative management center on measures to prevent intravascular sickling and to optimize cerebral blood flow and oxygen delivery. Angiography presents one of the initial difficulties encountered in the perioperative management of patients with sickle-cell disease and aneurysmal SAH because contrast agents may provoke intravascular sickling.[10] These patients require special evaluation and preparation. Before angiography the patient should be hydrated and, if necessary, partial exchange transfusion performed. Transfusion will reduce the amount of hemoglobin S to less than 50% and maintain the hematocrit at 30% to 35% (hemoglobin 9 to 11 gm/dL), which is the optimum range for cerebral blood flow (CBF).[158] Transfusion therapy (partial exchange trans-

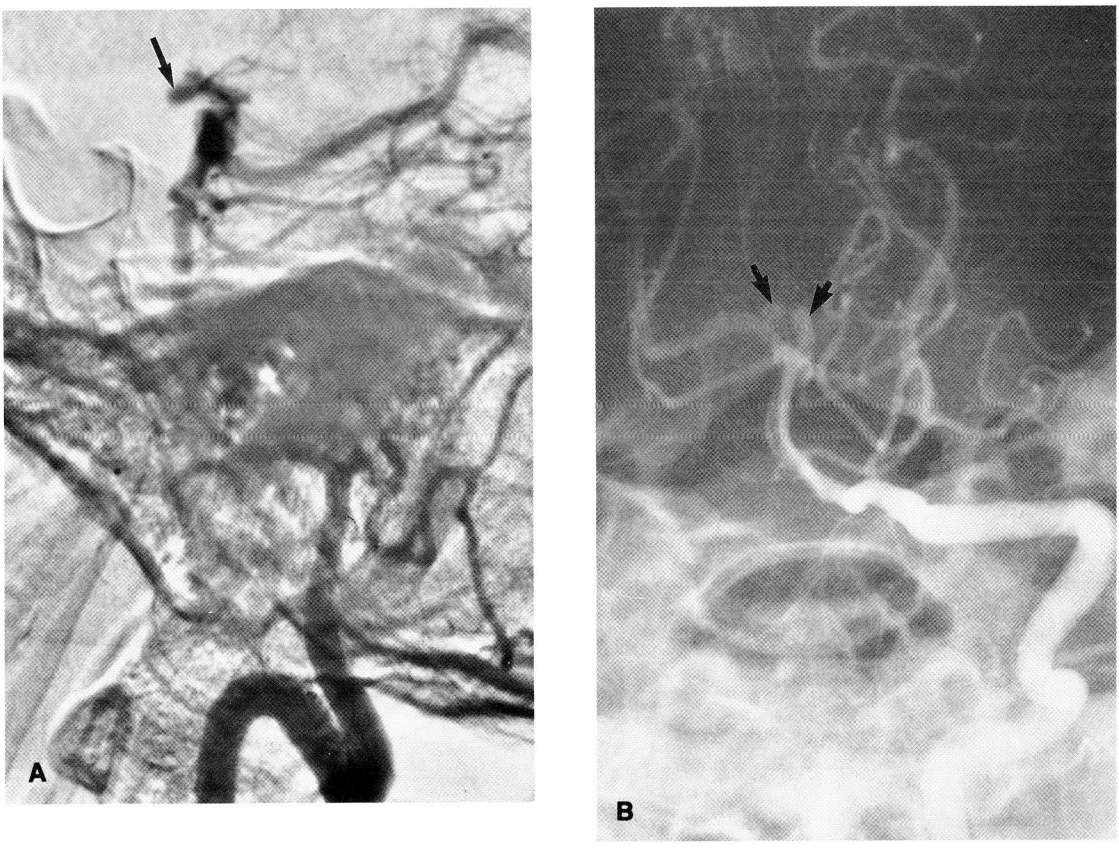


***Figure 16.*** *(A) Lateral and (B) AP vertebral angiogram demonstrates bilateral P1 segment PCA aneurysm (arrow) in this patient with sickle-cell anemia.*

fusion replaces some of the sickle cells with normal red blood cells (RBCs). This reduces the risk of intravascular sickling and increases oxygen delivery to brain tissue.

Hypoxemia, hypothermia, and acidosis (all of which precipitate sickling) frequently occur during anesthesia and in the immediate postoperative period. Therefore, patients should not receive respiratory-depressant drugs for preoperative sedation. Preinduction oxygen is administered for at least 5 minutes,[30,31,72] and hyperventilation is used to maintain a moderate alkalosis with a $pCO_2$ of 25 to 36 mm Hg. Anesthesia is maintained with a volatile agent that reduces hypocapnic vasoconstriction, thus sustaining good tissue perfusion.[155] Body temperature is maintained at 36.5° to 37.5°C, using a warming blanket, warmed intravenous fluid, and comfortable ambient temperature. Mean systemic blood pressure is sustained between 80 and 90 mm Hg during surgery. In the perioperative period, the blood pressure is maintained at a high level with aggressive volume replacement to reduce the potential for delayed ischemic complications of cerebral vasospasm.

In the critical immediate postoperative period, hemoglobin S should be assessed and blood transfusion therapy utilized to maintain the amount of hemoglobin S to less than 50%.

### *Surgical Treatment*

In contradistinction to the intensive medical surveillance and therapy to prevent intervascular sickling, the surgical treatment for these aneurysms, namely, neurosurgical dissection and clip ligation, does not differ from other saccular aneurysms. With proper medical initiatives, these patients can be treated with acceptable morbidity and mortality.[5,29,132]

## Neoplastic Aneurysms

### *Aneurysms Arising from Metastatic Disease*

Occasionally, patients with brain metastases develop intracranial hemorrhage secondary to neoplastic invasion of the arterial wall. The most frequent site of neoplastic aneurysms are the distal branches of the MCA. These aneurysms are usually small, single, and peripherally located. Metastatic tumors that may give rise to aneurysms include cardiac myxoma, choriocarcinoma, bronchogenic carcinoma, or undifferentiated carcinoma.

### *Clinical Features*

Cardiac myxoma may result in aneurysm formation as a sequel to symptomatic embolic cerebral infarction or from an asymptomatic embolus. Neurologic events (emboli or aneurysms) may occur in patients with cardiac myxoma even after successful removal of the cardiac tumor. A myxomatous aneurysm may hemorrhage, enlarge, or even stabilize. Some resolve spontaneously and others do so after removal of the cardiac tumor. The evolution of these aneurysms appears unaffected by chemotherapy, based on current evidence.[18,149] Most myxomatous aneurysms develop following invasion of the arterial wall by tumor, resulting in irregular dilatation of the arteries. Usually, these lesions are bilateral and are associated with multiple stenoses and occlusions of the vessel. The aneurysms are lobulated, gray-white swellings, usually less than 5 mm in diameter (but may be larger) and occur near arterial bifurcations.[167]

Cerebral choriocarcinoma should be suspected in women of childbearing age who present with acute or subacute neurologic symptoms and a history of recent pregnancy, abnormal vaginal bleeding, or pulmonary symptoms. The diagnosis is established by documenting rising titers of chorionic gonadotropin. Choriocarcinoma penetrates the vessel wall, disrupting the internal elastic lamina, and destroys the media. The intraluminal tumor embolus is usually associated with thrombus.[71,80,117,118,124]

### *Pathogenesis*

There are two suggested causes of aneurysm formation from metastatic tumors. One hypothesis suggests that the aneurysms are secondary to vessel obstruction by tumor emboli with subsequent perivascular damage and scarring. These pseudoaneurysms can be revealed after recanalization and restoration of the circulation.[171] A second hypothesis is that emboli lodge in the vessel and remain viable, the tumor cells subsequently penetrate the capillary endothelium and grow subintimally, destroying the arterial wall and causing fibroblastic proliferation.[123]

Histologic examination of these aneurysms may show occlusion of the vessel by tumor cell emboli, proliferation of tumor cells into the vessel walls, rupture of the internal elastic lamina,[144] and wall damage with aneurysmal dilatation. These findings are obviously consistent with either hypothesis.

The tumor emboli probably arrive via the pulmonary circulation, since there is a high incidence of metastasis to the lungs occurring prior to cerebral metastasis.[182] The emboli then proceed to the left ventricle and embolize cephalad to the brain.

## *Diagnosis*

The typical angiographic characteristics include peripheral filling defects or vessel occlusion from emboli and peripherally located saccular or fusiform aneurysms. These changes may be due to arterial obstruction with or without subsequent tumor growth. Bleeding secondary to rupture may obscure the aneurysms angiographically and pathologically, which, in part, may account for the paucity of tumor-induced aneurysms in the literature.[129]

## *Treatment*

Craniotomy and obliteration of the aneurysm is indicated for the patient with an enlarging myxomatous aneurysm or the patient with subarachnoid or intracranial hemorrhage (ICH) from a demonstrated myxomatous aneurysm. Surgical results in such patients are encouraging, although series are few and uncontrolled.[22,123,149] Given the lack of definitive data regarding the incidence and outcome of myxomatous aneurysms, patients with atrial myxomas, treated and untreated, should be followed for neurologic symptoms. Patients with neurologic symptoms should be evaluated by CT or MRI and cerebral angiography.

Craniotomy and obliteration of the aneurysm is also indicated for the patient who has an ICH and a ruptured aneurysm from choriocarcinoma, particularly if the hemorrhage is life-threatening. Following surgery, chemotherapy and radiation should be given. If the aneurysm is unruptured or without significant tumor mass, chemotherapy and radiotherapy are adequate treatment in some cases.[50,51] The usual regimen for choriocarcinoma with cerebral metastasis consists of chemotherapy with actinomycin D, methotrexate, and cyclophosphamide in combination with whole-brain radiation of 30 to 45 cGy.[111,112,159]

## *Brain Tumors and Intracranial Aneurysms*

Coexisting aneurysms have been described with meningiomas, gliomas, pituitary adenomas, craniopharyngiomas, neurinomas, and metastases. The usual locations are the internal carotid and anterior communicating arteries. The high incidence of multiple aneurysms in association with meningiomas prompted Jimenez et al to suggest a dysgenetic factor.[79] Local circulatory changes might account for internal carotid artery aneurysms in association with skull base tumors, such as meningiomas and pituitary adenomas. MCA aneurysms have a higher incidence ipsilateral to neoplasms, presumably related to increased regional blood flow.[138] MCA aneurysms are more common with convexity tumors, but less so in basal tumors. This proportion is reversed with internal carotid artery aneurysms.[138] The presenting symptoms usually result from the tumor. When benign tumors are associated with aneurysms, both lesions

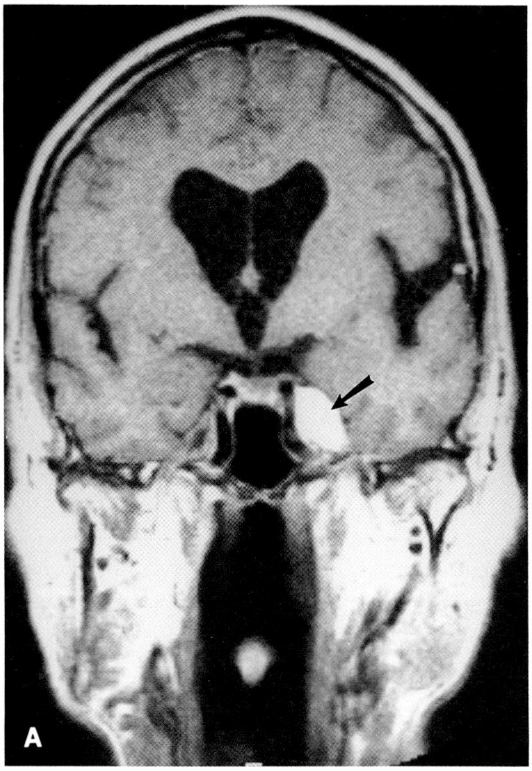


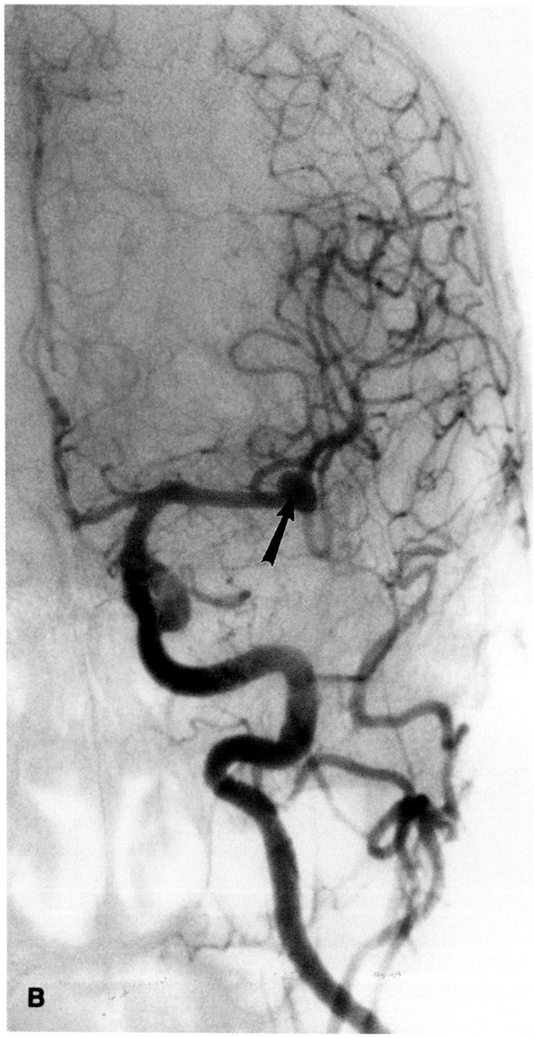


*Figure 17.* ***(A)*** *Coronal contrast-enhanced CT demonstrates an enhancing mass in the left cavernous sinus (arrow).* ***(B)*** *AP left carotid angiogram shows a small MCA aneurysm (arrow). At surgery the intracavernous lesion proved to be a Schwannoma that was completely removed, and the aneurysm was clipped.*

should be treated at the same operative procedure, if technically feasible (Figure 17).

## Inflammatory Aneurysms

Inflammatory aneurysms are rare and are usually associated with systemic arterial disease. The inflammatory response is cytologically indolent compared to bacterial aneurysms, and the aneurysms tend to be peripheral, multiple, and nonsaccular.

### *Systemic Lupus Erythematosus*

Cerebral arteritis is relatively uncommon with systemic lupus erythematosus (SLE), with a frequency ranging from 6% to 13%[43] and involves primarily small cerebral arteries (<2 mm diameter).[147] Large- and medium-vessel disease is rare.[42] Although subarachnoid hemorrhage (SAH) occurs in 30% of cases of SLE with neurologic involvement at autopsy, it is usually due to extension of ICH from rupture of a small vessel into the parenchyma. Nevertheless, few reported cases of intracranial aneurysm are associated with SLE. One of the earliest was that of Harvey et al[64] of a small ruptured aneurysm and cerebral hemorrhage, with evidence of arteritis at autopsy.

Ferris described focal area of fibrinoid necrosis and elastic tissue disruption, particularly at bifurcations of the internal and external carotid artery, and multiple intracranial aneurysms in a patient with SLE. These aneurysms were on branches of the MCA.[44] He describes another patient with multiple focal aneurysms of the superior cerebellar artery, posterior cerebral, thalamoperforating, and anterior choroidal arteries. This patient also had multiple aneurysmal dilitations of the MCA. The patient had presented with an SAH.[44] Multiple aneurysms have also been described in another patient with SLE by Taveras and Wood.[179]

### *Pathologic Findings*

A case study with clinicopathologic correlation in a patient with SLE and SAH due to a ruptured fusiform aneurysm of the posterior communicating and adjacent posterior cerebral artery provides some analysis of the pathologic findings in aneurysms associated with SLE. There was extensive transmural and lesser perivascular inflammation of the vessels at and around the site of rupture with fragmentation of the elastic lamina and marked focal subintimal proliferation. The inflammatory cells were chiefly lymphocytes with some polymorphonuclear leukocytes. There was no evidence for an infectious etiology.[83]

## *Polyarteritis Nodosa*

The etiology of polyarteritis nodosa is still obscure. However, the disease has been related to hypersensitivity to drugs,[176] and respiratory tract infections, especially streptococcal.[115,150] Immunohistochemical studies and other techniques lend weight to an immunologic hypothesis in the pathogenesis of polyarteritis nodosa.[136]

### *Pathology*

Polyarteritis nodosa is characterized by segmental degeneration and inflammation of medium and small arteries.[8]

Two complications of the pathologic process contribute to the clinical picture: thrombosis and the formation of aneurysms.[176] Infarctions due to thrombosis may result in acute and sometimes fatal clinical sequelae; small infarctions with mild acute symptoms may lead to progressive destruction of the involved organ. The development of multiple aneurysms with a predilection for medium-sized arteries, especially at bifurcations, is a characteristic feature. In patients with aneurysms, rupture with consequent hematoma is a continuous threat and is sometimes fatal.[192]

### *Diagnosis*

The diagnosis of polyarteritis nodosa is suggested by the complex of symptoms and the periodic exacerbations of its chronic course. Histologic examination of subcutaneous nodules and muscle biopsy specimens demonstrates changes in medium and small arteries. However, skin lesions occur in only some of the cases—about 25% according to Slinger and Starck[165]—and do not always show specific histologic features. Muscle biopsy may be used but is often uninformative.[103,165]

Cerebral angiography may show fusiform and racemose aneurysms of small peripheral intracranial arteries. These aneurysms, frequently multiple, may resemble a bunch of small grapes.[93]

In postmortem series, aneurysms have been demonstrated in extracerebral, intracerebral, and intraspinal vessels.[56,133] Symptoms and signs related to cerebral arteritis in polyarteritis nodosa include attacks of migraine like headache and vertigo, transient strabismus, loss of consciousness, facial paresis, and paresis of the limbs.[93]

## *Treatment*

Treatment with anticoagulants might be considered in patients with thrombosis,[36] but the presence of aneurysms strongly contraindicates such treatment; angiography is thus important for determining cases in which anticoagulants might be given. Corticosteroid therapy may be followed by regression of the vascular changes.[93] The prognosis in polyarteritis nodosa is poor, usually with a relatively short survival time.[176]

## Aortitis (Pulseless Disease, Takayasu's Disease)

In 1908, Takayasu[175] reported the case of a young female with a unique arteriovenous anastomosis in the retina. The 1948, Shimizu and Sano[162] noted specific symptoms consisting of disturbed blood circulation in the upper half of the body with absent or diminished arterial pulse in the upper limbs and head. They termed this "pulseless disease," an occlusive disease of chronic, nonspecific arteritis of unknown etiology in young females that mainly affects the aortic arch and its major branches and the pulmonary artery.

Takayasu arteritis is more common than previously suspected in North America and is not restricted to any one racial group.[59] Clinically, pulseless disease includes the following triad; absence of radial pulsation, hypersensitive carotid sinus reflex, and hypotensive ophthalmoangiopathy.[101]

### Diagnosis

Diagnosis of Takayasu's arteritis is often delayed, with a median delay of 18 months reported in a Mayo clinic report.[59]

Cerebral angiography may demonstrate irregular dilatation of the carotid arteries or narrowing of its branches such as the MCA. Other angiographic findings include dilatation of the aortic root, narrowing of the origins of both carotid arteries, and beading of the descending aorta.[87]

### Clinical Features

Patients may present with nonvascular (arthralgias, fever, weight loss) or vascular symptoms such as arm claudication and hypertension due to renal artery stenosis. Most patients have multiple vascular bruits or absent pulses. Laboratory findings include anemia and elevations of erythrocyte sedimentation rate and positive C-reactive protein.[101] Almost all patients have multiple sites of arterial involvement documented by angiography with various combinations of stenosis, luminal irregularity, and aneurysm formation. Patients with cerebrovascular disease may have aneurysms, minor stroke, or intermittent neurologic dysfunction.[148] Aneurysms in pulseless disease occur mostly in females, age 26 to 55 years. Virtually all of the aneurysms occur in the posterior circulation, usually at the basilar artery bifurcation.[76,91] In a 1972 review of 77 cases of pulseless disease, Sano and Saito[156] found no clinical or radiologic evidence of intracranial aneurysmal formation or SAH. Subsequently, reports of saccular aneurysms coincident with Takayasu's disease have been limited. In a report of 9 patients with 15 intracranial aneurysms, there were 8 females and only one male, ranging in age from 26 to 64 years. Among these 15 intracranial aneurysms, 9 originated from the vertebrobasilar circulation and the other 6 from the internal carotid circulation.[101]

### Pathogenesis

Pathologic changes are restricted to the media and adventitial layers of the vessel wall and are indistinguishable from those of giant-cell or temporal arteritis. The aortic arch and its major branches and the pulmonary arteries show a panarteritis with giant-cell granuloma.[102]

Autopsy findings in two patients with intracranial aneurysms and Takayasu's disease showed no evidence of arteritis in the intracranial vessels in either patient, and no pathologic changes in the intracranial arteries adjacent to the aneurysms. The intracranial aneurysms in Takayasu's disease are thought to be due to high arterial pressure or hemodynamic stress through patent brachiocephalic vessels.[102]

Clinical evidence indicates that these aneurysms gradually increase in size over a few years, compressing neighboring structures and then rupturing through the friable wall.[102]

### *Treatment*

Takayasu's arteritis is treatable with corticosteroids and surgical vascular reconstruction[59] (e.g., extracranial-intracranial bypass procedures using saphenous vein graft). If left untreated, 75% of patients die within 2 years.[49,87]

Successfully treated patients may show a return of the erythrocyte sedimentation rate to normal and resolution of the symptoms. Response to corticosteroid treatment is usually very good, with dramatic improvement in nonvascular symptoms and return of pulses in 50% of patients within absent pulse prior to treatment.[59] Angiography may show improvement in the appearance of the arteries and resolution of arterial wall irregularities. Therefore, early diagnosis and vigorous immunosuppression is warranted to improve outcome in this rare and often fatal vascular disease.[87]

Operative treatment of nonspecific aortoarteritis remains controversial and little information is available on the results of vascular reconstruction in this disease. In cases of pulseless disease, even if there are no signs of aneurysmal rupture, one should endeavor to find intracranial aneurysmal lesions, because aneurysmal rupture is often fatal. If pulseless disease is associated with a ruptured intracranial aneurysm, surgical treatment for the aneurysm should be carried out insofar as the patient's general condition allows for the operation. Very few aneurysms have been successfully clipped, and the operative mortality rate is significant.[76,91]

## *Giant-Cell Arteritis*

Involvement of the intracranial arteries in giant-cell arteritis is rare, although giant-cell arteritis (temporal arteritis) affects not only the temporal artery, but may involve other vessels. Giant-cell arteritis usually causes an occlusive change in the arteries, and aneurysmal dilatation of the affected vessel is rarely seen.[70,89,107,185]

Reports of intracranial aneurysms in giant-cell arteritis have involved the circle of Willis,[107,185] ACA and MCA, [70,89] and basilar and posterior cerebral arteries.[107] Multiple aneurysms have also been described.[55,70,107]

### *Pathology*

One report of a surgically obtained specimen from a patient with an aneurysm of the MCA induced by giant-cell arteritis described by Kozuka et al[89] consisted of an aneurysmal dome and the granulation tissue attached to the aneurysm. Granulation tissue had replaced the muscular wall of the aneurysm, and the internal elastic lamella had completely disappeared, but the inflammatory infiltration was scarce in other parts of the aneurysmal wall. In the granulation tissue adjacent to the aneurysm, there was marked infiltration of plasma cells, lymphocytes, polymorphonuclear cells, and macrophage-phagocytosed hemosiderin. Many multinucleated cells of foreign body type were also found, and there were fragments of degenerated elastic fibers.

Elastic tissue stain disclosed a destroyed arterial wall buried in the granulation tissue. The internal elastic lamella was severely wrinkled and partially disrupted. The muscular wall was completely replaced by granulation tissue, including many multinucleated giant cells, and the lumen of the artery was so narrow that the vessel was scarcely identified by hematoxylin and eosin stain. Granulation tissue was seen inside as well as outside the lumen formed by elastic lamella.[89]

### *Treatment*

Giant-cell arteritis is treatable by corticosteroids. The aneurysms may be treated by craniotomy and clip ligation, if approachable.

## Summary

Nonsaccular aneurysms present an unusual diagnostic and therapeutic challenge for neurosurgery. Our knowledge of these lesions has continued to improve with an increasing diagnostic capability. Timely reviews are necessary to keep us abreast of advancements in the management of these lesions.

## References

1. Aarabi B. Traumatic aneurysms of brain due to high-velocity missile head wounds. *Neurosurgery.* 1988;22:1056–1063.
2. Acosta C, Williams PE Jr, Clark K. Traumatic aneurysms of the cerebral vessels. *J Neurosurg.* 1972; 36:531–536.
3. Ahuja GK, Jain N, Vijayaraghavan M, et al. Cerebral mycotic aneurysms of fungal origin. *J Neurosurg.* 1978;49:107–110.
4. Andoh T, Sakai N, Yamada H, et al. Fusiform and dissecting aneurysm of the vertebrobasilar systems: differential diagnosis [in Japanese]. *No Shinkei Geka.* 1991;19:327–336. English abstract.
5. Anson JA, Koshy M, Ferguson L, et al. Subarachnoid hemorrhage in sickle-cell disease. *J Neurosurg.* 1991;75:552–558.
6. Aoki N, Sakai T. Rebleeding from intracranial dissecting aneurysms in the vertebral artery. *Stroke.* 1990;21:1628–1631.
7. Araki C, Handa H, Handa J, et al. Traumatic aneurysm of the intracranial extradural portion of the internal carotid artery: report of a case. *J Neurosurg.* 1965;23:64-67.
8. Arkin A. A clinical and pathological study of periarteritis nodosa. *Amer J Pathol.* 1930;6:401–426.
9. Asari S, Nakamura S, Yamada O, et al. Traumatic aneurysms of peripheral cerebral arteries [in Japanese]. *No To Shinkei.* 1970;28:793–805. English abstract.
10. Barrow DL, Oyesiku NM. Pathogenesis of sickle-cell anemia and aneurysm. *J Neurosurg.* 1992;76: 1050–1051. Letter.
11. Barrow DL, Prats AR. Infectious intracranial aneurysms: comparison of groups with andwithout endocarditis. *Neurosurgery.* 1990;27:562–572.
12. Bell WE, Butler C II. Cerebral mycotic aneurysm in children: two case reports. *Neurology.* 1968;18: 81–86.
13. Benoit BG, Wortzman G. Traumatic cerebral aneurysms: clinical features and natural history. *J Neurol Neurosurg Psychiatr.* 1973;36:127–138.
14. Berger MS, Wilson CB. Intracranial dissecting aneurysms of the posterior circulation: report of six cases and review of the literature. *J Neurosurg.* 1984;61:882–894.
15. Birley JL, Trotter W. Traumatic aneurysm of the intracranial portion of the internal carotid artery. *Brain.* 1928;51:184–208.
16. Bohmfalk GL, Story JL, Wissinger JP, et al. Bacterial intracranial aneurysm. *J Neurosurg.* 1978; 48:369–382.
17. Bollinger O. Ueber traumatische Spat-Apoplexie. Ein Beitrag zur Lehre von der Hirnerschutterung. In: Virchow R, ed. *Internationale Beitrage zurr Wissenschaftlichen Medicine Festschrift.* Berlin, Germany: Hirschwald; 1981;2:457–470.
18. Branch CL Jr, Laster DW, Kelly DL Jr. Left atrial myxoma with cerebral emboli. *Neurosurgery.* 1985; 16:675–680.
19. Braun J, Gdal-On M, Goldsher D, et al. Traumatic carotid aneurysm secondary to cavernous sinus penetration by wood: CT features. *J Comput Assist Tomogr.* 1987;11:525–528.
20. Brenner H. Frontale schädelspaltung mit traumatischem aneurysma der arteria pericallosa. *Acta Neurochir (Wien).* 1962;10:145–152.
21. Buckingham MJ, Crone KR, Ball WS, et al. Traumatic intracranial aneurysms in childhood: two cases and a review of the literature. *Neurosurgery.* 1988;22:398–408.
22. Burton C, Johnston J. Multiple cerebral aneurysms and cardiac myxoma. *N Engl J Med.* 1970;282:35–36.
23. Burton C, Velasco F, Dorman J. Traumatic aneurysm of a peripheral cerebral artery: review and case report. *J Neurosurg.* 1968;28:468–474.
24. Cantu RC, LeMay M, Wilkinson HA. The importance of repeated angiography in the treatment of mycotic-embolic intracranial aneurysms. *J Neurosurg.* 1966;25:189–193.
25. Capanna AH. Traumatic intracranial aneurysm and Gradenigo's syndrome secondary to gunshot wound. *Surg Neurol.* 1984;22:263–266.
26. Caplan LR, Baquis GD, Pessin MS, et al. Dissection of the intracranial vertebral artery. *Neurology.* 1988;38:868–877.
27. Cates JE, Christie RV. Subacute bacterial endocarditis: a review of 442 cases treated in 14 centres appointed by Penicillin Trials Committee of the Medical Research Council. *Q J Med.* 1951;20: 93–130.
28. Chadduck WM. Traumatic cerebral aneurysm due to speargun injury: case report. *J Neurosurg.* 1969; 31:77–79.
29. Chalif DJ, Decker RE. Intracranial aneurysms in sickle-cell anemia. *J Neurosurg.* 1992;76:1051–1052. Letter.
30. Close RA, Buchheit WA. The management of ruptured intracranial aneurysm in sickle-cell anemia: case report. *J Neurosurg.* 1977;47:761–765.
31. Coplans M. Sickle cell problems—anaesthetics. *Proc R Soc Med.* 1974;67:1072–1073.
32. Cosgrove GR, Villemure JG, Melançon D. Traumatic intracranial aneurysm due to arterial injury at surgery. *J Neurosurg.* 1983;58:291–294.
33. Courville CB. Traumatic aneurysm of an intracranial artery: description of lesion incident to a shotgun wound of the skull and brain. *Bull Los Angeles Neurol Soc.* 1960;25:48–54.
34. Cressman MR, Hayes GJ. Traumatic aneurysm of the anterior choroidal artery: case report. *J Neurosurg.* 1966;24:102–104.
35. Day AL. Extracranial-intracranial bypass grafting in the surgical treatment of bacterial aneurysms: report of two cases. *Neurosurgery.* 1981; 9:583–588.
36. Dines DE. Polyarteritis nodosa: report of a patient receiving long-term anticoagulant therapy. *JAMA.* 1964;189:156–158.

37. Drake CG. Subdural hematoma from arterial rupture. *J Neurosurg.* 1961;18:597–601.
38. Dratz HM, Woodhall B. Traumatic dissecting aneurysm of left internal carotid, anterior cerebral and middle cerebral arteries. *J Neuropathol Exp Neurol.* 1947;6:286–291.
39. Duan GS. Traumatic intracranial aneurysm: report of 2 cases [in Chinese]. *Chung-Hua Shen Ching Ching Shen Ko Tsa Chih.* 1981;14:208–209.
40. Eguchi T, Nakagomi T, Teraoka A. Treatment of bilateral mycotic intracavernous carotid aneurysms: case report. *J Neurosurg.* 1982; 56:443–447.
41. Eichler A, Story JL, Bennett DE, et al. Traumatic aneurysm of a cerebral artery: case report. *J Neurosurg.* 1969;31:72–76.
42. Ellis SG, Verity MA. Central nervous system involvement in systemic lupus erythematosus: a review of hemopathologic findings in 57 cases, 1955-1977. *Semin Arthritis Rheum.* 1979;8:212–221.
43. Feldges A, Nau HE, Reinhardt V. Two cases of sudden death by rupture of traumatic and bacterial aneurysms. *Intensive Care Med.* 1989;15:400–402.
44. Ferris EJ. Arteritis. Angiography. In: Newton TH, Potts DG, eds. *Radiology of the Skull and Brain.* St. Louis, Mo: CV Mosby Co; 1974;2:2583–2585.
45. Fleischer AS, Patton JM, Tindall GT. Cerebral aneurysms of traumatic origin. *Surg Neurol.* 1975; 4:233–239.
46. Foote RA, Reagan TJ, Sandok BA. Cerebral arterial lesions resulting from inflammatory emboli. *Stroke.* 1978;9:498–503.
47. Frazee JG, Cahan LD, Winter J. Bacterial intracranial aneurysms. *J Neurosurg.* 1980;53:633–641.
48. Friedman AH, Drake CG. Subarachnoid hemorrhage from intracranial dissecting aneurysm. *J Neurosurg.* 1984;60:325–334.
49. Friedrich H, Laas J, Waltherbusch G, et al. Extra-intracranial bypass procedure with saphenous vein grafts. *Thorac Cardiovasc Surg.* 1986;34:57–62.
50. Fijuwara T, Mino S, Nagao S, et al. Metastatic choriocarcinoma with neoplastic aneurysm cured by aneurysm resection and chemotherapy: case report. *J Neurosurg.* 1992;76:148–151.
51. Fukamachi A, Tamura M, Kawafuchi J, et al. [Case of cerebral metastasis of chorioepithelioma successfully treated by combination therapy] [in Japanese]. *Clin Neurol (Tokyo).* 1972;12:297–304.
52. Fukushima T, Yamamoto M, Tomonaga M. Vertebral dissecting aneurysms associated with medial mucoid degeneration. Case report and review of the literature. *Neurol Med Chir (Tokyo).* 1986;26:888–894.
53. Gallina E, Gallo O, Boccuzzi S, et al. Intracranial post-traumatic aneurysm of the internal carotid artery as a cause of epistaxis: considerations on 2 cases [in Italian]. *Acta Otorhinolaryngol Ital.* 1990;10: 607–613. English abstract.
54. Greenlee JE, Mandell G. Neurological manifestations of infective endocarditis: a review. *Stroke.* 1973;4:958–963.
55. Griffin J, Price DL, Davis L, et al. Granulomatous angiitis of the central nervous system with aneurysms on multiple cerebral arteries. *Trans Am Neurol Assoc.* 1973;98:145–148.
56. Griffith GC, Vural IL. Polyarteritis nodosa: a correlation of clinical and postmortem findings in 17 cases. *Circulation.* 1951;3:481–491.
57. Haddad FS, Haddad GF, Taha J. Traumatic intracranial aneurysms caused by missiles: their presentation and management. *Neurosurgery.* 1991;28: 1–7.
58. Hadley MN, Spetzler RF, Martin NA, et al. Middle cerebral artery aneurysm due to *Nocardia asteroides*: case report of aneurysm excision and extracranial-intracranial bypass. *Neurosurgery.* 1988;22:923–928.
59. Hall S, Barr W, Lie JT, et al. Takayasu Arthritis: a study of 32 North American patients. *Medicine (Baltimore).* 1985;64:89– 99.
60. Hamm KD, Pothe H, Steube D, et al. Traumatic infraclinoid aneurysms [in German]. *Neurochirurgia (Stuttg).* 1988;31:88–92. English abstract.
61. Handa J, Shimizu Y, Matsuda M, et al. Traumatic aneurysm of the middle cerebral artery. *AJR.* 1970; 109:127–129.
62. Hansmann GH, Schenken JR. Melitensis meningoencephalitis: mycotic aneurysm due to Brucella Melitensis var. porcine. *Am J Pathol.* 1932;8:435–444.
63. Harrison MJ, Hampton JR. Neurological presentation of bacterial endocarditis. *Br Med J.* 1967; 2:148–151.
64. Harvey AM, Schulman LE, Tumulty PA, et al. Systemic lupus erythematosus: review of the literature and clinical analysis of 138 cases. *Medicine (Baltimore).* 1954;33:291–437.
65. Hassler O. Medial defects in the meningeal arteries. *J Neurosurg.* 1962;19:337–340.
66. Hatanaka K, Yutani C, Fujieda T, et al. Polymyositis associated with dissecting aneurysms of arteries and cerebral hemorrhage. *Acta Pathol Jpn.* 1986;36:1217–1223.
67. Hayashi A, Oda M, Sekino T, et al. Traumatic aneurysm occurring after surgical procedure of large cerebral aneurysm [in Japanese]. *No Shinkei Geka.* 1986;14:881–885. English abstract.
68. Hebbel RP, Boogaerts MAB, Eaton JW, et al. Erythrocyte-adherence to endothelium in sickle-cell anemia: a possible determinant of disease severity. *N Engl J Med.* 1980;302:992–995.
69. Heidelberger KP, Layton WM Jr, Fisher RG. Multiple cerebral mycotic aneurysms complicating post-traumatic pseudomonas meningitis: case report. *J Neurosurg.* 1968;29:631–635.
70. Hinck VC, Carter CC, Rippey JG. Giant cell (cranial) arteritis: a case with angiographic abnormalities. *AJR.* 1964;92:769–775.
71. Hisanaga M, Kawai S, Maekawa M, et al. Neoplastic aneurysms due to cerebral metastasis of choriocarcinoma: report of two cases [in Japanese]. *Neurol Med Chir (Tokyo).* 1988;28:398–403. English abstract.
72. Homi J, Reynolds J, Skinner A, et al. General anaesthesia in sickle-cell disease. *Br Med J.* 1979;1: 1599-1601.
73. Horten BC, Abbott GF, Porro RS. Fungal aneurysms in intracranial vessels. *Arch Neurol.* 1976; 33:577–579.
74. Hosoda K, Fujita S, Kawaguchi T, et al. Spontaneous dissecting aneurysms of the basilar artery presenting with a subarachnoid hemorrhage: report of two cases. *J Neurosurg.* 1991;75:628–633.
75. Ide Y, Watuka Y, Onita T, et al. A case of iatro-

genic traumatic intracranial aneurysm [in Japanese]. *No Shinkei Geka.* 1987;15:1353–1359. English abstract.
76. Imaizumi S, Nagamine Y, Nakamura N, et al. Aneurysm of anterior communicating artery associated with aortitis syndrome: a treated case by aneurysmal neck clipping [in Japanese]. *No Shinkei Geka.* 1982:10:449–455. English abstract.
77. Jakobsson KE, Carolsson C, Elfverson J, et al. Traumatic aneurysms of the cerebral arteries: a study of five cases. *Acta Neurochir (Wien).* 1984;71:91–98.
78. Jenewein K, Pirker E, Furtschegger A, et al. Injuries of the intracranial arteries in the angiogram: ROFO. 1989:151:706–712. English abstract
79. Jimenez JP, Goree JA, Parker JC Jr. An unusual association of multiple meningiomas, intracranial aneurysm, and cerebrovascular atherosclerosis in two young women. *AJR.* 1971;,112:281–288.
80. Jones HR Jr, Siekert RG, Geraci JE. Neurologic manifestations of bacterial endocarditis. *Ann Intern Med.* 1969;71:21–28.
81. Karsner HT. *Acute Inflammations of Arteries.* Springfield, Ill: Charles C. Thomas; 1947:16.
82. Katz RI, Goldberg HI, Selzer ME. Mycotic aneurysm: case report with novel sequential angiographic findings. *Arch Intern Med.* 1974;134: 939–942.
83. Kelley RE, Stokes N, Reyes P, et al. Cerebral transmural angiitis and ruptured aneurysm. *Arch Neurol.* 1980;37:526–527.
84. Kieck CF, de Villiers JC. Vascular lesions due to transcranial stab wounds. *J Neurosurg.* 1984;60: 42–46.
85. Kikuchi K, Watanabe K, Sugawara A, et al. Multiple fungal aneurysms: report of a rare case implicating steroid as predisposing factor. *Surg Neurol.* 1985;24:253–259.
86. Kitani R, Itouji T, Noda Y, et al. Dissecting aneurysms of the anterior circle of Willis arteries: report of two cases. *J Neurosurg.* 1987;67:296–300.
87. Kohrman MH, Huttenlocher PR. Takayasu arteritis. A treatable cause of stroke in infancy. *Padiatr Neurol.* 1986;2:154–158.
88. Kojima T, Waga S, Furuno M. Fracture of the sella turcica. *Neurosurgery.* 1985;16:225–229.
89. Kozuka S, Iguchi I, Furuse M, et al. Cerebral aneurysm induced by giant cell arteritis: a case report. *Angiology.* 1979;30:131–137.
90. Kuhn RA, Kugler H. False aneurysms of the middle meningeal artery. *J Neurosurg.* 1964;21:92–96.
91. Kumagai Y, Sugiyama H, Nawata H, et al. Two cases of pulseless disease with cerebral aneurysm. [in Japanese]. *No Shinkei Geka.* 1981;9:611–615. English Abstract.
92. Kunze ST, Schiefer W. Angiographic demonstration of a dissecting aneurysm of the middle cerebral artery. *Neuroradiology.* 1971;2:201–206.
93. Leonhardt ETG, Jokobson H, Ringqvist OTA. Angiographic and chinicophysiologic investigation of a case of polyarteritis nodosa. *Am J Med.* 1972; 53:242–256.
94. Leys D, Lesoin F, Pruvo JP, et al. Bilateral spontaneous dissection of extracranial vertebral arteries. *J Neurol.* 1987;234:237–240.
95. Maillo A, Diaz P, Morales F. Dissecting aneurysm of the posterior cerebral artery: spontaneous resolution. *Neurosurgery.* 1991;29:291–294.
96. Markwalder VH, Huber P. Aneurysmen der meningeal arterien. *Schweiz Med Wochenschr.* 1961:91:1344–1347.
97. Martin EM, Hummelgard AB. Traumatic aneurysms. *J Neurosci Nurs.* 1986;18:89–94.
98. Martinez SN, Bertrand C, Thierry A. False post-traumatic aneurysm. [in French]. *Can J Surg.* 1966;9:397–402. English Abstract.
99. Mas JL, Bousser MG, Corone P, et al. Dissecting aneurysm of the extracranial vertebral arteries and pregnancy. [in French]. *Rev Neurol (Paris).* 1987; 143:761–764. English Abstract.
100. Masana Y, Taneda M. Direct approach to a traumatic giant internal carotid artery aneurysm associated with a carotid-cavernous fistula: case report. *J Neurosurg.* 1992;76:524–527.
101. Masuzawa T, Kurokawa T, Oguro K, et al. Pulseless disease associated with multiple intracranial aneurysms. *Neuroradiology.* 1986;28:17–22.
102. Masuzawa T, Shimabukuro H, Sato F, et al. The development of intracranial aneurysms associated with pulseless disease. *Surg Neurol.* 1982;17:132–136.
103. Maxeiner SR Jr, McDonald JR, Kirklin JW. Muscle biopsy in the diagnosis of periarteritis nodosa: an evaluation. *Surg Clin N Am.* 1952;32:1225–1233.
104. Meguro K, Rowed DW. Traumatic aneurysm of the posterior inferior cerebellar artery caused by fracture of the clivus. *Neurosurgery.* 1985;16:666–668.
105. Michel D, Pialat J, Antoine JC, et al. Dissecting aneurysm of the intracranial vertebral artery: a clinicopathologic case report [in French]. *Rev Neurol (Paris).* 1988;144:25–31. English Abstract.
106. Mielke B, Weir B, Oldring D, et al. Fungal aneurysm: case report and review of the literature. *Neurosurgery.* 1981;9:578–582.
107. Milgram JW, Stecher K Jr. Idiopathic arteritis with multiple intracranial aneurysms. *Angiology.* 1974;25:89–119.
108. Mokri B, Piepgras DG, Houser OW. Traumatic dissections of the extracranial internal carotid artery. *J Neurosurg.* 1988;68:189–197.
109. Molinari GF, Smith L, Goldstein MN, et al. Pathogenesis of cerebral mycotic aneurysms. *Neurology.* 1973;23:325–332.
110. Molinari GF. Septic cerebral embolism. *Stroke.* 1972;3:117–122.
111. Momma F, Beck H, Miyamoto T, et al. Intracranial aneurysm due to metastatic choriocarcinoma. *Surg Neurol.* 1986;25:74–76.
112. Montaut J, Hepner H, Tridon P, et al. Aspects pseudo-vasculaires des méstastases intracraniennes des choiro-épitheliomes. *Neurochirurgie.* 1971;17: 119–128.
113. Morawetz RB, Karp, RB. Evolution and resolution of intracranial bacterial (mycotic) aneurysms. *Neurosurgery.* 1984;15:43–49.
114. Moskowitz MA, Rosenbaum AE, Tyler HR. Angiographically monitored resolution of cerebral mycotic aneurysms. *Neurology.* 1974;24: 1103–1108.
115. Moskowitz RV, Baggenstoss AH, Slocumb CH. Histopathologic classification of periarteritis nodosa: a study of 56 cases confirmed at necropsy. *Proc Staff Meet Mayo Clin.* 1963;38:345–357.
116. Nagao S, Kinugasa K, Bukeo T, et al. Giant, fusiform and dissecting aneurysms at the vertebro-basi-

lar junction: report of five cases and their clinical pathophysiological aspects. [in Japanese]. *No Shinkei Geka.* 1987;15:1093–1100. English Abstract.

117. Nakagawa Y, Tashiro K, Isu T, et al. Occlusion of cerebral artery due to metastasis of chorioepithelioma. Case report. *J Neurosurg.* 1979;51: 247–250.
118. Nakahara T, Nonaka N, Kinoshita K, et al. Subarachnoid hemorrhage and aneurysmal change of the cerebral arteries due to metastases of chorioepithelioma. [in Japanese]. *Neurol Surg (Tokyo).* 1975;3:777–782. English Abstract.
119. Nakao S, Nakayama H, Ueba T, et al. Ruptured dissecting aneurysm of the vertebral artery missed by initial angiography: case report. [in Japanese]. *No Shinkei Geka.* 1992;20:475–479. English Abstract.
120. Nakata Y, Shionoya S, Kamiya K. Pathogenesis of mycotic aneurysm. *Angiology.* 1968;19:593–601.
121. Nakazawa T, Saito A, Watanabe K, et al. Dissecting aneurysms of the anterior cerebral artery: report of a case. [in Japanese]. *No Shinkei Geka.* 1984;12: 1211–1216. English abstract.
122. Nakstad P, Nornes H, Hauge HN. Traumatic aneurysms of the pericallosal arteries. *Neuroradiology.* 1986;28:335–338.
123. New PFJ, Price DL, Carter B. Cerebral angiography in cardiac myxoma. *Radiology.* 1970;96:335–345.
124. Noterman J, Verhest A, Baleriaux D, et al. A ruptured cerebral aneurysm from choriocarcinomatous origin: a case report and a review. *Neurosurg Rev.* 1989;12:71–74.
125. O'Connell BK, Towfighi J, Brennan RW, et al. Dissecting aneurysms of the head and neck. *Neurology.* 1985;35:993–997.
126. Ojemann RG, Fisher CM, Rich JC. Spontaneous dissecting aneurysm of the internal carotid artery. *Stroke.* 1972;3:434–440.
127. Ojemann RG, Heros RC, Crowell RM. *Surgical Management of Cerebrovascular Disease,* 2nd edition. Baltimore, Md: Williams & Wilkins; 1988: 337–346.
128. Ojemann RG. Infectious intracranial aneurysms. In: Fein JM, Flamm ES, eds. *Cerebrovascular Surgery.* New York, NY: Springer-Verlag; 1984; 3:1047-1060.
129. Olmstead WW, McGee TP. The pathogenesis of peripheral aneurysms of the central nervous system: a subject review from the AFIP. *Radiology.* 1977; 123:661–666.
130. Onishi H, Ito H, Kuroda E, et al. Intracranial mycotic aneurysm associated with transsphenoidal surgery to the pituitary adenoma. *Surg Neurol.* 1989; 31:149–154.
131. Overton MC III, Calvin TH Jr. Iatrogenic cerebral cortical aneurysm: case report. *J Neurosurg.* 1966; 24:672–675.
132. Oyesiku NM, Barrow DL, Eckman JR, et al. Intracranial aneurysms in sickle-cell anemia: clinical features and pathogenesis. *J Neurosurg.* 1991;75;356–363.
133. Parker HL, Kernohan JW. The central nervous system in periarteritis nodosa. *Proc Staff Meet Mayo Clin.* 1949;24:43–48.
134. Parkinson D, West M. Traumatic intracranial aneurysms. *J Neurosurg.* 1980;52:11–20.
135. Parkinson D. Surgical management of traumatic aneurysms. In: Schmidek HH, Sweet WH, eds. *Operative Neurosurgical Techniques, Indications, Methods and Results.* New York, NY: Grune & Stratton; 1982;2:941-947.
136. Paronetto F. Systemic nonsuppurative necrotizing angiitis. In: Miescher, PA, Müller-Eberhard, HJ, eds. *Textbook of immunopathology.* New York, NY: Grune & Stratton; 1969;2:722.
137. Paullus WS Jr, Norwood CW, Morgan HW. False aneurysm of the cavernous carotid artery and progressive external ophthalmoplegia after trans- sphenoidal hypophysectomy: case report. *J Neurosurg.* 1979;51:707–709.
138. Pia HW, Obrador S, Martin JG. Association of brain tumors and arterial intracranial aneurysms. *Acta Neurochir (Wien).* 1972;27:189–204.
139. Pilz P, Hartjes HJ. Fibromuscular dysplasia and multiple dissecting aneurysms of intracranial arteries: a further cause of moyamoya syndrome. *Stroke.* 1976;7:393–398.
140. Powars D, Imbus C. Cerebral vascular accidents in sickle-cell anemia. *Tex Rep Biol Med.* 1981;40:293–303.
141. Pozzati E, Giuliani G, Poppi M, et al. Blunt traumatic carotid dissection with delayed symptoms. *Stroke.* 1989;20:412–416.
142. Pozzati E, Tognetti F, Padovani R, et al. Association of cerebral mycotic aneurysm and brain abscess. *Neurochirurgia (Stuttg).* 1983;26:18–20.
143. Pruitt AA, Rubin RH, Karchmer AW, et al. Neurological complications of bacterial endocarditis. *Medicine (Baltimore).* 1978;57:329–343.
144. Pullar M, Blumbergs PC, Phillips GE, et al. Neoplastic cerebral aneurysm from metastatic gestational choriocarcinoma: case report. *J Neurosurg.* 1985;63:644–647.
145. Quattrocchi KB, Nielsen SL, Poirier V, et al. Traumatic aneurysm of the superior cerebellar artery: case report and review of the literature. *Neurosurgery.* 1990;27:476–479.
146. Roach M, Drake CG. Ruptured cerebral aneurysms caused by microorganisms. *N Engl J Med.* 1965; 273:240–244.
147. Robbins SL, Cotran RS. *Pathologic Basis of Disease.* 2nd edition. Philadelphia, Pa: WB Saunders; 1979:593-594.
148. Robbs JV, Human RR, Rajaruthnam P. Operative treatment of nonspecific aortoarteritis (Takayasu's arteritis). *J Vasc Surg.* 1986;3:605–616.
149. Roeltgen DP, Weimer GK, Patterson LF. Delayed neurologic complications of left atrial myxoma. *Neurology.* 1981;31:8–13.
150. Rose GA, Spencer H. Polyarteritis nodosa. *Q J Med.* 1957;26:43–81.
151. Rout D, Sharma A, Mohan PK, et al. Bacterial aneurysms of the intracavernous carotid artery. *J Neurosurg.* 1984;60:1236–1242.
152. Rumbaugh CL, Bergeron RT, Kurze T. Intracranial vascular damage associated with skull fractures: radiographic aspects. *Radiology.* 1972;104:81–87.
153. Sadar ES, Jane JA, Lewis LW, et al. Traumatic aneurysms of the intracranial circulation. *Surg Gynecol Obstet.* 1973;137:59–67.
154. Salmon JH, Blatt ES. Aneurysm of the internal carotid artery due to closed trauma. *J Thorac Cardiovasc Surg.* 1968;56:28–32.
155. Sampson I, Pratila M, Pratila SV. Anesthetic man-

agement of cerebral aneurysmectomy in a sickle cell anemia patient. *Mt Sinai J Med (NY).* 1982;49: 326–328.
156. Sano K, Saito I. Pulseless disease. Summary of our experiences and studies. *Schweiz Arch Neurol Neurochir Psychiatr.* 1972;111:417–433.
157. Sasaki O, Ogawa H, Koike T, et al. A clinicopathological study of dissecting aneurysms of the intracranial vertebral artery. *J Neurosurg.* 1991;75:874–882.
158. Schmalzer EA, Lee JO, Brown AK, et al. Viscosity of mixtures of sickle and normal red cells at varying hematocrit levels: Implications for transfusion. *Transfusion.* 1987;27:228–233.
159. Seigle JM, Caputy AJ, Manz HJ, et al. Multiple oncotic intracranial aneurysms and cardiac metastasis from choriocarcinoma: case report and review of the literature. *Neurosurgery.* 1987;20:39–42.
160. Sekino H, Katoh Y, Kanki T, et al. Iatrogenic traumatic intracranial aneurysm. Case report [in Japanese]. *Neurol Med Chir (Tokyo).* 1985; 23:945–951. English Abstract.
161. Shigemori M, Shirahama M, Hara K, et al. Traumatic aneurysms of intracranial internal carotid arteries: case reports [in Japanese]. *Neurol Med Chir (Tokyo)* 1982;22:241–247. English Abstract.
162. Shimizu K, Sano K. Pulseless disease. *Rinsho Geka (Tokyo).* 1948;3:377–396.
163. Shimoji T, Bando K, Nakajima K, et al. Dissecting aneurysm of the vertebral artery: report of seven cases and angiographic findings. *J Neurosurg.* 1984; 61:1038–1046.
164. Sklar EM, Quencer RM, Bowen BC, et al. Magnetic resonance applications in cerebral injury. *Radiol Clin North Am.* 1992;30:353–366.
165. Slinger WN, Starck V. Cutaneous form of polyarteritis nodosa: report of a case. *Arch Derm Syph.* 1951;63:461–468.
166. Smith RR, Parent D, Miller JD. Spontaneous and traumatic carotid artery dissections. *Contemp Neurosurg.* 1984;6:1–8.
167. Stehbens WE. Etiology of intracranial berry aneurysms. *J Neurosurg.* 1989;70:823–831.
168. Stehbens WE. The pathology of intracranial arterial aneurysms and their complications. In: Fox JL, ed. *Intracranial Aneurysms.* New York, NY: Springer-Verlag; 1983;I:272-357.
169. Steiner H, Lammer J, Kleiner R, et al. Dissecting aneurysm of cerebral arteries in congenital vascular deficiency. *Neuroradiology.* 1986;28:331–334.
170. Steinmetz H, Heiss E, Mironov A. Traumatic giant aneurysms of the intracranial carotid artery presenting long after head injury. *Surg Neurol.* 1988; 30:305–310.
171. Stoane L, Allen JH Jr, Collins HA. Radiologic observations in cerebral embolization from left heart myxomas. *Radiology.* 1966;87:262–266.
172. Suwanwela C, Suwanwela N, Charuchinda S, et al. Intracranial mycotic aneurysms of extravascular origin. *J Neurosurg.* 1972;36:552–559.
173. Sypert GW, Young HF. Ruptured mycotic pericallosal aneurysm with meningitis due to Neisseria meningitidis infection. *J Neurosurg.* 1972;37:467–469.
174. Takahashi A, Suzuki J, Sugawarra T, et al. Detachable balloon treatment of vertebral fusiform aneurysms [in Japanese]. *No Shinkei Geka.* 1988; 16(suppl 5):639–646. English Abstract.
175. Takayasu M. A case of strange changes in the central retinal vessels. *Jpn J Ophthalomol.* 1908;12: 554-555.
176. Talbott JH, Ferrandis RM. *Collagen Diseases.* New York, NY: Grune & Stratton; 1956.
177. Tanabe H, Manno T, Tanobe Y, et al. Dissecting aneurysm of the vertebral artery: report of two cases and review of the literature [in Japanese]. *No Shinkei Geka.* 1988;16:1405–1410. English Abstract.
178. Tani S, Funahashi K, Hashimoto T, et al. Traumatic aneurysm of the posterior inferior cerebellar artery [in Japanese]. *No Shinkei Geka.* 1982;10: 423–427. English Abstract.
179. Taveras JM, Wood EH. *Diagnostic Neuroradiology,* 2nd edition. Baltimore, Md: Williams & Wilkins; 1976;2:1041.
180. Van Damme H, Martin D, Stassen MP, et al. Spontaneous dissection of the internal carotid artery: report on 7 cases and a review of the literature [in French]. *J Mal Vasc.* 1990;15:14–22. English Abstract.
181. Van de Kelft E, Kunnen J, Truyen L, et al. Postpartum dissecting aneurysm of the basilar artery. *Stroke.* 1992;23:114–116.
182. Vaughan H Jr, Howard RG. Intracranial hemorrhage due to metastatic chorionepithelioma. *Neurology.* 1962;12:771–777.
183. Venger BH, Aldama AE. Mycotic vasculitis with repeated intracranial aneurysmal hemorrhage: case report. *J Neurosurg.* 1988;69:775–779.
184. Visudhiphan P, Bunyaratevej S, Klhantanaphar S. Cerebral aspergillosis: report of three cases. *J Neurosurg.* 1973;38:472–476.
185. Wagenvoort CA, Harris LE, Brown AL Jr, et al. Giant-cell arteritis with aneurysm formation in children. *Pediatrics.* 1963;32:861–867.
186. Wakai S, Yoshimasu N, Eguchi T, et al. Traumatic intracavernous aneurysm of the internal carotid artery following surgery for chronic sinusitis. *Surg Neurol.* 1980;13:391–394.
187. Wang AN, Winfield JA, Güçer G. Traumatic internal carotid aneurysm with rupture into the sphenoid sinus. *Surg Neurol.* 1986;25:77–81.
188. Wautier J, Pintigny D, Maclouf J, et al. Release of prostacyclin after erythrocyte adhesion to cultured vascular endothelium. *J Lab Clin Med.* 1986;107: 210–215.
189. Weinstein JM, Rufenocht DA, Parrtington CR, et al. Delayed visual loss due to trauma of the internal carotid artery. *Arch Neurol.* 1991;48:490–497.
190. Weir B, MacDonald N, Mielke B. Intracranial vascular complications of choriocarcinoma. *Neurosurgery.* 1978;2:138–142.
191. Weir B. *Aneurysms Affecting the Nervous System.* Baltimore, Md: Williams & Wilkins; 1987:147.
192. Wever GK, Perry IH. Periarteritis nodosa: report of a case with fatal perirenal hemorrhage. *JAMA.* 1935;104:1390–1395.
193. Yamashita M, Tanaka K, Matsuo T, et al. Cerebral dissecting aneurysms in patients with moyamoya disease. *J Neurosurg.* 1983;58:120–125.
194. Yamaura A. Diagnosis and treatment of vertebral aneurysms. *J Neurosurg.* 1988;69;345–349.
195. Yokota H, Tazaki H, Murayama K, et al. Traumatic cerebral aneurysm: 94 cases from the literature and 5 cases observed by the authors [in Japanese]. *No Shinkei Geka.* 1983;11:521–528. English Abstract.

196. Yonas H, Agamanolis D, Takaoka Y, et al. Dissecting intracranial aneurysms. *Surg Neurol.* 1977; 8:407–415.
197. Yoshimoto T, Kamiyama H, Abe H, et al. Proximal clipping and bypass between bilateral vertebral arteries using a radial arterial graft for treatment of a dissecting aneurysm of the vertebral artery. *Surg Neurol.* 1991;36:476–481.
198. Zervas NT, Liszczak TM, Mayberg MR, et al. Cerebrospinal fluid may nourish cerebral vessels through pathways in the adventitia that may be analogous to systemic vasa vasorum. *J Neurosurg.* 1982;56:475–481.
199. Ziment I, Johnson BL Jr. Angiography in the management of intracranial mycotic aneurysms. *Arch Int Med.* 1968;122:349–352.

# CHAPTER 13

# Unruptured Aneurysms, Multiple Aneurysms, Familial Aneurysms, and Aneurysms in Pregnancy

Richard Leblanc, MSc, MD, FRCSC

## Incidental and Multiple Aneurysms

The rupture of a cerebral aneurysm often is a catastrophic event that frequently affects people in their most productive time in life, when their family responsibilities are greatest. Many patients die before they reach a hospital, others die following admission to the hospital, and many of the survivors are disabled permanently. The mortality and morbidity associated with surgery of cerebral aneurysms is a function of the severity of the subarachnoid hemorrhage (SAH) that it produces, reflected by the clinical grade of the patient at the time of admission. Patients with unruptured aneurysms are generally in good neurologic condition, and surgery can be quite safe. Therefore, it is desirable to identify unruptured aneurysms and treat them before they rupture.

### *Incidental Aneurysms*

#### *Incidence*

Small, unruptured cerebral aneurysms are common after age 45. McCormick and Acosta-Rua found 55 aneurysms greater than 2 mm in largest diameter in 1,673 unselected autopsies (3.3%).[29] The premortem diagnosis of unruptured aneurysm has become more common with the use of computed tomography (CT) scanning, and magnetic resonance imaging (MRI) and angiography (MRA). These diagnostic modalities are used in patients who might not have undergone angiography in the past for relatively minor complaints (Figure 1).

#### *Presentation*

##### Nonspecific Complaints

Unruptured aneurysms can produce nonspecific complaints such as headache or dizziness. They also may produce specific complaints not related to the aneurysm itself, such as a seizure or an episode of transient ischemic attacks (TIAs) from associated carotid disease (Figure 2).

##### Specific Complaints

Patients may present with specific complaints related to the mass effect of the aneurysm on neighboring structures. Carotid aneurysms can produce well-recognized syndromes when (1) they compress the third, fourth, sixth, and sensory branches of the first and second divisions of the trigeminal (V)

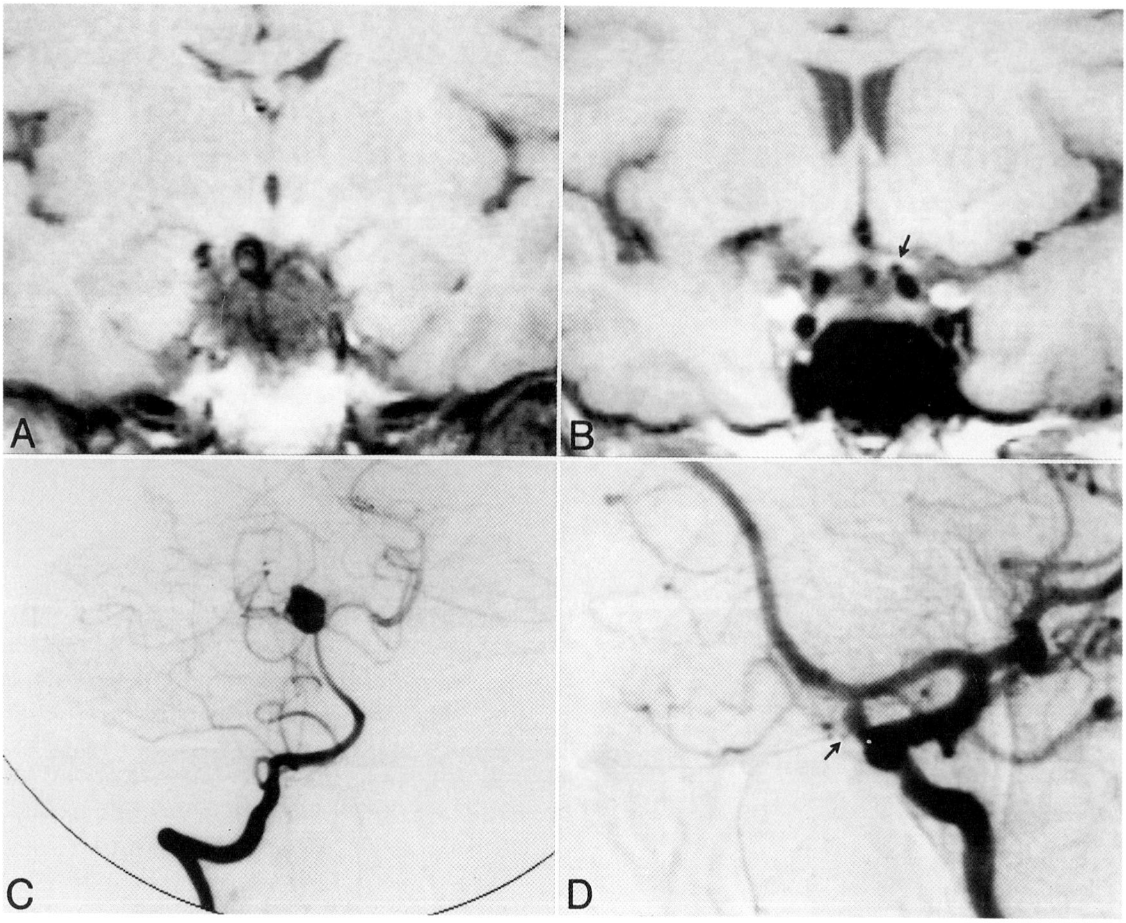


*Figure 1. MRI (**A,B**) and right vertebral and left ICA angiograms, oblique view (**C,D**) of a 42-year-old woman who underwent MRI examination following a noctural seizure. No cause for her seizure was identified, and it has not recurred. MRI demonstrated a large basilar bifurcation aneurysm (**A**), confirmed by vertebral angiography (**C**). Angiography also disclosed a small aneurysm at the origin of the left ophthalmic artery (**D, arrow**), which can be appreciated, in retrospect, in the coronal MRI (**B, arrow**). A small infundibular dilatation of the origin of the left posterior communicating artery is also seen in **D**. Both aneurysms were treated uneventfully.*

nerve within the cavernous sinus; (2) when they compress the optic (II) nerve and chiasm, as frequently occurs with aneurysms at the origin of the ophthalmic artery; or (3) when posterior communicating artery aneurysms compress the oculomotor (III) nerve. An abducens (VI) nerve palsy can be produced by aneurysms of the anterior-inferior cerebellar artery (AICA) or by basilar artery aneurysms arising at that level.[2]

A giant aneurysm can compress the brain or brain stem, mimicking a tumor, or obstruct cerebrospinal fluid (CSF) pathways, producing obstructive hydrocephalus (Figure 3). A large paraclinoid carotid aneurysm also can produce neuroendocrine disturbances from interruption of the hypothalamic-pituitary axis (Figure 4). A large cerebral aneurysm can produce TIAs in the absence of atherosclerotic narrowing, likely from embolization of platelet aggregates submitted to turbulent flow within the sac.[10] With the exception of a posterior communicating artery aneurysm producing an oculomotor nerve palsy, specific, nonhemorrhagic complaints related to the cerebral aneurysm usually are seen with a large or giant aneurysm within CT and MRI resolutions.

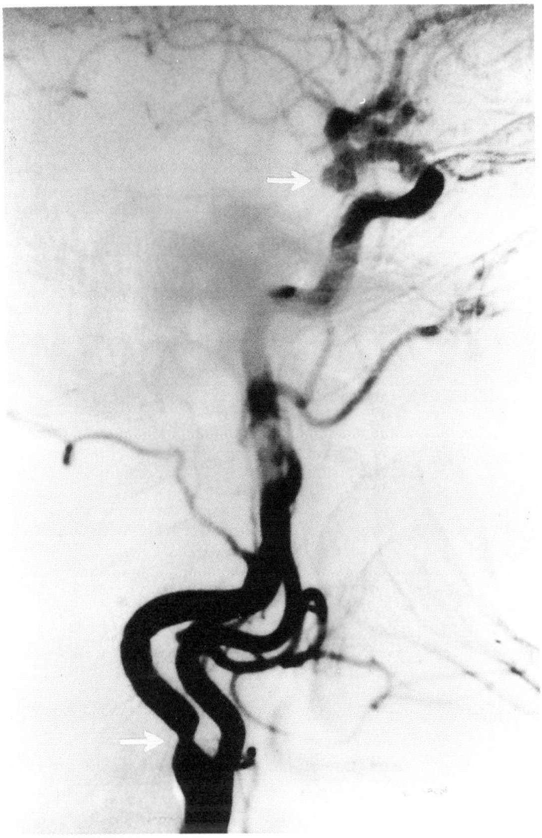

*Figure 2. Left carotid angiogram of a 58-year-old woman with a prolonged reversible ischemic neurologic deficit producing transient dysphasia, demonstrating 80% stenosis of the origin of the ICA (lower arrow) and an aneurysm originating at the level of the anterior choroidal artery (upper arrow).*

Cerebral aneurysms can be associated, perhaps causally, with other cerebrovascular pathology. Aneurysms are not infrequently seen in moyamoya disease and in association with cerebral arteriovenous malformations (AVMs), where they develop in response to hemodynamic stresses.[20] In moyamoya disease, stenosis and occlusion of the supraclinoid carotid artery results in redistribution of flow to the infraclinoid carotid circulation and to the vertebrobasilar system, precipitating the genesis of carotid-cavernous and basilar artery aneurysms. Similarly, patients with an AVM frequently have small, flow-related aneurysms on the arteries supplying the lesion. These flow-related aneurysmal dilatations are not true saccular aneurysms, but the latter also can be associated with cerebral AVM (Figure 5).[21]

Cerebral aneurysms can be found prior to rupture in patients at high risk of cerebral aneurysm, such as patients with familial aneurysms, polycystic kidney disease, or coarctation of the aorta.[19,27,28] Although aneurysms can be associated with Ehlers-Danlos syndrome, the cerebrovascular lesion most frequently seen in this condition is a carotid-cavernous fistula.[17] Unruptured, multiple cerebral artery (MCA) aneurysms can be found during the investigation of SAH.

## *Sex and Site*

A review of 3 large series encompassing 95 patients with 115 incidental aneurysms (21% multiple) reveals a clear female preponderance of up to 2:1, and a clear preference for the internal carotid artery (ICA).[15,44,53] It should be noted, however, that vertebral artery angiography was not routinely performed in the past for nonspecific complaints because many of the patients were assessed at a time when posterior fossa aneurysms were believed to be inoperable.

## *Risk of Rupture*

### Size

The risk of a cerebral aneurysm rupture is related to the aneurysm size and to the life expectancy of the patient.[24,29]

In a controversial study, Wiebers et al followed 65 patients with 81 unruptured aneurysms until death or for at least 5 years.[53] Fifty-three patients had a single aneurysm, and 12 had 2 or more. No ruptures were observed in 44 patients with aneurysms that measured less than 1 cm in diameter, while 8 of the 29 patients with aneurysms measuring greater than 1 cm experienced rupture, half within 10 weeks of diagnosis. Many investigators believe the 10-mm threshold for rupture is

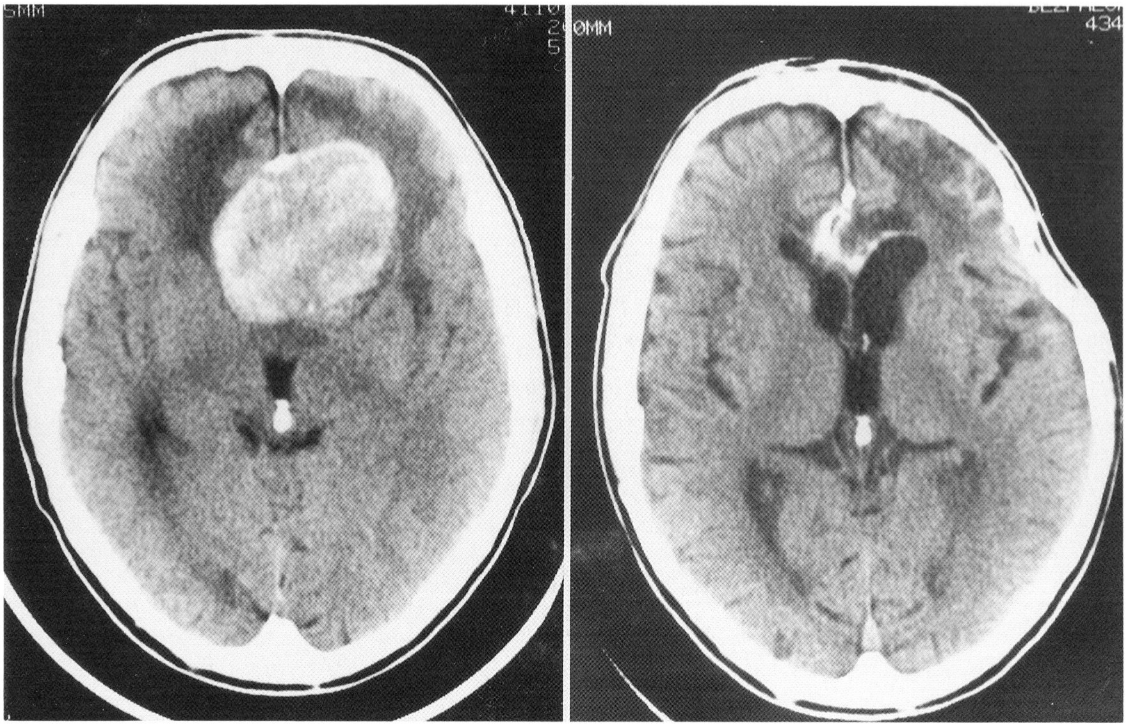

*Figure 3. Preoperative (left) and postoperative (right) noninfused CT scans of a 72-year-old man with subacute onset of psychomotor retardation and mutism demonstrating a giant aneurysm originating from the left pericallosal artery. Angiography also demonstrated a second aneurysm of the anterior commmunicating artery, a dural AV fistula, and a parasagittal meningioma. Angiography demonstrated luxuriant filling from the MCA distribution across the anterior borderzone into the ACA distribution, allowing the pericallosal artery to be clipped and the aneurysm to be excised except for some remnants of the capsule adherent to vital structures. The patient made a full recovery.*

overly generous; in an autopsy-based study, McCormick and Acosta-Rua found that only 3% of aneurysms smaller than 5 mm had ruptured, compared to 41% of 6–10 mm aneurysms (Figure 6)[29]. They observed that angiography overestimated the size of an aneurysm by an average of 30%, and concluded that a 5-mm aneurysm at autopsy would be 6–7 mm at angiography. This morphologic threshold of 5 mm for rupture (angiographic threshold 6-7 mm) is in keeping with a mean size of rupture ranging from 5–8 to 7–10 mm in large series.[11]

## Age

The risk of a cerebral aneurysm rupture is approximately 2% per year; it has also been estimated that rupture will produce death or disability in 64% to 82% of patients.[6,16] Population-based studies have reported a risk of death or disability of over 70%.[37,39] The lifetime risk of a cerebral aneurysm rupture can be calculated by the formula:

$$1-(1-R)^{L}$$

where R is the annual probability of rupture (0.02) and L is the life expectancy.[24] The lifetime risk of death or disability, therefore, can be calculated by the formula:

$$[1-(1-R)^{L}]M$$

where M is the risk that rupture will produce death or disability (Figure 7).

From these formulas it can be calculated that a patient with an unruptured aneurysm whose life expectancy is 20 years has a 33%

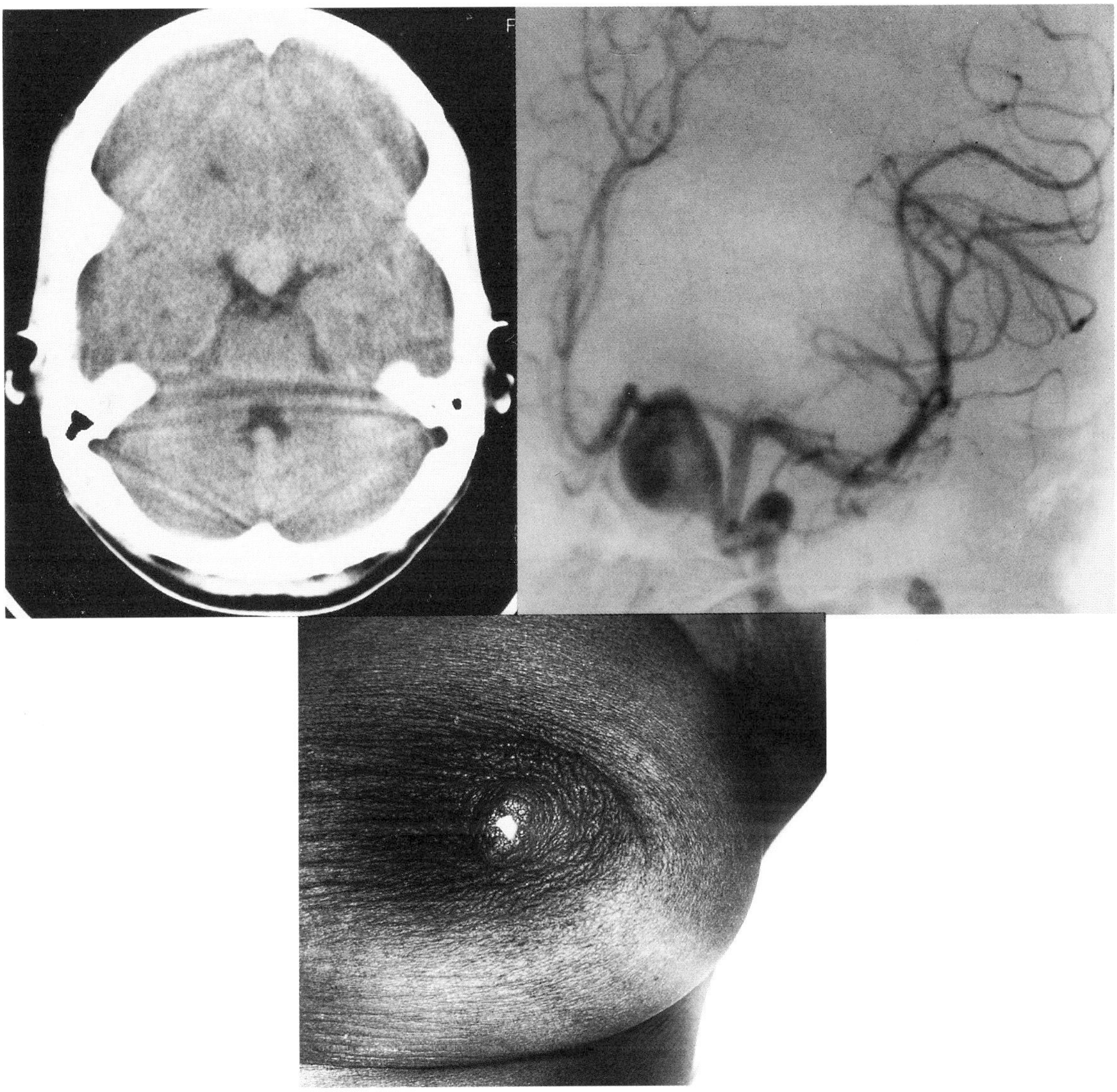

***Figure 4.*** *Noninfused CT and left carotid angiogram of a 42-year-old woman with galactorrhea and hyperprolactinemia. The large aneurysm originating at the level of the ophthalmic artery had compressed the hypothalamus, producing the neuroendocrine disturbance. A second aneurysm of the anterior choroidal artery, not seen on this angiogram, was found at surgery. Both aneurysms were clipped and there was a complete resolution of her symptoms and hormonal imbalance.*

risk of rupture and a 21% to 27% chance of dying or of becoming incapacitated.

### Arterial Hypertension

Arterial hypertension seems intuitively to be a significant risk factor for cerebral aneurysm rupture. However, the data are controversial and contradictory, and the weight of published evidence fails to support this contention. Many workers have failed to demonstrate an over-representation of arterial hypertension in patients with cerebral aneurysms,[1,29] and a multivariate analysis of 65 patients with unruptured aneurysms did not identify arterial hypertension as a factor related to eventual rupture.[53] Nonetheless, cerebral aneurysm rupture carries a higher mortality when complicated by arterial hypertension,[34] and if patients with hyperten-

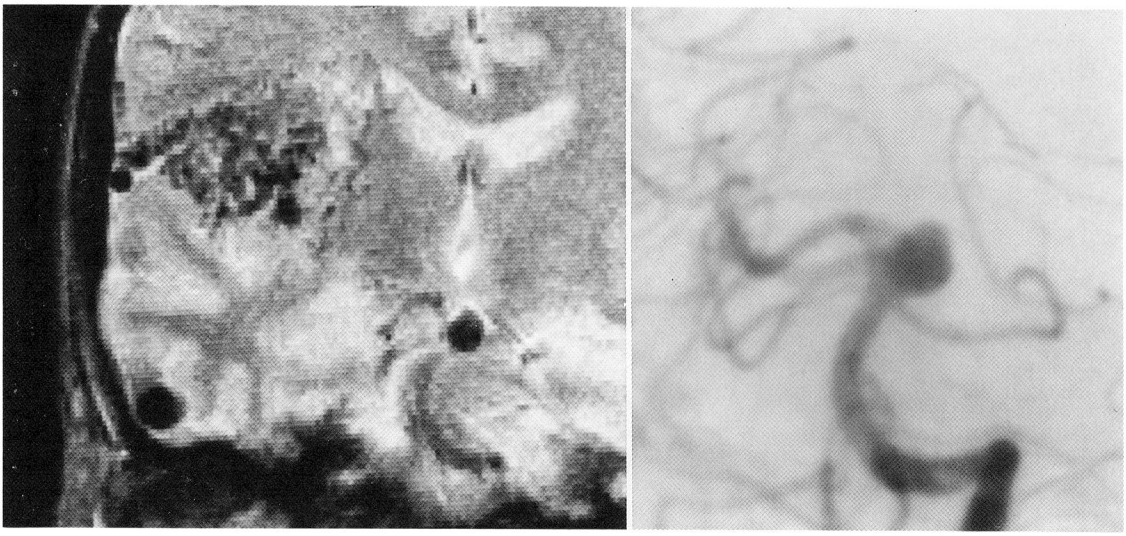

*Figure 5. MRI (left) and vertebral angiogram (right) of a 50-year-old man with a remote intracranial hemorrhage demonstrating the AVM in the right sylvian region and an aneurysm of the left superior cerebellar artery. (From Leblanc et al with permission.[21])*

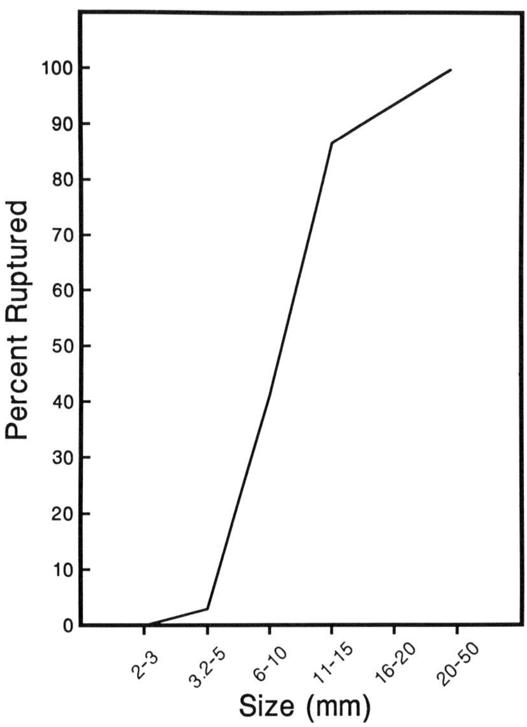


*Figure 6. Influence of size on the risk of rupture of a cerebral aneurysm. Visual display of data from McCormick and Acosta-Rua with permission.[29] This graph illustrates that the risk of a cerebral aneurysm rupture is a function of its size and that rupture is unusual when the aneurysm is smaller than 5 mm.*

sion are not at an increased risk of rupture, rupture is more likely to be fatal in these patients. Therefore, the presence of arterial hypertension in a patient with an incidental aneurysm is further incentive to treat it.

## *Treatment*

Surgery of unruptured, nongiant aneurysms can be accomplished with little or no mortality and infrequent morbidity,[7,15,44,45] while withholding surgery can result in death or disability in a significant proportion of patients. Many, including the author, would recommend that surgery seriously be considered for incidental aneurysms larger than 5 mm, especially in hypertensive patients. This is especially so for unruptured aneurysms producing an acute oculomotor nerve palsy, which the author treats most expediently, as it is believed to be a sign of aneurysm enlargement and impending rupture. The age of the patient is only a relative factor in relation to life expectancy and general medical condition. Even older patients can benefit from surgery, as this can generally be accomplished with little or no mortality and morbidity.

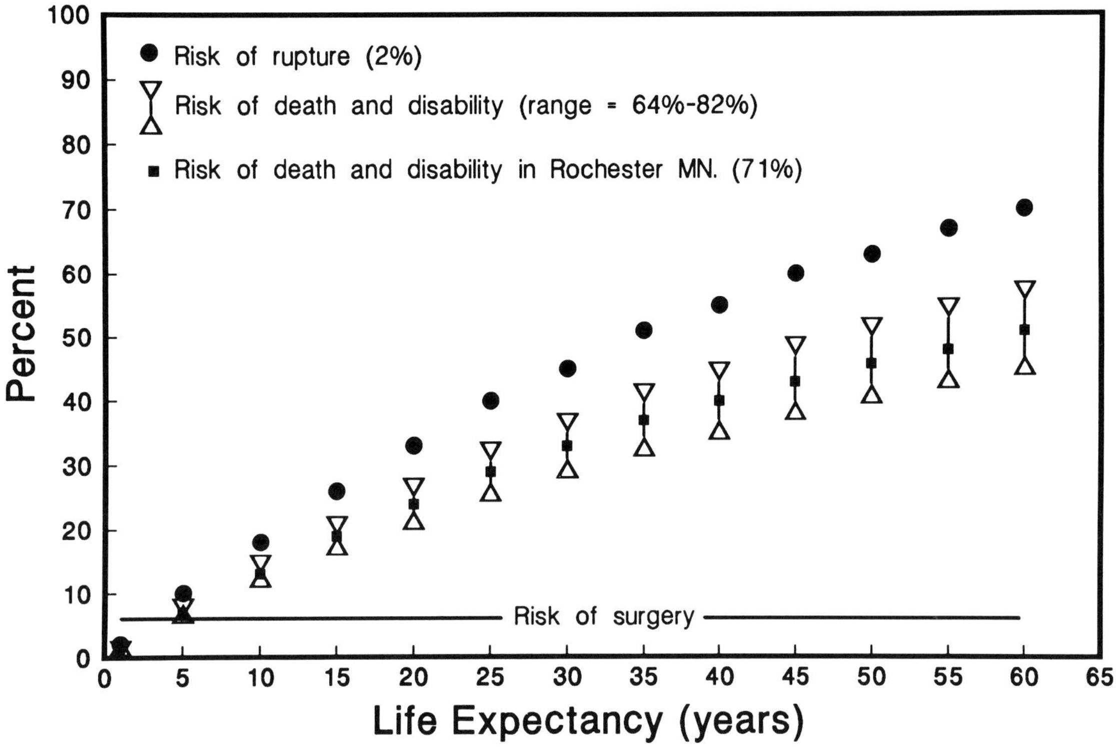


*Figure 7. Risk of a cerebral aneurysm rupture and risk that rupture will produce death and significant neurologic disability as a function of life expectancy. The risk of rupture of 2% per year generally is accepted.[24] The risk of death and disability ranges from 54% to 82% for each rupture according to Drake,[6] and Kassell and Drake,[16] and has been measured for a given population by Phillips et al.[39] The risk of surgery of an incidentally discovered aneurysm of 6% is from Wirth et al.[55] This graph illustrates that the risk of death and disability from an incidental aneurysm rupture is a function of the life expectancy of the patient.*

Unruptured giant aneurysms frequently are diagnosed when they compress the cranial nerves in their vicinity. All giant aneurysms thus discovered should be explored, as a clippable aneurysm neck frequently will be identified.[5] In cases where the aneurysm cannot be clipped or when surgery cannot be undertaken for other reasons, percutaneous techniques such as intravascular obliteration of the aneurysm, occlusion of its parent vessel, or placement of intravascular thrombogenic coils should be considered. It remains unclear, however, if such techniques will result in the detumescence of the aneurysm, relief of pressure symptoms, or even prevent eventual rupture.

## *Special Considerations*

Patients with severe cardiovascular and respiratory disease, those with malignancy, or those with the human immunodeficiency virus should probably not undergo craniotomy to treat an incidentally discovered aneurysm. The risk of rupture is low in these patients because of limited life expectancy.

Unruptured aneurysms associated with a ruptured AVM present an interesting challenge. The resection of an AVM associated with a nonflow-related, true saccular aneurysm, on the same vascular system, can precipitate rupture of the latter as the AV shunt is obliterated,and the flow is diverted toward the aneurysm. It is therefore wise to clip these aneurysms prior to excision of the AVM.[49] If the aneurysm is on a vascular distribution inaccessible at the same craniotomy, it should be treated at a later date once the patient has recovered from the initial surgery.[49]

Aneurysms originating from the intracavernous portion of the ICA frequently are diagnosed when they produce oculomotor disturbances, visual loss, or facial pain. These lesions are as likely to regress as to progress. It has been suggested that treatment should be reserved for unruptured aneurysms originating from the anterior genu of the carotid siphon and extending into the subarachnoid space, for aneurysms producing severe ipsilateral pressure symptoms, or for aneurysms with radiologic evidence of enlargement.[25] These aneurysms can be treated by direct surgery or by intravascular techniques.[14]

## Multiple Cerebral Aneurysms

### *Incidence*

Unruptured aneurysms discovered during the investigation of one that has ruptured are diagnosed on angiographs in 14% to 19% and at autopsy in 23% to 28% of patients with an aneurysmal SAH.[26] Angiography therefore underestimates the true incidence of aneurysm multiplicity because (1) complete angiography is sometimes not performed, (2) small aneurysms may not be demonstrated, and (3) multiple aneurysms may be more frequently fatal than single ones.

### *Multiplicity*

It is estimated that 80% of patients with multiple aneurysms have 2 aneurysms, 13% have 3, 5% have 4, and 1% have 5 or more aneurysms.[13,30,31] Alternatively, 15% of patients have 2 aneurysms, 3.5% have 3, and 1.4% have 4 or more (Figure 8).

A female preponderance has been reported in up to 70% of cases of multiple aneurysms, and a 2.4:1 ratio of females over males was reported in the Cooperative Study of Intra-

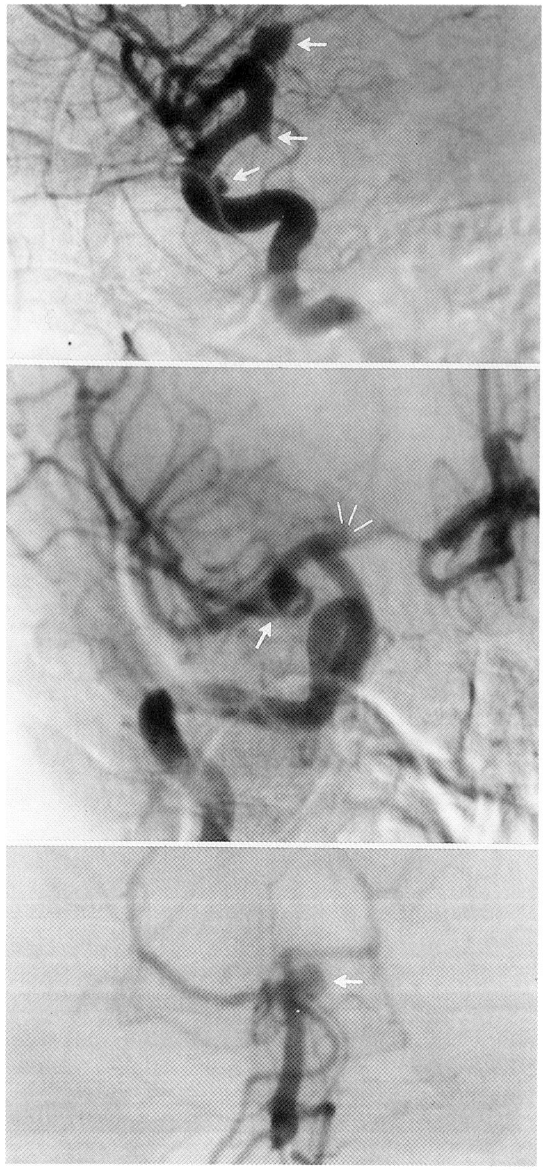

***Figure 8.*** *Cerebral angiogram of a 55-year-old woman who presented to the hospital 1 week after loss of consciousness. The noninfused CT scan was normal. Left ICA angiography* ***(top)*** *demonstrated a small aneurysm within the cavernous sinus, a small aneurysm at the origin of the posterior communicating artery, and a larger aneurysm at the origin of first segment of the ACA. A right ICA angiogram* ***(middle)*** *demonstrated a small aneurysm at the origin of the first segment of the ACA and a larger aneurysm at the bifurcation of the MCA. A left vertebral angiogram* ***(bottom)*** *demonstrated an aneurysm at the origin of the left SCA. All aneurysms, except the cavernous one, were clipped without incidence. At surgery, it was demonstrated that the left ACA aneurysm had bled.*

cranial Aneurysms and Subarachnoid Hemorrhage.[13,26,30,31,38]

## Aneurysm Sites

Multiple intracranial aneurysms involve the ICA in over half the cases, the MCA in one-quarter, and the anterior cerebral artery in one-eighth. The posterior circulation is involved in one-sixteenth of cases. The latter figure is probably an underestimate because the studies on which these figures are based did not routinely include vertebrobasilar angiography.[13,30]

The Cooperative Study addressed the location of multiple aneurysms in detail.[26] If 2 aneurysms are present, they will be contralateral in about half the cases but involve the anterior and posterior circulation only 1 time in 20. Given a posterior circulation aneurysm, a second aneurysm is likely to be on the ICA half of the time. Anterior communicating artery aneurysms are less likely to be associated with a second aneurysm than are ICA and MCA aneurysms; if a second aneurysm is present, it is most likely on the MCA. With an ICA aneurysm, there is a 50% chance that a second aneurysm will also be on an ICA, most likely on the contralateral one; with an MCA aneurysm, a second aneurysm most likely will be on the ICA.

The posterior communicating arteries, the MCAs, and the ICAs are the most likely sites of occurrence, in that order, for symmetric aneurysm pairs.

## Risk of Rupture

The risk of rupture of an intact aneurysm discovered during the investigation of SAH approximates 2% per year. Mount and Brisman, in a review of 4 studies, found a 10% rupture rate with 40% fatality over 5 years.[30] Moyes found a 27.6% rupture rate over a period of 1–10 years, and Winn estimated a bleeding rate of 1% to 2.2% per annum.[12,31] Heishanen initially found a rupture rate of 11.5%, with 57% fatality over 10 years. However, continued observation over the[13] subsequent 10 years indicated an increasing risk of rupture with the passage of time.[12]

The increasing risk of rupture over time has been noted by others.[7] Mount observed that a patient is never risk free; one of his cases died of an SAH after 23 years of followup.[5,30] The larger the aneurysm, the higher is the likelihood that it will rupture, but even small aneurysms are prone to rupture. Mount observed a 3-mm aneurysm that had produced a fatal hemorrhage, and Winn found that half of the multiple aneurysms that eventually bled were 5 mm or smaller.[30,54] Further, patients with multiple aneurysms found after one has ruptured have a higher risk of bleeding from a second aneurysm than patients with multiple aneurysms in whom none has bled.

## Treatment of Multiple Aneurysms

The advent of operative microsurgical techniques has caused a definite change in the attitude of neurosurgeons with regard to the treatment of multiple cerebral aneurysms. Prior to the 1970s, most authorities recommended that multiple aneurysms or even ruptured aneurysms not be treated surgically; others recommended clipping the unruptured aneurysm only if it was accessible, *en passant*, during the treatment of a ruptured one.

With prolonged followup indicating that the risk of rupture of a previously intact aneurysm increases unacceptably with time, and with the use of the operative microscope, this attitude changed. Current opinion favors the treatment of all accessible aneurysms at the same time as the treatment of the ruptured aneurysm, and the treatment of remaining aneurysms with a second craniotomy.[7,12,30,45]

## Timing of Surgery and Factors Related to Outcome

The *en passant* treatment of unruptured aneurysms is associated with low mortality and morbidity; complications are related to the clipping of the ruptured aneurysm and not the unruptured ones. The treatment of intact aneurysms frequently can be accomplished with no mortality and low morbidity because the sac is usually resilient and its dissection easy. Morbidity is related to the size of the aneurysm, to the complexity of its neck, to its accessibility, and to the amount of retraction necessary to expose it. Interestingly, one study found that surgery of multiple familial aneurysms may be associated with higher morbidity than surgery of nonfamilial ones, as is the treatment of multiple aneurysms presenting with cerebral ischemia.[55]

Mount and Brisman saw no mortality and 2% to 3% morbidity with the delayed treatment of multiple aneurysms.[30] Similarly, Drake and Girvin had no mortality and only 2 cases with deficits in 91 electively treated patients with multiple aneurysms.[7] Samson et al had no mortality or significant morbidity in 50 patients submitted to elective craniotomy for the treatment of multiple aneurysms.[45] Wirth et al, however, observed a 6% incidence of morbidity without fatality in 107 patients treated at 12 institutions.[55] It should be remembered that this low mortality and morbidity was achieved by treating the multiple aneurysms in a delayed fashion or on an elective basis. This is in keeping with the findings of Paterson and Bond who observed that early surgery in patients with multiple aneurysms was associated with a poor outcome and that one surgery had a worse outcome than staged procedures.[38]

The ruptured aneurysm usually can be readily identified by angiography and CT or MRI scanning. The CT will frequently reveal (1) focal accumulation of blood in the anterior hemispheric fissure, sylvian fissure, or pericarotid cisterns, suggesting an anterior communicating artery, MCA, or ICA aneurysm rupture respectively, or (2) a hematoma in the orbitofrontal region or in the temporal lobe, suggesting an anterior communicating artery or MCA aneurysm. On angiography, the larger aneurysm, the one that is multilobed, or the one associated with focal vasospasm usually is the one that has bled. Treatment is then directed at this aneurysm, and unruptured aneurysms that are accessible *en passant* can be treated at the same time. Contralateral aneurysms or aneurysms not reached by the initial exposure can be treated electively at a second stage once the patient has recovered from the initial hemorrhage and surgery.

## Familial Aneurysms and Aneurysms Associated with Inherited Diseases

The identification of patients with familial cerebral aneurysms, or cerebral aneurysms associated with familial conditions, such as polycystic kidney disease, is important. These conditions suggest a possible genetically determined etiology for cerebral aneurysms, perhaps related to a mesenchymal defect affecting the wall of cerebral blood vessels, and family members at risk can be diagnosed before aneurysms they harbor rupture.

### *Familial Cerebral Aneurysms*

#### *Incidence and Inheritance*

The incidence of familial cerebral aneurysms is probably underestimated. More cases are being documented because of greater access to medical imaging and to tertiary medical centers, and because easier communication between centers facilitates the epidemiologic recording of familial cerebral aneurysms.[22]

The inheritance pattern for familial aneurysms is unknown. Both autosomal-dominant (Figure 9) and recessive[3] multifactorial transmission patterns have been postulated. Cerebral aneurysms occur in association with autosomal-dominant disorders, such as polycystic kidney disease and Marfan's syndrome,[9] and with autosomal-recessive disorders such as Type IV Ehlers-Danlos syndrome and pseudoxanthoma elasticum.[27] A cluster of families with cerebral aneurysms has been identified in the Saguenay-Lac-St-Jean region of Canada, from 2 ancestral couples: 1 couple was married in Quebec City in 1660, and the other couple was married in La Pocatière in 1760.[3]

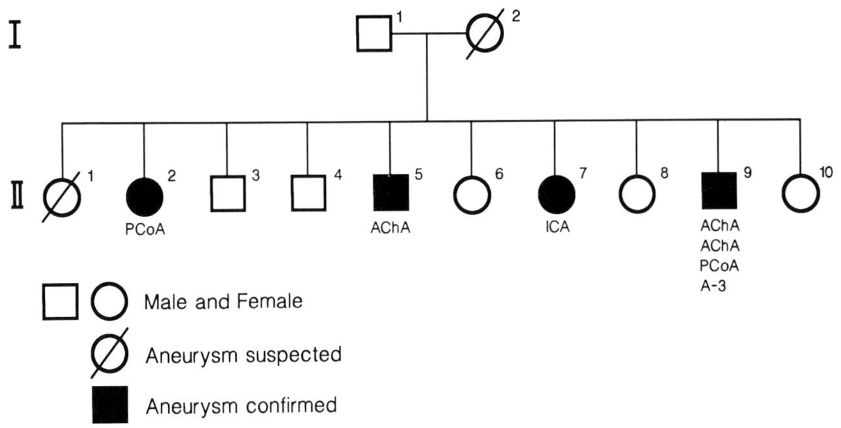


*Figure 9. Pedigree of a family with cerebral aneurysms. I-2 was a 39-year-old woman who sought medical advice because of an acute, sudden, severe headache. While being examined the headache recurred and she died rapidly. II-1 died under similar circumstances. II-2 had a proven, ultimately fatal, SAH from an angiographically demonstrated posterior communicating artery aneurysm. II-5 died following the rupture of an angiographically proven anterior choroidal artery aneurysm; II-7 died following a proven SAH from an angiographically-demonstrated carotid bifurcation aneurysm; II-9 had a documented SAH associated with a pericallosal, posterior communicating, and bilateral anterior choroidal artery aneurysms. The pattern of inheritance in this family suggests an autosomal-dominant transmission. (From Lozano and Leblanc, with permission[27]).*

## *Biologic Characteristics of Familial Cerebral Aneurysms*

The author's institution undertook a multivariate, computer-aided analysis of 243 aneurysms in 177 patients from 74 families and compared them to the 2,627 sporadic aneurysm cases reported by the Cooperative Study.[27] We identified a parent-child relationship in 56 patients and a relationship between 2 or more siblings in 129 patients. There was a similar incidence of multiplicity in the familial and sporadic cases, and there was a similar female to male ratio in both groups.

Familial aneurysms rupture at a younger age, the peak incidence of rupture being in the fifth decade in familial cases and the sixth decade in sporadic ones. By the fifth decade, 70% of familial aneurysms have ruptured versus 40% of the sporadic cases. The average age at the time of rupture of familial aneurysms is 42.3 years, compared to 51.4 years in the sporadic cases.

Sibling pairs are more than twice as likely to have their aneurysms rupture in the same decade as patients with sporadic aneurysms; aneurysms in identical twins rupture within 2–5 years of each other.

Half of familial aneurysms arise from the ICA, and one-quarter each arise from the MCA, anterior cerebral artery (ACA), and anterior communicating artery. A minority originate on the vertebrobasilar system. Familial aneurysms occur less frequently on the anterior communicating artery than do sporadic ones. Siblings are more than twice as likely to have aneurysms at the same or at mirror sites than patients with sporadic aneurysms; all identical twins reported had aneurysms at identical or mirror sites. Familial basilar aneurysms have the highest probability of rupture (100%), followed by anterior communicating and posterior communicating aneurysms (80% each). Familial MCA aneurysms, at 65%, have the lowest frequency of rupture. These biologic characteristics suggest that familial cerebral aneurysms may be determined genetically.

## *Biologic Markers*

The possibility that familial cerebral aneurysms may be determined genetically, and the desirability of identifying familial members at risk, short of angiography, has led to the study of possible biologic markers for familial cerebral aneurysms.

### Tissue Antigens

Human leukocyte antigens (HLA), residing on the short arm of chromosome 6, have been associated with specific diseases. This association most frequently results from a disorder of the immunologic system, but can also reflect the coinheritance of HLA loci and genes responsible for particular diseases. It has been suggested that cerebral aneurysms are associated with specific HLA loci, most notably HLA A-28, B-7, and DR-2, which would support a possible genetic etiology for cerebral aneurysms, perhaps related to a gene encoded on chromosome 6.

Ostergaard et al suggested that HLA B-7 and DR-2 may be over-represented in patients with cerebral aneurysms.[34] Norrgård et al were unable to confirm these results but observed an increased incidence of HLA A-28 in sporadic aneurysm patients, and an under representation of HLA B-40 in familial aneurysm patients.[36] Others have been unable to confirm the results of either of these laboratories.[46]

If specific antigens or inheritance of a specific HLA pattern is associated with cerebral aneurysms, then HLA-typing of relatives of patients with familial cerebral aneurysms might identify those at risk of having these lesions. To test this hypothesis, the author typed the HLA profile of 2 families with cerebral aneurysms.[23] No specific HLA pattern was observed that correlated with the presence of cerebral aneurysms. Although HLA B-7 and DR-2 were present in patients with aneurysms, they were also present in patients with negative angiograms and were absent in two patients with multiple aneurysms. HLA A-28 was absent in all individuals. Mellergårdet et al in a similar study found HLA B-7 expressed in five of six individuals with a cerebral aneurysm and in six of nine nonaffected relatives.[35] The author therefore concludes that HLA-typing is not sufficient to identify or exclude family members at risk of having cerebral aneurysms.

### Collagen

The demonstration that Ehlers-Danlos syndrome Type IV is caused by a relative deficiency in Type III collagen, and the demonstration that patients with Ehlers-Danlos syndrome can harbor cerebral aneurysms, suggests that aneurysms may be associated with a relative deficiency of Type III collagen.[32,43] If so, beside implying a possible genetically determined etiology for cerebral aneurysms, the demonstration of Type III collagen deficiency in family members might identify those at risk of harboring an aneurysm.

To test the hypothesis that cerebral aneurysms are associated with a deficiency of Type III collagen, the author cultured skin fibroblasts from a patient with three cerebral aneurysms whose mother and sister also had cerebral aneurysms, and in patients with multiple aneurysms.[23] The author was not able to observe a relative deficiency in Type III collagen in skin fibroblasts from these aneurysm patients compared to control cell lines. Therefore, he was unable to support the hypothesis that familial cerebral aneurysms are caused by a relative deficiency of Type III collagen, or that the demonstration of a relative deficiency of Type III collagen can identify relatives at risk of having a cerebral aneurysm. These results do not, however, rule out the possibility of a more subtle defect in the collagen metabolism in aneurysm patients.

## *Investigation of Family Members*

It has been recommended, and it has been the author's practice, to offer four-vessel cerebral angiography in siblings of patients with a documented familial occurrence of cerebral aneurysms. This has proven to be logistically difficult and time consuming.

Applying the formula for the lifetime risk of death or disability from a ruptured aneurysm:

$$[1-(1-R)^L]M$$

and multiplying the result by the hypothetic risk of a family member harboring an aneurysm at—for example, one in four and one in two—one obtains a graph that indicates a relatively low probability of grave consequences from a ruptured aneurysm in this patient population, especially at the lower incidence of inheritance (Figure 10). Nonetheless, patients who have seen two or more family members die or rendered disabled from a cerebral aneurysm frequently are not reassured by such statistics.

The author has not found CT or MRI useful in reassuring these patients since negative studies do not rule out the presence of an aneurysm. In these troubled patients, cerebral angiography has been carried out with little or no mortality or morbidity, and some aneurysms have been identified and treated without complications. It is therefore the author's practice to inquire into the possibility of a family history of cerebral aneurysm, to endeavor to document these from hospital records when such a possibility is suggested, and to be available for discussion with concerned relatives.

If all families with cerebral aneurysm had the inheritance pattern suggested in Figure 9, one could be quite forceful in recommending angiography and eventual surgery. This is not always the case, and the risk of aneurysm in an individual family member remains un-

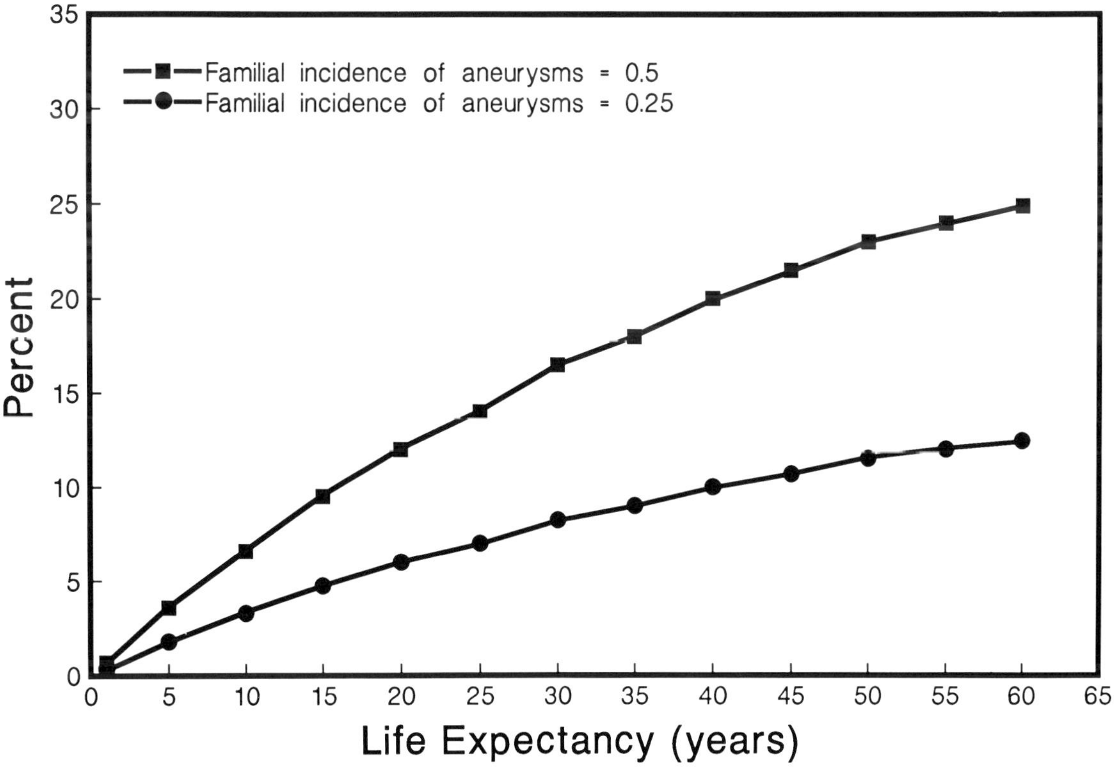


*Figure 10. Estimated risk of death or disability from the rupture of a familial-inherited cerebral aneurysm for hypothetic familial incidence rates of 50% and 25% as a function of life expectancy. This graph illustrates that the possible benefits of elective angiography in patients with possible familial aneurysms is a function of the incidence of aneurysms and the life expectancy of the patient.*

known. The possible benefits counterbalancing the small risk of elective angiography are the demonstration of an aneurysm that can be treated prior to rupture and reassurance if an aneurysm is absent. The risks of angiography, which is a logistically formidable undertaking if large populations are to be screened, may in the future be obviated by the development of magnetic resonance angiography (MRA). The sensitivity and specificity of MRA in cerebral aneurysms is discussed in detail in Chapter 3 of this book.

## *Aneurysms Associated with Familial Conditions*

### *Cerebral Aneurysms and Polycystic Kidney Disease*

Adult polycystic kidney disease (APKD) is an autosomal, dominantly inherited disorder arising from a defect that maps to chromosome 16. This disorder has extrarenal manifestations including cardiac valve abnormalities, thoracic aortic aneurysms, and cerebral aneurysms. The latter can be present in up to 30% to 40% of APKD patients. The pathogenesis of cerebral aneurysms in APKD is unknown. As the majority of APKD patients will become hypertensive during their illness, it is possible that aneurysms develop as a result of the effect of arterial hypertension on the cerebrovascular wall.

However, not every APKD patient with cerebral aneurysms is hypertensive, and it is unclear whether hypertension in itself is sufficient to produce cerebral aneurysms.[28] The occurrence of cerebral aneurysms in patients with APKD may simply reflect the inheritance of a disorder that affects the cerebral vasculature as well as other tissues of mesenchymal origin. If this is the case, hypertension could be considered a factor aggravating a congenital predisposition to aneurysm formation.

Cerebral aneurysms in APKD patients occur more commonly in males than in females by a ratio of 2.5 to 1, in marked contrast to sporadic aneurysms, which occur more commonly in females.[28] Aneurysms associated with APKD rupture at a younger age than sporadic aneurysms and three quarters of all APKD-associated aneurysms rupture by age 50, compared to less than half of sporadic aneurysms.[28] Aneurysms occur more frequently on the MCA in APKD patients than they do in sporadic cases.[28] Very interestingly, there does not appear to be an increased incidence of multiple aneurysms in APKD patients. This observation is especially pertinent because it has been suggested that multiplicity of cerebral aneurysms is related to arterial hypertension.[1,33] If this is the case, APKD should be associated with an over-representation of multiple cerebral aneurysms.

Further, it seems commonly to be held that cerebral aneurysms in APKD develop as the result of arterial hypertension. In their study the authors found that cerebral aneurysms coexist with APKD in the absence of arterial hypertension in one fourth of the cases, and in a systematic, angiographic study of 17 asymptomatic APKD patients from 10 families, 7 patients were identified with an unruptured aneurysm: 2 were hypertensive, 5 were not.[28,50] Studies are in progress at several centers to prospectively assess the prevalence of cerebral aneurysms in APKD patients using MRA (Awad et al, personal communication).

#### Screening of APKD Patients for Cerebral Aneurysms

Levey et al used decision analysis to assess whether or not patients with APKD should undergo routine cerebral angiography and eventual surgery if an aneurysm was demonstrated.[24] They used 0.3 as the probability of an APKD patient harboring an aneurysm, 0.02 as the annual probability of rupture of an aneurysm in APKD patients, and 0.25–0.55 as the probability of death or disability should an APKD-associated aneurysm rupture. Using 0.01% and 1% as the risks of a grave complication from arteriography and surgery, respectively, they concluded that the threshold age below which patients would gain 1 year of life expectancy by opting for angiography and surgery is 33 years. However, as discussed above, it is likely that Levey et al underestimate the risk of death or significant disability following aneurysm rupture. This pushes forward the age at which angiography and eventual surgery would be of benefit in APKD patients. Furthermore, clusters of APKD families with cerebral aneurysms have been reported,[8] so that the risk of aneurysm in these families may be higher than the 30% used by Levey et al.

### *Collagenous Vascular Diseases and Cerebral Aneurysms*

Cerebral aneurysms have been described in association with Marfan's syndrome, with pseudoxanthoma elasticum, and with Type IV Ehlers-Danlos syndrome.[4,35,48] The demonstration that Ehlers-Danlos syndrome is associated with a relative deficiency in Type III collagen, and the demonstration that such patients can harbor cerebral aneurysms, suggested that cerebral aneurysms may also be associated with a relative deficiency in Type III collagen. However, a critical review of the literature reveals that the most common lesions associated with Ehlers-Danlos syndrome Type IV are extracerebral, usually carotid-cavernous fistulas; given the relatively high incidence of cerebral aneurysm in the general population, it may not be unusual to encounter cases in which both conditions coexist statistically and not biologically. Furthermore, we have demonstrated that normal Type III collagen levels can exist in patients with familial and multiple aneurysms who would be expected to express a Type III collagen deficiency were it of etiologic importance.[23] These findings do not exclude the possibility of more subtle defects in the collagen molecule that might contribute to aneurysm formation either in familial or sporadic cases.

The investigation and treatment of Ehlers-Danlos Type IV patients who have a proven SAH can be quite formidable: angiography, because of the fragility of the blood vessels, can be associated with significant morbidity and mortality, as can major intracranial procedures directed at the dissection and clipping of the fragile and friable vascular tissue. The successful use of endovascular techniques to treat carotid-cavernous fistulas in patients with Ehlers-Danlos Type IV has been reported.[47] Whether these techniques would be useful in the treatment of unsupported cerebral aneurysms within the subarachnoid space remains to be demonstrated.

## Aneurysmal Subarachnoid Hemorrhage in Pregnancy

### *Incidence and Presentation of Ruptured Aneurysm in Pregnancy*

Up to 10% of maternal deaths are due to cerebral hemorrhage, many caused by a ruptured aneurysm. As other more treatable and preventable conditions associated with maternal death come under medical control, the relative importance of aneurysm rupture in pregnancy increases.[41,52]

A ruptured aneurysm will complicate from 1 in 2,000 to 1 in 10,000 pregnancies,[52] and up to one-fifth of all aneurysms will rupture in pregnancy or in the early postpartum period.[42] Approximately 40% of aneurysms rupture during the first pregnancy, 20% during the second pregnancy, 10% during the third pregnancy, and 25% during the fourth or subsequent pregnancies.[52] The authors treated a 27-year-old woman whose aneurysm bled during the last trimester of her sixth pregnancy, the five previous ones having been uneventful.

The manifestations of aneurysmal SAH are no different in a pregnant patient. The risk increases with advancing age and with each trimester (Figure 11), perhaps in response to alterations in blood volume accompanying pregnancy or in response to hormonal alterations.[4,41,42,52]

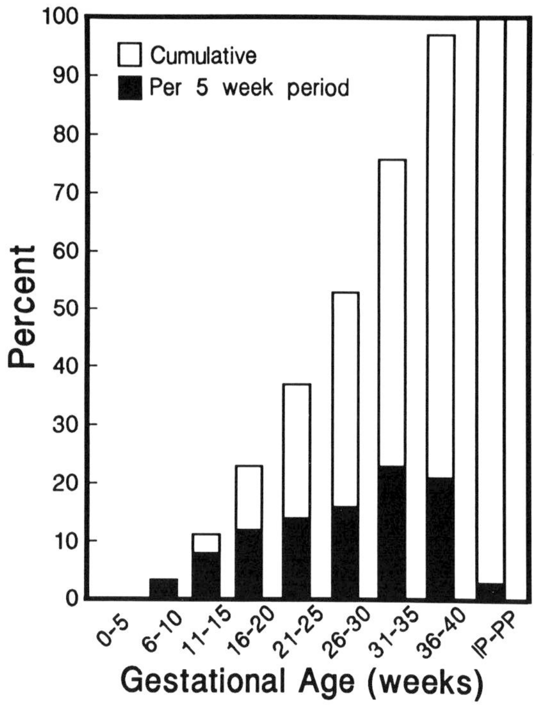


*Figure 11. Visual display of data reported by Robinson et al illustrating the increased risk of aneurysm rupture as a function of the gestational age and that interpartum or early postpartum (IP-PP) rupture is unusual. From reference 41.*

Some investigators found that the ICA is more frequently affected in pregnant patients while others found that aneurysms occur at the same site in pregnant and nonpregnant patients.[4,41]

## Diagnosis

The diagnosis of aneurysmal SAH in the pregnant patient is achieved as in the nonpregnant patient by lumbar puncture, CT scanning, and cerebral angiography. As multiple aneurysms have been documented in pregnant patients,[41] angiography should be complete and not limited to the vessel from which the ruptured aneurysm is believed to originate from based on previous CT scan. Appropriate shielding of the uterus should be performed compulsively, and should be documented during radiologic procedures on pregnant patients.

The differential diagnosis of aneurysmal SAH in the pregnant patient is the same as in the nonpregnant patient with the exception that the pregnant patient can also have a cerebral hemorrhage related to eclampsia, or related to the presence of a metastatic chorionepithelioma.[40]

## Natural History

The natural history of a ruptured aneurysm in a pregnant patient is similar to that of the nonpregnant patient. It is associated with high mortality and morbidity with the added burden of fetal wastage. Of 8 unclipped aneurysms in pregnant women followed by Robinson et al, 5 rebled and only 3 patients were well at followup.[41] Rebleeding occurs during the same pregnancy in up to half of the patients whose aneurysms are unclipped and more than half of these will die.[4] Rebleeding is more frequent within the first 2 weeks of hemorrhage, in the subsequent weeks prior to delivery, in the postpartum phase, and with subsequent pregnancy, in that order.[53] Few aneurysms rupture during labor or delivery.[4]

## Treatment

The surgical management of a ruptured aneurysm in the pregnant patient offers a clear benefit to both mother and child. In a review of the literature, Dias et al found maternal and fetal death rates of 11% and 5% respectively in patients undergoing surgery, versus 63% and 27% respectively in nonoperated patients.[4] Regression analysis, controlling for clinical grade and other covariants, found that the significant better outcome for the operated mother persisted, although a clear advantage for the fetus was not demonstrated, perhaps because of the small number of cases available for study.

### *Management*

A pregnant patient with aneurysmal SAH should be treated as if she were not pregnant. If the aneurysm ruptures near or at term, caesarean section immediately followed by craniotomy can be performed.[52] If the aneurysm ruptures before the fetus is capable of surviving without the use of a respirator, or if an unruptured aneurysm is discovered during pregnancy, the aneurysm is treated and the pregnancy is allowed to take its course.[52] If a ruptured aneurysm is believed to be unclippable and nontreatable by other means such as endovascular techniques, and rupture occurs early in pregnancy, a therapeutic abortion can be recommended in the hope of minimizing the risk of rerupture with its attendant high mortality and morbidity.[52] A patient whose aneurysm is unclippable or otherwise untreatable should be counseled against subsequent pregnancies.

A followup angiogram should be obtained following the clipping of an aneurysm in pregnant patients if there is any question whatsoever that the aneurysm might be partially clipped; a partially clipped aneurysm can increase dramatically in size during the course of the pregnancy.[51] If the aneurysm is found to be partially clipped, a more adequate clipping should be performed before delivery.

Pharmacologic adjuncts to the surgical treatment of ruptured aneurysms should be used with caution in the pregnant patient. Most notably, antifibrinolytic agents may be associated with increased thrombotic problems, and diuretics can produce severe fetal dehydration. It is probably wiser to avoid systemic hypotension during the treatment of the aneurysm if the fetus is in utero, with satisfactory control for the dissection and clipping of the aneurysm being achieved with the use of a temporary clip on the parent vessel. One should avoid volume expansion and induced arterial hypertension, if possible, in the event of cerebral vasospasm. It has not been established that calcium antagonists such as nimodipine are free of adverse effects to fetal development. They should be used in pregnancy only after careful assessment of their potential benefits versus their potential risk to the fetus. The use of nimodipine in the lactating mother is not advised.[18]

### *Delivery*

There is no evidence that a caesarean section has any advantages either for the mother or the child over an assisted vaginal delivery with a shortened second stage of labor using forceps. Certainly, if the aneurysm has been clipped during pregnancy, a vaginal delivery is preferred if there are no obstetric contraindications. This would seem to be the case also for patients with an unclipped aneurysm that had ruptured initially in the first or second trimester and that has not rebled in the interval. However, patients whose aneurysm ruptured in the third trimester and remains unclipped should probably be delivered by caesarean section.

## References


1. Andrews RJ, Spiegel PK. Intracranial aneurysms: age, sex, blood pressure and multiplicity in an unselected series of patients. *J Neurosurg.* 1979; 51:27–32.
2. Barnett HJM. Some clinical features of intracranial aneurysms. *Clin Neurosurg.* 1969;16:43–72.
3. Cantin L, Mathieu J, Debraekeleer M, et al. Anévrysmes intracrâniens familiaux: étude de 9 familles saguenéenes. *Can J Neurol Sci.* 1988;15:194–195. Abstract.
4. Dias MS, Sekhar LN. Intracranial hemorrhage from aneurysms and arteriovenous malformations during pregnancy and puerperium. *Neurosurgery.* 1990; 27:855–866.
5. Drake CG. Giant intracranial aneurysms: experience with surgical treatment in 174 patients. *Clin Neurosurg.* 1979;26:12–95.
6. Drake CG. Management of cerebral aneurysm. *Stroke.* 1981;12:273–283.
7. Drake CG, Girvin JP. The surgical treatment of subarachnoid hemorrhage with multiple aneurysms. In: Morley TP, ed. *Current Controversies in Neurosurgery.* Philadelphia, Pa: WB Saunders; 1976:274–278.
8. Fehlings MG, Gentili F. The association between polycystic kidney disease and cerebral aneurysms. *Can J Neurol Sci.* 1991;18:505–509.
9. Finney HL, Roberts TS, Anderson RE. Giant intracranial aneurysm associated with Marfan's syndrome. *J Neurosurg.* 1976;45:342–347.

10. Fisher M, Davidson RI, Marcus EM. Transient focal cerebral ischemia as a presenting manifestation of unruptured cerebral aneurysms. *Ann Neurol.* 1980; 8:367–372.
11. Ferguson GG, Peerless SJ, Drake CG. Natural history of intracranial aneurysms. *New Engl J Med.* 1981; 305:99. Correspondence.
12. Heiskanen O. Risk of bleeding from unruptured aneurysms in cases with multiple intracranial aneurysms. *J Neurosurg.* 1981;55:524–526.
13. Heishanen O, Marttila I. Risk of rupture of a second aneurysm in patients with multiple aneurysms. *J Neurosurg.* 1970;32:295–299.
14. Inoue T, Rhoton A Jr, Theele D, et al. Surgical approaches to the cavernous sinus: a microsurgical study. *Neurosurgery.* 1990;26:903–932.
15. Jain KK. Surgery of intact intracranial aneurysms. *J Neurosurg.* 1974;40:495–498.
16. Kassell NF, Drake CG. Timing of aneurysm surgery. *Neurosurgery.* 1982;10:514–519.
17. Kissel P, Arnould G, André GM. Incidence des accidents vasculaires cérébraux au cours des conjonctivo-dysplasies héréditaires. *J Genet Hum.* 1972; 20:151–167.
18. Krogh CME, Gillis MC, Bisson R, eds. ***Compendium of Pharmaceutics and Specialties.*** Ottawa, Canada: The Canadian Pharmaceutical Association; 1991: 791.
19. LeBlanc FE, Charrette EP, Dobell ARC, et al. Neurological complications of aortic coarctation. *Canad Med Assoc J.* 1968;99:299–303.
20. Leblanc R. Cerebral amyloid angiopathy and moyamoya disease. *Neurosurg Clin No Am.* In press.
21. Leblanc R, Levesque M, Comair Y, et al. Magnetic resonance imaging of cerebral arteriovenous malformations. *Neurosurgery.* 1987;21:15–20.
22. Leblanc R, Lozano AM. Graves' disease and subarachnoid hemorrhage: a possible familial association. *Can J Neurol Sci.* 1987;14:638–641.
23. Leblanc R, Lozano AM, Van der Rest M, et al. Absence of collagen deficiency in familial cerebral aneurysms. *J Neurosurg.* 1989;70:837–840.
24. Levey AS, Pauker SG, Kassirer JP. Occult intracranial aneurysms in polycystic kidney disease. *N Engl J Med.* 1983;308:986–994.
25. Linskey ME, Sekhar LN, Hirsch WL Jr, et al. Aneurysms of the intracavernous carotid artery: natural history and indications for treatment. *Neurosurgery.* 1990;26:933–938.
26. Locksley HB. Natural history of subarachnoid hemorrhage, intracranial aneurysms and arteriovenous malformations. Report on the Cooperative Study of Intracranial Aneurysms and Subarachnoid Hemorrhage, Section V, Part I. *J Neurosurg.* 1966;25:219–239.
27. Lozano AM, Leblanc R. Familial intracranial aneurysms. *J Neurosurg.* 1987;66:522–528.
28. Lozano AM, Leblanc R. Cerebral aneurysms and polycystic kidney disease. *Can J Neurol Sci.* In press.
29. McCormick WF, Acosta-Rua GJ. The size of intracranial saccular aneurysms: an autopsy study. *J Neurosurg.* 1970;33:422–427.
30. Mount LA, Brisman R. Treatment of multiple aneurysms: symptomatic and asymptomatic. *Clin Neurosurg.* 1974;21:166–170.
31. Moyes PD. Surgical treatment of multiple aneurysms and of incidentally-discovered unruptured aneurysms. *J Neurosurg.* 1971;35:291–295.
32. Neil-Dwyer G, Bartlett JR, Nicholls AC, et al. Collagen deficiency and ruptured cerebral aneurysms: A clinical and biochemical study. *J Neurosurg.* 1983; 59:16–20.
33. Østergaard JR, Bruun-Petersen G, Lamm LU. HLA antigens and complement types in patients with intracranial saccular aneurysms. *Tissue Antigens.* 1986; 28:176–181.
34. Østergaard JR, Høg E. Incidence of multiple intracranial aneurysms: influence of arterial hypertension and gender. *J Neurosurg.* 1985;63:49–55.
35. Mellergård P, Ljunggren B, Brandt L, et al. HLA-typing in a family with six intracranial aneurysms. *Br Neurosurg.* 1989;3:479–485.
36. Norrgård O, Beckman G, Beckman L, et al. Genetic markers in patients with intracranial aneurysms. *Hum Hered.* 1987;37:255–259.
37. Pakarinen S. Incidence, aetiology, and prognosis of primary subarachnoid haemorrhage. *Acta Neurol Scand Suppl.* 1967;43(suppl 29).
38. Paterson A, Bond MR. Treatment of multiple intracranial arterial aneurysms. *Lancet.* 1973; 1:1302–1304.
39. Phillips LH II, Whisnant JP, O'Fallon WM, et al. The unchanging pattern of subarachnoid hemorrhage in a community. *Neurology.* 1980;30:1034–1040.
40. Pool JL, Potts DG. Aneurysms and arteriovenous anomalies of the brain. New York, NY: Harper & Row.
41. Robinson JL, Chir B, Hall CJ, et al. Subarachnoid hemorrhage in pregnancy. *J Neurosurg.* 1972;36:27–33.
42. Robinson JL, Hall CS, Sedzimir CB. Arteriovenous malformations, aneurysms and pregnancy. *J Neurosurg.* 1974;41:63–70.
43. Rubinstein MK, Cohen NH. Ehler-Danlos syndrome associated with multiple intracranial aneurysms. *J Neurology.* 1964;14:125–132.
44. Salazar JL. Surgical treatment of asymptomatic and incidental intracranial aneurysms. *J Neurosurg.* 1980; 53:20–21.
45. Samson DS, Hodosh RM, Clark WK. Surgical management of unruptured asymptomatic aneurysms. *J Neurosurg.* 1977;46:731–734.
46. Schievink WI, De Waal LP, Hageman LM, et al. Intracranial aneurysm and HLA-DR2. *J Neurol Neurosurg Psychiatry.* 1988;51:883. Letter.
47. Schievink WI, Piepgras DG, Earnest F IV, et al. Spontaneous carotid-cavernous fistulae in Ehlers-Danlos syndrome Type IV. *J Neurosurg.* 1991;74: 991–998.
48. Shigemori M, Shirahama M, Tokutomi T, et al. Familial intracranial aneurysms associated with rare cerebrovascular anomalies: case reports. *Neurol Med Chir (Tokyo).* 1982;22:77–80.
49. Suzuki J, Onuma T. Intracranial aneurysms associated with arteriovenous malformations. *J Neurosurg.* 1979;50:742–746.
50. Wakabayashi T, Fujita S, Ohbora Y, et al. Polycystic kidney disease and intracranial aneurysms: early angiographic diagnosis and early operation from the unruptured aneurysm. *J Neurosurg.* 1983;58:488–491.
51. Weir BKA, Drake CG. Rapid growth of residual

aneurysmal neck during pregnancy. *J Neurosurg.* 1991;75:780–782.

52. Wiebers DO. Subarachnoid hemorrhage in pregnancy. *Semin Neurol.* 1988;8:226–229.
53. Wiebers DO, Whisnant JP, O'Fallon WM. The natural history of unruptured intracranial aneurysms. *N Engl J Med.* 1981;304:696–698.
54. Winn HR, Almaani WS, Berga SL, et al. The long-term outcome in patients with multiple aneurysms. *J Neurosurg.* 1983;59:642–651.
55. Wirth FP, Laws ER Jr, Piepgras D, et al. Surgical treatment of incidental intracranial aneurysms. *Neurosurgery.* 1983;12:507–511.

# CHAPTER 14

# Results and Complications of the Surgical Management of Intracranial Aneurysms

Jacques J. Morcos, MD, and Roberto C. Heros, MD

Aneurysmal subarachnoid hemorrhage (SAH) afflicts from 4.0 to 23.9 persons per 100,000 population each year,[57] and in North America it kills or disables 18,000 individuals yearly.[46] After the ictus strikes, 83% survive long enough to be taken to a hospital.[46] Without treatment, 4.1% will rebleed on the first day, then 1.5% daily for two weeks.[45] By 6 months, 50% would have rebled,[41] and the risk stabilizes at 3% per year thereafter.[41,42] By 10 years, 18% would be functional survivors, 8% disabled, and 74% dead.[43]

Despite major advances in acute care management, diagnostic neuroimaging, interventional neuroradiology, microneurovascular techniques, and neurologic rehabilitation, no more than 33% of currently afflicted patients achieve a functional outcome, while 29% die.[57]

Table 1 lists in chronologic order all the factors involved, to various degrees, in determining the ultimate prognosis of the patient presenting with subarachnoid hemorrhage. These determinants of overall "management outcome" are quite more encompassing than the more discrete factors that determine "surgical outcome." Clinical series that tend to focus on surgical results skew favorably the overall picture, in that both preoperative mortality and preoperative morbidity that contraindicates surgery are unaccounted for. This is illustrated in Table 2, which lists some major clinical series that have evaluated management and/or surgical outcome. In most respects, comparing results between series can be misleading; the very characteristics that influence outcome differ widely among the series and relate mostly to time and manner of patient selection.

Table 3 summarizes the direct causative factors of management morbidity and mortality that apply to ruptured aneurysms at any location.

This chapter will address the issue of surgical outcome only as it relates to surgical technique. The pitfalls of intracranial aneurysm surgery, as they pertain to particular aneurysm locations, will be expanded on. The tabulated results following each section represent the collective surgical experience of the senior author over the past 12 years. The policy of late surgery (days 10–14) was generally followed until the mid-1980s with a policy of early surgery (days 0–3) in force for "good"-grade patients thereafter.

**TABLE 1**
**Subarachnoid Hemorrhage—Prognostic Factors**

I. Demographics
- Age
- Sex

II. Medical Background

III. State on Admission
- Time from hemorrhage
- Neurologic grade
- Hemodynamic status

IV. CT Findings
- Intracerebral hemorrhage
- Intraventricular hemorrhage
- Fisher's grade
- Hydrocephalus

V. Angiographic Findings
- Aneurysm characteristics
  Site
  Size
  Multiplicity
  Type (mycotic, traumatic, etc.)
- Vasospasm
- Collateral network

VI. Surgical Factors
- Time from hemorrhage
- Neurologic grade at time of surgery
- Hemodynamic status at time of surgery
- Conceptual planning of operation
- Technical difficulty of operation

## Anterior Circulation Aneurysms

### *Petrous and Carotid-Cavernous Aneurysms*

The relatively benign natural history of these lesions, their difficult location at the base of the skull, the favorable results obtained by treating the symptomatic lesions with proximal carotid ligation (with or without bypass grafting, depending on tolerance to occlusion) are all factors that have prompted the senior author to treat most of these lesions either conservatively or by carotid occlusion. Generally we believe that only significant clinical symptoms or radiographic evidence of aneurysmal growth warrants therapeutic intervention. A full discussion of the indications, techniques, results, and complications of proximal carotid ligation with or without bypass grafting is outside the scope of this chapter and is addressed adequately by previous reports.[25,44,56,78,90,92,96]

The senior author has no personal experience with direct intracranial surgery of petrous aneurysms, but the obvious surgical challenge lies in obtaining safe and adequate exposure. A detailed knowledge of anatomic landmarks of the petrous region is essential to prevent injury to the acoustic apparatus and the facial nerve while drilling.[82] Failure to recognize and obliterate an opened eustachian tube can lead to postoperative cerebrospinal fluid (CSF) leak.[82] Being commonly fusiform, these aneurysms are likely to require resection and interposition grafting,[82,85] and we would agree with full heparinization of the patient during the period of occlusion to prevent thromboembolic phenomena.[85]

Only four of the authors' patients with intracavernous aneurysms have been subjected to intracranial surgery. The aneurysms have been small and located in the distal segment of the intracavernous carotid, readily accessible through the superior approach to the cavernous sinus advocated by Dolenc.[22] Although we remove epidurally the pterion and most of the lesser wing of the sphenoid down to the base of the anterior clinoid process, we do not favor completing the removal of the clinoid epidurally as indicated by Dolenc because of our apprehension of possible aneurysmal rupture prior to securing distal carotid control, as previously described.[38,65] We open the dura in a standard fashion and remove the last portion of the anterior clinoid intradurally. We have experienced one case of postoperative ipsilateral blindness that remained unexplained despite immediate re-exploration. Conceivably, direct optic nerve damage at the level of the optic foramen could have occurred due to either electrocoagulation of the dorsal dura after removal of the anterior clinoid tip or to the drilling of the optic strut between artery and nerve. We believe that the optic canal must be drilled completely to allow full mobilization of the optic nerve, as also applies for paraclinoid aneurysms. Damage to the oculo-

TABLE 2
**Surgical Treatment: Recent Morbidity/Mortality Figures**

| | | Management | | Surgical | | |
|---|---|---|---|---|---|---|
| **Clinical Series** | **Number of patients** | **Morbidity** | **Mortality** | **Morbidity** | **Mortality** | **Remarks** |
| Yoshimoto et al[101] 1979 | 1,000 | Not available | | 8.4% | 6.4% | • 982 ruptured<br>18 unruptured<br>• All grades<br>• Random admission times |
| Sundt et al[87] 1982 | 722 | 10%<br><br>G1* 3%<br>G2 16% | 17%<br><br>6%<br>11% | 12%<br><br>G1 2%<br>G2 7% | 4%<br><br>2%<br>4% | • 544 ruptured<br>178 unruptured<br>• All grades<br>• Random admission times |
| Ropper and Zervas[76] 1984 | 112 | 20% | 11% | Not available | | • All ruptured<br>• Only "good" grades<br>• Random admission times |
| Ljunggren et al[58] 1985 | 251 | 19% | 39% | 20% | 5% | • All ruptured<br>• All grades<br>• Immediate admission<br>• Preadmission deaths accounted for |
| Rosenørn et al[77] 1987 | 1,076 | 27% | 45.5% | 36% | 23% | • Prospective study<br>• All ruptured<br>• All grades<br>• Random admission times |
| Disney, Weir and Petruk[20] 1987 | 437 | Yrs 68–77:24%<br>Yrs 77–85:23% | 47%<br>38% | Yrs 68–77:17.9%<br>Yrs 78–85:14.1% | 19%<br>11% | • All ruptured<br>• All grades<br>• Admission within 2 days of SAH<br>• Compares two eras |
| Chyatte, Fode and Sundt[16] 1988 | 244 | 13% | 23% | 14% | 15% | • All ruptured<br>• All grades<br>• Admission within 3 days of SAH |
| Öhman and Heiskanen[63] 1989 | 216 | AS** 3%<br>IS 16%<br>LS 7% | 6%<br>6%<br>13% | AS 3%<br>IS 16%<br>LS 8% | 6%<br>1.5%<br>4.7% | • Prospective randomized study<br>• All ruptured<br>• Only grades 1–3<br>• Admission within 3 days from SAH |
| Cooperative study[46,47] 1990 | 3,521 | 16% | 26% | 18% | 14% | • Prospective study<br>• All ruptured<br>• All grades<br>• Admission within 3 days from SAH |
| Lee[54] 1991 | 780 | Not available | | 2.7% | 4% | • 745 ruptured<br>35 unruptured<br>• All grades<br>• Random admission times |

* Botterell grade
** AS = Acute surgery (0-3 days)
IS = Intermediate surgery (4-7 days)
LS = Late surgery (> 7 days)

**TABLE 3**
**Subarachnoid Hemorrhage—Causes of Management Morbidity and Mortality**

I. Effects of the Initial Bleed

II. Vasospasm

III. Rebleeding

IV. Hydrocephalus

V. Seizures

VI. Other Medical Complications
  a. Cardiac abnormalities
  b. Electrolyte disturbance
  c. Thrombophlebitis and pulmonary embolism
  d. Systemic infection

VII. Surgical Complications
  a. Intraoperative
    - Rupture
    - Arterial occlusion
    - Perforator injury
    - Distal embolization
    - Direct neural injury
  b. Postoperative
    - Intracranial hemorrhage
    - Delayed ischemic deficits
    - Systemic complications
    - Incomplete clipping

motor (III), trochlear (IV), and abducens (VI) nerves is usually related to excessive packing of the cavernous sinus.

## *Paraclinoid Aneurysms*

The nomenclature of aneurysms arising in this region can be confusing. As reported by Day,[19] it is convenient to classify these aneurysms, when feasible, according to their arterial branching site within a segment. Thus, the opthalmic segment may give rise to either a true carotid ophthalmic or to a superior hypophyseal artery aneurysm, the latter being designated as "paraclinoid" (when growing ventral to the carotid and lateral to the sella), and "suprasellar" (when growing and displacing the chiasm medially). For purposes of simplicity, we have called all these aneurysms "paraclinoid," although we are keenly aware of the importance of precise preoperative recognition of the relationship of the aneurysmal neck to the clinoid and the ophthalmic artery.[38]

Patient positioning for surgery is crucial with these aneurysms. If they are flush with skull base, the authors prefer to flex the neck slightly rather than tilt the head back as for deep- seated aneurysms. A double advantage is (1) reduction of cavernous sinus bleeding, and (2) better visualization of the anterior clinoid region. We value greatly the ability to alternate between a frontal and a temporal line of vision for optimal clip placement, and therefore to perform a widely based pterional craniotomy. The head is turned no more than 20 degrees for optimal visualization of the opticocarotid cistern. Adequate exposure is so crucial with these aneurysms that skull base surgeons such as Al-Mefty[3,83] have used a tailored orbitocranial approach to these and similar complex aneurysms of the anterior circulation. We have had no reason to modify our current pterional approach.

The senior author has discussed in detail the surgical techniques involved in the exposure of paraclinoid aneurysms.[65] The authors routinely obtain proximal control of the carotid in the neck for large and giant aneurysms and an argument could be made for including some small aneurysms in this selection. We recently encountered a small aneurysm that we felt did not warrant proximal control. It was pointing upward and anteromedially under the anterior clinoid process, the erosion of which was not recognized preoperatively. Drilling of the clinoid resulted in massive hemorrhage that could not be controlled adequately. (The details of the case are reported elsewhere.[50]) Damage to the optic nerves is one of the major concerns with direct surgery in this area. As previously reported, we have had several instances of lost vision as a result of these operations.[38,65] As discussed under cavernous aneurysms, coagulation of the dura at the optic foramen can result in direct damage to the nerve if the bony optic roof is defective. We currently coagulate the flap of dura only away from the optic canal and complete the bony removal medially to the optic nerve so as to allow its medial mobilization in cases of giant aneurysms. Any remaining sharp edge of dura or bone in this location can serve as a fulcrum against which the optic nerve could be damaged when retracted medially. Utmost care should be taken when introducing the drill bit between the carotid and the optic nerve to remove the remnants of the optic strut. We routinely use a high-speed air drill, first with a cutting and then with a diamond bit. The generous medial bony removal can result in entering the ethmoidal cells and a potential cerebrospinal fluid (CSF) leak. We seal the area with fat or muscle, preferably covered by fibrin glue. An interesting report describes a case of tension pneumocephalus that complicates clipping of a carotid ophthalmic artery aneurysm, secondary to drilling of the planum sphenoidal.[4] Occlusion of the ophthalmic artery is another potential cause of visual loss. Hamby[35] and Adson[1] reported a low rate of visual loss when the ophthalmic artery was occluded. Indeed, none of our patients who underwent intentional ophthalmic artery occlusion as part of aneurysm trapping lost vision. A decade ago, we were using visual evoked potentials for these aneurysms; however, we have abandoned this technique because when the changes are recognized, the damage has usually occurred and is already irreversible.

The authors routinely use intraoperative electroencephalogram (EEG) when prolonged temporary carotid occlusion is expected or necessary, although the limitation to the number of leads that can be used around the surgical site weakens the validity of the technique. We rely more heavily on a preoperative determination of tolerance to temporary balloon occlusion with the patient fully awake.[27]

Direct injury to the oculomotor nerve and, on one occasion, the abducens nerve has been encountered with excessive packing of the cavernous sinus, in particular when the paraclinoid aneurysm is partly intracavernous. The Dolenc technique[22] of gentle minimal packing with Surgicel™ (Johnson & Johnson, New Brunswick, NJ) helps to avoid this complication, which fortunately has usually been reversible.

Finally, in reference to clipping, kinking of the parent artery is a serious problem, especially with giant aneurysms. The neck is usually broader in the direction of the carotid artery and one should attempt clipping parallel to it. Intraoperative angiography is very helpful in assessing carotid patency in time for corrective measures to be instituted.[8] When multiple clips are necessary, one should avoid optic nerve impingement and use the shortest possible clips to avoid placing blindly their tips in the cavernous sinus and causing oculomotor damage. Fox[28] recently reported on eight cases of ventral (paraclinoid) carotid artery aneurysms and recognized that a wide atherosclerotic base causing clip slippage and a partial intracavernous location are the main reasons for incomplete clipping and repeated surgery. Reviewing 14 patients with carotid ophthalmic artery aneurysms using the combined epidural and subdural direct approach, Dolenc[22] encountered two deaths, one due to pulmonary embolus and one due to gastrointestinal (GI) bleeding; three patients had transient visual symptoms, and obliteration of the aneurysm was achieved in all patients.

Table 4 summarizes the principal surgical pitfalls, and Table 5 reports the senior author's results with these aneurysms.

## *Supraclinoid Aneurysms*

In addition to posterior communicating, anterior choroidal, and carotid bifurcation aneurysms, this section will include aneurysms arising from the ventral wall of the carotid artery, excluding the ones arising from the ophthalmic segment, although a preoperative distinction is frequently impossible, especially when the ophthalmic segment is short.

Ventral wall aneurysms are frequently globular, and proximal control in the neck may be necessary with large aneurysms obscuring the ophthalmic segment. It is even sometimes necessary to drill part of the anterior clinoid to mobilize the optic nerve partially (as was described for paraclinoid aneurysms). A fenestrated right-angle Sugita clip has become essential for proper clipping of many of these

TABLE 4
**Paraclinoid Aneurysms**
**Surgical Pitfalls**

- Poor patient positioning: avoid neck extension
- Lack of proximal control
- Excessive dural coagulation over optic nerve
- Insufficient drilling of optic canal
- Poor clip application
- Blind use of larger clips
- Excessive packing of cavernous sinus

aneurysms, with the blades invariably applied parallel to the carotid artery. As with paraclinoid aneurysms, the authors frequently use the technique described by Samson and Batjer[81] of proximal forced suctioning of the carotid artery after complete trapping of the aneurysm and find it very helpful with "soft" aneurysms; this technique has not eliminated the need for aneurysmorrhaphy in calcified and partially thrombosed aneurysms. Occasionally the authors have encountered an atherosclerotic plaque at the neck of the aneurysm, making dissection more treacherous. We recently created a tear at such a site, and pushing the aneurysm away from the carotid artery to control the bleeding resulted in further widening of the tear. We resorted to using a circumferential Sundt type of clip to control the bleeding and had to include the choroidal artery in the clip, resulting in an infarct in the anterior choroidal distribution with a serious hemiparesis. Cooper[17,18] used anterior choroidal ligation for the treatment of Parkinson's disease and reported a low 20% incidence of serious neurologic deficits, explained by Rhoton[72] on the basis of rich but very variable collateral blood supply from other internal carotid, posterior cerebral,

TABLE 5
**Paraclinoid Aneurysms**
**Results of Direct Surgery**

| Size | Number | Good | Poor* | Dead |
|---|---|---|---|---|
| Giant | 42 | 39 | 2 | 1 |
| <25 mm | 41 | 38 | 2 | 1 |
| Total | 83 | 77 | 4 | 2 |

*In two cases the poor result was due to ipsilateral blindness.

posterior communicating, and middle cerebral artery branches.

In contrast to ophthalmic segment aneurysms, posterior communicating artery aneurysms project posteriorly, posterolaterally, or laterally. Therefore, one of the main problems is premature rupture with retraction of the deep aspect of the temporal lobe. When these aneurysms point straight laterally and are not associated with a third nerve palsy, we assume that they are pointing over, rather than under, the fold of tentorium and therefore that the dome may be adherent to the temporal lobe. In these cases we make a point during patient positioning of not turning the head more than 20 degrees contralaterally to obtain preliminary carotid control by a simple subfrontal exposure without temporal retraction. Once the carotid artery is exposed, another dangerous maneuver is to retract it medially, as many of these ruptured aneurysms develop adhesions laterally between their dome and either the temporal lobe or the tentorial edge. To avoid rupture, we prefer rotating the microscope medially, looking into the opticocarotid cistern and retracting the carotid laterally toward the dome to identify the posterior communicating artery, which invariably is proximal to the aneurysm. Only the "shoulder" of the origin of the posterior communicating artery needs to be visualized and, provided the clip is placed parallel to the posterior communicating artery, occlusion should not result. A clip too long and too medially placed can occlude the posterior communicating artery or its perforators more distally, and, if applied in the lateral direction can include the oculomotor nerve.

With anterior choroidal artery aneurysms, the same factors of premature rupture and inappropriate clipping apply. An additional pitfall is failure to identify and include inadvertently in the clip a duplicate anterior choroidal artery, the incidence of which may be as high as 4%.[72,79]

With carotid bifurcation aneurysms, the authors prefer a wide frontal and temporal exposure to be able to dissect behind the aneurysm and apply the clip from both the medial and the lateral direction with minimal aneurysmalmanipulation. The major pitfall is occlusion of the perforators usually originating from the initial portion of A1 and M1. In addition, some important perforators arise from the back wall of the distal internal carotid and from the anterior choroidal artery and run behind, and sometimes adherent to, the back wall of the aneurysm. Long clips can occlude either the recurrent artery of Heubner's, which is usually parallel to the A1 deep to the carotid artery, or the basal vein of Rosenthal, which originates deep to the carotid bifurcation. The wide exposure allows a multidirectional view of important perforators. In addition, the longest axis of the aneurysm is usually parallel to the A1 and M1 and a wide exposure is essential for clip application in that direction. It is hazardous and unnecessary to attempt the complete exposure of the dome, as the relevant anatomy is all located at the base. A wide opening of the sylvian fissure is essential for these aneurysms and helps in recognizing such rare anomalies as a duplicated middle cerebral artery which, if unrecognized because of insufficient exposure, could be inadvertently included in the clip.

Tables 6 and 7 summarize, respectively, the surgical pitfalls and the senior author's results with these aneurysms.

TABLE 6
**Supraclinoid Carotid Aneurysms Surgical Pitfalls**

1. Poor positioning with excessive head rotation
2. Insufficiently wide craniotomy for bifurcation aneurysms
3. Premature rupture from temporal retraction
4. Retraction of carotid away from adherent dome
5. Use of excessively long clips and blind clip application with damage to:
   - Posterior communicating artery or its perforators
   - Anterior choroidal or its perforators
   - Recurrent artery of Heubner's
   - Oculomotor nerve
   - Basal vein of Rosenthal
6. Application of clip perpendicular to long axis of neck on bifurcation aneurysms
7. Insufficient opening of sylvian fissure for bifurcation aneurysms
8. Damage to a duplicated M1 artery

## *Anterior Cerebral Aneurysms*

It is convenient to think of these aneurysms as belonging to one of three categories: proximal anterior cerebral (A1), anterior communicating artery complex, or distal anterior cerebral aneurysms. The latter type has been subdivided by some authors[64] into infracallosal, genu, and supracallosal aneurysms.

A1 aneurysms are usually related to perforating arteries, and the most important technical challenge is to preserve these vessels. Given adequate collateral circulation, the origin of the aneurysm can be temporarily trapped between the origin of the A1 and the anterior communicating artery for relatively long periods of time, even permanently if necessary, provided that the important perforators that usually come from the origin of the A1 are preserved. Occasionally the recurrent artery of Heubner's comes from the distal A1 and must also be preserved. The situation is different, of course, if there is no contralateral A1 and a patent anterior communicating artery; then the ipsilateral A1 must be treated as an end artery, and clipping with preservation of the parent vessel becomes imperative. One should also be aware of other anatomic variations (such as an infraoptic course of the A1 or a duplication).

Anterior communicating artery complex

TABLE 7
**Supraclinoid Carotid Aneurysms—Surgical Results**

| Size | Number | Good | Poor | Dead |
|---|---|---|---|---|
| Giant | 12 | 9 | 2 | 1 |
| < 25 mm | 123 | 117 | 6 | 0 |

aneurysms present several potential problems. The first major pitfall is premature rupture during the subfrontal retractionstage, prior to obtaining proximal control, in particular when the aneurysm points downward and the dome is attached by adhesions to the tuberculum sella or to the chiasm. In these instances, the senior author retracts only laterally and minimally and exposes the aneurysmal complex by subpial dissection through the gyrus rectus.

The major problem with anterior communicating artery aneurysms is damage to, or occlusion of, perforating vessels. These generally originate from the dorsal aspect of the anterior communicating artery and the proximal A2 and run backward upwardly to the hypothalamic area. The recurrent artery of Heubner's usually takes origin from the initial segment of A1. Therefore, circumferential dissection of the entire aneurysmal complex is essential to prevent this complication. The authors prefer to obtain control of the ipsilateral A1 and A2 and then also the contralateral A1. Unless the aneurysm is pointing downward and stuck to the tuberculum sellae, we prefer using Poletti's technique[70] of approaching the aneurysm from a temporal direction by achieving slightly more generous bony removal of the temporal bone behind the pterion and obtaining a more direct upward line of vision from underneath the aneurysmal complex and identifying easily the contralateral A1. When the aneurysm is stuck to the base, the contralateral A1 needs to be exposed from a more frontal direction or, if the aneurysm is large, from behind the aneurysmal complex, a difficult approach because of the perforators in this area. Visualizing the opposite A2 is usually more difficult, particularly with large aneurysms. The surgeon may have to accept an inadequate temporary clip placement that may incorporate the contralateral A2, until the aneurysm is completely freed. Once the contralateral A2 is visualized properly, the clip can be readjusted. If there is difficulty
dissecting the ipsilateral A2 from the ipsilateral neck of the aneurysm, a fenestrated clip may be very helpful. In a report of three patients sustaining symmetrical bilateral infarctions in the territories of Heubner's artery,[32] temporary clipping of both A1s, deliberate intraoperative hypotension, acute surgery, and the presence of thick and diffuse SAH were all implicated in the pathogenesis.

Another major pitfall is lack of appreciation of the frequent anatomic variations that occur frequently in this area. The most dangerous anomaly is the presence of three different A2s indicating generally that the pericallosal and callosomarginal arteries on one side take origin directly from the anterior communicating artery. Alpers and Berry[2] demonstrated this anomaly in 8% of normal brains. Unsuspecting the presence of the third A2, the surgeon may clip the aneurysm after freeing two A2s, incorporate the third A2 in the clip, and realize it only after the patient wakes up with a significant deficit (as happened in one of our cases).[34] Kwak and Suzuki demonstrated anomalies of the circle of Willis in about 60% of cases of aneurysms of the anterior communicating artery; 90% of these patients had unilateral hypoplasia of the A1.[51,52] In addition, about 9% of 296 cases of anterior communicating artery aneurysms had either fenestration of the anterior communicating artery or more than two anterior cerebral arteries. This reflects on the choice of side of approach for aneurysms in this location. Yasargil[100] almost always adopts the right side. The authors generally prefer the side of the dominant A1 to ensure proximal control. As the dome generally points toward the opposite hemisphere, this approach avoids encountering the aneurysmal dome first. The disadvantage is damage to the remaining intact gyrus rectus in cases where there is already a hematoma in the opposite frontal lobe. For this reason, we attempt to minimize the amount of retraction and brain resection on the side of the exposure. In their 38 anterior cerebral artery aneurysm cases, Awad and Little[6] approached always from the right side, except in the presence of a hypoplastic right A1 and a dome projecting to the right.

The authors invariably use the pterional approach for anterior communicating aneurysms and have had no experience with the anterior interhemispheric approach advocated by Suzuki[89] and others. This approach achieves complete visualization and control of both A1s and A2s. The shortcomings are opening the frontal sinus and possibly sacrificing both olfactory tracts, although the latter is claimed to have occurred in only 20% of cases.[89]

Distal anterior cerebral artery aneurysms are approached by most surgeons through an interhemispheric route through a small frontal craniotomy. The first major pitfall is trying to open the interhemispheric fissure with an aneurysm that is stuck through adhesions to the cingulate gyrus, resulting in premature rupture at the dome. Therefore, the authors rely on subpial dissection through the cingulate gyrus when the aneurysm appears to be adherent. The other pitfall is lack of proximal control, because the proximal A2 hides beneath the genu of the corpus callosum and may be difficult to visualize, particularly if the craniotomy is too posteriorly located.

Anatomic variations in this area are also notoriously treacherous. Ohno[64] reported the largest series of distal anterior cerebral artery aneurysms and noted the coexistence of multiple aneurysms in 42.9% of cases. Associated local vascular anomalies included azygoüs anterior cerebral, a single pericallosal artery, an early origin of the callosomarginal artery, and a bihemispheric anterior cerebral artery. Due to their depth, the infracallosal aneurysms were approached antegradely through the interhemispheric approach. The genu and supracallosal types were adequately approached retrogradely. The same authors noted a tendency of these aneurysms to bleed at smaller critical sites. Due to their rarity, aneurysms beyond the region of the genu should raise the suspicion of mycotic or traumatic origin or of an unusual arterial loop.[10] Giant pericallosal aneurysms are even more of a rarity, and Maiuri et al[61] reported the eighth such case in the literature. The authors' series contains only one giant aneurysm.

**TABLE 8**
**Anterior Cerebral Aneurysms**
**Surgical Pitfalls**

A. Proximal Anterior Cerebral
- Lack of appreciation of vascular anomalies

B. Anterior Communicating Region
- Approach from the "wrong" side
- Premature rupture of aneurysms adherent to tuberculum
- Lack of control of contralateral A1
- Incomplete aneurysmal exposure
- Occlusion of or injury to perforators Heubner's artery
- Lack of appreciation of vascular anomalies

C. Pericallosal Aneurysms
- Posterior placement of craniotomy with lack of proximal control
- Premature rupture from interhemispheric retraction
- Inclusion of major efferent vessel in the clip

Tables 8 and 9, respectively, summarize the surgical pitfalls and the senior author's results with anterior cerebral aneurysms.

## *Middle Cerebral Aneurysms*

Middle cerebral aneurysms (MCAs) can be approached in three ways. The first is the proximal trans-sylvian approach, which requires a simple pterional craniotomy with thorough removal of the pterion, particularly posteriorly. After the optic nerve and carotid artery have been exposed, the sylvian fissure is opened from medially to laterally following the M1 to the aneurysm. The main advantage

**TABLE 9**
**Anterior Cerebral Aneurysms**
**Surgical Results**

| Size | Number | Good | Poor | Dead |
|---|---|---|---|---|
| **A. Anterior Communicating Aneurysms** | | | | |
| Giant | 5 | 4 | 1 | 0 |
| < 25 mm | 115 | 99 | 14 | 2 |
| **B. Pericallosal Aneurysms** | | | | |
| Giant | 1 | 1 | 0 | 0 |
| < 25 mm | 11 | 11 | 0 | 0 |
| Total | 132 | 115 | 15 | 2 |

is ensuring early proximal control. However, there are several problems with this approach. MCAs are large and often point anteriorly, therefore obstructing the view to the M1 and rendering application of the retractors more difficult. In addition, opening the sylvian fissure can lead to premature rupture of the dome if adherent to the frontal or the temporal lobes. By nature of this approach, and despite a wide opening of the sylvian fissure, it is more difficult to dissect thoroughly the posterior aspect of the aneurysm and the divisions of the M2. One is restricted to applying the clip from anteriorly, not necessarily the ideal direction. However, this is the best approach for aneurysms of the M1, which are proximal to the insula, or M1 bifurcation aneurysms, when the M1 segment is short. Due to its simplicity, the authors also use this approach for most small, unruptured aneurysms where opening the sylvian fissure is a clean and straightforward maneuver.

The second is the lateral trans-sylvian approach. Here the sylvian fissure is first opened laterally and the distal divisions followed proximally to the base of the aneurysm. Small arterial branches can serve as guides if the fissure is difficult to find. The main advantage of this approach is that it provides prompt access to the complicated distal and dorsal anatomy of the aneurysm. The disadvantage is not having early proximal control unless one follows the divisions proximally to the base of the aneurysm and then finds the distal M1 before proceeding to dissect the aneurysm thoroughly. Another disadvantage is the potential for injuring sylvian veins. This approach is valuable only when the aneurysm is at, or distal to the insula.

The third approach is through the superior temporal gyrus; the authors have previously reported on this technique and its results.[39] A small portion of the superior temporal gyrus in its most anterior aspect is resected and the sylvian fissure is entered at a depth of about 2 cm. This avoids injury to the sylvian veins and is a quick approach to the deeper part of the fissure. The dissection then proceeds from lateral to medial. Excellent visualization of the dorsal and distal portion of the aneurysm complex is obtained, allowing circumferential freedom for clip application. This approach preserves the sylvian veins but involves cortical resection and therefore a potential for subsequent seizures. The shortcoming of lacking early proximal control can be avoided by dissecting free the distal M1 as soon as the base of the aneurysm is reached. The bone flap has to be larger inferiorly and posteriorly, compared with the other two approaches.[39] For the authors, approach through the superior temporal gyrus is preferred in patients with a temporal lobe hematoma and patients in acute surgery, particularly with large aneurysms. It is not suited for short M1s or for aneurysms arising proximally to the lumen of the insula.

The major problem with MCAs is incorporation or occlusion by the clip of a main division or a distal perforator. Umansky et al[94] reported that the incidence of the "classical" middle cerebral artery bifurcation was no more than 66% in 104 studied hemispheres. The M1 itself was fenestrated, duplicated, or arose as an accessory from the A1 segment in 4% of the cases. The distal perforators can originate not only from the M1 but also from the early part of the major divisions. The latter condition is more common when the M1 is shorter.

MCAs often acquire large necks and become multilobular, so that perfect clip application is difficult. They may need multiple clips lodged through the fenestration of other clips. Large calcified aneurysms may require aneurysmorrhaphy, and temporary occlusion of the MCA is obviously much less tolerated than that of the proximal carotid. Friedman[29] recently reported on the use of intraoperative somatosensory evoked potential monitoring in 53 MCA procedures and found it to be a very valuable adjunct to alert the surgeon in time to the danger of ischemia and to allow its reversal by maneuvers such as adjusting the clip, removing temporary clips and inducing hypertension after aneurysm trapping. Patterns of change also correlated with the presence or absence of postoperative neurologic deficits.

Giant MCAs have presented particular difficulties, and the authors have reported on the poor prognosis of patients presenting with massive cerebral edema despite good technical results.[37] Another pitfall is distal embolization from a calcified base at the time of clip application, a complication potentially preventable by aneurysmorrhaphy and plaque removal.

When the MCA has to be occluded with giant aneurysms and a bypass graft to the distal circulation is needed, the authors recommend use of a vein graft, with its capacity for immediate large flow, rather than a superficial temporal artery bypass. One has to be careful when choosing as the recipient a division branch that has not been occluded by the clip.

Tables 10 and 11, respectively, summarize the surgical pitfalls and the senior author's results with MCAs.

TABLE 11
**Middle Cerebral Aneurysms**
**Surgical Results**

| Size | Number | Good | Poor | Dead |
|---|---|---|---|---|
| Giant | 26 | 21 | 4 | 1 |
| < 25 mm | 110 | 97 | 7 | 6 |
| Total | 136 | 118 | 11 | 7 |

# Posterior Circulation Aneurysms

## *Top of the Basilar*

Although the top of the basilar is the most common posterior circulation location, unfortunately it is the most difficult as well. After relying for many years on the subtemporal approach, the senior author has come to prefer, and use more frequently, the "combined" pterional-anterior temporal approach. The standard pterional approach is felt to be too confining because frequently it limits working space to the opticocarotid cistern.

With the subtemporal approach, the authors prefer a wide-based subtemporal craniotomy exposing all of the superior aspect of the zygoma and reaching the middle fossa floor. This provides a wide angle of vision from anterior to posterior and freedom to work on both sides of the oculomotor (III) nerve, sometimes preserving it by leaving it attached to the retracted uncus. The major strength of this approach is the good visualization of the posterior aspect of the aneurysm and the important perforators. The major shortcoming is the restricted lateral line of vision it provides, making it difficult to visualize the opposite P1 with large aneurysms. This lack of visualization can lead to a poor clip application, with occlusion of the opposite P1 or, more commonly, one of its important perforators. The senior author has encountered two instances of bilateral oculomotor nerve palsies incurred by this approach, with the contralateral palsy due to a perforator injury and resulting ischemia to the oculomotor nucleus. The senior author has also produced other "perforator syndromes," which he has ascribed to the occlusion of perforators at the origin of the opposite P1. This approach is best suited for relatively low-lying aneurysms. Very low aneurysms can be reached by extending the exposure with a division of the tentorium posterior to oculomotor nerve and resection of the anterior medial aspect of the petrous pyramid, as recommended by Kawase.[48] High-lying aneurysms require a substantial amount of temporal retraction. The senior author frequently resects the anterior-inferior aspect of the temporal lobe in those instances, or when the anterior temporal fossa is deep. This minimizes the

TABLE 10
**Middle Cerebral Aneurysms**
**Surgical Pitfalls**

- Choosing the "wrong" approach
- Lack of proximal control with the lateral approaches
- Lack of complete circumferential exposure of the aneurysm and occlusion of important branches or perforators
- Kinking of divisions with clip
- Distal embolism
- Inappropriate bypass graft: use of small donor vessel or anastomosis to "wrong" division

need for temporal retraction and so far has not resulted in an increase in the incidence of postoperative epilepsy, although we do not have sufficient long-term follow up data to make a definite statement to this effect.

The combined pterional-anterior temporal approach adds a more anterior angle of vision, making visualization of the opposite P1 easier. This is a deeper and technically more demanding approach. The authors carry the skin incision just in front of the tragus, below the zy-goma. The latter is exposed completely by dissecting the temporalis fascia with the skin flap at the area of the "fat pad" above the zygoma in order to preserve the frontalis nerve. We cut the attachments of the temporal muscle superiorly anteriorly (and also partially inferiorly) along the superior aspect of the zygoma so as to allow a posterior rather than an inferior retraction of the muscle, avoiding the creation of a bulk over the zygoma. The sylvian fissure is opened widely to the first bifurcation of the MCA, allowing posterior retraction of the temporal tip. With the freedom of microscope movement, one can alternate between a lateral view of the perforators of the posterior aspect of the aneurysm and a more anterior view of the contralateral P1. There is always the danger of creating a tear in a dried-up carotid artery as it sometimes needs to be retracted. In the authors' experience, the incidence of postoperative cranial nerve III palsy has dropped from about 50% for the subtemporal approach to about 20% with this approach. An additional advantage of the width of this approach is the opportunity it gives for clipping multiple aneurysms of the anterior aspect of the circle of Willis. Occasionally the question arises of transecting a hypoplastic posterior communicating artery to improve visualization of a basilar tip aneurysm, especially when this approach is used with a high-lying aneurysm. A recent report[71] describes the occurrence of a tuberothalamic infarct subsequent to such a maneuver, despite seemingly preserved perforators, and warns against its indiscriminate use.

For high-basilar-tip aneurysms accompanied by a short intracranial internal carotid artery, a combination that makes standard approaches difficult, Ikeda[40] combines two previously described skull base techniques into an orbitozygomatic temporopolar approach in two patients. With this approach, the surgeon acquires an upward and oblique view of the aneurysm from below and can access aneurysms located higher than 10 mm above the interclinoid line. The authors have had no experience with this or similar skull base approaches to the basilar tip.

With all approaches the major problem of perforator occlusion is compounded by the presence of large aneurysms, where occlusion of one of the two P1s or of the top of the basilar artery is more likely because of the wider neck. The clip tends to slip down to the top of the basilar. On a few occasions the authors have mistaken the opposite superior cerebellar artery for the P1 and incorporated inadvertently the latter in the clip; fortunately, the mistake was recognized by thorough inspection after clipping, an essential step with these as with any other aneurysms. It should be noted here that this thorough inspection refers only to the region of the neck, where all the important surgical anatomy is located. As is the case with carotid bifurcation aneurysms, it is unnecessary to dissect out all of the dome of basilar aneurysms, even after clipping. With large aneurysms such unnecessary dissection may cause parenchymal damage to the mesencephalon and to important diencephalic structures. Giant aneurysms in this location are even more dreaded and the senior author has had success with only two of seven giant aneurysms clipped in this location. The surgeon frequently has to resort to indirect procedures involving basilar occlusion for these lesions, but even in the best hands the results leave much to be desired.[68]

Intraoperative aneurysmal rupture is obviously a dreaded complication in this location, for it compounds the risk of perforator injury, and temporary occlusion of the proximal basilar and both P1s in the confined space of the interpeduncular cistern is very difficult.

Reporting on 50 basilar bifurcation aneurysms treated acutely in the first week, Peerless et al[67] attributed immediate postoperative deficits to perforator injury in 11 patients, intraoperative rupture and inadequate neck clipping in 3, retraction edema in 1, epidural hematoma in 1, and aneurysmal rupture prior to tourniquet application in 1. Thirteen patients recovered completely within several weeks; 10 patients had delayed ischemic deficits attributed to vasospasm, 3 of whom made a complete recovery. Timing of the procedure did not seem to affect the results. In a sobering article,[9] Batjer and Samson analyze their surgical failures with 126 patients with distal basilar artery aneurysms. They had 8% mortality and 11% permanent neurologic disability and ascribed the causes of failed management to the initial hemorrhage, timing errors, conceptual errors, technical errors, delayed ischemic deficits, hypertensive hypervolemic therapy, and bad luck.

## *Posterior Cerebral Aneurysms*

Aneurysms of the P1 segment are frequently related to the junction with the posterior communicating artery. These are adequately approached through a combined pterional-anterior temporal approach. The incidence of fusiform aneurysms in this area seems particularly high, reported to be from 10%[31,69] to 45%.[15] Trapping of these aneurysms is usually well tolerated. The authors have had good results in all three cases treated in that fashion, even when the posterior communicating artery was incorporated in the clip. Other authors have had similarly good results.[23,73,86,100]

More distally located aneurysms are better approached subtemporally. They are frequently adherent to the parahippocampal gyrus, and we do not hesitate to resect a small amount of brain in this area to expose the aneurysm subpially and prevent premature rupture during temporal retraction. To avoid injury to the vein of Labbé when it is in the way, we prefer resecting part of the inferior temporal gyrus on either side of the vein to preserve it. We had good results in two casesthat were trapped; in a third case, incorporation of the thalamogeniculate perforators resulted in a thalamic infarct with a major postoperative pain syndrome as well as hemihypesthesia. Chang[15] also encountered some instances of postoperative contralateral hemiparesis, homonymous hemianopsia, hemihypesthesia, and ipsilateral oculomotor nerve palsy in a series of 10 patients.

In view of the generally good track record of trapping procedures, the value of routine cerebral revascularization for unclippable aneurysms at this location is hard to establish. The problem is that so far there is no good intraoperative way of selecting the few patients who will develop hemianopsia from insufficient collaterals after P1 occlusion. Preoperative testing by balloon occlusion may be helpful in this respect. When trapping procedures are undertaken, every effort should be made to avoid including any of the geniculostriate arteries in the trapped segment. If such arteries arise from the aneurysmal segment, it may be safer to do only a proximal occlusion and depend on retrograde flow to supply the geniculostriates.

## *Superior Cerebellar Aneurysms*

Superior cerebellar aneurysms are relatively straightforward since they are not directly related to crucial perforators. The combined pterional-anterior temporal approach is quite adequate for these aneurysms. The major pitfall is tearing of the aneurysm neck as one separates the superior cerebellar artery (SCA) and the posterior cerebral artery (PCA) from the aneurysm. In one of our cases this necessitated incorporation of the superior cerebellar artery in the clip without neurologic sequelae. One of our patients died from a giant SCA aneurysm. The error was in approaching the aneurysm through a standard pterional approach, which limited the surgeon's working line of vision to the opticocarotid cistern; opening the applicator forcibly to disengage the clip resulted in a major tear of the junction of the anterior cerebral and the internal carotid artery. This area was atherosclerotic and became quite "dried" during the exposure.

## Basilar Trunk Aneurysms

Very high trunk aneurysms can be approached by the anterior subtemporal route, sometimes using Kawase's modification by drilling some of the superior anterior aspect of the petrous pyramid, the so-called modified middle fossa approach. Most, however, have to be approached transtentorially using a subtemporal approach. The major pitfall is damage to the vein of Labbé and excessive temporal retraction; therefore, better exposure can be obtained with some modification. The first option is to use a combined subtemporal suboccipital approach with division of the junction of the transverse and sigmoid sinuses, provided there is good venous outflow contralaterally. Thus the cerebellum can be retracted backward after dividing the tentorium completely from lateral to medial. Solomon and Stein[84] reported on nine such cases. The other modification is to combine the subtemporal approach with a generous transmastoid, presigmoid exposure and divide the superior petrosal sinus to allow posterior retraction of the transverse-sigmoid junction. This approach offers a slightly more anterior angle of vision and preserves the major venous sinuses; however, it requires more bone drilling and familiarity with temporal bone anatomy, if the hearing apparatus and the facial (VII) nerve are to be preserved. The authors find the third modification, Giannotta's retrolabyrinthine trans-sigmoid approach,[33] to be relatively confining and prefer to use it only for small aneurysms.

Potential complications with all these approaches are related to direct damage to the lower cranial nerves, particularly the facial and vestibulocochlear nerve complex. Other problems relate to the anatomy of the aneurysm and the relation of the neck to the important basilar artery branches.

## Vertebrobasilar Junction Aneurysms

Vertebrobasilar junction aneurysms can be approached similarly to basilar trunk aneurysms, or, alternatively, by a suboccipital approach. The authors have described a far lateral occipital approach for these aneurysms.[36] A "lazy-S"-shape incision is made in the suboccipital region. After exposing the vertebral artery over the arch of C1, a lateral suboccipital craniectomy is carried through the foramen magnum to the occipital condyle. C1 is removed far laterally to the lateral mass. The approach allows a lateral angle of vision without the need for brain stem retraction. The major problems relate to damage to the cranial nerves. We prefer to work in the space between the spinal accessory (XI) nerve inferiorly and glossopharyngeal (IX) and vagal (X) nerve complex superiorly because of the width of this space. In our experience, the facial and vestibulocochlear (VIII) nerve complex is more sensitive to injury than the lower cranial nerves although, of course, major lower cranial nerve injury is more life threatening. We prefer utilizing the space just inferior to the facial and vestibulocochlear nerve complex to visualize the aneurysm, but applying the clip through the lower wider space obliquely to the line of vision. In addition to problems related to the approach, the anatomy of the aneurysm itself is usually complex. These aneurysms, as noted by Campos et al,[13] frequently arise in relation to a fenestration of the origin of the basilar artery. They are frequently bilobar and even trilobar and call for ingenuity in designing a clipping stratagem. Fortunately there are no major perforating vessels in this area. The main pitfall is kinking or occlusion of the basilar artery itself. Intraoperative aneurysmal rupture in this area is very difficult to control because of the relative inaccessibility for temporary clipping of the contralateral vertebral artery.

According to Yamaura et al,[99] the risk of serious morbidity for these as well as for aneurysms of the posterior inferior cerebellar artery–vertebral artery (PICA-VA) complex correlates with how close they are to the midline and how far they are from the clivus. No one has accumulated enough surgical experience with these rare lesions to establish a standard treatment, but it may be that, as Salcman et al note,[80] contralateral and translabyrinthine approaches could render these distances less relevant.

### *Vertebral Artery Aneurysms*

Most vertebral artery aneurysms arise at the origin of the PICA. The authors approach them through a regular suboccipital approach without expanding the craniotomy as far laterally as we would do for a vertebrobasilar junction aneurysm. Often the aneurysm is seen immediately upon opening the dura. The main pitfalls relate to occlusion of the PICA and the distal vertebral artery, which could be obscured by large aneurysms. Almost invariably the aneurysm is anterior to the PICA, but the latter may take origin from the base of large aneurysms, making it difficult to exclude it from the clip. In addition, the lower cranial nerves and the hypoglossus nerve can be intermingled with the neck and will need careful separation prior to clipping.

A report of six unclippable vertebral aneurysms treated by therapeutic occlusion of the proximal vertebral artery[98] underlines the importance of the PICA. All three cases that were clipped proximally to the PICA either developed a Wallenberg's syndrome or their aneurysm failed to thrombose because of persistent retrograde flow. All three patients who were clipped distal to the PICA origin or in whom the PICA was absent had no complications. This finding stresses the importance of a very careful preoperative angiographic assessment of each vertebral artery separately to study the collateral network.

### *Peripheral PICA Aneurysms*

Despite their rarity, the authors have had considerable experience with peripheral PICA aneurysms.[11,60] Most are located distal to the tonsillomedullary segment of the PICA, which ends at the choroidal point. By that time, all the important medullary perforators have been given,[55] allowing a safe simple ligation and excision of the aneurysm with its parent vessel distal to that point (if, for technical reasons, the aneurysm cannot be clipped effectively). In the more proximal segments of the PICA (anterior medullary, lateral medullary, tonsillomedullary), any necessary resection should be accompanied by microvascular reconstruction, a technique first reported by Dolenc[21] and subsequently used in one of our cases.[60] The major pitfall with distal PICA aneurysms is premature rupture due to their adherence to the tonsil that is being retracted. In those instances, we prefer subpial exposure through the tonsil. One should not forget that, compounding their rarity, these aneurysms can be located extracranially, even below the level of C1,[80] and can be missed entirely on acursory examination of the angiogram. Also, it must be emphasized that whenever a peripheral PICA aneurysm is suspected because of the pattern of hemorrhage seen on the CT scan, both vertebral arteries must be injected during the arteriogram. If one is satisfied with a single vertebral injection with retrograde opacification of the contralateral vertebra, one can miss a peripheral PICA aneurysm on the opposite side.[11]

Tables 12 and 13, respectively, summarize the surgical pitfalls and the senior author's results with posterior circulation aneurysms.

## Failed Aneurysm Surgery

Drake[24] reviewed the reasons for reoperation in 115 aneurysms and identified three causes: (1) clipping had been judged impractical or dangerous, (2) the clip had been applied improperly, or (3) carotid ligation without intracranial exploration was the therapy of choice. By reoperation he was able to achieve obliteration of 89% of these aneurysms. Suzuki[88] reported a 7% incidence of incomplete surgical obliteration of aneurysms, although postoperative angiography was done in only 70% of cases. The natural history of these incompletely clipped aneu-

TABLE 12
**Vertebrobasilar Aneurysms**
**Surgical Pitfalls**

A. Basilar Bifurcation
- Choice of approach
- Perforator injury
- P-1 occlusion
- Unnecessary exposure of dome
- Oculomotor damage

B. Posterior Cerebral
- Excessive temporal retraction
- Injury to vein of Labbé
- Thalamogeniculate occlusion

C. Superior Cerebellar
- Rupture at the neck from manipulation
- Oculomotor damage

D. Basilar Trunk
- Choice of approach
- Excessive temporal retraction
- Damage to vein of Labbé
- Cranial nerve damage

E. Vertebrobasilar Junction
- Choice of approach
- Fenestrations
- Basilar occlusion
- Cranial nerve damage
- Lack of control

F. Vertebral and PICA
- Cranial nerve damage
- PICA occlusion

rysms was addressed by Feuerberg et al,[26] who found them in 3.8% of treated patients with a rebleeding rate of 0.4% to 0.8% per year compared to 0.02% per year for satisfactorily clipped aneurysms.

The natural history of aneurysms treated by indirect surgical methods or inadequate direct clipping was estimated by several reports.[25,30,44,78,90–93,96] Expanding on the techniques, complications, and results of these methods is beyond the scope of this chapter. Table 14 is a composite summary of the various estimated figures for rebleeding rates. Two recent papers report on optochiasmal arachnoiditis and gauze-induced granuloma as uncommon but serious complications of aneurysm wrapping.[14,62]

## Long-Term Sequelae: Cognition and Epilepsy

For the aneurysm patient, the fight for survival does not end with a technically successful operation. Ranging from mild to devastating, the neuropsychological effects can interfere significantly with social functioning. Several studies have shown that the cursory outpatient examination of the surviving patient does not reflect the extent of "true" neurologic deficits. Eleven of 37 patients, judged by their neurosurgeon to have achieved a "good" outcome, were found with careful psychometric testing to have a poor neuropsychological outcome.[12] The alarming 83% incidence reported by Ljunggren[59] has not been reproduced by others. The relationship be-

TABLE 13
**Vertebrobasilar Aneurysms—Surgical Results**

| Location | Size | Number | Good | Poor | Dead |
|---|---|---|---|---|---|
| Basilar Top | Giant | 7 | 2 | 3 | 2 |
| | < 25 mm | 56 | 48 | 7 | 1 |
| PCA | Giant | 7 | 6 | 1 | 0 |
| | < 25 mm | 6 | 5 | 1 | 0 |
| SCA | Giant | 2 | 1 | 0 | 1 |
| | < 25 mm | 6 | 6 | 0 | 0 |
| Trunk | Giant | 2 | 1 | 1 | 0 |
| | < 25 mm | 5 | 4 | 1 | 0 |
| Vertebral and PICA | Giant | 5 | 3 | 1 | 1 |
| | < 25 mm | 17 | 16 | 1 | 0 |
| Total | | 113 | 92 | 16 | 5 |

TABLE 14
**Ruptured Aneurysms: Estimated Rebleeding Rates Versus Treatment Method**

| | Untreated[42] | Wrapping[93] | Carotid Ligation[92] | ACA* Ligation[91,92] | Incomplete Clipping[26] | Satisfactory Clipping[26] |
|---|---|---|---|---|---|---|
| Early rebleeds (< 6 months) | 50% | 86% | 4.4%–8.8% | 3.9% | *** | 0 |
| Late rebleeds (> 6 months) | 3%/year | 1.5%/year | 1%/year | 1%/year | 0.4%–0.8%/year | 0.02%/year |
| rebleeds that are fatal | 66%–78% | 90%** | 66%–80% | 77% | *** | *** |

* Anterior cerebral artery ligation for AcomA aneurysms
** Probably an overestimate, due to under-reporting of minor rebleeds
*** Insufficient data

tween cognitive deficits and radiographic abnormalities is unclear. One year after subarachnoid hemorrhage, the presence of infarction on CT scan seemed to correlate well with the type and degree of psychological abnormalities, according to one report.[95] According to another,[75] which found a one-third incidence of MRI or psychological abnormalities in a population of treated aneurysm patients with no obvious neurologic deficits, the degree of tissue loss seen on MRI did not correlate with cognitive dysfunction. As to the role aneurysm location plays in giving rise to a particular pattern of cognitive deficits, particularly with anterior communicating artery aneurysms, most studies support the concept of some form of "toxic" brain impairment sustained as a direct effect of the initial bleed or the surgical intervention.[7,53,74] Cognitive deficits are not, by and large, aneurysm site-specific. The role surgery plays in altering the nature or severity of the initial injury is unclear.

The role of prophylactic anticonvulsant therapy with aneurysmal hemorrhage continues to be controversial. Keränen et al[49] report a 14% incidence of late seizures with a mean latency of 8.4 months in 177 patients. He identifies an MCA location, presence of a large intracerebral hematoma, postoperative spasm with ischemic infarction, and shunt-dependent hydrocephalus as the main risk factors. Another report[66] finds a less than 3% incidence of late epilepsy, two-thirds of which had predisposing epileptogenic factors prior to the hemorrhage, and argues against the routine use of prophylactic anticonvulsants.

# Conclusion

Since Dott planned the first direct intracranial attack on a ruptured aneurysm in 1931, challenges have accrued in conjunction with technical demands. Weir[97] has adequately outlined the windows of opportunity in the management of this treacherous disease. This chapter has focused on a small yet crucial part of the overall management strategy: the appraisal and avoidance of surgical pitfalls. Devastated by an intracranial hemorrhage, the last thing a patient needs is added insult from surgical intervention. Short of being able to prevent all aneurysmal ruptures, only through refinement of concepts,[5] judgment, and techniques can we hope to pursue refinement in management results.

# References


1. Adson AW. Surgical treatment of vascular diseases altering the function of the eyes. *Trans Am Acad Ophthalmal.* 1942;46:95–111.
2. Alpers BJ, Berry RG. Circle of Willis in cerebral vascular disorders. *Arch Neurol.* 1963;8:398–402.
3. Al-Mefty O, Smith RR. Tailoring the cranio-orbital approach. *Keio J Med.* 1990;39:217–224.
4. Asai A, Yamada H, Tsutsumi K, et al. Tension pneumocephalus after clipping of a carotid-ophthalmic artery aneurysm via an interhemispheric approach: case report. *Neurosurgery.* 1988;23:650–654.
5. Ausman JI, Diaz FG, Malik GM, et al. Management of cerebral aneurysms: further facts and additional myths. *Surg Neurol.* 1989;32:21–35.
6. Awad IA, Little JR. Perioperative management and outcome after surgical treatment of anterior cerebral artery aneurysms. *Can J Neurol Sci.* 1991; 18:120–125.

7. Barbarotto R, De Santis A, Laiacona M, et al. Neuropsychological follow-up of patients operated for aneurysms of the middle cerebral artery and posterior communicating artery. *Cortex.* 1989;25: 275–288.
8. Barrow DL, Boyer KL, Joseph GJ. Intraoperative angiography in the management of neurovascular disorders. *Neurosurgery.* 1992;30:153–159.
9. Batjer HH, Samson DS. Causes of morbidity and mortality from surgery of aneurysms of the distal basilar artery. *Neurosurgery.* 1989;25:904–916.
10. Becker DH, Newton TH. Distal anterior cerebral artery aneurysm. *Neurosurgery.* 1979;4:495–503.
11. Beyerl BD, Heros RC. Multiple peripheral aneurysms of the posterior inferior cerebellar artery. *Neurosurgery.* 1986;19:285–289.
12. Bornstein RA, Weir BKA, Petruk KC, et al. Neuropsychological function in patients after subarachnoid hemorrhage. *Neurosurgery.* 1987; 21:651–654.
13. Campos J, Fox AJ, Viñuela F, et al. Saccular aneurysms in basilar atery fenestration. *AJNR.* 1987; 8:233–236.
14. Chambi I, Tasker RR, Gentili F, et al. Gauze-induced granuloma ("gauzoma"): an uncommon complication of gauze reinforcement of berry aneurysms. *J Neurosurg.* 1990;72:163–170.
15. Chang HS, Fukushima T, Takakura K, et al. Aneurysms of the posterior cerebral artery: report of ten cases. *Neurosurgery.* 1986;19:1006–1011.
16. Chyatte D, Fode NC, Sundt TM Jr. Early versus late intracranial aneurysm surgery in subarachnoid hemorrhage. *J Neurosurg.* 1988;69:326–331.
17. Cooper IS. Surgical alleviation of Parkinsonism: effects of occlusion of the anterior choroidal artery. *J Am Geriatr Soc.* 1954;2:691–718.
18. Cooper IS. Surgical occlusion of the anterior choroidal artery in Parkinsonism. *Surg Gynecol Obstet.* 1954;99:207–219.
19. Day AL. Clinicoanatomic features of supraclinoid aneurysms. *Clin Neurosurg.* 1990;36:256–274.
20. Disney L, Weir B, Petruk K. Effect on management mortality of a deliberate policy of early operation on supratentorial aneurysms. *Neurosurgery.* 1987;20: 695–701.
21. Dolenc V. End-to-end suture of the posterior inferior cerebellar artery after the excision of a large aneurysm: case report. *Neurosurgery.* 1982; 11:690–693.
22. Dolenc V. A combined epi- and subdural direct approach to carotid-ophthalmic artery aneurysms. *J Neurosurgery.* 1985;62:667–672.
23. Drake CG. The treatment of aneurysms of theposterior circulation. *Clin Neurosurg.* 1979;26: 96–144.
24. Drake CG, Freidman AH, Peerless SJ. Failed aneurysm surgery: reoperation in 115 cases. *J Neurosurg.* 1984;61:848–856.
25. Dyste GN, Beck DW. De Novo aneurysm formation following carotid ligation: case report and review of the literature. *Neurosurgery.* 1989;24:88–92.
26. Feuerberg I, Lindquist C, Lindqvist M, et al. Natural history of postoperative aneurysm rests. *J Neurosurg.* 1987;66:30–34.
27. Fox AJ, Viñuela F, Pelz DM, et al. Use of detachable balloons for proximal artery occlusion in the treatment of unclippable cerebral aneurysms. *J Neurosurg.* 1987;66:40–46.
28. Fox JL. Microsurgical treatment of ventral (paraclinoid) internal carotid artery aneurysms. *Neurosurgery.* 1988;22:32–39.
29. Friedman WA, Chadwick GM, Verhoeven FJS, et al. Monitoring of somatosensory evoked potentials during surgery for middle cerebral artery aneurysms. *Neurosurgery.* 1991;29:83–88.
30. Fujiwara S, Fujii K, Nishio S, et al. Long-term results of wrapping of intracranial ruptured aneurysms. *Acta Neurochir (Wien).* 1990;103:27–29.
31. Fukamachi A, Hirato M, Wakao T, et al. Giant serpentine aneurysm of the posterior cerebral artery. *Neurosurgery.* 1982;11:271–276.
32. Fukamachi A, Horikoshi T, Nagaseki Y, et al. Symmetrical bilateral low-density lesions in the areas of supply by Heubner's arteries after aneurysm surgery. *Acta Neurochir (Wien).* 1987;84:89–92.
33. Giannota SL, Maceri DR. Retrolabyrinthine transsigmoid approach to basilar trunk and vertebrobasilar artery junction aneurysms. *J Neurosurg.* 1988;69:461–466.
34. Gibbons K, Hopkins LN, Heros RC. Occlusion of an "accessory" distal anterior cerebral artery during treatment of anterior communicating artery aneurysms: report of two cases. *J Neurosurg.* 1991; 74:133–135.
35. Hamby WB. *Intracranial aneurysms.* Springfield, Ill, Charles C Thomas; 1952:230.
36. Heros RC. Lateral suboccipital approach for vertebral and vertebrobasilar artery lesions. *J Neurosurg.* 1986;64:559–562.
37. Heros RC, Kolluri S. Giant intracranial aneurysms presenting with massive cerebral edema. *Neurosurgery.* 1984;15:572–577.
38. Heros RC, Nelson PB, Ojemann RG, et al. Large and giant paraclinoid aneurysms; surgical techniques, complications and results. *Neurosurgery.* 1983;12:153–163.
39. Heros RC, Ojemann RG, Crowell RM. Superior temporal gyrus approach to middle cerebral artery aneurysms: technique and results. *Neurosurgery.* 1982;10:308–313.
40. Ikeda K, Yamashita J, Hashimoto M, et al. Orbitozygomatic temporopolar approach for a high basilar tip aneurysm associated with a short intracranial internal carotid artery: a new surgical approach. *Neurosurgery.* 1991;28:105–110.
41. Jane JA, Kassell NF, Torner JC, et al. The natural history of aneurysms and arteriovenous malformations. *J Neurosurg.* 1985;62:321–323.
42. Jane JA, Winn HR, Richardson AE. The natural history of intracranial aneurysms: rebleeding rates during the acute and long term period and implication for surgical management. *Clin Neurosurg.* 1976;24:176–184.
43. Jennett B, Galbraith S. *An Introduction to Neurosurgery.* 4th ed. Chicago, Ill: Year Book Medical Publishers; 1983:187.
44. Jha AN, Butler P, Lye RH, et al. Carotid ligation: what happens in the long term? *J Neurol Neurosurg Psychiatry.* 1986;49:893–898.
45. Kassell NF, Torner JC. Aneurysmal rebleeding: a preliminary report from the Cooperative Aneurysm Study. *Neurosurgery.* 1983;13:479–481.
46. Kassell NF, Torner JC, Haley EC Jr, et al. The International Cooperative Study on the Timing of Aneurysm Surgery, I: overall management results. *J Neurosurg.* 1990;73:18–36.
47. Kassell NF, Torner JC, Jane JA, et al. The Inter-

national Cooperative Study on the Timing of Aneurysm Surgery, II: surgical results. *J Neurosurg.* 1990;73:37–47.
48. Kawase T, Toya S, Shiobara R, et al. Transpetrosal approach for aneurysms of the lower basilar artery. *J Neurosurg.* 1985;63:857–861.
49. Keränen T, Tapaninaho A, Hernesniemi J, et al. Late epilepsy after aneurysm operations. *Neurosurgery.* 1985;17:897–900.
50. Korosue K, Heros RC. "Subclinoid" carotid aneurysm with erosion of the anterior clinoid process and fatal intraoperative rupture. *Neurosurgery.* 1992;31:356–360.
51. Kwak R, Niizuma H, Hatanaka M, et al. Anterior communicating artery aneurysms with associated anomalies. *J Neurosurg.* 1980;52:162–164.
52. Kwak R, Suzuki J. Correlation of anterior communicating artery aneurysm with blood circulation at the anterior part of the circle of Willis and its vascular anomalies. *Phronesis.* 1974;11:407–417.
53. Laiacona M, De Santis A, Barbarotto R, et al. Neuropsychological follow-up of patients operated for aneurysms of anterior communicating artery. *Cortex.* 1989;25:261–273.
54. Lee KC. Surgery of intracranial aneurysms at Yonsei University: 780 cases. *Keio J Med.* 1991; 40:1–5.
55. Lister JR, Rhoton AL Jr, Matsushima T, et al. Microsurgical anatomy of the posterior inferior cerebellar artery. *Neurosurgery.* 1982;10:170–199.
56. Little JR, Rosenfeld JV, Awad IA. Internal carotid artery occlusion for cavernous segment aneurysm. *Neurosurgery.* 1989;25:398–404.
57. Ljunggren B, Brandt L, Säveland H, et al. Management of ruptured intracranial aneurysms: a review. *Br J Neurosurg.* 1987;1:9–32.
58. Ljunggren B, Säveland H, Brandt L, et al. Early operation and overall outcome in aneurysmal subarachnoid hemorrhage. *J Neurosurg.* 1985; 62:547–551.
59. Ljunggren B, Sonesson B, Säveland H, et al. Cognitive impairment and adjustment in patients without neurological deficits after aneurysmal SAH and early operation. *J Neurosurg.* 1985;62:673–679.
60. Madsen JR, Heros RC. Giant peripheral aneurysms of the posterior inferior cerebellar artery treated with excision and end-to-end anastomosis. *Surg Neurol.* 1988;30:140–143.
61. Maiuri F, Corriero G, D'Amico L, et al. Giant aneurysm of the pericallosal artery. *Neurosurgery.* 1990;26:703–706.
62. McFadzean RM, Hadley DM, McIlwaine GG. Optochiasmal arachnoiditis following muslin wrapping of ruptured anterior communicating artery aneurysms. *J Neurosurg.* 1991;75:393–396.
63. Öhman J, Heiskanen O. Timing of operation for ruptured supratentorial aneurysms: a prospective randomized study. *J Neurosurg.* 1989;70:55–60.
64. Ohno K, Monma S, Suzuki R, et al. Saccular aneurysms of the distal anterior cerebral artery. *Neurosurgery.* 1990;27:907–913.
65. Ojemann RG, Heros RC, Crowell RM. ***Surgical Management of Cerebrovascular Disease.*** 2nd ed. Baltimore, Md: Williams & Wilkins; 1988: 199–216.
66. O'Laoire SA. Epilepsy following neurosurgical intervention. *Acta Neurochir (Wien)* Suppl. 1990; 50:52–54.
67. Peerless SJ, Nemoto S, Drake CG. Acute surgery for ruptured posterior circulation aneurysms. *Adv Tech Stand Neurosurg.* 1987;15:115–129.
68. Pelz DM, Viñuela F, Fox AJ, et al. Vertebrobasilar occlusion therapy of giant aneurysms. *J Neurosurg.* 1984;60:560–565.
69. Pia HW, Fontana H. Aneurysms of the posterior cerebral artery: locations and clinical pictures. *Acta Neurochir (Wien).* 1977;38:13–35.
70. Poletti CE. A temporal approach to anterior communicating artery aneurysms: technical note. *J Neurosurg.* 1989;71:144–146.
71. Regli L, de Tribolet N. Tuberothalamic infarct after division of a hypoplastic posterior communicating artery for clipping of a basilar tip aneurysm: case report. *Neurosurgery.* 1991;28:456–459.
72. Rhoton AL Jr, Fujii K, Fradd B. Microsurgical anatomy of the anterior choroidal artery. *Surg Neurol.* 1979;12:171–187.
73. Rice BJ, Peerless SJ, Drake CG. Surgical treatment of unruptured aneurysms of the posterior circulation. *J Neurosurg.* 1990;73:165–173.
74. Richardson JTE. Performance in free recall following rupture and repair of intracranial aneurysm. *Brain Cogn.* 1989;9:210–226.
75. Romner B, Sonesson B, Ljunggren B, et al. Late magnetic resonance imaging related to neurobehavioral functioning after aneurysmal subarachnoid hemorrhage. *Neurosurgery.* 1989;25:390–397.
76. Ropper AH, Zervas NT. Outcome 1 year after SAH from cerebral aneurysm: management morbidity, mortality, and functional status in 112 consecutive good-risk patients. *J Neurosurg.* 1984; 60:909–915.
77. Rosenørn J, Eskesen V, Schmidt K, et al. Clinical features and outcome in 1076 patients with ruptured intracranial saccular aneurysms: a prospective consecutive study. *Br J Neurosurg.* 1987; 1:33–46.
78. Roski RA, Spetzler RF, Nulsen FE. Late complications of carotid ligation in the treatment of intracranial aneurysms. *J Neurosurg.* 1981;54:583–587.
79. Saeki N, Rhoton AL Jr. Microsurgical anatomy of the upper basilar artery and the posterior circle of Willis. *J Neurosurg.* 1977;46:563–578.
80. Salcman M, Rigamonti D, Numaguchi Y, et al. Aneurysms of the posterior inferior cerebellar artery-vertebral artery complex: variations on a theme. *Neurosurgery.* 1990;27:12–21.
81. Samson DS, Batjer HH. ***Intracranial Aneurysm Surgery: Techniques.*** Futura Publishing Company; Mount Kisco, Ny: 1990:51.
82. Sekhar LN, Estonillo R. Transtemporal approach to the skull base: an anatomical study. *Neurosurgery.* 1986;19:799–808.
83. Smith RR, Al-Mefty O, Middleton TH. An orbitocranial approach to complex aneurysms of the anterior circulation. *Neurosurgery.* 1989; 24:385–391.
84. Solomon RA, Stein BM. Surgical approaches to aneurysms of the vertebral and basilar arteries. *Neurosurgery.* 1988;23:203–208.
85. Spetzler RF, Fukushima T, Martin N, et al. Petrous carotid-to-intradural carotid saphenous vein graft for intracavernous giant aneurysm, tumor, and occlusive cerebrovascular disease. *J Neurosurg.* 1990; 73:496–501.
86. Sundt TM Jr. Surgical technique for giant intra-

cranial aneurysms. *Neurosurg Rev.* 1982; 5:161–168.
87. Sundt TM Jr, Kobayashi S, Fode NC, et al. Results and complications of surgical management of 809 intracranial aneurysms in 722 cases. *J Neurosurg.* 1982;56:753–765.
88. Suzuki J, Kwak R, Katakura R. Review of incompletely occluded surgically treated cerebral aneurysms. *Surg Neurol.* 1980;13:306–310.
89. Suzuki J, Mizoi K, Yoshimoto T. Bifrontal interhemispheric approach to aneurysms of the anterior communicating artery. *J Neurosurg.* 1986;64:183–190.
90. Swearingen B, Heros RC. Common carotid occlusion for unclippable carotid aneurysms: an old but still effective operation. *Neurosurgery.* 1987; 21:288–295.
91. Taylor W, Miller JD, Todd NV. Long-term outcome following anterior cerebral artery ligation for ruptured anterior communicating artery aneurysms. *J Neurosurg.* 1991;74:51–54.
92. Todd NV. Aneurysm rebleeding after treatments that leave the aneurysm sac patent. *Br J Neurosurg.* 1990;4:373–379.
93. Todd NV, Tocher JL, Jones PA, et al. Outcome following aneurysm wrapping: a 10-year follow-up review of clipped and wrapped aneurysms. *J Neurosurg.* 1989;70:841–846.
94. Umansky F, Dujovny M, Ausman JI, et al. Anomalies and variations of the middle cerebral artery: a microanatomical study. *Neurosurgery.* 1988;22: 1023–1027.
95. Vilkki J, Holst P, Ohman J, et al. Cognitive deficits related to computed tomographic findings after surgery for a ruptured intracranial aneurysm. *Neurosurgery.* 1989;25:166–172.
96. Weil SM, van Loveren HR, Tomsick TA, et al. Management of inoperable cerebral aneurysms by the navigational balloon technique. *Neurosurgery.* 1987;21:296–302.
97. Weir BKA. The management of intracranial aneurysms: prospects for improvement. *Clin Neurosurg.* 1988;34:154–160.
98. Yamada K, Hayakawa T, Ushio Y, et al. Therapeutic occlusion of the vertebral artery for unclippable vertebral aneurysm: relationship between site of occlusion and clinical outcome. *Neurosurgery.* 1984;15:834–838.
99. Yamaura A, Ise H, Makino H. Radiometric study on posterior inferior cerebellar aneurysms with special reference to accessibility by the lateral suboccipital approach. *Neurol Med Chir (Tokyo).* 1981; 21:721–723.
100. Yasargil MG. *Microneurosurgery.* New York, NY: Theime-Stratton. 1984.2:
101. Yoshimoto T, Uchida K, Kaneko U, et al. An analysis of follow-up results of 1000 intracranial saccular aneurysms with definitive surgical treatment. *J Neurosurg.* 1979;50:152–157.

# Index

Page numbers for tables, figures, and illustrations are in ***boldface italics***.

# Previously Published Books in the *Neurosurgical Topics* Series

*Management of Posttraumatic Spinal Instability*
Edited by Paul R. Cooper, MD

*Malignant Cerebral Glioma*
Edited by Michael L.J. Apuzzo, MD

*Intracranial Vascular Malformations*
Edited by Daniel L. Barrow, MD

*Neurosurgical Treatment of Disorders of the Thoracic Spine*
Edited by Edward C. Tarlov, MD

*Contemporary Diagnosis and Management of Pituitary Adenomas*
Edited by Paul R. Cooper, MD

*Complications of Spinal Surgery*
Edited by Edward C. Tarlov, MD

*Neurosurgical Aspects of Epilepsy*
Edited by Michael L.J. Apuzzo, MD

*Complications and Sequelae of Head Injury*
Edited by Daniel L. Barrow, MD

*Practical Approaches to Peripheral Nerve Surgery*
Edited by Edward C. Benzel, MD

*Cerebrovascular Occlusive Disease and Brain Ischemia*
Edited by Issam A. Awad, MD

*Neurosurgery for the Third Millennium*
Edited by Michael L.J. Apuzzo, MD

*Degenerative Disease of the Cervical Spine*
Edited by Paul R. Cooper, MD

*Surgery of the Cranial Nerves of the Posterior Fossa*
Edited by Daniel L. Barrow, MD

*Spinal Trauma: Current Evaluation and Management*
Edited by Gary L. Rea, MD, and Carole A. Miller, MD

For order information call (708) 692-9500.